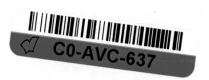
C0-AVC-637

Handbook of
Behavioral Neurobiology

Volume 9
Developmental
Psychobiology and
Behavioral Ecology

HANDBOOK OF BEHAVIORAL NEUROBIOLOGY

General Editor:
Norman T. Adler
University of Pennsylvania, Philadelphia, Pennsylvania

Editorial Board:

Mortimer Appley	Richard Held	Michael Menaker
Elliott M. Blass	James L. McGaugh	Mortimer Mishkin
Robert Capranica	Paul McHugh	Eliot Stellar
Vincent G. Dethier	Peter Marler	Richard Thompson
Robert W. Goy		

Volume 1   Sensory Integration
Edited by R. Bruce Masterton

Volume 2   Neuropsychology
Edited by Michael S. Gazzaniga

Volume 3   Social Behavior and Communication
Edited by Peter Marler and J. G. Vandenbergh

Volume 4   Biological Rhythms
Edited by Jürgen Aschoff

Volume 5   Motor Coordination
Edited by Arnold L. Towe and Erich S. Luschei

Volume 6   Motivation
Edited by Evelyn Satinoff and Philip Teitelbaum

Volume 7   Reproduction
Edited by Norman T. Adler, Donald Pfaff, and Robert W. Goy

Volume 8   Developmental Psychobiology and Developmental Neurobiology
Edited by Elliott M. Blass

Volume 9   Developmental Psychobiology and Behavioral Ecology
Edited by Elliott M. Blass

A Continuation Order Plan is available for this series. A continuation order will bring delivery of each new volume immediately upon publication. Volumes are billed only upon actual shipment. For further information please contact the publisher.

Handbook of
Behavioral Neurobiology

Volume 9
Developmental Psychobiology and Behavioral Ecology

Edited by

Elliott M. Blass

Johns Hopkins University
Baltimore, Maryland

1988

PLENUM PRESS • NEW YORK AND LONDON

Library of Congress Cataloging in Publication Data

Developmental psychobiology and behavioral ecology.
  (Handbook of behavioral neurobiology; v. 9)
  Includes bibliographies and index.
  1. Developmental psychobiology. 2. Animal behavior. I. Blass, Elliott M., 1940–
II. Series. [DNLM: 1. Animals—growth & development. 2. Behavior, Animal. 3. Fetal
Development. W1 HA511 v.9/QL751 D4895]
QL763.D48   1988   599′.051   87-38501
ISBN 0-306-42728-1

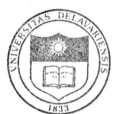

QL
763
.D48
1988

© 1988 Plenum Press, New York
A Division of Plenum Publishing Corporation
233 Spring Street, New York, N.Y. 10013

All rights reserved

No part of this book may be reproduced, stored in a retrieval system, or transmitted
in any form or by any means, electronic, mechanical, photocopying, microfilming,
recording, or otherwise, without written permission from the Publisher

Printed in the United States of America

To my children,
David and Joshua Blass

IBBH9116

Contributors

JEFFREY R. ALBERTS, *Department of Psychology, Indiana University, Bloomington, Indiana*

ANNE A. ARBERG, *Department of Psychology, University of North Carolina, Chapel Hill, North Carolina*

ELLIOTT M. BLASS, *Department of Psychology, Johns Hopkins University, Baltimore, Maryland*

STEPHEN C. BRAKE, *Department of Developmental Psychobiology, New York State Psychiatric Institute, College of Physicians and Surgeons, Columbia University, New York, New York*

GORDON M. BURGHARDT, *Departments of Psychology and Zoology, Graduate Program in Ethology (Life Sciences), University of Tennessee, Knoxville, Tennessee*

ROBERT COOPERSMITH, *Department of Psychobiology, University of California, Irvine, California*

CATHERINE P. CRAMER, *Department of Psychology, Dartmouth College, Hanover, New Hampshire*

MYRON A. HOFER, *Department of Developmental Psychobiology, New York State Psychiatric Institute, College of Physicians and Surgeons, Columbia University, New York, New York*

JERRY A. HOGAN, *Zoology Laboratory, University of Groningen, A.A. Haren 9750, The Netherlands, and Department of Psychology, University of Toronto, Toronto, Canada*

WARREN G. HOLMES, *Department of Psychology, University of Michigan, Ann Arbor, Michigan*

INGRID B. JOHANSON, *Department of Psychology, Florida Atlantic University, Boca Raton, Florida*

PRISCILLA KEHOE, *Department of Psychology, Trinity College, Hartford, Connecticut*

ANDREW P. KING, *Department of Psychology, Duke University, Durham, North Carolina*

MICHAEL LEON, *Department of Psychobiology, University of California, Irvine, California*

DAVID B. MILLER, *Department of Psychology, University of Connecticut, Storrs, Connecticut*

SCOTT R. ROBINSON, *Laboratory for Psychobiological Research, Departments of Psychology and Zoology, Oregon State University, Corvallis, Oregon*

HARRY SHAIR, *Department of Developmental Psychobiology, New York State Psychiatric Institute, College of Physicians and Surgeons, Columbia University, New York, New York*

WILLIAM P. SMOTHERMAN, *Laboratory for Psychobiological Research, Departments of Psychology and Zoology, Oregon State University, Corvallis, Oregon*

LESLIE M. TERRY, *Department of Psychology, Duke University, Durham, North Carolina*

MEREDITH J. WEST, *Department of Psychology, University of North Carolina, Chapel Hill, North Carolina*

PAULINE YAHR, *Department of Psychobiology, University of California, Irvine, California*

Preface

The previous volume in this series (Blass, 1986) focused on the interface between developmental psychobiology and developmental neurobiology. The volume emphasized that an understanding of central nervous system development and function can be obtained only with reference to the behaviors that it manages, and it emphasized how those behaviors, in turn, shape central development.

The present volume explores another natural interface of developmental psychobiology; behavioral ecology. It documents the progress made by developmental psychobiologists since the mid-1970s in identifying capacities of learning and conditioning in birds and mammals during the very moments following birth—indeed, during the antenatal period. These breakthroughs in a field that had previously lain dormant reflect the need to "meet the infant where it is" in order for behavior to emerge. Accordingly, studies have been conducted at nest temperature; infants have been rewarded by opportunities to huddle, suckle, or obtain milk, behaviors that are normally engaged in the nest. In addition, there was rejection of the excessive deprivation, extreme handling, and traumatic manipulation studies of the 1950s and 1960s that yielded information on how animals could respond to trauma but did not reveal mechanisms of normal development. In their place has arisen a series of analyses of how naturally occurring stimuli and situations gain control over behavior and how specifiable experiences impose limitations on subsequent development. Constraints were identified on the range of interactions that remained available to developing animals as a result of particular events.

Along with the increased experimental success has come a new awareness on the part of psychologists of other ways to reveal the behavior of animals, namely, through ethology and behavioral ecology. These disciplines, among others, have made available for proximal analyses the strategies used by animals at different times and in different situations during their life cycle and provide means of assessing how these strategies may be directly influenced by developmental events. Stated differently, rich social interactions that are determined by preweaning factors became accessible for developmental analyses.

Coincident with psychobiologists' turning to naturalistic phenomena for analyses was an awareness by behavioral ecologists that an understanding of evolutionary (ultimate) mechanisms could not be complete without an understanding of how proximate factors determine the behaviors in question. It was no longer sufficient simply to identify classes of strategies and behavioral patterns used toward an end; it was necessary to identify the affordances provided by the environment and the animals means of interacting with them. Stated differently, attention became focused more narrowly on particular niches occupied by an animal at different times and on the tactics used to exploit each niche. And in keeping with Tinbergen's prescient advice (*The Study of Instinct,* 1951), all camps recognized that to ignore influences cast during development was to travel at risk.

Thus, the present volume. It offers theoretical and empirical discussions of the interface between the development of behavior and environments that afford natural interactions. It is written by scientists whose own research reflects an appreciation of the concerns and nuances of both developmental psychobiology and behavioral ecology. All of the authors responded warmly to my challenge of producing an interdisciplinary text that reflects the infant's sophistication, its rich natal (and prenatal) habitat, and the often enduring influences of negotiations with its immediate and changing niches.

Furthermore, as shown in the chapters by Coopersmith and Leon, by Kehoe, and by Yahr, sophisticated questions concerning events that occur naturally can provide rich information concerning neural, neurochemical, and hormonal processes and functions in ways that simply had not been available in the mid-1970s. These chapters reflect the startling technical progress attained in these disciplines and the wealth of information now available for the study of central function. They also reflect the sophisticated understanding of behavioral systems used under natural circumstances that can be articulated experimentally by psychobiologists with sufficient precision to allow an empirical interface with the new technologies.

This volume and its predecessor acknowledge the coming of age of developmental psychobiology as an independent discipline that systematically analyzes the demands placed on animals at various developmental points and the changes in these demands with time, maturation, growth, and experience. Although of one basic theme, the text is of two sections. The first four chapters, by Alberts and Cramer, West *et al.,* Hogan, and Burghardt, are basically theoretical. Each chapter provides different but complementary perspectives of the demands on infants during development, the various strategies used to meet these demands by different vertebrates, and the perceptual and motivational changes that may occur in the infant as a result of these interactions.

The other chapters look specifically at different niches occupied during development and adjustments to that ambience (e.g., fetal life—Smotherman and Robinson); behaviors that characterize the early period (e.g., suckling—Brake, Shair, and Hofer); general processes (e.g., conditioning—Johanson and Terry); and outcomes (e.g., kin selection—Holmes; imprinting—Miller). As mentioned above, Coopersmith and Leon focus on neural changes during conditioning; Kehoe on opioids and development; and Yahr on hormonal and behavioral influences on the CNS and behavioral sexual differentiation. Obviously, there are overlaps among certain themes, and as editor, I have attempted to integrate them.

The opening chapter by Alberts and Cramer provides the volume with its intellectual setting. They write of the different habitats that infants simultaneously occupy, the different support systems available in each habitat, the infants' task in each one, the reinforcing stimuli of each respective habitat, and the immediate and longer term influences exerted by each habitat during the infant's passage. The approach dispenses with the vague and cumbersome notions of environments that leave the infant passive and at their mercy. With their ideas on both specialized and general responses to specialized and differing habitats, the authors point the way to focal, specific, and nonrandom classes of interactions between the infant and specific portions of its setting.

These ideas are advanced further by West, King, and Arberg, who advocate investigating exogenetic forms of heredity. This approach is especially compelling for the study of development during the nesting period, when the amount of environmental variability is so very much lower than after weaning. With eloquence West, King, and Arberg argue that the highly specialized, relatively restricted classes of behavior that altricial infants present at birth and during the nesting period reflect the stability of the species nest relative to the wider fluctuations in the environments in which nests are constructed. Environmental vagaries and variabilities are reduced by specialized parental feeding and nurturing behaviors that mesh with the infant's own correlated specializations. The mesh, as emphasized in these initial chapters, gives rise to the infant's discovering the regularities and idiosyncracies of its own particular sets of niches and habitats.

Hogan's chapter focuses on the changes in the infant that reflect specific classes of interactions. Following lines of classic ethological theory, Hogan offers a contemporary position on the integration of sensory, motor, perceptual, and motivational systems. Through a series of thought and empirical experiments, Hogan demonstrates the independence of each system and illustrates steps that are sufficient to synthesize the independent systems. Some of the steps are not immediately apparent, and Hogan clarifies their subtlety. In some instances, the player actively manipulates specific aspects of its niche; in other cases, a more passive attitude is taken. Hogan therefore provides a theoretical framework that permits the specification and testing of conceptual changes (which are reflected in behavioral changes) following different categories of sensory and motor experiences during ontogeny. As will be seen, the value of Hogan's program as a heuristic extends beyond the ontogenetic framework.

A different tack is taken by Burghardt, who provides lessons from a comparative behavior approach. Burghardt grapples with the knotty evolutionary problem of play and its origins. His argument is that play can be understood from the perspective of peripheral energetics and does not have to be understood as a higher order behavior with certain ultimate functions that have yet to be determined. Peripheral explanations may have considerable heuristic value for understanding other, seemingly radical changes in the reptilian and avian–mammalian grades, as well as for seemingly discontinuous developmental phenomena (motor patterns, for example; Thelen, 1985)

Burghardt's sensitizing us to the tasks faced by infant reptiles and amphibia, raised in a liquid medium, helps prepare us for Smotherman and Robinson's chapter on when mammals also live in a liquid medium, namely, as fetuses. Through a series of creative and precise experiments, the authors reveal very sophisticated sensorimotor, perceptual, and conditioning capacities of the fetus. The fetus is responsive to external events; indeed, it influences them, actively through swallowing, passively through hormonal secretions (which help determine the characteristics of its immediate neighbors). The fetus can learn, and this information appears to carry over into postnatal life. This chapter, in particular, could not have been written 5 years ago. It may represent a watershed in developmental psychobiology, as it provides investigators with the possibility of studying the differentiation and integration of behaviors (and their underlying neurologies) at the time of their earliest expression.

Pauline Yahr's chapter also focuses on the fetal period and evaluates events during that time that uniquely determine gender and its derivative behavioral expressions. She demonstrates time-linked responses of fetuses and, later, infants to their changing hormonal-behavioral environments. This is a very powerful analysis that may serve as a model for the multilevel analyses of habitat–mechanism–neural alteration, morphological, and behavioral changes. Yahr demonstrates these classes of changes at each level and prepares us for the next two chapters, which first thoroughly describe mechanisms of conditioning and then neural modifications that reflect the actions of conditioning systems.

Johanson and Terry address the process of conditioning during infancy and its ramifications. They demonstrate that, when certain boundary conditions are met (e.g., high ambient temperature and stimulation), infant rats, among others, on the day of birth exhibit classical and operant conditioning that is remarkably similar to that of adults. That the boundary conditions mimic those provided by the mother in the nest expands the opportunities for conditioning influencing immediate consequences (e.g., activation by the odor of milk) and long-term consequences (e.g., on male sexual behavior). The power of their analysis offers hope for what seemed an impossibility 5 years ago—technological and theoretical bases for identifying classes of events—sensory, perceptual, and motor, and their underlying associative mechanisms that shape behavior during development. My own feeling is that the possibilities for modification are remarkably few, probably restricted to the activities specified by Johanson and Terry (e.g., suckling and huddling) but that, within these activities, their concomitant rewards and limited motor patterns, a very broad spectrum of stimuli will be able to gain control over specific classes of motor acts (see Hogan's chapter).

Whereas Johanson and Terry have gained experimental control over vital behaviors as they appear spontaneously in the nest, Coopersmith and Leon reveal that this type of control can be brought into the service of analyzing natural events that determine neural structure and possibly function (also see Pedersen, Greer, and Shepherd, in the previous volume on this point). Coopersmith and Leon used state-of-the-art anatomical techniques to identify specific changes on the glomerular portion of the olfactory bulb in infant rats that were smelling a certain odor. The particularity of the stimulus reflects its previously having been paired with the type of excitatory stimulation normally provided by the mother on nest entry. Thus, the neurology of conditioning and excitation is now able to move apace with the behavioral advances.

Kehoe's chapter demonstrates another powerful system that participates in conditioning and in various infantile coping behaviors. She shows the advanced functional development of the endogenous opioid systems, their availability to the animal as potential mediators of positive affect, and also their participation in naturally occurring stressful situations (e.g., individual or group separation from the mother). Kehoe's analysis expands into broader motivational issues of the circumstances under which circulating levels of opioids may be enhanced by exposure to conditioned stimuli and how these elevated levels, in turn, sustain preferences for the conditioned stimuli. By conditioning infants during the quiet of opioid administration, Kehoe demonstrates convincingly that conditioning can occur in rats during periods of quiescence as well as during periods of excitation, as documented by Johanson and Terry. In addition to providing a new substrate for functional central analyses, Kehoe suggests a third class of reinforcers: nonopioid and nonexcitatory. Her data suggest that the thermotactile qualities of the mother operate through nonopioid channels and, indeed, appear to negate elevated levels of circulating opioids.

The chapter by Brake, Shair, and Hofer fractionates suckling—on the surface, a simple behavior—into its component parts and demonstrates the integration and contribution of each of these components to attachment, facilitation of milk let-down and milk withdrawal. The authors point out the complexity of the mother as a suckling stimulus, a supplier of milk and stimulation. This maternal habitat is likewise defined by the particular actions of the infant and the various behaviors and strategies that it uses to manipulate the mother, thereby maximizing milk yield. The niche has a third dimension: time, as suckling is embedded in the larger sleep–wake cycle. We will progress on the development of conditioning in the nest setting only to the extent that we solve the problems raised in this chapter on the circumstances that allow the infant to quickly emerge from sleep and then quickly lapse back into sleep, having obtained milk and information about the circumstances in which milk is provided.

The final two chapters, by Holmes and by Miller, focus on outcomes as well as mechanisms. Both authors come from the perspective of well-defined phenomena as they occur in the field. In powerful analyses, they scrutinize in the field and the laboratory the classes of developmental and proximal circumstances that gave rise to their respective phenomena. Holmes writes of kin selection as an exemplar of how familiarity influences different classes of social interactions, including altruistic behavior, cooperative defenses of territory, and mate selection, as well as influences of strangers on pregnancy and puberty onset. These are rich literatures that share the common perceptual event of the recognition of family (possibly self) and the recognition of "not-family." Using Belding ground squirrels as subjects, Holmes shows how kin recognition—in this species, at least—reflects the animal's experience with conspecifics during development. The mechanisms naturally at play here appear, on the surface, to have many of the temporal qualities of those identified experimentally in laboratory analyses in the preceding chapters. They provide, therefore, a rich bioassay for studying the ontogeny of conditioning and its lasting memory from both behavioral and neuroanatomical perspectives.

Miller's chapter brings us full circle. We started broadly theoretically and then focused on particular niches, behaviors, or mechanisms. Miller's approach epitomizes the classic ethological analysis of studying the very classes of stimuli and their quantitative manipulations, that give rise to behaviors as they naturally occur. This is the clearest analysis of exogenetic factors as they influence behavior. Miller eschews studies of imprinting behavior that have historically selected stimuli out of convenience rather than from the natural context in which imprinting occurs. The latter kind of analysis, although the more demanding, is the one of choice. One can only agree with Miller and train the next generation of developmental psychobiologists to bring the powerful "psychological" concepts and paradigms to the service of phenomena as they occur in their natural (or closely approximated) niches, as exemplified by the authors in this volume.

It remains for me to thank each of the contributors publicly for their enthusiasm in undertaking this volume, and for their good cheer and reflection in responding to my editorial queries, prods, and suggestions. As before, I close on a personal developmental note. This text is dedicated to my children, David and Joshua, whose own development has always been a great education for me. They taught with clarity how their nestmates (parents) could influence their behavior and, with equal clarity, the limitations of these influences. That these lessons were also taught with grace and joy have made them so much the more enjoyable and memorable.

ELLIOTT M. BLASS

Contents

CHAPTER 5

The Uterus as Environment: The Ecology of Fetal Behavior 149

William P. Smotherman and Scott R. Robinson

CHAPTER 6

Sexual Differentiation of Behavior in the Context of Developmental
Psychobiology 197

Pauline Yahr

CHAPTER 7

Learning in Infancy: A Mechanism for Behavioral Change during
    Development 245

Ingrid B. Johanson and Leslie M. Terry

CHAPTER 8

The Neurobiology of Early Olfactory Learning 283

Robert Coopersmith and Michael Leon

CHAPTER 9

CHAPTER 10

CHAPTER 11

Warren G. Holmes

CHAPTER 12

David B. Miller

Ecology and Experience
Sources of Means and Meaning of Developmental Change

Jeffrey R. Alberts and Catherine P. Cramer

Introduction

Two worlds merge in the perspective we take for this chapter. One world is derived from behavioral ecology, the other from the discipline of developmental psychobiology. Their amalgamation provides a particularly rich view of behavioral development, one that we believe can stimulate the formulation and testing of new concepts and hypotheses.

Behavioral ecology draws on the relationship between organism and environment. Ecological perspectives focus on specific environmental features and organismic characteristics, and they emphasize functional relations between the two. Such perspectives constitute a central, indispensable theme in evolutionary, adaptationist thinking.

Developmental psychobiology reveals changes during development in the organization of behavior, which unlocks a world of sensory development, physiology, motivation, motor development, learning, and other underlying behaviorally relevant processes.

Together, these two perspectives provide breadth and depth for the analysis of behavior. With them, we are better attuned to the external events that impinge on an organism and the internal changes derived from the sensory and neural

Jeffrey R. Alberts   Department of Psychology, Indiana University, Bloomington, Indiana 47405. Catherine P. Cramer   Department of Psychology, Dartmouth College, Hanover, New Hampshire 03755.

JEFFREY R. ALBERTS
AND CATHERINE P.
CRAMER

transduction of the events. The developmental aspects of psychobiology are particularly important here, because sensory, motor, and neural functions change considerably during early life, a fact implying that the internal world of experience changes correspondingly. In addition, there is widespread evidence for the general rule that sensory and neural function during early life are a formative influence on the development of perceptual systems (see Hogan, Chapter 3). Generally speaking, research in behavioral ecology emphasizes the external factors, and research in developmental psychobiology emphasizes the internal ones.

In the subtitle of this chapter, we also refer to "means and meaning." These terms represent two goals of empirical science. First, empirical investigations are often designed to identify and clarify mechanisms. In the context of this chapter, we will view these mechanisms as the *means* by which developmental change is realized. A second goal of empirical investigation is to explore conceptual and theoretical issues, thereby enhancing the *meaning* of the data. In the context of this chapter, developmental psychobiology provides much of the empirical analysis that elucidates the mechanisms of developmental change (means), whereas behavioral ecology accounts for much of the conceptual framework (meaning).

The organization of this chapter tracks the developing mammal's journey through a fixed sequence of habitats. We deal with four definable habitats, which are depicted in Figure 1. The Norway rat *(Rattus norvegicus)* serves as our primary example, but we believe that most of the general ideas and ontogenetic patterns discussed in this treatment are relevant, if not directly applicable, to other mammalian species.

Figure 1A illustrates several rat fetuses in place in the uterine horns. We will

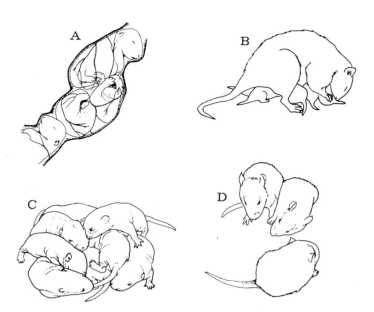

Figure 1. Four habitats in rat development. (A) The uterine habitat. (B) The mother as habitat. (C) The huddle as habitat. (D) The coterie or social group.

discuss the uterine environment as a habitat for fetal life and will describe behavior within it. Next, we will examine the universal mammalian phenomenon of maternal care and will evaluate how the mother's body and behavior constitute a distinct habitat, prominent during early postnatal life (Figure 1B). The huddle as habitat is depicted in Figure 1C, and we will discuss the pile of siblings in the nest as an important physical and social environment for the developing animal. The fourth habitat is the social coterie (represented in Figure 1D), which provides a habitat containing important elements for social and physical development as well as sexual maturation. (This range of habitats is not completely inclusive, but it represents common mammalian processes.)

ONTOGENETIC NICHES IN MAMMALIAN DEVELOPMENT

MAKING A LIVING: ADDRESS AND OCCUPATION

Ecology and adaptation are *relational* concepts. Both involve relations between organism and environment; as psychobiologists, our emphasis naturally is on the *organism* in relation to its environment. When these perspectives of ecology and adaptation are applied jointly to developmental questions, they become powerful tools for elucidating mechanism because ontogenesis involves marked changes in both the organism and its environments.

We shall consider an organism's immediate environment the "address" at which it lives. This address can be located in space and time and can be described in terms of its temperature, humidity, light level and cycle, energy sources and their distribution, as well as other basic environmental parameters. In a word, *address* equals *habitat*.

Behavioral ecology also helps us to focus on what an animal *does* in relation to its environment; that is, it points toward the animal's "occupation." The primary occupation of every animal is to "make a living" (adapt and survive) in its immediate environment. Thus, *occupation* equals *niche*.

Concepts of behavioral ecology, such as habitat and niche (address and occupation), help clarify the distinctions and interrelations between the physical environment (habitat) and the adapted organism in that environment (niche). We shall apply both concepts to the developmental sequences in the early life of mammals.

MAKING A MAMMAL: ADAPTATION AND ANTICIPATION

There is sensational diversity among the more than 4,000 kinds (species) of mammalian life forms. We mammals exist at every latitude on the planet, inhabiting the oceans (whales and seals), the air (bats), and the land (rodents, ungulates, and primates). Mammalian niches are highly varied and contain a wide range of diets, feeding strategies, social organizations, and life spans.

With such divergence, dispersal, and diversification, what makes the mammals a meaningfully unified group? All mammals share as characteristics: internal fertil-

JEFFREY R. ALBERTS
AND CATHERINE P.
CRAMER

ization, lactation, suckling behavior, and postnatal parental care. We think it is significant that the defining attributes of mammals nearly all pertain to developmental processes. Indeed, one unifying dimension of the mammals is that we share a common ontogenetic heritage. Fetal, newborn, infant, and juvenile mammals each inhabit distinctly different worlds, and each address requires a different occupation. In effect, the developing mammal occupies a predictable, discrete series of niches during its early life.

ADAPTATION DURING DEVELOPMENT. It is the offspring's "job" to make a living at its current address. In more traditional parlance, there is selection pressure for adaptive specializations to the habitat. An offspring's mode of adaptation (strategy) determines its specific occupation.

Physiologists such as E. F. Adolph (1968) have done elaborate analyses of the function and development of regulatory systems (e.g., heart, kidney, and temperature regulation) and have emphasized that the immature animal is not incomplete, it is different. The Russian physiologist Peter Anokhin (1964) proposed that infantile preadaptive systems are a general determinant of ontogenesis. Evolutionary theorists such as Williams (1966) remind us that the immature organism is specifically adapted to its environments as a result of natural selection, which exerts its force at each point in development, not just on the so-called final, adult product. Ethologists have long documented and studied various forms of infantile adaptations (Tinbergen, 1960). In addition to sensory, neural, physiological, and behavioral strategies, specific adaptive types of learning have been proposed for the immature organism (Alberts, 1987; Alberts and Gubernick, 1985; Johnston, 1985; West, King, and Arberg, Chapter 2).

ANTICIPATION DURING DEVELOPMENT. The young, rapidly developing offspring has a problem that the adult does not. In addition to its job of "being an infant" (i.e., adapting to an infantile niche, where, for example, food is sucked out of a teat, and efficient intestines are specialized for picocytosis, the digestion of fluid substrates), there is a *second occupation*. The developing organism also has the job of *anticipating the future niches* that it will encounter and preparing itself for the changes needed for successful adaptation. Thus, while exclusively suckling, many animals display tooth eruption and drastic alterations in the lining and the functional characteristics of the entire gastrointestinal tract (e.g., Henning, 1981), which will be needed in relation to an imminent but subsequent habitat and a different feeding niche (solid food).

CONCEPTS OF ONTOGENETIC NICHE AND ADAPTATION IN MAMMALIAN DEVELOPMENT

The concept of ontogenetic adaptation has received a good deal of attention in recent years (e.g., Alberts and Gubernick, 1985; Galef, 1981; Gould, 1977; Oppenheim, 1981). Much of our previous discussion in this chapter has been built around some of the basic tenets derived from the concept. That is, we have been viewing mammalian development as a process driven by dual forces: adaptation to the immediate environment and preparation for the next environment.

West, King, and Arberg (Chapter 2) have woven a timely and important perspective on the role of the ontogenetic niche, which they define as "the set of ecological and social circumstances surrounding organisms engaged in the business of development." Their view includes the idea that one of the roles of the niche is to be a formative force, which is passed on from generation to generation. That is, these authors show niche as a potential form of inheritance, a nongenetic structure but inherited as surely as genes. This "exogenetic inheritance" creates continuous, transgenerational legacies.

Together, the concepts of ontogenetic adaptation and ontogenetic niche create a thoroughly ecological perspective on development. Such a perspective is central to a psychobiological approach. Indeed, the present volume is a formal statement of the intimate connections between behavioral ecology and developmental psychobiology.

UTERUS AS HABITAT

All animals begin life before birth (or hatching), so we begin by examining the prenatal environment for clues and insights into the roots of developmental processes. Because this chapter is focused on mammals' development, we will therefore focus on their living conditions before birth, although similar analyses are available for oviparous species and other forms. Our analysis will begin around the time of the onset of behavior. Although behavioral onset is an ill-defined landmark, it puts us within the prenatal period and helps avoid an infinite regression into earlier and earlier ontogenetic antecedents (see Smotherman & Robinson, Chapter 5).

THE UTERUS AS LIFE SUPPORT SYSTEM

Despite the vast diversity and the enormous range of habitats occupied by adult mammals, all fetal mammals reside at a similar uterine address before birth. Nevertheless, the uterus is not to be considered a completely stable environment for the embryo or fetus. During the course of prenatal development, the uterus undergoes numerous chemical and mechanical transformations. In the case of some larger mammals, only a single individual is carried per pregnancy, but most mammals bear multiple offspring with each parity. In these more common species, such as the Norway rat, both uteri are occupied by fetuses during their gestation. Within this tubular world, early life is established and maintained.

Each individual fetus is attached to the uterine wall at a single point, via its *placenta*. The placenta is the avenue of physical exchange between the fetus and the mother. Their shared blood supply carries in and out all nutrients, oxygen, and wastes. During most of early fetal development, the placenta envelopes each fetus, apparently preventing direct contact. Between embryonic Days 15 and 17, the placentas recede until they each become a disc against the uterine wall; thus the physical buffer between fetuses is removed.

Each fetus is tethered to its placenta and the uterus by the *umbilical cord,* a flexible conduit of arterial and venous circulation. Fetal movements are permitted but limited by the umbilical cord. The chorion and the amnion are extraembryonic membranes that comprise specialized, fluid-filled sacks within which a fetus resides. The amniotic fluid around each fetus helps create a space in which the fetus can move and also serves as a reservoir for excreted waste. Later in gestation, when fluid volume diminishes and viscosity increases, the remaining fluid serves as a lubricant and facilitates movement. The uterus shows enormous elasticity as it transforms from "a string of pearls" (when it contains young fetuses) to a taut-walled, cylindrical tube just before term.

LIFE IN THE UTERINE WORLD

Our brief description of the uterus as a life support system provides an overview of some of the basic structural features of the world of the fetus. Smotherman and Robinson (Chapter 5) provide a more detailed and expert review of the uterine environment. We shall complete our abbreviated rendition to allow for a chronological coverage of the perinatal period.

The intrauterine world is commonly characterized as a dark, warm, silent environment, protected and buffered from extrinsic influences. Implied here are homogeneous conditions, continuously bland and undisturbed, perhaps fundamentally comfortable. Most mammals are born at immature stages of sensory development (e.g., sealed ears and eyes). Immaturity often implies lack of function, which can foster the question of whether fetal sensory systems actually transduce much stimulation (experience) at all.

Contrary to some traditional views, empirical studies of intrauterine conditions have revealed numerous forces of change and environmental fluctuation. Moreover, fetal sensory-perceptual systems, though incompletely developed, may be "functionally tuned" to receive particularly important environmental information. Fetal behavior, like postnatal behavior, can be examined for specific adaptive specializations that serve to help the organism both adjust to its immediate, proximate environment and prepare itself for an imminent change in its ontogenetic niche. Perceptions of smells, tastes, sounds, and tactile and vestibular events in the uterus can directly affect fetal behavior. These fetal responses can assist in ongoing adjustments to the uterine environment, and they can constitute useful practice for the sensory systems as preparation for later functional demands. Some stimuli, initially experienced *in utero,* will be encountered in postnatal life, so this type of early experience can serve as very specific preparation for later adaptation.

BEGINNINGS OF BEHAVIOR: FIRST MOVEMENTS. All vertebrate embryos that have been studied (including lampreys, sharks, amphibians, reptiles, birds, and mammals) exhibit the same type of initial muscular contraction pattern: slow, arrhythmic contractions in the anterior trunk region (Bekoff, 1985). These primary movements, called *head flexures,* occur spontaneously, in the absence of any known external stimulus. Debates continue over whether these are myogenically or neurally mediated movements (see Bekoff, 1985), but it is clear that this is an evolutionarily conservative pattern. Locomotor development in vertebrates is a story of species' specializations superimposed on templates of phylogenetic regularities.

Movements of the limbs, when they first appear, are coupled with trunk movements and do not appear independently (Hamburger, 1963). This obligatory coupling appears to result from a simultaneous activation of limb and trunk muscles by common input. Subsequent development of the limb movements involves integration and coordination between and within limbs.

In mammals, the development of interlimb coordination begins prenatally, first between homologous limbs (e.g., forelimb–forelimb) and then between homolateral limbs (right or left forelimb–hindlimb pairs) (Bekoff and Lau, 1980). Interlimb patterns typical of postnatal walking have been reported in fetal kittens (Windle and Griffith, 1931) and other mammals.

Although prenatal movements are constrained by umbilicus, placenta, and surrounding membranes, they are functionally important in the maintenance of flexible joints. The neuromuscular blockade of embryonic movements in chicks leads to fixed, immobilized joints (Drachman and Coulombre, 1962). One or two days' early paralysis leads to immobilization of the neck, legs, and toes. Similar effects have been noted in human fetuses, immobilized by maternal alcoholism (Walker and Quarles, 1962).

Fetal Respiratory Movements. Liggins (1972) stated a general, cross-species rule, that from midgestation on, fetuses display respiratory movements. Fetal respiratory movements are irregular and shallow; there is no air, only fluid to be moved. The inertial mass of the fluid must limit fetal respiratory movements, and only small volumes of fluid are moved.

Two functions are ascribed to fetal breathing movements. First, the fluid shifts distend the lungs and stimulate their growth. Supporting this hypothesis are instances in which nervous system abnormalities that impaired prenatal breathing were associated with small lungs, which were functionally inadequate to support extrauterine life (Liggins, 1972). Prenatal breathing is also believed to provide valuable "practice" that facilitates the performance of a complex neuromuscular action, needed immediately and continuously after parturition. In some species, respiratory movements are correlated with organized behavioral states. Human fetuses are believed to display breathing movements during periods of REM sleep, but not during quiet sleep or wakefulness.

Developmentalists interested in primacy often note that the very first movements made during embryogenesis are "spontaneous." Motor neurons can establish functional connections with muscle tissue before synaptogenesis with sensory afferents, providing a natural output-only motor system. Nevertheless, sensorimotor organization develops early as well.

Circadian Rhythmicity. Recent evidence indicates that the fetus's biological clock begins oscillating before birth, at least 3 days before the rat's 22-day gestation is complete. Reppert and Schwartz (1983) injected 2-deoxyglucose into pregnant mothers at different times of day. The isotope is taken up by brain cells in both the mother and the fetuses, so that the marker measures the circadian rhythms of pacemaker cells in mother and fetuses simultaneously. The fetuses proved to be synchronized to the rhythm of the mother. However, the basis of the fetal rhythms is not light passing through the mother's abdomen. Some mothers were blinded early in pregnancy and were placed in an environment with a reversed light–dark cycle. The rhythms of blind mothers remained on the original schedule, and their fetuses were synchronized to the mother, rather than to the outside world. Although it is clear that the fetus uses a maternal signal as *Zeitgeber,* the nature of the message has not yet been identified (Reppert, 1985).

The functional significance of prenatal rhythmicity remains indefinite. It may have preparatory usefulness, as a foundation for entrainment or maintenance by the mother's behavior after birth. It has also been suggested that fetal circadian rhythms are responsible for the timing of birth. In sheep, fetal adrenal secretions initiate labor. Pacemaker cells of the hypothalamus may regulate the adrenal control of labor, allowing the fetuses to time their departure from the uterine habitat and their arrival at their next address.

Numerous behavioral and physiological rhythms do not coalesce or become entrained to adultlike patterns until later in postnatal life (Allen and Kendall, 1967; Asano, 1971; Kittrell and Satinoff, 1986; Levin and Stern, 1975; Okada, 1971). To date, there has been little effort to analyze the intrinsic or extrinsic factors that support and regulate the development of these biorhythms.

BEGINNINGS OF EXPERIENCE: PRENATAL SENSORY-PERCEPTUAL FUNCTION. Although we can create a detailed, quantitative profile of the environmental parameters that exist *in utero* and give precise accounts of how the uterus functions as a fetal life-support system, these facts reveal little about the nature of fetal life—from the fetus's point of view.

To appreciate the development of behavior, there are at least two aspects of habitat that are critical to understand. One is the physical environment that provides stimulation of various kinds to the developing organism. We have already outlined some of important ecological parameters of the prenatal environment. *Experience* of the habitat is the second critical aspect necessary for understanding the extrinsic influences of the environment, particularly its behavioral consequences. If we know that the fetus is unable to detect particular features of its environment because it lacks sensory systems for certain classes of cues or because its immature sensoria are insensitive to the available levels of stimulation, then we can conclude that certain classes of stimulative experience are not directly relevant to development. However, we are well aware of the determinative, formative, and regulatory effects of experience on the development of behavior and the nervous system, effects that can begin at any point of sensory function, including before birth. To answer fully questions about the life in the uterine world we must know (a) what is present in the environment and (b) what information is available from the environment to the living, responsive organisms within it.

There is a regular sequence of onset of sensory function in the laboratory rat (see Alberts, 1984, for a review and discussion of the supporting data), which appears to be shared by all vertebrates. Gottlieb (1971) first published his meticulous review and synthesis of sequences of the onset of sensory function in a broad range of species. On the basis of his analysis of behavioral, histological, and physiological evidence, Gottlieb concluded that there may be a fixed sequence of functional onset that is common to all vertebrates. From this analysis can be derived several general rules or "principles" of sensory development (Alberts, 1984), which appear to have considerable cross-species validity. Thus, in analyzing the development of behavior in relation to sensory development in the rat, we may be addressing issues of considerable generality in mammalian development.

How can we learn about sensory function in a fetus? What is known about the prenatal development of sensory function? What do the data tell us about fetal experience during the prenatal period? Over the years, a variety of techniques have been developed by which living fetuses can be exposed to the observations and manipulations of experimenters (see Smotherman and Robinson, Chapter 5). When appropriate care is taken, the fetus remains viable and robust for substantial periods of time and, in certain preparations, can be replaced in the mother's body and permitted to develop to term. With such preparations, it has been found that the fetus displays unconditioned, reliable behavioral responses to suprathreshold sensory stimuli, allowing experimenters to study prenatal sensory function. Changes in fetal activity in response to an experimentally provoked stimulation reveals fetal perception of the cue. In addition, there are a variety of anatomical, morphological, and physiological measures that can be used to assess the function of immature sensory systems (see Gottlieb, 1971). With such methodological approaches, we can derive a psychobiological picture of the fetal world.

Integrative reviews of the sequence of onset of sensory function in the albino rat indicate that tactile perception, vestibular function, thermal sensitivity, olfaction, and taste all begin before birth (Alberts, 1984; Gottlieb, 1971). Tactile sensitivity is usually studied by providing gentle, punctate stimulation to discrete parts of a fetus and observing movement responses. Figure 2 shows the development of regional sensitivity to tactile stimulation across the body of a fetal rat from embryonic Days 16–20 (Narayanan, Fox, and Hamburger, 1971). It seems likely that, late in gestation, with the decreases in amniotic fluid, crowding in the uteri, and recession of the placenta, the fetuses stimulate and maintain in each other useful levels of movements.

Vestibular sensitivity is also present in fetuses. This fact has puzzled some workers, who imagined that amniotic fluid might create a condition of weightless buoyancy. Nevertheless, even in neutral buoyancy, gravitational forces are present, and it is possible that the vestibular mechanisms respond to geomagnetic forces. More important, probably, by late gestation amniotic fluid volume is greatly diminished, and the mother's movements alone provide linear and angular accelerations. Thus, we can safely judge the uterine environment as containing vestibular cues.

To date, only one study has evaluated vestibular sensitivity in newborns that were deprived of vestibular cues during gestation. The Soviet biosatellite *Cosmos 1514* carried 10 pregnant rats, exposing them and their fetuses to microgravity

JEFFREY R. ALBERTS
AND CATHERINE P.
CRAMER

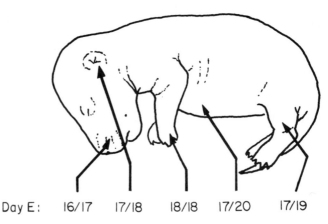

Day E: 16/17 17/18 18/18 17/20 17/19

Figure 2. Regional sensitivity to tactile stimulation in the fetal rat. There is a general rostral-to-caudal progression of tactile sensitivity that begins around embryonic Day 16 (about 6 days before birth in the rat). The numerical values shown in this figure indicate the prenatal ages on which 50% or more of the fetuses tested by Narayanan, Fox, and Hamburger (1971) displayed a response to punctate tactile stimulation on each body area shown.

conditions from embryonic Days 13 to 18. Pups born on earth, 4 to 5 days after the spaceflight, evidenced vestibular sensitivity in tests of righting, negative geotaxis, and a head of nystagmus to angular motion (Alberts, Serova, Keefe, and Apanesenko, 1985).

Vestibular function is implicated in fetal behavior crucial for the transition from prenatal to postnatal life. Figure 3 is based on some of Tinbergen's classic work (1960) on herring gulls, in which he observed egg shifting within nests. He collected data on the orientation of marked eggs, noting that the parents periodically shifted or rotated each egg around its longitudinal axis. We have redrawn some of Tinbergen's data, showing the recorded orientations of eggs across 400 repeated observations of eight eggs. The summary diagram on the right-hand side of Figure 3 shows that the egg shifting results in fairly regular and random orientations over time.

The left-hand portion of the figure, in contrast, shows the orientations of the chick's pip hole, as it initiates its emergence from the egg. Tinbergen found that nearly every chick in 43 observations pipped at the top of the egg. In fact, nearly half of all pip holes were located at the highest point in the upper quadrant. Tinbergen offered the likely, but tentative, conclusion that the chick's vestibular sense determines its pipping orientation. Tinbergen's finely detailed analysis addresses the anomalous concentration of pip holes at the very base of the egg as a possible "illusion" created by the mechanics of the chick's vestibular organ.

The Chemical Senses in Utero. Little is known about the initial onset of function for either olfaction or taste, although it appears that both are among the early-developing systems. It is also clear that both modalities undergo considerable postnatal maturation (Alberts, 1984). Chemosensitivity *in utero* is an aquatic feat. Although the developing olfactory system is preparing for continuous nasal respiration in air, it begins by transducing chemical cues in amniotic fluid. There is evidence from behavioral (Pedersen and Blass, 1982) as well as from 2-deoxyglucose autoradiographic techniques (see Pedersen, Greer, and Shepherd, 1986) for prenatal olfactory function.

Bradley and Mistretta (1973) conducted elegant studies of *in utero* taste function in sheep. With surgically implanted flow transducers, they monitored fetal swallowing *in utero* and found that they could modify rates of fetal swallowing by changing the chemical environment. When sucrose was injected into the amniotic fluid, swallowing rates increased.

Earlier, we described some of the functions of fetal swallowing in altering the uterine environment. Ingestion of amniotic fluid is one way of creating room for growth and movement *in utero;* it also provides some nutrient and aids gastrointestinal development. To the extent that active chemical senses either stimulate swallowing or provide generally arousing stimulation that activates behavior, including swallowing, such sensory function stimulates or augments a critical behavior. Indeed, without the tongue movements associated with fetal swallowing, development of the palate can be impaired (Walker and Quarles, 1962).

The Thermal Environment in Utero. The body temperature of the mother fluctuates with a circadian rhythm. In sheep, the daily temperature change is about 1°C. In rats, with a higher metabolic rate, the changes are even more dramatic. Prenatal temperature sensitivity in rats has not been studied, but there is evidence of fetal temperature responses in other organisms. Fetal sheep change their gross

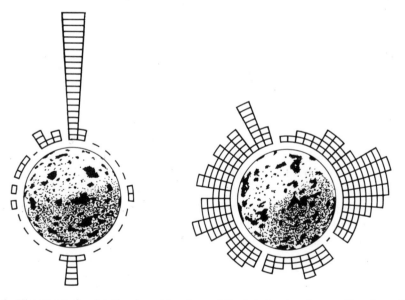

Figure 3. Histograms showing the skewed locations of the hole in pipped eggs of herring gulls (left drawing), which can be contrasted with the random position tracked on marked eggs of the same type before pipping (see Tinbergen, 1960 for a description of these field studies). Each rectangle surrounding the eggs indicates an observation. Vestibular cues are apparently used by the prenatal gull chicks to direct their pipping activities against gravity. Before hatching, the parents shift the eggs frequently and continuously.

activity levels in response to changes in temperature. Some fetuses show small variations in metabolic heat production in response to changes in environmental temperature.

Audition during Prenatal Life. In rats, the prenatal environment is probably silent to the fetuses; the onset of auditory function does not occur until well after birth. Nevertheless, in a variety of more precocial species, prenatal auditory experience can influence perinatal behavior. Unborn chicks and ducklings can hear the mother's vocalizations as well as those of their unhatched nestmates through the shells. Such stimulation can synchronize their hatching activities. Gottlieb (1975) made the extraordinary revelation that prenatal auditory self-stimulation (hearing its own vocalizations) is a necessary precursor to normal, species-typical discrimination of maternal calls.

More recently, the existence of rich and functionally significant prenatal auditory experiences has been documented for human infants. The findings of DeCasper and Fifer (1980) include demonstrations that infants detect and learn the identity of their mother's voice while *in utero.* Auditory preference tests, administered soon after birth, reveal preferences for the sound of their own mother's voice compared to that of another female reading an identical passage from a children's book. Miller (Chapter 12) provides a thoughtful review of some of the relevant literature on early acoustic experiences.

MOTHER AS HABITAT

The infant's passage through the birth canal is a sudden and dramatic change of address. Before birth, although surrounded by the mother, the fetus is only indirectly influenced by the mother's behavior. However, after birth, the mother's actions can be more specifically directed toward her young and can become the central feature of their ontogenetic ecology. As an integral element of the postpartum habitat, she continues to serve as a buffer between the young and the larger environment, but now as much via her behavior as via her physiology and morphology. For example, although no longer encased within her uteri, altricial young continue to depend on the warmth provided by contact with the dam. Similarly, if housed in a burrow, the young's only access to environmental *Zeitgebers* continues to be through social contact with their mother. Thus, as the young mammal develops between fetal and independent life, its habitat is defined largely by the characteristics and actions of other individuals. In this section, we consider the features of the habitat derived from the mother, that is, the nursing habitat; in the next section we consider the littermates, that is, the huddle habitat.

MOTHER AS LIFE SUPPORT SYSTEM

The rat dam prepares for parturition by building a nest and by licking her anogenital region and spreading amniotic fluid across her ventrum (Rosenblatt and Lehrman, 1963). As each pup is born, she licks it, both cleaning the pup and providing it with tactile stimulation. Without tactile stimulation, as many as 40% of newborn rats do not survive. Within an hour after the birth of the last pup, the dam begins nursing. During their first few days together, she spends 60%–80% of her time with the pups, most of it nursing. Her nursing bouts are only occasionally interrupted when she must leave the nest for routine foraging activities. Over the first two weeks, these times away from the litter gradually increase in frequency and duration. As shown in Figure 4, maternal nest time declines, although the amount of milk transferred increases, during Days 11–15.

A typical nursing bout begins when the dam enters the nest, often stepping on the pups as she gathers them together and licks their anogenital regions. Within 2 minutes, she assumes a nursing posture, arching over the litter, as she continues licking them. To suckle, the pups must actively seek and attach to available nipples, because there is little or no direction provided by the dam. About 5–20 minutes after they attach, the pups receive their first milk letdown (Grosvenor and Mena, 1974), in which a finite quantity of milk (averaging 0.1 cc) is released to each nipple. A period of quiescence lasting 3–5 minutes is then followed by another letdown episode. The bout ends with the dam leaving the nest, usually after 30–45 minutes and 8–10 milk letdowns in 10-day-old litters.

Throughout this series of interactions, the dam provides several vital commodities to her young. The most important of these is undoubtedly milk, which constitutes the sole source of both food and fluid intake during the first 17 days. She is also their primary avenue for gaining heat (although they have the ability to generate some warmth themselves via brown adipose tissue and, additionally, have some very elegant mechanisms for retaining heat, to be described later). On a more subtle level, the mother continues her preparturition functions of removing wastes and providing protection within the nest. Thus, although the pups are no longer housed within her body, she continues to envelop them within an intricate structure of interactions that achieves essentially the same complete transfer of energy and support. The pattern of these interactions supplies to the offspring a variety of "punctuated" experiences. Milk comes in discrete ejections, and licking is provided during several bouts per day; thermotactile stimulation is regular but peri-

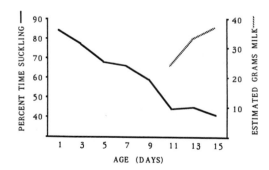

Figure 4. Time spent by lactating rats with their litters and estimated milk transferred to pups during the first 2 weeks postpartum, illustrating increasing feeding efficiency (more milk intake per unit time suckling) during this period (redrawn from Grota and Ader, 1969, and Babicky, Ostadalova, Parizek, Kolar, and Bibr, 1970).

odic and changes with each postural adjustment by the mother and the litter. Such punctuations may provide opportunities for the formation of regular and predictive associations or relations among stimuli and experience.

ADAPTING TO THE NURSING WORLD

In no case are the pups simply passive recipients of the maternal resources; they have specific behavioral adaptations to increase the utility of each of these functions. They stimulate the dam to enter the nest and retrieve them, particularly with ultrasonic cries when isolated or cold (e.g., Noirot, 1968; Allin and Banks, 1971). Her milk letdowns are induced by the tactile stimulation of sucking, which initiates the neuroendocrine arc culminating in oxytocin release (Brake, Shair, and Hofer, Chapter 10). The pups can modulate their intake of the available milk by varying negative pressure on the nipple as they extract milk or by increasing the incidence of nipple-shifting (Cramer and Blass, 1983). Finally, the pups do not soil the nest but instead contribute to the dam's fluid balance via urine reclamation, thus indirectly providing more resources for themselves (Alberts and Gubernick, 1983). All of these feats require that the infant be able to perceive, to some degree, both internal state and environmental conditions. We begin with an assessment of those abilities.

SENSORY-PERCEPTUAL SYSTEMS. The tactile stimulation received by the pups at birth is immediate and intense. As the mother removes the amniotic sac and umbilical cord, most of the pup's body is licked and stimulated. This process is repeated, to a lesser extent, when the mother manipulates the pups in her paws and licks their anogenital region before nursing. Moore and her colleagues have described an interesting variation in this stimulation. They observed that mother rats lick anogenital (AG) areas of their males offspring three times more than they lick the AG areas of female littermates (Moore and Morelli, 1979). This gender difference in maternal licking is controlled by the hormonal status of the infant. Male pup urine contains androgen-dependent chemicals that produced increased licking (Moore, 1984). Castrated males are licked at the low female rates. Female pups either anointed with male urine or given injections of testosterone, are licked at rates equivalent to those for male pups.

As they contact the mother's body to nurse, the pups no doubt feel her fur, which contrasts with their own furless skin. When they contact the nipple, the tactile stimulation on their snouts guides the movements leading to attachment. Finally, the oral sensations of the extended teat in the mouth are of sufficient importance to the pup so that they have reinforcing value in their own right (Kenny and Blass, 1977). Also, in the process of suckling, pups probably receive vestibular stimulation, both from turning as the mother licks them and during the course of nipple attachment and nursing, which they do from an inverted position underneath the mother.

The olfactory stimuli with which the infant rat is confronted at birth change dramatically from the relatively slow-changing liquid-borne scents *in utero* to the rapidly fluctuating volatiles available in the nest. In addition to the odors from birth fluids, the pup immediately encounters scents from the mother's saliva, as well as whatever residual odors from her excreta that are retained on her skin and fur. The pups use these odors to guide them in their search for nipples (Teicher and Blass, 1976, 1977).

Pedersen *et al.* (1986) suggested, on the basis of recent studies with radioactive uptake markers, that odors are processed by accessory olfactory bulb during the prenatal period, whereas the anatomically adjacent but separate main olfactory bulb appears to be the active mechanism for postnatal olfactory transduction. These authors discussed the possibility that associative mechanisms mediate the transition from accessory to main olfactory function, and they speculated on various levels of neural control, within both the olfactory bulb and the amygdala, on which this transition might occur.

Gustatory experience is surprisingly rich, even within the confines of the nest. Nursing, including nonnutritive suckling, occupies much of the pups' time. This activity is organized around oral and gustatory stimulation. There is evidence that, by the end of the 2nd week, the pup's gustatory abilities allow it to detect in the mother's milk specific chemical clues typical of her diet (Galef and Henderson, 1972). Pups are capable of tasting solutions of quinine and salt as early as 5 days of age; however, in the suckling situation, with the nipple extended far back in the mouth, the opportunity to taste the milk may not occur during the first week or so (Kehoe and Blass, 1985). Pups may nonetheless be able to sense volatile flavors during this time. By day 15, certainly, they show evidence of sensing and responding to gustatory cues in the milk determined by the mother's diet (Galef and Sherry, 1973).

MOVEMENTS IN THE NURSING HABITAT. Among the first obviously functional motions made by neonatal rats are the head movements as they scan the mother's body before locating and attaching to a nipple. Figure 5 is a fine-grain analysis of these scanning movements, made by a 3-day-old pup, along the ventrum of an anesthetized dam (MacFarlane, Pedersen, Cornell, and Blass, 1983). Beyond attachment, pups respond to a milk letdown by emitting a "stretch" response, in which the limbs are extended and the head is pulled perpendicular to the back (Lincoln, Hill, and Wakerly, 1973; Vorherr, Kleeman, and Waverly, 1967). This behavior may function to increase the ease and rapidity with which milk can be extracted during the few seconds in which it is available in the teat. During milk letdown, the pups' sucking becomes rhythmic, and the negative pressure on the nipple increases (Brake, Shair, and Hofer, Chapter 10). After a few seconds, presumably when the milk is depleted, the pups release the stretch and return to their resting posture and nonnutritive sucking pattern.

Until about 2 weeks of age, rat pups suckling the nipples of anesthetized dams remain attached to a single nipple for hours on end. After 2 weeks of age, they begin shifting from nipple to nipple (Hall, Cramer, and Blass, 1977). The incidence of nipple-shifting increases with age and with level of deprivation and occurs most prominently immediately after each milk letdown (Cramer, Blass, and Hall, 1980).

JEFFREY R. ALBERTS
AND CATHERINE P.
CRAMER

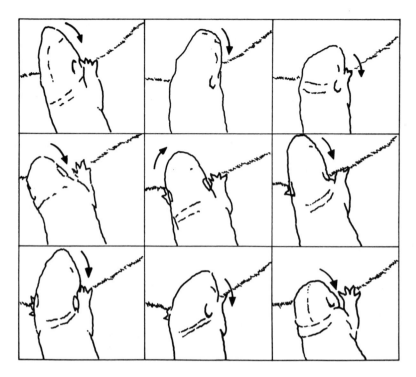

Figure 5. Movements of a 7-day-old rat pup in the process of locating the nipple of an anesthetized dam. Each panel represents a single frame from a videorecording (Adapted from Pedersen and Blass, 1983).

In addition to the motions used in reattachment, nipple-shifting requires that the pup release the nipple, push itself away, and move to an alternative site.

LEARNING IN THE NURSING NICHE

The milk, warmth, and tactile stimulation that the dam provides her young during the nursing period not only are important for the pups' immediate survival but may also provide a context for experiential plasticity. Mother–infant interaction represents a dynamic process, changing over the course of development. The situational demands placed on both mother and young are altered as the pups mature. In the terminology outlined above, the niche of a 1-day-old pup is very different from that of a 20-day-old pup, both because the pup itself has grown and its morphology has changed and because the dam's responses to those changes are reflected in the interaction. For example, the modest thermoregulatory capabilities of a hairless newborn, with a large surface-to-mass ratio and an inability to generate much heat independently, require a regular pattern of maternal contact in which the pups can derive warmth from the dam. As well, it requires behavioral mechanisms for the pups to retain that increased thermal gain from the dam. Older pups, with a smaller surface-to-volume ratio, more adultlike physiological thermoregulatory mechanisms, and a good coat of fur, no longer require supplemental warming by the dam. In fact, the interaction may be limited by excessive heat exchange

(Leon, Croskerry, and Smith, 1978), creating a situation in which the pup must invoke alternative strategies for inducing the dam to nurse if it is to receive adequate nutrition.

In adapting to such changing features of the habitat, pups may also acquire information or skills that can be used in another, similar context. The nursing interaction, in particular, has proved to be an arena for several specific forms of learning. An excellent example of this process is the olfactory control of nipple location. Although pups will suckle the normal nipples of anesthetized dams, they fail to attach if the nipples have been washed (Teicher and Blass, 1976). Suckling can be reinstated by coating the nipple with an extract of the wash or with rat pup saliva. The critical component of pup saliva appears to be dimethyl disulfide, which itself initiates suckling when applied to washed nipples (Pedersen and Blass, 1982). At first glance, this would seem to be a relatively hard-wired system, with a particular compound controlling the complex motivated behavior. However, in a subsequent series of studies, Pedersen and Blass and their colleagues found several experiential mechanisms involved in specifying the stimuli that came to elicit the first and succeeding nipple attachments.

The first nipple attachment is normally elicited by amniotic fluid (Teicher and Blass, 1977). Amniotic fluid would seem an unusual stimulus for a behavioral system resistant to experience. First, the composition of amniotic fluid is continuously altered by fetal swallowing and excretion. Second, changes in maternal hormonal state alter amniotic fluid as parturition nears. Because amniotic fluid is a plasma filtrate, its composition and properties probably reflect the mother's diet. Finally, amniotic fluid is probably the first major olfactory stimulus that is experienced *in utero* (as a fluid) and *ex utero* (as volatiles from the nest area saturated with birth fluids; Pedersen and Blass, 1982).

Based on these observations, Pedersen and Blass (1982) altered the olfactory composition of the amniotic fluid by introducing citral, a tasteless, lemon-scented compound into each amniotic sac. Pups exposed both pre- and immediately postnatally to citral did not suckle normal nipples but instead attached to washed nipples scented with citral. Either pre- or postnatal citral alone did not result in this effect. Thus, a behavior that appears to have a primary function in one niche can contribute to the expression of another behavior in the next niche. In this case, the swallowing of amniotic fluid (which promotes normal gastrointestinal functions and helps regulate the uterine volume of amniotic fluid) and the activation provided by the mother at parturition (which is hygienic and promotes infant breathing and elimination) are critical events in the determination of the stimuli that subsequently elicit nipple attachment.

Activation that occurs in the normal nest situation in the days following birth may also provide a basis for plasticity. Stimulation normally occurs when the pups are in close contact with an odor source, the nipple. Because the presence of an odor during stimulation in the nest predicts that odor (usually pup saliva) on the nipple, the opportunity for Pavlovian conditioning may exist in the mother–infant niche. In support of such a notion, Pedersen, Williams, and Blass (1982) demonstrated that 2-day-old pups stimulated in the presence of an odor (e.g., citral) attached to washed nipples in the presence of that odor. An odor elicited attachment only if it was experienced during stimulation; neither odor alone in the absence of stimulation nor stimulation in the absence of the odor was sufficient for attachment. Thus, the licking behavior of the dam could serve both the primary function of eliciting urination (and aiding her subsequent fluid balance) and the secondary function of being a conditioned stimulus for the unexpected learning of the attachment cue. In fact, Pedersen *et al.* have suggested that this may be the mechanism by which a pup makes the transition from attaching to amniotic fluid (which does not contain dimethyl disulfide) to attaching to pup saliva.

In a further extension of this olfactory pairing paradigm, Fillion and Blass (1986b) demonstrated that adult male responsiveness to estrous odors is determined by infantile experience with apparently similar (Fillion and Blass, 1986a) odors on the maternal ventrum that elicit suckling. Adult male rats reared by mothers whose nipple and vaginal odors were altered with citral, and that therefore presumably never experienced normal nipple and vaginal odors, were slow to mate with normal estrous females, but they mated readily when such females were citral-scented. Males reared without citral mated in the opposite pattern, and males reared by dams whose backs were citral-scented mated as readily with either type of female. Thus, the responsiveness to an odor resulting from specific early adaptations to the nest environment can extend even to a different context much later in life.

A second example of a behavior that may have both an immediately adaptive and an anticipatory function is nipple shifting. The proximate function of nipple-shifting behavior seems to be to increase milk intake during a suckling bout, as relative intake is highly correlated with the amount of nipple shifting (Cramer and Blass, 1983). Nipple-shifting behavior seems to be somewhat responsive to environmental conditions. Normally, rats are raised in litters of 8–10 with 12 nipples available, leaving 2–4 nipples unsuckled after each milk letdown. Pups' opportunity to nipple-shift can be enhanced by reducing the number of pups to 5, thus leaving 7 nipples unsuckled after each letdown. Conversely, nipple-shifting opportunity can be decreased by reducing the number of pups to 5 but also reducing the number of nipples to 4. In this situation, virtually no nipples with remain unsuckled, as it is unlikely that a letdown will occur unless all four nipples are being suckled. When pups are raised from Days 5 to 20 in these conditions, they show alterations in both the incidence and the patterns of nipple shifting when tested on Day 21 (Cramer, Pfister, and Haig, 1986). As is shown in Figure 6, normal pups routinely shift 2 to 3 times per letdown, but they are essentially random in their choice of "new" versus "visited" nipples. Pups raised in litters of 5 with 12 nipples shift not only more frequently but also with greater accuracy, particularly in the later shifts. Pups raised in litters of five with four nipples shift infrequently, and when they do shift, they are essentially at chance. Thus, pups adapt to the number of nipples available to them and their littermates with appropriate levels and accuracy of nipple shifting.

There are interesting commonalities between the task demands during nipple-

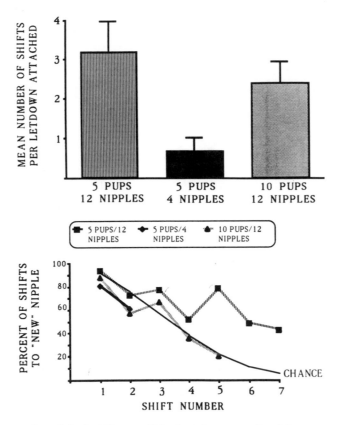

Figure 6. Mean number of nipple shifts per milk letdown (upper panel) and the percentage of shifts to a previously unsuckled nipple (lower panel) following rearing with a high density (5 pups with 12 nipples), a normal density (10 pups with 12 nipples) or a low density (5 pups with 4 nipples) of teats available. All pups were tested at Day 20 with a 12-nipple anesthetized dam as stimulus. The chance line in the lower panel is derived from Mellgren, Misasi, and Brown's estimate (1984) of the likelihood of foraging in previously visited patches in the absence of memory.

shifting behavior and those during adult foraging, at least as the latter is modeled in the radial maze (Olton and Samuelson, 1976). The maze simulates foraging patterns by requiring animals to retrieve food pellets from the ends of arms radiating from a central platform, much as a free-living rat would need to sample a variety of distant potential food sites. To maximize intake in the radial maze, a rat must (a) choose and run down a specific arm to a food well that contains a single pellet; (b) remove the pellet; and (c) avoid returning to that arm and instead visit the rest of the nondepleted arms. To maximize intake while suckling, an infant rat must (a) locate and attach to a nipple; (b) remove the finite amount of milk available; and (c) avoid returning to that nipple and shift to other nipples. Given these similarities, differential opportunities to nipple-shift during ontogeny could alter performance in the eight-arm radial-maze task after weaning (Cramer *et al.*, 1986). Figure 7 depicts this analogy between the challenge of foraging in a field of nipples and the challenge of a radial maze. Again, shifting opportunity was enhanced over normal

JEFFREY R. ALBERTS
AND CATHERINE P.
CRAMER

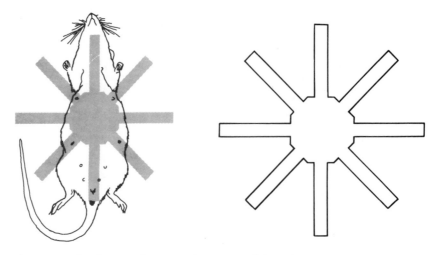

Figure 7. A comparison between the maternal ventrum and the eight-arm radial maze. Both represent a spatial array of discrete food sites, which can be depleted by a single visit.

(10 pups with 12 nipples) by reducing litters to 5 pups with 12 nipples and was decreased by reducing both litters to 5 pups and number of nipples to 4. Beginning at Day 25, the rats were separated from their dams and began daily maze testing.

Rats reared in litters of 5 with 12 nipples performed as well as normal rats. Thus, enhanced opportunity to nipple-shift does not improve performance. It could be that the amount of shifting provided in the normal nest is both necessary and sufficient, or the performance of both of these groups may have reflected a ceiling effect in the sensitivity of the maze paradigm. In marked contrast, however, rats reared in litters of five with four nipples performed very poorly, requiring three times the number of trials to reach criterion. These differences in peformance could not be attributed to differences in body weight, maternal care, or competition. Pups whose suckling experience was limited to anesthetized, oxytocin-induced dams, with all of these variables held constant, showed the same shifting-related variation in their acquisition of the spatial maze task (Cramer *et al.,* 1986). Thus, diminishing the opportunity to sample freely among nipples in the next situation compromised performance in a different task with different geometrical but similar demand qualities.

HUDDLE AS HABITAT

For the first 2 weeks postpartum, pups live in a pile or cluster called the *huddle* (Figure 1C). The huddle habitat provides continuous, direct physical contact with littermate siblings. In addition, the mother spends much of each day in the nest with them and contributes her own forms of stimulation, described in the previous section. Thus, the huddle constitutes a major aspect of the infant rat's habitat during early postnatal life. In this section, we examine the nature of this habitat and the pup's life in it. Huddling is also seen in adult animals, and we will briefly consider this phenomenon as a means of comparison and for developmental continuity.

21

ECOLOGY AND
EXPERIENCE

ECOLOGICAL SIGNIFICANCE OF HUDDLING BY ADULTS

There are in the ecological literature a number of studies addressing the role of huddling among adult organisms of many diverse species. In fact, even species in which the adults tend to live solitary lives often adopt more intimate arrangements with conspecifics during colder months (Hart, 1971). Huddling in furred animals provides each participant with a localized area of thicker insulation and reduces heat loss by conduction to colder surfaces. The general conclusion derived from this work is that huddling is an ecologically significant defense against cold (Whittow, 1971). But as we will see, there have been questions concerning whether huddling by infant mammals can be understood in the same terms as huddling by adults.

ALLOMETRIC IMPERATIVES

Size is an aspect of infancy and development frequently overlooked in behavioral analyses. We can, however, draw directly from morphological and physiological studies in which dimensional analyses called *scaling* or *allometry* (e.g., Schmidt-Nielsen, 1984) have contributed importantly to our understanding of the functional constraints on organisms.

Numerous characteristics of the rat pup can be understood as a function of its diminutive size. One physiologically significant consequence of small size is a correspondingly large surface–mass ratio. The importance of this parameter is apparent in terms of body temperature regulation: the rate of heat loss is a direct function of surface–mass. Small objects have larger surface–mass ratios than do larger ones.

The parameters of heat production differ between immature and adult rats, a situation typical of nearly all mammals, including humans. For its size, the infant produces less and loses more body heat that does the adult (Taylor, 1960). Thermogenesis by shivering is absent in the infant, and the limits of metabolic heat production are below those of the adult. Furthermore, heat loss is rapid in pups because they lack insulative fur and subcutaneous fat and cannot exert control over vascular flow (Hull, 1973).

The pups' small size (and large surface–mass ratio), their lack of subcutaneous fat, their hairlessness, and other physical characteristics together conspire to make the individual pup extremely vulnerable to temperature challenges, especially loss of body heat. As a result many writers have termed the infant rat *poikilothermic,* thereby likening the process of body temperature regulation in this small mammal to that in a reptile. In this regard, the significance of the huddle as a habitat can be appreciated.

JEFFREY R. ALBERTS
AND CATHERINE P.
CRAMER

PHYSIOLOGICAL CONSEQUENCES OF HUDDLING BY PUPS: TEMPERATURE REGULATION AND ENERGY CONSERVATION. By clumping together, pups reduce their exposed, heat-dissipating body surface, thereby decreasing their surface–mass ratio. Heat loss is significantly reduced, and huddling pups display higher body temperatures than nonhuddling littermates during periods of maternal absence (Alberts, 1978). Thus, we can derive two quite different views of the infant rat in terms of its thermal vulnerability. The isolated pup is far more fragile and poikilothermic than the pup in its "natural environment" (i.e., the huddle).

Rectal temperature is the most commonly used estimate of average "body temperature." This and other regional measures reflect, at best, the difference between the heat produced and the heat lost; they reveal little about the specific thermal strategies used.

Metabolic rate, measured in terms of oxygen consumption, is a more direct and global account of an organism's thermal strategy. Oxygen consumption can be translated into heat production or energy use. By combining such measures of metabolic effort with temperature data, we can derive a fairly complete picture of an animal's efforts and their thermal consequences.

The effect of huddling on metabolic rate (e.g., Alberts, 1978; Cosnier, 1965; Taylor, 1960) is the opposite of what would be predicted if rat pups were truly poikilothermic or, more accurately, ectothermic. Metabolic rate in an ectotherm is a direct function of ambient temperature. In contrast, pups in huddles are warmer than singletons, and they reduce their metabolic rates as one would expect of an adult. Metabolically, the huddle behaves much as does a single organism that is the size of the group, rather than as do the single organisms that comprise the group. The metabolic savings derived from huddling are formidable: without augmentation by nest insulation, a huddle of eight pups allows each pup save as much as 40% of its metabolic energy in the process of thermal maintenance. This savings, in effect, increases the limited nutritive resources (mother's milk) available. That is, pups can channel the nutritive energy from mother's milk into processes of growth and development. With increase in size, the development of fur, the deposition of fat, and other thermal capacities and defenses, the pups eventually are emancipated from the stiff challenges that appear to constrain them to the nest and the huddle.

REGULATORY BEHAVIOR IN THE HUDDLE. The important physiological consequences of huddling are not simply the result of piling bodies on one another. The infants actively participate in maintaining and regulating the huddle. They exchange positions frequently and interact to produce an effective form of "group regulatory behavior." The huddle acts as an adjustable unitary body, actively compensating for changes in ambient temperature. Arranged loosely in warm temperatures and tightly cohesive in the cold, the huddle expands and contracts, as its members maximize and minimize the heat-dissipating surface area of the clump (Alberts, 1978).

The huddle is a special habitat, and the infant pups display corresponding specializations by which they earn their living in it. Pups exchange positions in the huddle and, in effect, share the costs of exposure to the cool air and the benefits of insulation derived during the group activity (Alberts, 1978). Most of these behavioral mechanisms of thermoregulation have been studied in experimental tests of isolated litters, but the flow of pups within the huddle and the regulation of huddle size also occur in a seminatural habitat, in synchrony with maternal behavior (Addison and Alberts, 1980).

SENSORY EXPERIENCE IN THE HUDDLE. From the pups' point of view, postnatal life involves barrages of stimuli of greater scope and intensity than those experienced *in utero*. Sensory maturation progresses rapidly, so we assume that the pups' perceptual world is both broadening and deepening with the simultaneous expansion of sensory modalities, increased sensitivity, discriminability, and experience (Alberts, 1984).

The huddle is a source of rich and varied sensory input and of motoric opportunities even for the altricial neonate. Tactile stimulation abounds, for the huddle is usually a tightly packed mass of squirming bodies. At birth, the pups are hairless and thus receive and provide direct cutaneous stimulation. The mother's body is furry and warm. It is more appropriate to discuss *thermotactile* stimulation in the nest because the pups' contact behavior invariably involves heat exchanges (Alberts, 1978; Hull, 1973; Leon *et al.,* 1978; Mount, 1960). Rat pups are strongly attracted to sources of thermotactile stimulus and actively maintain contact with them, whether animate or inanimate. Their behavior in this regard is reminiscent of the dramatic responses to sources of warm, soft "contact comfort" displayed by Harlow and Harlow's infant monkeys (1962).

The movements of the pup throughout the huddle require vestibular and proprioceptive feedback. The constant agitation and reorganization of the huddle produced by the movement of 8–12 bodies in a mass is undoubtedly a source of vestibular stimulation.

The close physical interactions in the huddle bring many sources of olfactory and gustatory experiences to the pups. Gregory and Pfaff (1971) were among the first to show that rat pups become sensitive to nest odors early in life. Pups inspire olfactorily rich air from the bodies of their sibs, and from the first days of life, they scan and olfactorily explore the nest and their mother's body. Beyond the textures and tastes experienced during nursing, direct observations of litters have generated catalogs of the range and number of items that are orally sampled by the pups (Galef, 1979; Melcer and Alberts, 1985). These include the paws, tails, ears, and fur of themselves and their littermates, as well as the excretions available on virtually every portion and orifice of the mother's body. Figure 8 provides an overview of the rat pup's typical gustatory experience during the first two weeks of postnatal life, at least as it occurs in a typical tub cage in the laboratory. How "natural" are these experiences? That is, do the data in Figure 8 resemble conditions for feral rats, or is the laboratory situation more varied or constrained? Unfortunately, we are unaware of comparable observations in the wild, so there is no definitive answer to this reasonable question. Nevertheless, it has been noted that the mother rats maintain a clean nest environment, by urinating and defecating outside

JEFFREY R. ALBERTS
AND CATHERINE P.
CRAMER

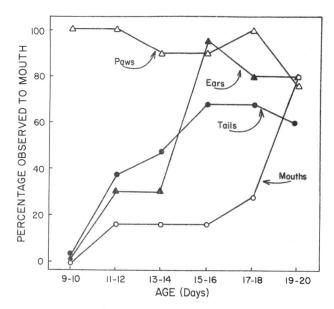

Figure 8. The gustatory experiences during early postnatal life in the rat include stimulation derived from mouthing body parts of the mother and the littermates. This graph illustrates the observed frequency of such mouthing activities in litters of rat pups from postnatal Day 9 to Day 20 (Melcer and Alberts, 1985).

the nest and by ingesting the pups' excreta (Galef, 1979; Gubernick and Alberts, 1983). Thus, it may be that the highly constrained nest in the laboratory is a reasonable facsimile of the gustatory conditions present in the wild.

There is good evidence that pups can detect acoustic cues before the point of ear opening, but the mechanical unsealing of the external auditory meatus produces an instant increase in sensitivity. Pups emit high-frequency vocalizations in the range of 40 kHz. These cries are commonly interpreted as representing "distress" vocalizations because they can be reliably elicited by decreasing the pup's temperature, and an isolated (and presumably distressed) pup rapidly loses heat. Hofer and Shair (1978) studied the ultrasonic emissions of 2-week-old pups. At this age, pups are far less thermally vulnerable; yet they emit cries when isolated. It appears that by 2 weeks of age, the pups clearly detect their separation from the familiar stimuli of the nest, such as the nest odors, and they respond with high-frequency calls. These presumably alert or attract the dam, and she can respond to the pup directly (Bell, 1974). (See Kehoe, Chapter 9, on the possible opioid mediation of this behavior.)

There are no clear demonstrations of the manner in which auditory perceptions may function during early life, although the sense is clearly functional. That is, there is no demonstrated role for auditory cues in the pups' world. Adult rats emit high-frequency vocalizations, but these have been documented only in adult–adult interactions, rather than in interactions with pups. It has been reported, however, that one of the critical stimuli that triggers the pup's initial egression from the nest into the world is movement cues provided by adult rats (Alberts and Leimbach, 1980), and these cues may be acoustic. Perhaps if researchers studied pup behavior under darkened conditions, thereby minimizing visual cues, we would be better attuned to the roles of auditory stimuli in the animal's world.

It is difficult to evaluate the likelihood and quality of typical visual stimulation during early life for the rat. As mentioned earlier, there is no "typical" site for natal nests, but in the wild, at least, they are probably in darkened areas. Rats frequently live in subterranean burrows where photic cues may be absent or very attenuated. Although there is a sizable literature on the consequences of different forms of visual stimulation and deprivation during early life (see Aslin, Alberts, and Pedersen, 1981), we will not dwell here on this indefinite aspect of the early life of the rat.

We have already discussed the way in which the mother and her behavior constitute a habitat for the pups. In the immediate postnatal period, maternal presence is nearly continuous. Beginning in the 2nd week, maternal presence in the nest becomes increasingly interrupted by periods of absence. Maternal nest bouts decrease both in frequency and in duration (Grota and Ader, 1969; Leon *et al.*, 1978; Plaut, 1974). The habitat is changing.

Despite the increasing absence of the dam, the huddle of pups maintains its coherence. Studies of the sensory controls of huddling in developing rat pups (Alberts, 1978; Alberts and Brunjes, 1978; Pfister and Alberts, 1983), indicate that, as maternal attendance is withdrawn, the maintenance of contact among the pups becomes more broadly controlled and takes on the additional strengths of filial attachments.

The infant rat's predominant organized behavioral activites—namely, suckling and huddling—accomplish two vital needs. Suckling brings nutritive energy into the organism, and huddling allows the infant rat to channel nutritive energy from the milk into processes of growth and development, rather than losing it to the environment. Together, growth and development lead to larger body size, the deposition of insulative subcutaneous fat, a fur coat, the autonomic control of blood vessel constriction, and greater powers of metabolic heat production. Thus, the juvenile produces and retains body heat more efficiently than its infantile counterpart. One consequence of its enhanced thermal capacities is that the pup can afford to leave the huddle and its physical contact with the dam. In fact, Leon *et al.* (1978) suggested that the enhanced thermogenic output of the huddle may literally drive the mother off the litter in order to prevent hyperthermia.

LEARNING IN THE HUDDLE HABITAT

One of the remarkable aspects of the developmental processes is the simultaneous occurrence of ontogenies at different levels of organization. Organismic development includes the developmental changes displayed by numerous integrated systems (e.g., musculoskeletal, central and peripheral nervous systems, gastrointestinal, sensory and behavioral). Many of the events that are integral to the huddle and the nest habitats work together in special concert that produces orderly changes in behavior that are relatively long-lasting. In this regard, the huddle becomes a learning milieu.

FILIAL PREFERENCES. Beginning around Day 15, rat pups exhibit a profound change in the nature of their huddling behavior. Although the contact behavior looks no different from that in the preceding periods, experimental studies of the sensory controls of huddling—especially the hierarchies of control—reveal fundamental discontinuities that have pointed the way to discoveries about natural sequences of learning that can affect the animal's lifetime social behaviors.

Day 15 marks a stage in rat development when heat and cues of contact comfort (furriness) are no longer the dominant forces determining approach and contact. Although warm, furry surfaces remain highly attractive, pups 15 days of age and older are more influenced by olfactory cues, specifically odors of their species (Alberts and Brunjes, 1978). This olfactory-guided huddling has been termed *filial huddling* because the defining cues appear to be olfactory signals of affiliation, and it is also a stimulus to which the animal attaches.

It was conceivable that the rat pups' tendency to affiliate with other rats was unlearned and preprogrammed, but Brunjes and Alberts (1979) found that they could reassign the rat pup's filial attractions by altering the social odors it experienced in the nest. By anointing the mother with an artificial odor and allowing her to interact with the pups in a motherly manner, the rat pups came to prefer the artificial to the natural rat odors. The ease with which pups' filial preference could be reassigned (Brunjes and Alberts, 1979) suggests that pups' normal preference may reflect certain nest experiences. In other words, rats exhibit a species-typical preference because they are reared in a species-typical environment.

It was important to examine the specificity of altered preferences. These experiments have been reviewed elsewhere (Alberts, 1984), so only the conclusions will be given here. First, it was found that the pups' altered preference was different from the kind that could arise from familiarization with a new odor. The "induced" preferences had a power greater than familiarization could bestow and, in fact, equaled the preference induced by a mother rat that huddled with, licked, and nursed the infant.

A series of "titration" studies was conducted to identify the events or contingencies that occur in the nest during mother–litter interactions, which induce the pup's olfactorily guided filial preferences. The test odors were associated with different kinds of experiences. For example, Odor A might be associated with a lactating, maternally responsive foster mother that nursed the test pups for a portion of each day, every other day, during the first 2 weeks of life. Odor B would be experienced equally, on the alternate days, in association with a maternally responsive foster mother that did *not* nurse the pups or provide milk. Then, on Day 15, when filial huddling is displayed, the pups were given preference tests designed to compare the relative strengths of filial attractions induced by different forms of odor–experience associations. The following kinds of experiences were assessed in different combinations: mere exposure to an odor (familiarization, or exposure learning), maternal care from a lactating foster mother, maternal care from a nonlactating foster mother, and contact with a warm, inanimate object. The conclusion from this study (Alberts and May, 1984) was that an odor experienced in association with *thermotactile stimulation* becomes a cue for filial attraction.

The "rewarding" nature of thermotactile stimulation was not surprising to discover, given the acknowledged salience of sources of warmth and insulation in the world of small, immature mammals. It was surprising, however, to discover that other sources of reward, such as the opportunity to suckle and the receipt of milk, had no measurable effect on the formation of filial huddling preferences. In one experiment, for instance, the pups formed equivalent filial preferences for each of two odors, one of which was associated with a lactating foster mother and the other with a heated tube.

Johanson and Terry (Chapter 7) provide other examples of how early experiences might establish in the neonate associations that enable certain stimuli to have "permissive" functions that can give conditional breadth or specificity to the infant's behavioral repertoire.

Coterie as Habitat

As the pups move into their 3rd week, they begin a process of achieving greater independence from maternal and filial resources. By this age, their sensory systems have all begun functioning, and their increased motoric competence allows them to emerge from the natal nest. In so doing, they usually first contact non familial conspecifics, that is, members of the coterie. These older rats can strongly influence the young, providing information about feeding sites and diet selection, and influencing the juveniles' rate of sexual maturation.

Taking on Life Support for Oneself

The amount of time the dam spends with her litter declines gradually but consistently from Day 20. As a result, the milk transferred from mother to young tapers off, and the pups cease suckling by Day 35. These trends are illustrated in Figure 9. Similarly, heat transfer and protection (in the form of retrieving and nest building) gradually disappear. In order to achieve a positive net energy flow, the pups must begin to exploit alternative resources. In particular, they must begin to ingest independently. Although some food may be available in the nest, the pups must eventually acquire food in the larger environment. This need presents a series of new challenges for the pups: what to eat and drink, where to find it, and how to avoid negative consequences (such as predation or poisoning) in the process. We will first consider behavioral adjustments to this new challenge that the pup makes based on its own individual experience, and then, we will turn to adaptations transmitted socially by other members of the coterie.

CONDITIONED ASPECTS OF FOOD RECOGNITION. In one recent set of experiments, litters were reared in cages that allowed the mother to feed freely but prevented the pups from sampling food (Melcer and Alberts, 1985). Then, in separate observational tests, pups were offered two cups, each containing an experimental diet. The substances were similar in texture and basic content and contained dis-

JEFFREY R. ALBERTS
AND CATHERINE P.
CRAMER

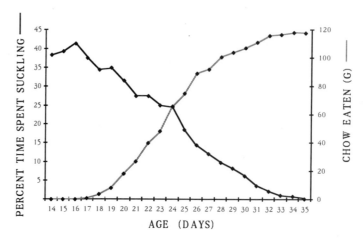

Figure 9. Daily time spent suckling and feeding and estimated chow eaten by pups during the weaning period (Thiels, Cramer, and Alberts, unpublished observations).

tinct, nonnutritive bread or peanut flavorants. Both were sweetened with saccharin; one was completely void calorically, and the other had a source of carbohydrate added, the taste of which was masked by the flavorant and the saccharin. Within 30 minutes, the food-naive rat pups showed their ability to learn which diet contained nutritive energy. Moreover, these pups showed evidence of rapid associative learning. The day after a 2-hour period of sampling the two diets, they were given an "extinction test" in which both diets were again presented, but both were calorically void. The new weanlings indicated that they had indeed learned which diet was associated with nutritive consequences because they preferred the flavor that had contained the calories during the initial exposure trial.

OTHER-ASSISTED SELF-REGULATION

Although such mechanisms for recognizing and rapidly exploiting food sources are undoubtedly useful to young juveniles, there are risks inherent in such a trial-and-error approach. For the weanling rat, one of the best sources of information about appropriate food sites and types is the adult members of the coterie, which, if they are surviving, must be adequately exploiting local conditions. Galef and his colleagues have described mechanisms by which rat pups could preferentially ingest the diet the adults are eating and reject the diets the adults are avoiding. Flavor cues transmitted via the dam's milk (and reflecting her diet) are preferred by weanling pups when they encounter those same flavors in their own food choices (Galef and Sherry, 1973). The social cues provided by either familial or nonfamilial coterie members also have a strong influence (Galef and Clark, 1971). Pups seeking their first meals have a strong tendency to approach adults at a distance from the nest site and to ingest the food available in the immediate vicinity of a feeding adult. Because different food sources are generally somewhat separate from one another, this tendency to eat primarily in the presence of adults is likely to result in the pup's ingesting the same diet.

This socially mediated choice of feeding sites may also extend to other activities, including exploration. Pups raised from before emergence in a seminatural environment with six distinct areas for food, water, and several types of ramps, tubes, and platforms were strongly influenced by the activity patterns of subadult rats (Hueston and Cramer, unpublished observations, 1986). Among litters with no subadults present, pups showed no initial preferences for particular areas. Except for time spent in the feeding area or in the nesting chamber, the pups were not strongly influenced by the presence of the dam. Among litters living with six subadults, the pups spent most of their item with the older coterie members, regardless of the particular activity available at that location. Further, the subadults avoided an area that had previously contained foul-tasting water, and the pups rarely entered that area, even though it currently contained sweetened water. Without coterie members present, the pups spent threefold the amount of time in the area with tainted water, relative to age-mates living with coterie members.

PLAY. One of the most commonly expressed types of social intercourse in young juveniles is play. Poole and Fish (1976), for example, suggested that two-thirds of the social interactions among juvenile rat pups are components of play fighting. Although even defining play has proved a problem (Fagen, 1981), a number of authors have suggested functions for the behavior that would fit it well within our framework of ontogenetically adapted behavior that also serves a preparatory function. For example, play may provide a pup with exercise or allow it to dissipate excess energy without incurring overt risk (e.g., Fagen and George, 1977; Harlow, 1969; Tinklepaugh, 1942). Also, in the current niche, the distinctive movements of play may serve to inhibit the aggressive responses of older coterie members and thus may protect a naive new inhabitant (Galef, 1985). A prominent hypothesis, which would come under our rubric of anticipatory function, is that play provides practice of skills that will become important in adult life (e.g., Aldis, 1975). Early play-fighting, for example, could be the basis for the subsequent prey-killing or intraspecific aggression (Bekoff, 1974), for the formation and maintenance of social bonds (Bekoff, 1978), or for communication skills (Symons, 1974). Burghardt (Chapter 4) discusses in more detail the role of play behavior in development.

ADULT INFLUENCES ON SEXUAL MATURATION. Once a young juvenile enters the coterie, its sexual development, like its feeding selections, are influenced by members of the social group. In fact, among house mice, the social environment appears to be the major factor determining the age at which a female reaches puberty (Vandenbergh, 1967; Vandenbergh, Drickamer, and Colby, 1972). (Most of this work has been done with *Mus musculus;* however, similar results have been obtained with other rodent species.) Female mice reared in the presence of a male reach puberty at an earlier age than those reared alone. Conversely, those reared in the presence of adult females have delays in the onset of puberty. Chemical stimuli, particularly those emanating from urine, play a significant role in the effect of males on female puberty. Contact stimuli from behavioral interactions also

JEFFREY R. ALBERTS
AND CATHERINE P.
CRAMER

appear to contribute to the phenomenon (Bronson and Maruniak, 1975; Drickamer, 1974a). Soiled bedding from a male produces an intermediate age of puberty onset, between the early puberty induced by actual male presence and the late puberty resulting from isolation rearing. The presence of a female showing male-like behavior (because of prenatal androgenization) also results in an intermediate age of puberty onset. However, when both male-soiled bedding and an androgenized female are present, the effect is equivalent to that produced by an adult male. Thus, both contact stimuli resulting from masculine behavior patterns and a chemical stimulus from males contribute to the timing of first estrus.

Puberty in young females is also modulated by cues emanating from the urine of other females (Vandenbergh *et al.*, 1972). Again, contact with adult females appears to be necessary for the pheromonal potency of female urine to be fully expressed (Drickamer, 1974b). Female urinary cues not only delay the onset of ovulation among juvenile females in the coterie, they also almost totally block any acceleratory action of a male.

Young males entering the coterie experience similar modulating social influences from conspecifics. The presence of adult female *Mus musculus* accelerates male sexual development, whereas the presence of an adult male inhibits sexual development in immature males (Vandenbergh, 1971). Bronson and Coquelin (1979) suggested that this female "priming" of males may function as a way for a female to increase the stimulation of her own ovulation via the increased "urinary potency" induced in the male. Given that complementary processes seem to be functioning in both sexes, with same-sex conspecifics delaying and opposite-sex conspecifics accelerating development, the argument could be extended to include males as well. Thus, at the same time an individual is being woven into the particular sexual fabric of the coterie by the gender of its members, it could be indirectly influencing its own sexual expression.

As we have considered adaptations and mechanisms in the coterie habitat, it has become clear to us that this period of ontogeny has received the least attention from developmental psychobiologists. Perhaps this is not surprising, in that our laboratory procedures do not generally allow animals to enter and live in (or disperse from) larger social groups. The three habitats we have previously discussed—uterus, mother, and huddle—are all accessible within the confines of a singly housed dam and her litter. Only a few studies (e.g., those by Galef and colleagues; see also Holmes, Chapter 11) have dealt with larger social contexts, and even these studies have been done within somewhat constrained conditions. Another potential source of this paucity of information is the heavy dependence of psychobiologists on laboratory rats and mice, animals whose naturally occurring group dynamics, particularly during the juvenile period, are sparsely documented (Barnett, 1975; Burghardt, Chapter 4; Calhoun, 1962).

Clearly, these are areas of inquiry requiring more work in the field tradition that use methods allowing for the examination of the intricacies of interaction within a natural context, and that include species with more defined social structures (e.g., the herds of large ungulates or the coteries of prairie dogs). Considerable progress has been made recently in work on juvenile social interactions in birds, and a similar approach to mammals could be very valuable. It is perhaps fitting that we end our tour of the interfaces between developmental psychobiology and behavioral ecology with a call for greater cooperation and coordination between these two endeavors (see Holmes, Chapter 11, for an example of the fruits of such collaboration).

Concluding Remarks

Our ecologically based tour of the rat's early life has taken us through a sequence of diverse environments: the prenatal world, the early postnatal settings of maternal behavior and sibling interactions, and finally, the "outside" world of independence and complex social interactions. We noted that this sequence is remarkable for its virtual universality across all placental mammal species. Adult mammals are found at many different addresses and have diverse occupations. Despite the diversity of the final adult addresses and occupations, all share similar beginnings, which highlights the fundamental pattern that is characteristic of and intrinsic in mammalian development.

One of the most exciting challenges facing contemporary students of behavioral development is to fashion novel perspectives and to explore the terrain that they define. This book contains numerous such exercises united around common themes of developmental psychobiology and behavioral ecology. The "ecological perspective" on development, as we have applied it in this chapter, can be used as a device to help focus attention on a variety of general ontogenetic issues. To illustrate this point, we will consider some examples.

Continuities and Discontinuities in Development

We have emphasized ecological differences that prevail in the various early habitats typical of mammalian development. In this sense, development occurs in contexts that change so suddenly and profoundly (e.g., with birth) that we speak of a sequence of different "worlds" that are experienced during early life. Though we recognize the stability of the sequence, these worlds do not appear to lie on a continuum, so we are inclined to focus on the *discontinuity*, say, between the prenatal milieu and that of the rat nest. Nevertheless, we recognize that there is utter continuity in the individual that proceeds from niche to niche, regardless of the differences that we ascribe to the transitions (see Fillion and Blass, 1985, 1986b). The value of this vocabulary, we think, is that it helps us to train our attention and to note factors that can be appreciated as continuous or discontinuous. Thus, the question is not whether development is a continuous or discontinuous process, but whether a specific feature displays continuity or discontinuity in organization or expression over specific periods of developmental time.

It may be easier for us to recognize dicontinuities in environment than in an individual; yet there are instances in which the environment remains constant and

JEFFREY R. ALBERTS
AND CATHERINE P.
CRAMER

the individual in it displays developmental discontinuity. One such example can be seen in the development of the sensory control of huddling.

Huddling among rats is a model of virtually complete developmental continuity. The rat pup is born into a huddle of littermates and it remains in that group continuously for the first couple of postnatal weeks. Even after weaning and leaving the maternal nest, the young rat is usually part of a larger social group, the colony in which contact interactions are a common and vital aspect of the social repertoire. Adult rats huddle with one another, choosing to rest and sleep in groups, even if abundant individual nesting opportunities are available. Huddling by adult rats is a lifelong activity.

The cues that attract rats to one another and maintain their contact behavior have been studied systematically in pups from about Day 5 to Day 20. At each age, huddling is under multisensory control (Alberts, 1978) but, interestingly, the organization of the sensory control of huddling changes considerably with age. For each age, it is possible to measure *hierarchies* of control for the range of cues that influence huddling. Huddling by young pups (e.g., 5- and 10-days), for instance, is most profoundly influenced by thermal cues. Although, thermal cues remain active and attractive, by Day 15 the influence of olfactory cues exceeds that of heat cues (Alberts and Brunjes, 1978). Similar changes occur in the salience of thermal and tactile controls of huddling (Pfister & Alberts, 1985). These findings demonstrate that continuity on one level of organization, in this case the developmental maintenance of huddling behavior, can be mediated by processes that involve *discontinuities* on another level of organization, namely the cues that control huddling. Indeed, profound changes in the underlying organization of huddling controls occur while the pups remain in the relatively constant environment of their natal nest.

HABITATS AS SOURCES OF STIMULATION

The themes of ecology and experience were used throughout this chapter to provide a broad conceptual framework for analyzing development, to generate testable hypotheses concerning proximate mechanisms that affect behavior, and to illuminate common patterns of behavioral organization during development. The combined forces of behavioral ecology and developmental psychobiology are a formidable mixture, one that has been successful and, in our opinion, has much to offer in the future. At this early phase in these joint ventures, it seems appropriate to discuss briefly the various ways in which the ecological analysis has affected the study of stimulative effects of experience during development.

We have derived from the ecological concepts of habitat and niche, the notion that at each stage in its development mammals are exposed to a predictable and common profile of environmental features. That is, each developmental habitat presents a constellation of stimuli that impinge on the fetus, newborn, juvenile, and so on. There are at least two types of stimulation that merit distinction. The more general type is any form of environmental input to which the organism responds (including responses that might be measurable primarily on a neuronal or cellular level). This type of input represents the form of stimulation that Gottlieb has discussed and analyzed in his seminal essays on stimulation and the development of neural and behavioral function (Gottlieb, 1973, 1976).

A second, relevant class of stimulation is the type that is the product of *sensory-perceptual transduction*. We consider the products of stimulation that activates sensory systems to constitute the raw materials of an animal's *experience*. In this realm, ecological concerns are an important guide to the selection of the stimuli to analyze, because if a sensory system processes special sensitivities or capacities, it is most likely that its specializations will be linked to stimulus characteristics that represent important features of the typical environment. But the ecological characteristics of a habitat are only part of the story of the analysis of experience. Developing animals undergo a specific sequence of sensory maturation (Gottlieb, 1971; Alberts, 1984). Thus, at any point in development (particularly early development), the input received from the environment (experience) is largely determined by the maturational status of the animal's sensory systems. It is not sufficient, therefore, to know all the stimulative parameters in an environment, because the organism's experience may well be impermeable to at least some of it.

There is a large and rich literature on the development of sensory function. Sensory stimulation can affect the functional status of sensory systems, the rate of their development, certain biases in their operating characteristics, and a host of other vital parameters. The traditions of developmental psychobiology provide an armamentarium for sophisticated and incisive analyses of such environment–organism relations that can add a great deal to the analysis of behavior, particularly in the study of proximate causation.

Another particularly strong set of analytical tools offered by developmental psychobiology is in the analysis of experiences that can form the basis of *learning*. Again, the traditions of developmental psychobiology contain a wealth of analytical tools for rigorous and useful analyses of numerous forms of learning. It is quite remarkable, we think, that our discussion of animal development in this chapter contains barely a single reference to the literature on the laboratory analysis of early learning, of which there is quite a large amount (for example, see reviews by Campbell, 1967, 1984; Campbell and Coulter, 1976). The major reason for this gap is that the laboratory studies have been aimed at phenomena that shed relatively little light on phenomena or processes that are readily interpretable in terms of stimulation or contingencies that are clearly typical of typical developmental habitats. Here, we believe, is an especially fruitful and promising area for joint concerns among developmental psychobiologists and behavioral ecologists.

ONTOGENETIC NICHE AND ONTOGENETIC ADAPTATION

An ecological perspective on development inevitably leads to a keener awareness of the *context* of development. And, in accordance with ecological parlance, this context is called the *habitat* or the *niche*. Again, this is a theme that we have exploited in this chapter. The concept of the *ontogenetic niche* is a special one because it proves to be extraordinarily changeable. Placed in its niche(s), the developing organism can be seen to have myriad characteristics that enable it to *adapt* to the special conditions around it, whether it be *in utero,* at the teat, in the nest, or emerging into the adult world.

The terms *niche* and *adaptation,* used ontogenetically, represent important and powerful ideas. Unfortunately, the terms *ontogenetic niche* and *ontogenetic adaptation* have also been subject to a wide variety of uses and misuses, which have led to serious confusion. It is beyond the scope of this chapter to review and discuss these issues; there are a number of essays that address the status of these concepts and their place in current developmental analyses (e.g., Alberts, 1987; Alberts and Gubernick, 1985; Galef, 1981; Oppenheim, 1981; Oppenheim and Haverkamp, 1986; West, King, and Arberg, Chapter 2).

In relation to our chapter, and as a preface to this book, it is instructive to note some selected ideas in ontogenetic thinking that we believe can be related directly and indirectly to the concepts of *niche* and *adaptation.* One important idea can be termed the *dual infant* (cf. Alberts, 1985), which refers to two dimensions of functional organization displayed by mammalian infants. First, the infant can be viewed as a specially adapted creature, possessing features by which it adapts to its current niche (this in itself is an important departure from the view that the infant is simply an incomplete adult). The second dimension of infantile organization is that the infant also possesses capabilities that it does *not* display and that, in fact, may be actively inhibited. Thus, maturation and the corresponding display of "emergent" capabilities can sometimes involve the disinhibition of capacities that have been in place, but that have not been used. Aspects of thermoregulation and motor components of locomotion and of sexual behavior are among the processes that have been discussed in this framework (see also Hogan, Chapter 3).

As far back as 1957, the noted physiologist E. F. Adolph promoted the notion that the developing infant has a "double vocation": it makes a living by being a successful (niche-adapted) infant, and simultaneously, it undergoes developmental changes that can be understood as preparation for undertaking the job of being an adapted adult (Adolph, 1968). We see this idea as very similar to our characterizations of "adaptation and anticipation," which we have used throughout this chapter.

Systemogenesis is a theoretical perspective promulgated by Peter Anokhin (1964), which relies explicitly on the demands of early postnatal life as the source of selection pressure for developmental rate and canalization. Anokhin expressed his theoretical views mostly in relation to the development of sensory systems, but the spirit of his perspective, which combines the concepts of the early niche, infantile adaptations to meet the special demands of the niche, and the evolution by natural selection of these adaptations, has been rather widely influential.

Overall, there probably has been more lip service paid to than empirical testing done on the ideas and hypotheses of ontogenetic adaptation (cf. Alberts, 1985, 1987). Although this may be acceptable for the time being, we would like to suggest that, if these ideas are to earn and retain the importance that they deserve, we should begin to formulate rigorous empirical approaches and standards for identifying and analyzing adaptation. Williams (1966), for example, discussed the value of distinguishing between two kinds of organismic adjustments that promote kinds of "goodness of fit" between organism and environment and that inspire the labeling of "adaptation" in interested and sometimes reverent observers. Williams's distinction was between the simple *adaptive response,* which refers to features that enhance an organism's fitness (regardless of its historical precursor) and *evolutionary adaptation,* which refers to a feature shaped by natural selection. This is an important biological distinction (discussed also by Darwin, 1871) between historical genesis and current utility. More meticulous attention to such fundamental distinctions, as well as modern variants that are shaping contemporary biological thought (e.g., Gould and Vrba, 1981), should be incorporated more widely and more frequently by developmental psychobiologists if this discipline is to enter the broader biological context and to maximize its possible contributions there. We hope this book in general and our chapter in particular will be part of a renewed wave of productive research and discussion.

Acknowledgments

Preparation of this chapter and the original research was supported by grants MH-28355 from the National Institute of Mental Health to Jeffrey R. Alberts and RII-850387 from the National Science Foundation to Catherine P. Cramer, and by a Faculty Fellowship to Catherine P. Cramer. We thank the editor, Elliott M. Blass, for his guidance, suggestions, and patience in the formulation of the chapter.

REFERENCES

Addison, K. S., and Alberts, J. R. *Patterns of mother-litter interaction in a semi-natural habitat.* Paper presented at the Annual Meeting of the International Society for Developmental Psychobiology, Cincinnati, 1980.

Adolph, E. F. *Origins of physiological regulations.* New York: Academic Press, 1968.

Alberts, J. R. Huddling by rat pups: Group behavioral mechanisms of temperature regulation and energy conservation. *Journals of Comparative and Physiological Psychology,* 1978, *92,* 231–240.

Alberts, J. R. Sensory-perceptual development in the Norway rat: A view toward comparative studies. In R. Kail and N. Spear (Eds.), *Comparative perspectives on memory development.* New York: Plenum Press, 1984.

Alberts, J. R. New views of parent-offspring relationships. In W. T. Greenough and J. M. Juraska (Eds.), *Developmental neuropsychobiology.* New York: Academic Press, 1985.

Alberts, J. R. Early learning and ontogenetic adaptation. In N. Krasnegor, E. M. Blass, M. A. Hofer, and W. Smotherman (Eds.), *Perinatal development: A psychobiological perspective.* Orlando, FL: Academic Press, 1987.

Alberts, J. R., and Brunjes, P. C. Ontogeny of thermal and olfactory determinants of huddling in the rat. *Journal of Comparative and Physiological Psychology,* 1978, *92,* 897–906.

Alberts, J. R., and Gubernick, D. J. Early learning as ontogenetic adaptation for ingestion by rats. *Learning and Motivation,* 1985, *15,* 334–359.

Alberts, J. R., and Leimbach, M. P. The first foray: Maternal influences on nest egression in the weanling rat. *Developmental Psychobiology,* 1980, *13,* 417–430.

Alberts, J. R., and May, B. Nonnutritive thermotactile induction of filial huddling in rat pups. *Developmental Psychobiology,* 1984, *17,* 161–181.

Alberts, J. R., Serova, L. V., Keefe, J. R., and Apanasenko, Z. Early postnatal development of rats derived from Cosmos 1514. *NASA Technical Memorandum* 88223, 1986, pp. 145–188.

Aldis, O. *Playfighting*. New York: Academic Press, 1975.

Allen, C., and Kendall, J. W. Maturation of the circadian rhythm of plasma corticosterone in the rat. *Endocrinology,* 1967, *80,* 926–930.

Allin, J. T., and Banks, E. M. Effects of temperature on ultrasound production by infant albino rats. *Developmental Psychobiology,* 1971, *4,* 149–156.

Anokhin, P. K. Systemogenesis as a general regulator of brain development. *Progress in Brain Research,* 1964, *90,* 50–86.

Asano, Y. The maturation of the circadian rhythm of brain norepinephrine and serotonin of the rat. *Life Science,* 1971, *10,* 883–894.

Aslin, R. N., Alberts, J. R., and Petersen, M. P. (Eds.). *Development of Perception,* Vol. 2. New York: Academic Press, 1981.

Babicky, A., Ostadalova, I., Parizek, J., Kolar, J., and Bibr, B. Use of radioisotope techniques for determining the weaning period in experimental animals. *Physiologia Bohemoslovaca,* 1970, *19,* 457–467.

Barnett, S. A. *The rat.* Chicago: University of Chicago Press, 1975.

Bekoff, A. Development of locomotion in vertebrates: A comparative perspective. In E. S. Gollin (Ed.), *The comparative development of adaptive skills: Evolutionary perspectives.* Hillsdale, N.J.: Erlbaum, 1985.

Bekoff, A., and Lau, B. Interlimb coordination in 20-day old rat fetuses. *Journal of Experimental Zoology,* 1980, *214,* 173–175.

Bekoff, M. Social play in mammals. *American Zoology,* 1974, *14,* 265–436.

Bekoff, M. Social play: Structure, function, and the evolution of a cooperative social behavior. In G. Burghart and M. Bekoff (Eds.), *The development of behavior: Comparative and evolutionary aspects.* New York: Garland Press, 1978.

Bell, R. W. Ultrasounds in small rodents: Arousal-produced and arousal producing. *Developmental Psychobiology,* 1974, *7,* 39–42.

Bradley, R. M., and Mistretta, C. M. Swallowing in fetal sheep. *Science,* 1973, *179,* 1016–1017.

Bronson, F. H., and Coquelin, A. The modulation of reproduction by priming pheromones in house mice: Speculations on adaptive function. In D. Muller-Schwartz and R. M. Silverstein, *Chemical signals.* New York: Plenum Press, 1979.

Bronson, F. H., and Maruniak, J. Male-induced puberty in female mice: Evidence for a synergistic action of social cues. *Biology of Reproduction,* 1975, *13,* 94.

Brunjes, P. C., and Alberts, J. R. Olfactory stimulation induces filial huddling preferences in rat pups. *Journal of Comparative and Physiological Psychology,* 1979, *93,* 548–555.

Calhoun, J. B. *The ecology and sociology of the Norway rat.* Public Health Service Publication No. 1008, Bethesda, Maryland, U.S. Public Health Service, 1962.

Campbell, B. A., and Coulter, X. The ontogenesis of learning and memory. In M. R. Rosenzweig and E. L. Bennett (Eds.), *Neural mechanisms of learning and memory* (pp. 209–235). Cambridge, MA:MIT Press, 1976.

Cosnier, J. *Le comportement du rat d'elevage.* Unpublished doctoral dissertation, University of Lyon, France, 1965.

Cramer, C. P., and Blass, E. M. Mechanisms of control of milk intake in suckling rats. *American Journal Physiology,* 1983, *245,* R154–R159.

Cramer, C. P., Blass, E. M., and Hall, W. G. The ontogeny of nipple-shifting behavior in albino rats: Mechanisms of control and possible significance. *Developmental Psychobiology,* 1980, *13,* 165–180.

Cramer, C. P., Pfister, J. F., and Haig, K. A. Experience during suckling alters later spatial learning. *Developmental Psychobiology,* in press.

Darwin, C. R. *The descent of man in relation to sex.* London: Murray, 1871.

DeCasper, A. J., and Fifer, W. P. Of human bonding: Newborns prefer their mothers' voices. *Science,* 1980, *208,* 1174–1176.

Drachman, D. B., and Coulombre, A. J. Experimental clubfoot and arthrogryposis multiplex congonita. *Lancet,* 1962, *2,* 523–526.

Drickamer, L. C. Contact stimulation, androgenized females and accelerated sexual maturation in female mice. *Behavioral Biology,* 1974a, *12,* 101.

Drickamer, L. C. Sexual maturation of female house mice: Social inhibition. *Developmental Psychobiology,* 1974b, *7,* 257.

Fagen, R. *Animal play behavior.* New York: Oxford University Press, 1981.

Fagen, R., and George, T. K. Play behavior and exercise in young ponies (*Equus caballus,* L.). *Behavior, Ecology, and Sociobiology,* 1977, *2,* 267–269.

Fillion, T. J., and Blass, E. M. Responsiveness to estrous chemostimuli in male rats (Rattus norvegicus) of different ages. *Journal of Comparative Psychology*, 1985, *99*, 328–335.

Fillion, T. J., and Blass, E. M. Infantile behavioral reactivity to oestrous chemostimuli in Norway rats. *Animal Behaviour*, 1986a, *34*, 123–133.

Fillion, T. J., and Blass, E. M. Infantile experience with suckling odors determines adult sexual behavior in male rats. *Science*, 1986b, *231*, 729–731.

Galef, B. G., Jr. Investigation of the functions of coprophagy in juvenile rats. *Journal of Comparative and Physiological Psychology*, 1979, *93*, 295–305.

Galef, B. G., Jr. The ecology of weaning: Parasitism and the achievement of independence by altricial mammals. In D. J. Gubernick and P. H. Klopfer (Eds.), *Parental care in mammals*. New York: Plenum Press, 1981.

Galef, B. G., and Clark, M. M. Parent-offspring interactions determine the time and place of first ingestion of solid food by wild rat pups. *Psychonomic Science*, 1971, *25*, 15–16.

Galef, B. G., and Henderson, P. W. Mother's milk: A determinant of the feeding preferences of weanling rat pups. *Journal of Comparative and Physiological Psychology*, 1972, *78*, 213–219.

Galef, B. G., and Sherry, D. F. Mother's milk: A medium for the transmission of cues reflecting the flavor of mother's diet. *Journal of Comparative and Physiological Psychology*, 1973, *83*, 374–378.

Gottlieb, G. Ontogenesis of sensory function in birds and mammals. In E. Tobach, L. R. Aronson, and E. Shaw (Eds.), *The biopsychology of development*. New York: Academic Press, 1971.

Gottlieb, G. Introduction to behavioral embryology. In G. Gottlieb (Ed.), *Studies on the development of behavior and the nervous system*, (Vol. 1). New York: Academic Press, 1973.

Gottlieb, G. Development of species identification in ducklings. I. Nature of perceptual deficit caused by embryonic auditory deprivation. *Journal of Comparative and Physiological Psychology*, 1975, *89*, 387–399.

Gottlieb, G. The role of experience in the development of behavior and the nervous system. In G. Gottlieb (Ed.), *Studies on the development of behavior and the nervous system* (Vol. 3). New York: Academic Press, 1976.

Gould, S. J., and Vrba, E. S. Exaptation—A missing term in the science of form. *Paleobiology*, 1982, *8*, 4–15.

Gregory, E., and Pfaff, D. Development of olfactory-guided behavior in infant rats. *Physiology and Behavior*, 1971, *6*, 573–576.

Grosvenor, C. E., and Mena, F. Neural and hormonal control of milk secretion and milk ejection. In B. L. Larson and V. R. Smith (Eds.), *Lactation: A comprehensive treatise*. New York: Academic Press, 1974.

Grota, L. J., and Ader, R. Continuous recording of maternal behavior in *Rattus norvegicus*. *Animal Behavior*, 1969 *17*, 722–729.

Gubernick, D. J., and Alberts, J. R. Maternal licking of young: Resource exchange and proximate controls. *Physiology and Behavior*, 1983, *31*, 593–601.

Hall, W. G., Cramer, C. P., and Blass, E. M. The ontogeny of suckling in rats: Transitions toward adult ingestion. *Journal of Comparative and Physiological Psychology*, 1977, *91*, 1141–1155.

Hamburger, V. Some aspects of the embryology of behavior. *Quarterly Review of Biology*, 1963, *38*, 342–365.

Harlow, H. F. Age-mate or peer affectional system. In D. Lehrman, R. Hinde, and E. Shaw (Eds.), *Advances in the study of behavior*, Vol. 2. New York: Academic Press, 1969.

Harlow, H. F., and Harlow, H. F. Social deprivation in monkeys. *Scientific American*, 1962, *207*, 137–146.

Hart, J. S. Rodents. In C. G. Whittow (Ed.), *Comparative physiology of thermoregulation*, Vol. 2. New York: Academic Press, 1971.

Henning, S. J. Postnatal development: Coordination of feeding, digestion, and metabolism. *American Journal of Physiology*, 1981, *241*, G199–214.

Hofer, M. A., and Shair, H. Ultrasonic vocalization during social interaction and isolation in 2 week old rats. *Developmental Psychobiology*, 1978, *11*, 495–504.

Hull, D. Thermoregulation in young mammals. In C. G. Whittow (Ed.), *Comparative physiology of thermoregulation*, Vol. 3. New York: Academic Press, 1973.

Johnston, T. D. Conceptual issues in the ecological study of learning. In T. D. Johnston and A. T. Pietrewicz (Eds.), *Issues in the ecological study of learning*. Hillsdale, N. J.: Erlbaum, 1985.

Kehoe, P., and Blass, E. M. Gustatory determinants of suckling in albino rats 5–20 days of age. *Developmental Psychobiology*, 1985, *18*, 67–82.

Kenny, J. T., and Blass, E. M. Suckling as an incentive to instrumental learning in preweanling rats. 'Science, 1977, 196, 898–899.

Kittrell, E. M. W., and Satinoff, E. Development of the circadian rhythm of body temperature in rats. Physiology and Behavior, 1986, 38, 99–104.

Leon, M., Croskerry, P. G., and Smith, G. K. Thermal control of mother-young contact in rats. Physiology and Behavior, 1978, 21, 793–811.

Levin, R., and Stern, J. Maternal influences on ontogeny of suckling and feeding rhythms in the rat. Journal of Comparative and Physiological Psychology, 1975, 89, 711–721.

Liggins, G. C. The fetus and birth. In C. R. Austin and R. V. Short (Eds.), Reproduction in mammals, Book 2: Embryonic and fetal development. New York: Cambridge University Press, 1982.

Lincoln, D. W., Hill, A., and Wakerly, J. B. The milk-ejection reflex of the rat: An intermittent function not abolished by surgical anesthesia. Journal of Endocrinology, 1973, 57, 459–476.

MacFarlane, B. A., Pedersen, P. E., Cornell, C. E., and Blass, E. M. Sensory control of suckling-associated behaviours in the domestic Norway rat, Rattus norvegicus. Animal Behavior, 1983, 31, 462–471.

Melcer, T., and Alberts, J. R. Recognition of food by "food-naive" weanling-age rat pups. Paper presented at meeting of the International Society for Developmental Psychobiology, Dallas, 1985.

Mellgren, R. L., Misasi, L., and Brown, S. W. Optimal foraging theory: prey density and travel requirements in Rattus norvegicus. Journal of Comparative Psychology, 1984, 98, 142–153.

Moore, C. Maternal contributions to the development of masculine sexual behavior in laboratory rats. Developmental Psychology, 1984, 17, 347–356.

Moore, C., and Morelli, G. A. Mother rats interact differently with male and female offspring. Journal of Comparative Physiology and Psychology, 93, 677–684.

Mount, L. E. The influence of huddling and body size on the metabolic rate of the young pig. Journal of Agricultural Sciences, Cambridge, 1960, 55, 101–105.

Narayanan, C. H., Fox, M. W., and Hamburger, V. Prenatal development of spontaneous and evoked activity in the rat (Rattus norvegicus albinus). Behaviour, 1971, 29, 100–131.

Niorot, E. Ultrasounds in small rodents. II. Changes with age in albino rats. Animal Behaviour, 1968, 17, 340–349.

Okada, F. The maturation of the circadian rhythm of brain serotonin in the rat. Life Sciences, 1971, 10, 77–86.

Olton, D. S., and Samuelson, R. J. Remembrance of places past: Spatial memory in rats. Journal of Experimental Psychology: Animal Behavior Processes, 1976, 2, 97–116.

Oppenheim, R. W. Ontogenetic adaptations and retrogressive processes in the development of the nervous system and behavior: A neuroembryological perspective. In K. Connelly and H. Prechtl (Eds.), Maturation and development: Biological and psychological perspectives. London: Spastica Society Publications, 1981.

Oppenheim, R. W., and Haverkamp, L. Early development of behavior and the nervous system: An embryological perspective. In E. M. Blass (Ed.), Handbook of behavioral neurobiology, Vol. 8: Developmental psychobiology and developmental neurobiology. New York: Plenum Press, 1986.

Pedersen, P. E., and Blass, E. M. Olfactory control over suckling in albino rats. In R. N. Aslin, J. R. Alberts, M. R. Petersen, (Eds.) Development of perception: Psychobiological perspectives, Vol. 1. New York: Academic Press, 1981. Also cited in Development of perception, 1981, 1, 359–381.

Pedersen, P. E., and Blass, E. M. Prenatal and postnatal determinants of the first suckling episode in the albino rat. Developmental Psychobiology, 1982, 15, 349–356.

Pedersen, P. E., Williams, C. L., and Blass, E. M. Classical conditioning of suckling behavior in three-day-old albino rats. Journal of Experimental Psychology: Animal Behavior Processes, 1982, 8, 329–356.

Pedersen, P. E., Greer, C. A., and Shepherd, G. M. Early development of olfactory function. In E. M. Blass (Ed.), Handbook of behavioral neurobiology, Vol. 8: Developmental psychobiology and developmental neurobiology. New York: Plenum Press, 1986.

Pfister, J. P., and Alberts, J. R. Development of thermotactile controls of huddling in the rat pup. Paper presented at the meeting of the International Society for Developmental Psychobiology, Hyannis, Massachusetts, 1983.

Plaut, S. M. Adult-litter relations in rats reared in single and dual-chambered cages. Developmental Psychobiology, 1974, 7, 111–120.

Poole, T. B., and Fish, J. An investigation of individual, age, and sexual differences in the play of Rattus norvegicus. Journal of Zoology, 1976, 179, 249–260.

Reppert, S. M. Annals of the New York Academy of Science, 1985, 162.

Reppert, S. M., and Schwartz, W. J. Science, 1983, 22, 969–971.

Rosenblatt, J. S., and Lehrman, D. S. Maternal behavior of the laboratory rat. In H. L. Rheingold (Ed.), *Maternal behavior in mammals.* New York: Wiley, 1963.

Schmidt-Nielson, K. *Scaling: Why is animal size so important?* New York: Cambridge University Press, 1984.

Symons, D. Aggressive play and communication in rhesus monkeys *(Macaca mulatta). American Zoologist,* 1974, *14,* 317–322.

Taylor, P. M. Oxygen consumption in new-born rats. *Journal of Physiology (London),* 1960, *154,* 153–168.

Teicher, M. H., and Blass, E. M. Suckling in newborn rats: Eliminated by nipple lavage, reinstated by pup saliva. *Science,* 1976, *193,* 422–425.

Teicher, M. H., and Blass, E. M. First suckling response of the newborn albino rat: the roles of olfaction and amniotic fluid. *Science,* 1977, *198,* 635–636.

Tinbergen, N. *The herring gull's world.* New York: Harper & Row, 1960.

Tinklepaugh, O. L. Social behavior of animals. In F. A. Moss (Ed.), *Comparative psychology* (2nd ed.) New York: Prentice-Hall, 1942.

Vandenbergh, J. G. Effect of the presence of a male on the sexual maturation of female mice. *Endocrinology,* 1967, *84,* 658.

Vandenbergh, J. G. The influence of the social environment on sexual maturation in male mice. *Journal of Reproduction and Fertility,* 1971, *24,* 383–390.

Vandenbergh, J. G., Drickamer, L. C., and Colby, D. R. Social and dietary factors in the sexual maturation of female mice. *Journal of Reproduction and Fertility,* 1972, *28,* 397.

Vorherr, H., Kleeman, C. R., and Lehman, E. Oxytocin-induced stretch reactions in suckling mice and rats: A semiquantitative bioassay for oxytocin. *Endocrinology,* 1967, *81,* 711–715.

Walker, B. E., and Quarles, J. Palate development in mouse foetuses after tongue removal. *Archives of oral biology,* 1962, *2,* 523–526.

Whittow, G. C. (Ed.) *Comparative physiology of thermoregulation* (Vol. 1). New York: Academic Press, 1971.

Williams, G. C. *Adaptation and natural selection.* Princeton, N.J.:Princeton University Press, 1966.

Windle, W. F., and Griffin, A. M. Observations on embryonic and fetal movements of the cat. *Journal of Comparative Neurology,* 1931, *52,* 149–188.

2

The Inheritance of Niches
The Role of Ecological Legacies in Ontogeny

MEREDITH J. WEST, ANDREW P. KING, AND ANNE A. ARBERG

EXOGENETICS: SEEING THE OBVIOUS

The study of genetics overshadows that of exogenetics for three reasons. First, no single unit of exogenetic inheritance exists. Even the most central feature of exogenetic inheritance, the concept of something "outside" the genes, lacks clarity. That something is the environment, but how do we define the environment? To some, the term stands for the complex of biotic elements that surrounds all organisms. To others, the term refers to a particular species' or population's habitat.

Lack of a name makes any concept easier to neglect. Dawkins's "meme" (1976) or Lumsden and Wilson's "culturgen" (1981) do not qualify as appropriate constructs for our purposes because they represent attempts to parallel cultural and morphological evolution. The objective here is to consider exogenetic inheritance from an ontogenetic, not a phylogenetic, perspective.

The study of exogenetics is also made more difficult by its external diversity of form across cultures: What do nest sites, territories, dominance ranks, dialects, food preferences, money, furniture, names, and family businesses have in common beyond their fate as examples of legacies? The material of biological inheritance is known, and the means by which its information is decoded has been worked out for many organisms, revealing common rules. The lack of a common foundational material and/or common rules for exogenetic inheritance makes its study appear

MEREDITH J. WEST   Department of Psychology, University of North Carolina, Chapel Hill, North Carolina 27514.   ANDREW P. KING   Department of Psychology, Duke University, Durham, North Carolina 27706.   ANNE A. ARBERG   Department of Psychology, University of North Carolina, Chapel Hill, North Carolina 27514.

more complex. Consult the card catalog in any university library, and before you will be a bewildering array of entries to cover the historical and modern laws pertinent to the inheritance and rights to succession of property for countries, cultures, and religions. Whether or not something can be passed on, to whom, and under what conditions represent important questions for every society.

And recurrent among the questions is the issue of an individual's "right" to wealth or property in relation to behavior: Merely because of kinship, should land and/or money remain in the possession of those who did not labor for it? Humans have answered this question differently at different times in different places. It is a question much like that underlying debates about the degree to which "nature" or "nurture" plays a deterministic role in development—a debate also centuries old. Is it, then, surprising that the subset of humans designated as scientists have yet to formulate "the" principles governing exogenetic inheritance?

Finally, the heavy hand of human habit has also hindered the study of exogenetics. We of the twentieth century now feel comfortable equating heredity and genes. This sense of comfort is not easily disturbed. To say a behavior or a trait is inherited is now taken to mean something quite concrete; it is to say that exploration (and possibly engineering) of only the genetic substrate is in order.

An issue embedded within this third problem is the "value" of the behavior and the consequences to humans of decisions about a behavior's ontogenetic status. When the behavior in question is the phototactic response of an insect, only a handful of experts might quarrel about the role of genetics and exogenetics. But when the behavior in question is IQ, the quarrel cannot be contained in the laboratory, and the harm done by insufficient analyses is immense. Thus, explorations into any form of inheritance can be intimidating.

THE SEMANTIC CONVERSION OF NATURE AND NURTURE

The phrase "nature and nurture" entered the language in 1582, the creation of a teacher named Richard Mulcaster (Teigen, 1984). He saw these entities as forces acting in harmony to advance a child's development: "Whereto natur(e) makes him [the boy] toward, but that nurtur(e) sets him foreward" (Mulcaster, 1582/1925, p. 39). Shakespeare and Carlyle used these words to put forth much the same view of ontogeny. It was Sir Francis Galton, as part of his analysis of English scientists, who cast the terms into different roles (Fancher, 1979):

> The phrase "nature and nurture" is a convenient jingle of words, for it separates under two distinct heads the innumerable elements of which personality is composed . . . When nature and nurture compete for supremacy on equal terms in the sense to be explained, the former proves the stronger. (Galton, 1874/1970, p. 12)

Mulcaster's friends became Galton's foes. In his transformation of the relationship between nature and nurture, Galton created a perception of the nature of the interaction between genes and experience that dominated science for many years. Much has been written about Galton's words: less has been said about the visual image implied, that of the "distinct heads" of nature and nurture. The picture it brings to mind is that of the compelling, ambiguous picture often labeled the "wife–mother-in-law" picture (Boring, 1930). Boring brought this "puzzle picture" to the attention of psychologists because it displayed a more complex form of a figure–ground illusion (see Super, 1981, for the use of another illusion in relation to culture). Other illusions typically involve alternating figure and ground perceptions based on a shared external contour, but in the case of Figure 1, "the two alternating figures interpenetrate each other spatially and there is no definite division of the field by a contour" (Boring, 1930, p. 444).

Nature and nurture also have a complex figure-and-ground relationship, and they often compete for equal attention, leading easily to Galton's perception of them as rivals:

> In the competition between nature and nurture, when differences in either case do not exceed those which distinguish individuals of the same race living in the same country under no very exceptional conditions, nature certainly proves the stronger of the two. (Galton, 1874/1970, p. 16)

Galton's use of the terms *competition* and the *stronger of the two* reveal his perceptual bias. But his words also explain why the concept of nature–nurture, like Boring's ambiguous picture, is so complex an illusion. Galton stated that he could

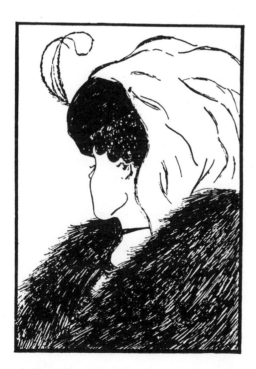

Figure 1. The wife–mother-in-law illusion. (From E. G. Boring, *American Journal of Psychology*, 1930, *42*, 444–445).

not predict developmental outcomes except in the case where countrymen possessed not only their countrymen's genes, but also their countrymen's country. Thus, although Galton declared nature normally to dominate, he assumed that the contributions of nature automatically depended on those of a particular environment: The English inherit English nurture along with English nature.

It is the interpenetrability of nature and nurture that Galton perceived. At other points in his treatise, he noted the lack of clear boundaries between nature and nurture and presented a unified, as opposed to competitive, view of them. In this regard, he cited Carlyle's prior use of the term *nurture* (1838/1937) and his own subscription to Carlyle's view that "an infant of genius is quite the same as any other infant, only that certain surprisingly favourable influences accompany him through life, especially through childhood, and expand him, while others lie closefolded and remain dunces" (Carlyle, pp. 93–94). Thus, Galton could see both sides of the nature–nurture illusion: he could see companions, and he could see competitors. But in the end, he saw only the latter view.

Boring (1930) introduced his "puzzle picture" as a means of studying the phenomenon of perceptual set because "neither figure is favored over the other" (p. 445), so that the experimenter has an opportunity to explore how words change what subjects see. We consider it critical that, when Galton introduced the terms, he also introduced a perceptual set. If we are told that nature and nurture compete, we look for divisibility; we look for the strong and the weak. But if we are told that they are part of one another, that neither exists without the other, we come to apprehend their composite design. It is the composite view of nature and nurture that Galton had seen but chose not to stress: the interpenetrability of species-typical genes and species-typical habitats.

A PLACE FOR NATURE AND NURTURE

We offer the term *ontogenetic niche* to capture the set of ecological and social circumstances that come with an organism's genes. The term *niche* is used by ecologists to specify both the physical habitat of a species and the role of the species in the ecological community. It gives the species' address and its occupation (J. Alberts, personal communication, 1987).

Given the disagreements that have been engendered by the terms *nature* and *nurture,* why risk additional unproductive debate by the addition of a niche? Three reasons motivate us. First, the major problem, as we see it, with the terms *nature* and *nurture* lies in specifying the relationship between them. To say nature and nurture "interact" is an agreeable but vague proposition that often does not lead to testable hypotheses. The time has come to find words, not diagrammatic arrows or numerical formulas, to capture the synergy of ontogeny. The ontogenetic niche is one means of stimulating the search for functional metrics of development, metrics that capture the translation of initial abilities into actual proficiencies.

A second source of motivation comes from observing the success of the niche in the science of ecology. Ecology seeks to understand the relationships between organisms and the resources that they need to survive. It is not the study of nature with a capital *N* or of its conservation. The closest parallel we know is to a discipline, formerly labeled a science, now an archaic college major: home economics. Home economics has gone the way of husbandry. The study of house, hearth, offspring, land, or livestock smacks of the mundane in a modern world. But when the home under study is not yours, mine, or ours, but everyone's, it is the very stuff of current science—it is ecology. Thus, ecology is the study of homes with a captial *H,* and it has much to teach us about how the different social relationships and interactions of individuals serve as higher order regulatory mechanisms.

Ecology confronts the same issues as homemakers: What are the dynamics of organism–resource interrelationships? Clean clothes no more find their way into drawers or hot food onto the table than do crickets appear at the mouths of gaping nestlings or leaves appear on the trees just as nests become of interest to predators. The providential appearance of any ecology, animal or human, is misleading. It is the same providential quality of exogenetic inheritance that may have fostered its neglect. We take for granted that genes inherit an environment and that that environment supports ontogeny. But the time has come to recognize and analyze these implicit assumptions—assumptions we have found ourselves forced to reformulate in our own research because animals do not "interact" with one another in the same way that statistical variables do (King and West, 1987).

We define the niche as that part of an animal's environment constituting its species-typical habitat. We exclude from consideration those parts of an animal's environment common to all organisms, the universal environment or ecotope (Hutchinson, 1978). Within this framework, the word *environment* is neither a synonym for *nurture* nor an antonym to *nature* or *genes.* Despite the word's frequent occurrence in the vocabulary of psychologists, it often qualifies as no more than jargon. And thus, part of our fascination with ecology's niche is frustration with psychology's environment, a problem many others are now addressing (see Johnston and Turvey, 1980; Schleidt, 1981, 1985) and a problem boldly confronted by psychologists such as Barker (1960), Brunswick (1955), and Stone (1943).

The final incentive to adding a niche is that many others have recognized the role of the inherited environment in ontogeny, although few have formally labeled it as a unit of heredity. Montagu (1959) stated the idea explicitly:

> The potentialities of each individual are dependent on genetic endowment, but these potentialities have a wider range than is generally observed, so that the environment which is a part of an individual's inheritance is also the means by which the heredity of an individual can be changed, modified, enlarged, and so on. (p. 109)

Others have come to the same conclusion (see especially Boyd and Richerson, 1985; Medawar and Medawar, 1983; Oppenheim, 1982; Oyama, 1982; Super and Harkness, 1981). But genes still reign supreme in most texts, and most dictionaries define them as "the" units of heredity. By giving the concept of exogenetic inheritance a formal name, but one easy to say, we hope to make its trip beyond the tip of the tongue as painless as possible.

THREE PERSPECTIVES ON NATURE–NURTURE–NICHE

The triadic form of nature–nurture–niche leads to at least three ways in which ontogenetic phenomena can be viewed (West and King, 1987). The niche represents a legacy, a link, and a way of life for its occupants.

It is the dependability of the niche in delivering certain resources to the young that makes it a legacy. Warburton (1955) once complained that genetic programs that explicitly excluded environmental feedback were "comparable to being sewn into one's winter underwear" (p. 136). The concept of the ontogenetic niche demonstrates why the young of so many species need no such preprovisioning: they inherit the senses and the surroundings to find what they need. The Gibsons' ecological approach to perception (J. Gibson, 1966, 1979; E. Gibson, 1969) offers, at present, the most powerful analogue for viewing the niche as a legacy because they developed their theories to deal with a similar problem, the nature of the mechanisms permitting accurate perception.

What the Gibsons proposed for theories of perception was a biologically and ecologically based taxonomy of the affordances of an animal's habitat. They showed that an animal's surroundings provide sure footing for perceiving. The need was not to search for the internal mechanisms to correct or protect the animal from the vagaries of an erratic environment, but to search for the behaviors used to explore and detect features of the niche and ways to measure and categorize the niches themselves. By so doing, they turned the study of perception inside out. Mace (1977) summed up the Gibsons' approach as "ask not what's inside your head, but what your head's inside of" (p. 43). When viewing the niche as a legacy, we say the same: Ask not what is inherited by genes, but what genes inherit.

The basic task of describing the ontogenetic environment has often followed rather than preceded attempts to study ontogeny by depriving the young of or enriching them with certain external influences. Although such manipulative approaches address the historically relevant question of the degree of interdependence of genetic and environmental mechanisms, they often only indirectly illuminate the normal processes of development. Few of the studies on the effects of sensory or social enrichment or deprivation in young animals provide meaningful details of what happens *during* treatment. What do animals do when isolated that their socially housed peers do not? How do young behave when in the presence of increased or decreased levels of particular forms of stimulation? Measuring the experience of early experience must become a preeminent practice.

Such a practice is called for to deal with two facets of ontogeny. First, it is clear that many animals can and do undergo different kinds of early experience and yet show similar adult phenotypes—there are multiple pathways to the same goal. But animals can also undergo different experiences and manifest different adult behaviors. Understanding which adult outcome occurs offers the opportunity to uncover the mechanisms underlying ontogenetic transitions (Meier, 1984).

The niche is also a link between generations. With this perspective, it is possible to see not only the ultimate dependence of the generations on one another, but their proximate dependence via mechanisms that promote orderly transitions in species-typical development for both adults and young. The niche is a link as well because many exogenetic legacies, such as nest sites, breeding grounds, food, and migration routes, require social interactions between parents and young in order for the resources to be used (Rheingold, 1963).

The study of the parent–offspring relationship in rodents offers diverse examples of the specificity and connectivity of the links. Galef and Wigmore (1983) revealed the wild Norway rat's nest site to be an "information center" in which members learn about potential sites for foraging that exist at some distance from the nest. Moore (1984) demonstrated that the mother rat's licking of her pups contributes to later sexual differentiation because the dams lick males more than females, discriminating chemical differences in the pups' urine. Alberts and Gubernick (1983) connected maternal licking and development even further by demonstrating that nursing dams replenish their loss of fluid and electrolytes by ingesting pup urine. And Pedersen and Blass (1982) demonstrated that odors experienced *in utero* and immediately after birth lead to nipple attachment by rat pups, thereby physically linking mother and young. And finally, Fillion and Blass showed that odors experienced while suckling facilitate the recognition of estrous females. Male rat pups denied experience with their dams' normal ventral odors show less reactivity to estrous females both in infancy (Fillion and Blass, 1986a) and in adulthood (Fillion and Blass, 1986b). Thus, there are links within links exposing the young to stimuli of future relevance when they initiate adult sexual behavior.

Links between parents and offspring or between offspring do not just happen. Members of both generations must act to realize their investments as parents or inheritances as offspring. The niche is thus a way of life and is the study of behavioral ecology. To illustrate the niche as a way of life, we consider the social and physical habitats inherited by the young of several different species. How do differences in their ontogenetic niches affect the offspring that inherit them? In particular, we are trying to begin to identify the overarching social mechanisms that affect an individual's development.

THE ACORN WOODPECKER: THE ROLE OF THE FAMILY TREE

Finding the center of the acorn woodpecker's physical niche is easy: this species congregates in family groups guarding granary trees in which they have drilled and filled up to 30,000 holes with acorns or other nuts. For a young woodpecker, the characteristics of this tree dictate much of its future. But finding the center of the woodpecker's social niche is more complex and has even more relevance to the young woodpecker's ontogeny (Stacey, 1979; Stacey and Koenig, 1984).

In this species, in certain geographical locations, the demographics of the social environment vary with the availability of food: in areas in which granaries remain plentiful, the setting saturates with successful breeders bequeathing to the young the problem of finding a reproductive vacancy. Given that the young cannot affect resource saturation before hatching, they must accommodate to the circumstances they inherit.

If a young acorn woodpecker is hatched in an area such as coastal California, where the food supply is plentiful and available nesting territories are few, then it will probably spend at least one and perhaps up to four to five years as a helper in its natal group. In this group will be one or more mature breeders of each sex and juveniles from past breeding seasons. These juveniles will help to raise the new brood by gathering food, defending the nest and the granary, drilling holes in the granary, increasing the supply of stored food, and fighting off predators. All of these activities contribute to the survival of the young helper, to the survival of the family, and to the survival of the species. But this "good fortune" of the species may lead to problems for any given individual young woodpecker. If the survival rate is high, then juveniles abound, and as breeding age approaches, competition for nest sites is an event of uncertain outcome for the individual.

Some juveniles will not be able to contribute any offspring to the extended family unless all breeders of the opposite sex die or move on. If its parents are young and healthy, then the juvenile must strike out on its own in order to make its genetic mark in the woodpecker world. Finding an unoccupied nesting site or fighting to fill a reproductive vacancy in another group may then be its legacy. If unsuccessful, it may return home to assume the role of "protector" of the collective family resources, postponing, perhaps indefinitely, its own opportunity to be a parent.

The role of "protector" provides a more indirect pathway toward reproductive success. If ecological constraints on new colonization and new breeding opportunities exist, then the juvenile bird can maximize its contribution by preserving and protecting the "family genes" (Stacey and Koenig, 1984). It may also receive the bonus of acquiring better parenting skills, which will, at some later time, enhance its reproductive success.

If, however, a young acorn woodpecker is born in an area such as New Mexico, where the food supply is more limited, a different future unfolds. If the supply of food is not sufficient to last a group during the winter, then that group must leave its territory in search of food. Nesting sites are then available for the juveniles of other groups. Juveniles spend fewer years serving as helpers in their natal groups, and group size is much smaller than in California (Stacey, 1979). But smaller group size means fewer helpers, and fewer helpers mean less food, often leading to winter dispersal and decreased chances of surviving the winter.

Thus, for the acorn woodpecker, the composite nature of the family tree, in nutritional and generational dimensions, affects the duties that the young come to perform, the choice of mate, and whether they mate at all. And where the family tree is geographically situated has overarching effects on the nature and timing of these occupational transitions in the lives of individual woodpeckers.

The center of the scrub jay's niche is even easier to locate because the social and physical cores converge on the family nest. And as for some of the woodpecker groups, the state of the nest at the time of an individual's hatching has much to say about how the young will spend their youth and adulthood. Most remain apprentices or helpers for at least 1 year, some for much longer, before leaving to form a new breeding pair or taking over reproductive duties at the natal nest. Jays with large extended families appear to thrive, a fact suggesting that the occupation of helper or surrogate parent has benefits for both the group and the individual. There are not only immediate advantages in terms of nest and territory defense, but also the intangible advantages of learning what to do when assuming the role of actual breeder. Breeding pairs produce more independent young if there are helpers in the nest, and breeders that have been helpers produce more nestlings than novice breeders (Woolfenden, 1975; Woolfenden and Fitzpatrick, 1984).

But any individual's chances for actual parenthood vary greatly, depending on the initial and continuing state of its extended family. Within the family, there is a dominance hierarchy headed by a male breeder. Linear dominance also exists among male and female helpers, age being the primary factor. Thus, the oldest helper should be the first to leave and set up its own breeding pair. But the dynamics are more complex. A younger helper may be displaced by an adopted helper, usually low in the chain, which may appear after the death of the same-sex breeder. This immigrant may then mate with its adoptive mother, thereby displacing the previously dominant male helpers.

Because males dominate females, a male juvenile may inherit the family nest after the death of its father. Its mother may then be forced to leave and mate with a lone male in another group. The possibility of such a legacy may explain the degree of helping among juveniles because jays are philopatric, and thus, the young have a vested interest in the protection of the nest and the territory. Families with older male helpers (older then 2 years) frequently have larger territories than those with older female or younger male helpers. The territorial expansion may be due in part to a more active territorial defense by males. It may also result in direct benefits for the older male helper, which may then be able to establish an ancillary territory and thus increase its potential breeding possibilities.

In another jay species, the Mexican jay, several nests may exist within the same family territory. These nests belong to members of the same family that have mated with immigrant birds. Juveniles may help in the nest of their parents, their grandparents, or their siblings. Although maintaining separate nests, they forage and defend as a group and may also help feed all the young in the unit. These birds thus also have a special interest in the protection of their territory because it is passed down through successive generations (Brown and Brown, 1981).

The woodpeckers, and especially the jays, illustrate a crucial point about exogenetic legacies: the continuing behavioral efforts demanded of both young and old to maintain their value. Unlike genes, which are the permanent possessions of progenitor and progeny, granary trees and family nests are of changing value depending greatly on the collective industry of their owners. The state of the granary tree is critical to opportunities for breeding and the survival of the young; so, too, the size of the jay's territory correlates with nestling success. Thus, in such species, behaviors must be transmitted as to how the legacies are to be maintained (e.g., how to drill holes, how to replace moldy nuts, how to drive off intruders, and how to attract mates). And it is the social obligation to shared family resources that makes the generationally intermediate role of helper seminal; it is a means to preserve exogenetic legacies. The young may be bequeathed a potentially supportive habitat, but its potential remains only that unless the young learn to exploit it. Exogenetic legacies are inherited, but they are also earned.

It is probably no phylogenetic coincidence that many human cultures also value and reward helping by the young by giving them precedence as legal heirs. A founder of the American jurisprudence system put it as follows:

> It is in accordance with the sympathies and reason of all mankind, that the children of the owner of property, which he acquired and improved by his own skill and industry, and by their association and labor, should have better title to it than the passing stranger. (Chester, 1982), p. 41)

THE COWBIRD: LIVING UP TO ITS GENETIC POTENTIAL

The most obvious exogenetic legacy of a mother cowbird to its offspring is also a nest, but in this case, it contains eggs of other species. Much effort precedes the choice of nest and the female lays many eggs. Ideally, female cowbirds get their offspring off to a good start by laying in a nest already containing an egg or two, ensuring that it will be actively attended, and with eggs slightly smaller than the egg containing the cowbird. The cowbird typically hatches first and, by virtue of being bigger than its foster siblings, can exploit its size and first-hatched status to thrive (King, 1978).

But beyond this inheritance, cowbirds would seem to inherit only an abundance of problems. Cowbirds can hatch into the nests of over 200 different subspecies, so that the natal niche is unpredictable and undependable as a means of acquiring species-typical behaviors. Cowbirds appear to possess no special adaptations and are no more or less successful nestlings than other "cross-fostered" young (Eastzer, Chu, and King, 1980). If anyone warranted Warburton's winter underwear, it would seem to be the cowbird. Given the differences in its natal niche compared to that of most vertebrate young, has the species evolved a comparatively reduced dependence on exogenetic heredity?

Cowbirds do not appear to be exceptions to many of the statements made here about exogenetic inheritance; the major difference is one of timing and type of inheritance. In this respect, the cowbird represents an excellent example of the need to consider transitions in the nature of niches, transitions common to many nonparasitic species that contribute to the realization of exogenetic and genetic inheritance (Alberts and Cramer, Chapter 1; Oppenheim, 1981).

That the cowbird begins life in a natal niche quite unlike the one that it inhabits as a juvenile is not really unusual for birds; it is the jay or the woodpecker that is unusual in remaining for so long with its parents. Transitions in habitat and social groups occur in many species. The cowbird is perhaps only a more obvious case of the discontinuities that characterize many species' social and ecological circumstances.

But to leave the nest is to enter a new stage of development in which new capabilities are required and in which old ones are no longer applicable. After their foster rearing, young cowbirds form flocks with other young and adult cowbirds. How do they "know" to do so? Why not remain socially and/or physically attached to their foster species? Do special recognition mechanisms help them to meet other cowbirds?—probably none more complex than those proposed by Holmes and Sherman (1983) for many species. Cowbirds become attracted to other cowbirds because they have evolved a need of the same kind of food, food found in only certain locations: in the case of cowbirds, insects found at the feet of ungulates or on their grazing grounds.

Thus, initial juvenile flock formation in cowbirds is a case of association mediated by attraction to a common need: food. It is undoubtedly aided by innate social affinities as well. Young cowbirds reliably appear at our aviaries when under 30 days of age with nothing more to attract them than the sights and sounds of other cowbirds. But our aviaries border pastureland and cows, so that it could be the coexistence of preferred food and preferred stimulation that produces the result. Our experience suggests that cowbirds find cowbirds easily. What appears to be difficult is living up to the genetic gifts of their parents, gifts that begin to develop at about this time—in particular, the male's ability to develop courtship songs and the female's capacity to discriminate among songs.

Male cowbirds that have never heard other cowbirds sing can produce and discriminate potent songs (King and West, 1977, 1986). Female cowbirds that have never heard adults sing can respond appropriately and selectively to conspecific song (King and West, 1977). To some, these data are sufficient to suggest that cowbirds are the only songbirds that do not require species-typical experience in order to develop normal song (Rothstein, Yokel, and Fleischer, 1985). But such an interpretation is wrong because it ignores the fact that ontogeny involves both the natural origins and the natural modifications of behavior. It also ignores the fact that the natal niches producing origins may be quite different from the juvenile niches that facilitate modifications.

Burghardt (1977) termed the conceptual confusion in the interpretation of ontogenetic data the difference between the "O" question (for origins) and the "M" question (for modification). He cautioned that the "processes involved in the developmental shaping of a behavior may have little in common with those subsequently altering such behavior" (p. 79).

And it is just this kind of confusion that has led to confusion about whether the cowbird learns its song by genetic or exogenetic means. Males may inherit a potentially rich genetic legacy, but realizing its value depends greatly on the subsequent behavior of the legatees in relation to the social circumstances surrounding them. And here, cowbirds are like jays or woodpeckers because precisely what surroundings they live in have much to say about later reproductive success.

A series of studies sensitized us to "O" versus "M" confusions. The clearest indication came from carrying the classic "deprivation" experiment to its functional conclusion. For many years, "Kaspar hausen" singers have been considered the genetic standard bearers for the study of birdsong, revealing to human listeners the "innate blueprint" provided by genes (Marler, 1982; Thorpe, 1961). Not only is the logic of such an experiment wrong; so is the typical methodology (West and King, 1985a). Isolation from song is usually confounded with isolation from social companions. Moreover, the experiment is often not carried out to its functional endpoint: How does the Kaspar hausen fare when faced with conspecifics?

We were empirically prodded to ask this question because our classic deprivation experiment yielded an odd result: the acoustically deprived males' songs were not worse than those of normally reared males, nor were they the same—they were "better"! We had tested the songs' potency by playing them back to receptive wild-caught females deprived of male company, and these females had responded twice as often to the songs of the acoustically naive males as to the songs of those with normal acoustic stimulation (King and West, 1977). Did the result mean that isolation from song was "good" for cowbirds? The finding seemed even odder given that song learning in the wild took place in a social setting containing singing adults. To understand this apparent anomaly, we took the next functional step: we asked if an acoustically naive male would be successful when actually courting females.

The songs of isolate males of many species have not been tested in a functional arena because of the often quite global pathogenic effects of social and acoustic isolation. But by being provided avian companions (sometimes other juveniles, sometimes females, and sometimes other species), cowbirds can be deprived of adult song and still be successfully tested for the functional end point of song development. In cowbirds, such individuals can settle into a captive colony under one important condition: that they do not sing their potent song to females in the presence of resident males. This is a condition that their previous isolate rearing has not prepared them for (preparing them perhaps in the opposite direction), thereby explaining the seemingly anomalous effect of naive song of "super normal" potency.

Thus, by observing captive colonies, we learned that, whereas males housed alone with females or heterospecifics can sing with impunity, new males in a social group cannot. A naive cowbird singing a potent song does not succeed in that context until it learns to behave effectively with the other males. Potency may be inherited, but the "right" to sing is not (West and King, 1980; West, King, and Eastzer, 1981). In cowbirds, the juvenile niche is a forum in which males learn the pragmatics of singing, which appears to be a performatory, if not sometimes martial, art. The juvenile niche also serves as an acoustic forum for modifying the exact acoustic content of song, making the male's song more geographically specific and more attractive to local females. Without such opportunities for modification, the genetically well-endowed male is actually poorly equipped because the songs it produces may be representative of the species but not optimized to a particular population or individual.

These studies, however, do more than show the need to answer the two kinds of ontogenetic questions. They emphasize the role of the particular ecological and social circumstances that surround maturing organisms. Our work has also shown that the presence of females is an especially important circumstance. In a series of studies, we documented the ways in which males modify what they sing as a function of the behavior of nonsinging female cowbird companions (King and West, 1983a; King, West, and Eastzer, 1980; West and King, 1985b; West, King, and Harrocks, 1983). What determines song modification is the dynamics not of one's auditory environment, but of one's audience. The cowbird's niche is a public arena.

Several studies revealed the potential power of the female as a silent partner in the process of song modification. First, we learned that adult eastern *Molothus ater ater* males would become bilingual only if housed with males *and* females from a geographically separate population of a second cowbird subspecies, *M.a. obscurus*, but not if housed with only *Molothus ater obscurus* males, a finding suggesting to us that the eastern adults required both the means (hearing *M.a. obscurus* song) and the motive (the female) to modify their singing.

Second, we studied naive eastern *M.a. ater* males housed for an entire year, with (1) other species; (2) adult eastern *M.a. ater* females; or (3) adult *M.a. obscurus* females. At the end of this period, the three groups of males (all obtained as eggs from the same colony and most likely full or half siblings) had developed structurally and functionally different vocal phenotypes, although none had ever heard another male sing (King and West, 1983a; West and King, 1985b).

The performance of the males with other species proved a convenient midpoint, as these males experienced abundant social and vocal stimulation from their starling or canary companions, but none of species-typical relevance. Their repertoires were diverse; they sang some protypical *M.a. ater* and *M.a. obscurus* song and some highly atypical song, including imitations of starling and canary vocalizations. The nonspecific nature of their repertoires highlighted the biasing effects of the females in the other two groups. The females' presence apparently produced local song differentiation: the males with *M.a. ater* females sang all *M.a. ater* songs; the *M.a. ater* males with *M.a. obscurus* females sang predominantly *M.a. obscurus* song, but some *M.a. ater* song. In nature, such differentiation is undoubtedly further facilitated by feedback from males serving as fellow performers and sometimes censors of what is sung.

As a further test of the effect of female stimulation, we explored the impact of females when appropriate auditory input *was* present (King and West, 1983a). Here, *M.a. ater* males were tutored with a potent *M.a. ater* song and were individually housed with *M.a. obscurus* females or nonconspecifics. Again, the males developed significantly different repertoires. Males with other species sang significantly more of the tutor song than did males with *M.a. obscurus* females. The males housed with these females sang reliably more original song, but songs that were functionally unattractive to *M.a. ater* females. Thus, even when males were given the acoustic means of learning, the behavior of the heterosubspecific female modified the outcome (West and King, 1985b).

All of the effects reported took place before the females displayed any breeding behavior at all, and thus, the data are based on songs measured and tested before the males had seen a female in a copulatory posture. The young males are apparently sensitive to stimulation from females from as early in development as they can sing (King and West, 1987). It is also important to say that however the females affected the differences in the structure and potency of the males' songs, they did *not* do it by singing. In the two experiments just reported, over 30,000 songs were recorded with an observer present; all were sung by males and none by females.

What was most visible about the vocal behavior of the males housed with the females in the aforementioned experiments was the number of songs and song attempts performed by males that were met with apparent indifference by the females. The seemingly indefatigable energy of the singing male stood in stark contrast to the passive posture of the "listening" female as, song after song, she stared straight ahead with not so much as a head turn toward her companion. Although we cannot yet specify how females communicate their likes and dislikes, their apparent inattention is quite likely a powerful social mechanism because it highlights the specific times when they do change their behavior by moving toward or away from the male, by moving their wing feathers, and by turning their heads. Because of the high incidence of no visible change in their behavior, when changes such as wing movements or approaches did occur, they had a high "signal-to-noise" ratio.

But why is it to the female's "advantage" to influence song development? Given that local females show a high level of intrasexual concordance in song perception, would not their individual efforts tend to homogenize song content among local males, thereby removing song content as a means of comparing males? Perhaps females "help" males learn to sing to enhance the female's ability to assess males. By stimulating males to sing the same song material, the females would then be able to make finer discriminations among males by judging how well the males sing a song the females know well. If males are to be "socially screened" in West-Eberhard's terms (1983), a screening based on the same material would appear to be most advantageous. Homogenization of song material might also have the effect of allowing females to assess males on other attributes, such as dominance status, that might be important indicators of a male's fitness.

The tutorial behavior of the female also brings us back to the original problem faced by the cowbird: How does it develop species-typical behavior, given it does not hatch into a nest with parents and peers of its own species? As our studies show, however, the cowbird inherits a juvenile niche containing other cowbirds, some of which may well be its own parents and/or siblings. Whether kin recognition occurs is not known; nor is it known whether related females or males associate with one another preferentially. But cowbirds may not have abdicated all parenting behaviors: care giving to the young may be carried out by a foster species, but culture giving may not be. The propensity of juvenile males to modify their song may then coincide in time with their contact with kin, an association that normally occurs earlier for other species.

These studies demonstrate the role of the inherited niche in quite a proximate sense. We now have evidence of the niche's impact at a more ultimate level. In all of our work on eastern *M.a. ater* cowbirds, we conceived of the female as a guide, in part because its own behavior appeared inflexible, even after considerable attempts to manipulate its innate preference (King and West, 1983b, 1987). But studies of a different population of cowbirds suggests that such inflexibility may be a local response to the specific properties of the inherited environment.

Recently, we tested the perceptual responsiveness and modifiability of *M.a. ater* females from a different part of this subspecies' range: females living in Oklahoma near the morphologically described subspecies border with *M.a. obscurus,* the southern subspecies. We asked the same questions we had asked of North Carolina *M.a. ater* females: First, would Oklahoma *M.a. ater* prefer their own population's song in comparison to *M.a. obscurus* song, and second, would Oklahoma females show a lack of perceptual modifiability if housed with *M.a. obscurus* males?

The results revealed differences between the two populations of the same subspecies. Wild-caught adult Oklahoma females demonstrated as statistically strong a preference for Oklahoma *M.a. ater* song as did North Carolina females for North Carolina *M.a. ater* song, compared to *M.a. obscurus* song. But when young and adult Oklahoma females were housed for nine months with *M.a. obscurus* males, they showed no preference for either *M.a. ater* or *M.a. obscurus* song; they had developed an apparently equal tolerance for the two subspecies variants (King, West, and Eastzer, 1986).

The Oklahoma and North Carolina populations that we compared differ in four ways: (a) the Oklahoma females live in populations that are much denser than those in North Carolina, (b) the Oklahoma birds live much closer to the subspecies border (250 miles compared to 1,500), (c) they represent part of the ancestral population for the species, whereas cowbirds have colonized North Carolina only since the mid-1940s (Potter and Whitehurst, 1981), and (d), the Oklahoma females live in the central as opposed to the peripheral part of the species range. How these ecological differences relate to the potential differences in modifiability is now the topic of our inquiries.

At this point, our working hypothesis is that Oklahoma females are more sensitive to song differences because the acoustic and social environment surrounding them is different from that of the North Carolina females. The songs of Oklahoma males are more stereotyped in terms of their rhythms and musical qualities—subtle differences to humans, but not to the female cowbirds (King *et al.,* 1986). In order for the females to make the finer discriminations, especially when judging more males (given the greater population density), early exposure and learning may be beneficial. The degree of fine discrimination required has thus led to a more flexible developmental program to "tune" the female's perceptual system to the sounds of her local population.

Wild-caught females from Oklahoma show preferences not only for local songs as opposed to songs from 250 miles away, but for songs of their own subspecies from 1,500 miles away as well: when tested for their responsiveness to North Carolina as opposed to Oklahoma song, they show a strong native bias. In contrast, North Carolina females exposed to the same contrast show no discrimination, responding equally to *M.a. ater* songs from several locations along the eastern coast or from the Oklahoma site. Because cowbirds are more sparsely settled in the East, local differentiation of songs may not have evolved to the point where early exposure can have any measurable effect. The capacity for subtle song discrimination and modification of song preferences may be latent or absent in eastern populations, but in any case, it is different within the same subspecies.

Thus, the females from Oklahoma tell us that ontogenetic programs for song perception may vary even within the same subspecies because the "environment" of a subspecies varies in both a social and a physical sense. Determining which features of an animal's surroundings are stable or labile may help us to predict the ecological circumstances that will favor one ontogenetic pattern over another. Such an analysis may also elucidate how different geographic addresses demand different divisions of labor within the same species. Whereas in the East the female cowbird appears to take the lead in guiding song development, in the West the male's influence appears to be preemptive. But in both cases, synergistic links between the sexes and the settings obtain.

HUMAN FAMILIES: CONFLUENT INHERITANCE

In much the same ways that woodpeckers, scrub jays, and cowbirds are shaped by the culture they inherit, humans also find themselves in quite different "nests." Much of what a human infant first experiences is determined by parental choice. Children are exposed to the foods their parents eat, hear the music that parents choose, meet the people that the family likes, wear the clothes that suit the parents' tastes, and live in rooms bearing the decorating biases of adults. In Rheingold and Cook's study (1975) of children's rooms in a university town in the 1970s, they found no weapons in the rooms of girls and no doll carriages or accessories in the rooms of boys. Given the supposedly "liberated" atmosphere of that decade, the data suggested a different atmosphere:

> Clear in the findings of this study was the extent to which the boys were provided with objects that encouraged activities directed away from home—toward sports, cars, animals, and the military—the girls, objects that encouraged activities directed toward the home—keeping house and caring for children. (p. 463)

None of these early unidirectional influences are unchangeable, but for most children, parents have the upper hand in fashioning children's physical and social environment for many years. Of more lasting importance than the nature of their rooms or toys may be the social nature of the family configuration they live in. Much has been written about the implications of being the oldest, the middle, or the youngest child. Researchers have linked possible differences in such areas as personality, academic achievement, and language development to birth order and the age difference between siblings (Altus, 1966; Zajonc and Markus, 1975). Zajonc (1986) related the decline in scholastic aptitude scores that occurred from 1962 to 1980 to the birth order of the test takers. The reversal in the decline of test scores began in 1980, at the time when children from smaller families became of test-taking age. The same trends toward higher scores were found for children in the elementary grades. If these data do point to important influences, then a child's college admission, career choice, and potential success in the "marketplace" may be affected by the number of siblings already in the family "nest" when he or she arrives.

Given the possibility of differences in such important skills, an important task becomes to find out how differences within the family structure proximately influence development. At present, a study is under way to examine families with one or two children, where the youngest child is under 12 months of age. The focus is on conversations between the mother and her child or children to give us a way of looking at both linguistic and social differences in the familial transmission of knowledge (Arberg and West, 1987).

Thus far, one-child families and two-child families seem quite different on even subtle measures of conversational style. In one-child families, mothers directed more speech to their babies, and infant vocalizations received more responses from the mothers. Vocal turn-taking, where mothers and babies participate in interactions thought to be important precursors to linguistic interactions, was frequent (Stern, 1977). The content of the speech involved the state of the infant or the state of the family, mothers routinely informing their infants that they "were really hungry," "were really sleepy," "liked eggs just like their daddy," or were "really excited about going on an outing."

In two-child families, both the type of speech and the dynamics of the interactions differed. If the infant and the sibling were close in age (a difference of less than 3 years), then conversation focused on and around the mother and the older sibling. Mothers spoke much less to the younger infant, and the older siblings rarely spoke to the infants at all. Compared to the one-child family, the younger infant overheard more speech but had much less speech directed to him or her. Moreover, when the infant vocalized, it was often not as a result of being addressed. The infant's vocalizations were also not acknowledged or answered, and turn taking seldom occurred. The most prevalent type of speech was information from the mother for the toddler—information about toys, family activities, names of objects, and instructions.

But when the older sibling was truly older, an age difference greater than 6 years, there was a different kind of family member present, a "helper" at the nest, if you will. The predominant interactional pair was the sibling and the infant. Moreover, the sibling talked to the young infant in much the same way that the mother did in the one-child families. The older sibling assumed what could almost be termed a surrogate-parent role toward the infant. The conversation was not only infant-directed, but also infant-focused. The older child used appropriate "baby talk," elicited vocalizations from the infant, and responded to vocalizations from the infant, thereby initiating a turn-taking role that seemed to maximize the infant's participation in the "conversation." The older child commiserated with the mother when the baby fussed, instructed the infant in "proper" behavior, and tried to convince the baby to eat its vegetables. Typical were comments like "Eat, little guy, so we can go bye-bye. No, don't chew with your mouth open."

What is the significance of these differences? In an immediate sense, the major difference may be in the changes they make in the life of the mother, freeing the mother with more widely spaced children to expand her horizons in ways that the mother of two children under 4 cannot as yet even imagine. And for the older sibling, the opportunity to experiment with a parental role is provided, but on a voluntary basis, a liberty denied actual parents. In a less immediate sense, the teaching provided by not two, but three parents may influence intelligence and language, as Zajonc proposed. However, the two-child families with closely spaced siblings may find themselves with children that can be friends and playmates in ways not possible for more widely spaced siblings and may thereby provide the siblings valuable experience in gaining social competence.

Family dynamics also affect basic patterns of interactions with the physical world. Following on Rheingold and Eckerman's charting (1970) of the maturation of infants' willingness to leave their mothers and to explore a strange environment, Samuels (1980) found that this willingness was even greater if there was an older sibling present. Infants were tested both with and without their older sibling. When the sibling was present, the infants were more willing to explore, ranged farther afield, spent less time with their mothers, and fussed less. In this situation, the sibling served as a facilitator—a link between the novel and the familiar. Looking longitudinally at infants with closely spaced or widely spaced older siblings, Teti, Bond, and Gibbs (1986) reported that infants with much older siblings received more stimulating intellectual and social experience, especially with respect to language mastery and knowledge of objects.

We cannot as yet attach short- or long-term implications to these differences. All we seek is to emphasize that there are differences, and that a newborn inherits these differences with the family. A baby can no more banish an older sibling than can the sibling "send back" the baby. The family is a package of influences. It is as much a biological and social resource as the granary tree or the scrub jay's territory.

The challenge now is to explore the nature of the "packaging." Birth-order differences constitute naturally occurring instances of varied kinds of "early experience." They merit the kind of scientific attention thus far accorded to more contrived human or animal environments or to satellite configurations such as day care (Belsky and Steinberg, 1978). It is the "home" environment that implicitly represents the standard against which these other settings are evaluated. And it is perhaps because that standard appears to be a moving target that the study of human ecology is so complex.

SUMMARY: SEEING THE OBVIOUS

A Thai proverb has it that "The fish is the last to see the water." The ontogenetic niche is clearly as critical to development as its conceptual cognates: nature and nurture. Why, then, has the idea not undergone the energetic scrutiny accorded "nature" and "nurture"? We suggest that part of this reason is that we share the fish's problem. Eisenberg (1971) put it as follows:

The challenge in understanding such interactions lies in overcoming the limitations of our own ingenuity in recognizing those aspects of the ubiquitous environment that we fail to see because they are ever present. (p. 523)

As a start, we propose the need not only for new words, but for new images to help our eyes adjust to a finer level of observation. Let us begin by replacing illusion with reality. Instead of Boring's puzzle picture, we offer an actual picture depicting organisms engaged in the business of development (Figure 2). It should be a thousand pictures, all depicting interpenetrating alliances among individuals and surroundings. Enough puzzles exist in Figure 2 to suit scientists of diverse persuasions and to make the study of exogenetics as fundamental as that of genetics.

And with respect to words, we argue that the triadic form used here is only a start, soon to be replaced by better descriptors. Gone is the era when sketches of ontogeny relying on the security of black-and-white strokes will suffice. The expositions of ontogeny now available as a result of the efforts of several generations of psychobiologists constitute a gallery of art with myriad images, each in its own way as compelling at that of the double helix. It is now up to us to find the words to animate the science and art of development.

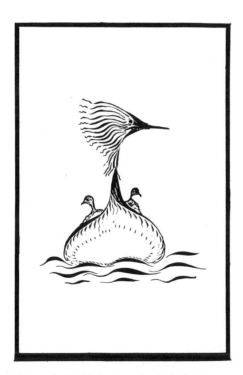

Figure 2. Untitled picture by Eddy Cobbiness.

Acknowledgments

We thank the National Science Foundation (BNS 84-0115), the National Institute of Neurological and Communicative Disorders and Stroke (1 KO1 NS00676-5), the University Research Council, and Sigma Xi for funds supporting some of the research described here.

REFERENCES

Alberts, J. R., and Gubernick, D. J. Reciprocity and resource exchange: A symbiotic model of parent-offspring relations. In L. A. Rosenblum and H. Moltz (Eds.), *Symbiosis in parent-offspring interactions.* New York: Plenum Press, 1983.

Altus, W. D. Birth order and its sequelae. *Science,* 1966, *151,* 44–49.

Arberg, A. A., and West, M. J. *Infant language environment with respect to birth spacing.* Unpublished manuscript, University of North Carolina, 1987.

Barker, R. G. Ecology and motivation. In M. R. Jones (Ed.), *Nebraska Symposium on Motivation,* Vol. 7. Lincoln: University of Nebraska Press, 1960.

Belsky, J., and Steinberg, L. D. The effect of day care: A critical review. *Child Development,* 1978, *49,* 929–949.

Boring, E. G. A new ambiguous picture. *American Journal of Psychology,* 1930, *42,* 444–445.

Boyd, R., and Richerson, P. J. *Culture and the evolutionary process.* Chicago: University of Chicago Press, 1985.

Brown, J., and Brown, E. Extended family in a communal bird. *Science,* 1981, *211,* 959–960.

Brunswick, E. The conceptual framework of psychology. In *International Encyclopedia of Unified Science.* Vol. 1, Pt. 2. Chicago: University of Chicago Press, 1955.

Burghardt, G. M. Ontogeny of communication. In T. E. Sebeok (Ed.), *How animals communicate.* Bloomington: Indiana University Press, 1977.

Carlyle, T. *Sartor resartus: The life and opinions of Herr Teufelsdrockh* (Ed. by C. F. Harrold). New York: Odyssey, 1838/1937.

Chester, R. *Inheritance, wealth, and society.* Bloomington: Indiana University Press, 1982.

Dawkins, R. *The selfish gene.* New York: Oxford University Press, 1976.

Eastzer, E. H., Chu, P. R., and King, A. P. The young cowbird: Average or optimal nestling? *Condor,* 1980, *82,* 417–425.

Eisenberg, L. Persistent problems in the study of the biopsychology of development. In E. Tobach, L. A. Aronson, and E. Shaw (Eds.), *The biopsychology of development.* New York: Academic Press, 1971.

Fancher, R. E. A note of the origin of the term "nature and nurture." *Journal of the History of Behavioral Science,* 1979, *15,* 321–322.

Fillion, T. J., and Blass, E. M. Infantile behavioural reactivity to oestrous chemostimuli in Norway rats. *Animal Behavior,* 1986a, *34,* 123–133.

Fillion, T. J., and Blass, E. M. Infantile experience with suckling odors determines adult sexual behavior in male rats. *Science,* 1986b, *231,* 729–731.

Galef, B. G., and Wigmore, S. W. Transfer of information concerning distant foods: A laboratory investigation of the "information-centre" hypothesis. *Animal Behavior,* 1983, *31,* 748–758.

Galton, F. *English men of science: Their nature and nurture* (2nd ed.). London: Frank Cass, 1874/1970.

Gibson, E. J. *Principles of perceptual learning and development.* New York: Appleton-Century-Crofts, 1969.

Gibson, J. J. *The senses considered as perceptual systems.* Boston: Houghton Mifflin, 1966.

Gibson, J. J. *The ecological approach to perception.* Boston: Houghton Mifflin, 1979.

Holmes, W. G., and Sherman, P. W. Kin recognition in animals. *American Scientist,* 1983, *71,* 46–55.

Hutchinson, G. E. *An introduction to population ecology.* New Haven, CN: Yale University Press, 1978.

Johnston, T. D., and Turvey, M. T. A sketch of an ecological metatheory for theories of learning. In G. H. Bower (Ed.), *The psychology of learning and memory.* New York: Academic Press, 1980.

King, A. P. *Factors affecting brood parasitism in the North American cowbird.* Unpublished doctoral dissertation. Cornell University, New York, 1978.

King, A. P., and West, M. J. Species identification in the N.A. cowbird: Appropriate responses to abnormal song. *Science,* 1977, *192,* 1002–1004.

King, A. P., and West, M. J. Epigenesis of cowbird song: A joint endeavor of males and females. *Nature*, 1983a, *305*, 704–706.

King, A. P., and West, M. J. Female perception of cowbird song: A closed developmental program. *Developmental Psychology*, 1983b, *16*, 335–342.

King, A. P., and West, M. J. The experience of experience: An exogenetic program for social competence. In P. P. G. Bateson and P. H. Klopfer (Eds.), *Perspectives in ethology*, Vol. 7. New York: Plenum Press, 1986.

King, A. P., and West, M. J. Different outcomes of synergy between song production and song perception in the same subspecies *(Molothrus ater ater)*. *Developmental Psychobiology*, 1987, *20*, 177–187.

King, A. P., and West, M. J. Searching for the functional origins of song in eastern brown-headed cowbirds. *Animal Behavior*, in press.

King, A. P., West, M. J., and Eastzer, D. H. Song structure and song development as potential contributors to reproductive isolation in cowbirds. *Journal of Comparative Physiology and Psychology*, 1980, *94*, 1028–1036.

King, A. P., West, M. J., and Eastzer, D. H. Female cowbird song perception: Evidence for different developmental programs within the same subspecies. *Ethology*, 1986, *72*, 89–98.

Lumsden, C., and Wilson, E. O. *Genes, mind, and culture*. Cambridge: Harvard University Press, 1981.

Mace, W. M. James J. Gibson's strategy for perceiving: Ask not what's inside your head, but what your head's inside of. In R. Shaw and J. Bransford (Eds.), *Perceiving, acting, and knowing: Toward an ecological psychology*. Hillsdale, NJ: Erlbaum, 1977.

Marler, P. Some ethological implications for neuroethology: The ontogeny of birdsong. In J. P. Ewert, R. R. Capranica, and D. J. Ingle (Eds.), *Advances in vertebrate neuroethology*. New York: Plenum Press, 1982.

Medawar, P. B., and Medawar, J. S. *Aristotle to zoos: A philosophical dictionary of biology*. Cambridge: Harvard Univesity Press, 1983.

Meier, G. W. Behavioral development: A goal-directed dialogue. *Developmental Psychobiology*, 1984, *17*, 573–586.

Montagu, A. *Human heredity*. Cleveland: World Publishing, 1959.

Moore, C. L. Maternal contributions to the development of masculine sexual behavior in laboratory rats. *Developmental Psychobiology*, 1984, *17*, 347–356.

Mulcaster, R. *Mulcaster's elementarie*. London: Clarendon Press, 1582/1925.

Oppenheim, R. W. Ontogenetic adaptations and retrogressive processes in the development of the nervous system and behaviour: A neuroembryological perspective. In K. J. Connolly and H. F. R. Prechtl (Eds.), *Maturation and development: Biological and psychological perspectives*. Philadelphia: J. B. Lippincott, 1981.

Oppenheim, R. W. Preformation and epigenesis in the origins of the nervous system and behavior: Issues, concepts, and their history. In P. P. G. Bateson and P. H. Klopfer (Eds.), *Perspectives in ethology*, Vol. 5, *Ontogeny*. New York: Plenum Press, 1982.

Oyama, S. A reformulation of the idea of maturation. In P. P. G. Bateson and P. H. Klopfer (Eds.), *Perspectives in ethology*, Vol. 5, *Ontogeny*. New York: Plenum Press, 1982.

Pedersen, P. E., and Blass, E. M. Prenatal and postnatal determinants of the 1st suckling episode in albino rats. *Developmental Psychobiology*, 1982, *15*, 349–355.

Potter, E. F., and Whitehurst, G. T. Cowbirds in the Carolinas. *Chat*, 1981, *45*, 57–68.

Rheingold, H. L. (Ed.). *Maternal behavior in mammals*. New York: Wiley, 1963.

Rheingold, H. L. and Cook. K. V. The contents of boys' and girls' rooms as an index of parents' behavior. *Child Development*, 1975, *46*, 459–463.

Rheingold, H. L., and Eckerman, C. O. The infant separates himself from his mother. *Science*, 1970, *168*, 78–83.

Rothstein, S. I., Yokel, D. A., and Fleischer, R. C. Social dominance, mating, and spacing systems, female fecundity, and vocal dialects in captive and free-ranging brown-headed cowbirds. In R. J. Johnston (Ed.), *Current ornithology*, Vol, 3. New York: Plenum Press, 1985.

Samuels, H. R. The effect of an older sibling on infant locomotor exploration of a new environment. *Child Development*, 1980, *51*, 667–669.

Schleidt, W. M. The behavior of organisms, as it is linked to genes and populations. In P. P. G. Bateson and P. K. Klopfer (Eds.), *Perspectives in ethology*, Vol. 4, *Advantages of Diversity*. New York: Plenum Press, 1981.

Schleidt, W. M. Learning and the description of the environment. In T. D. Johnston and A. T. Pietrewicz (Eds.), *Issues in the ecological study of learning*. Hillsdale, NJ: Erlbaum, 1985.

Stacey, P. B. Habitat saturation and communal breeding in the acorn woodpecker. *Animal Behavior,* 1979, *27,* 1153–1166.

Stacey, P. B., and Koenig, W. D. Cooperative breeding in the acorn woodpecker. *Scientific American,* 1984, *251,* 114–121.

Stern, D. *The first relationship: Infant and mother.* Cambridge: Harvard University Press, 1977.

Stone, C. P. Multiply, vary, let the strongest live and the weakest die—Charles Darwin. *Psychological Bulletin,* 1943, *40,* 1–24.

Super, C. M., and Harkness, S. Figure, ground, and gestalt: The cultural context of the active individual. In R. M. Lerner and N. A. Busch-Rossnagel (Eds.), *Individuals as producers of their development: A life-span perspective.* New York: Academic Press, 1981.

Teigen, K. H. A note on the origin of the term "nature and nurture": Not Shakespeare and Galton, but Mulcaster. *Journal of The History of Behavioral Science,* 1984, *30,* 363–364.

Teti, D. M., Bond, L. A., and Gibbs, E. D. Sibling created experiences: Relationships to birth-spacing and infant cognitive development. *Infant Behavior and Development,* 1986, *9,* 27–42.

Thorpe, W. H. *Bird-song: The biology of vocal expression in birds.* London: Cambridge University Press, 1961.

Warburton, F. E. Feedback in development and its evolutionary significance. *American Naturalist,* 1955, *89,* 129–140.

West, M. J., and King, A. P. Enriching cowbird song by social deprivation. *Journal of Comparative Physiology and Psychology,* 1980, *94,* 263–270.

West, M. J., and King, A. P. Learning by performing: An ecological theme for the study of song learning. In T. D. Johnston and A. T. Pietrewicz (Eds.), *Issues in the ecological study of learning.* Hillsdale, NJ: Erlbaum, 1985a.

West, M. J., and King, A. P. Social guidance of song learning by female cowbirds: A test of its functional significance. *Zeitschrift Tierpsychologie,* 1985b, *70,* 225–235.

West, M. J., and King, A. P. Settling nature and nurture into an ontogenetic niche. *Developmental Psychobiology,* 1987, *20,* 549–562.

West, M. J., King, A. P., and Eastzer, D. H. The cowbird: Reflections on development from an unlikely source. *American Scientist,* 1981, *69,* 57–66.

West, M. J., King, A. P., and Harrocks, T. H. Cultural transmission of cowbird song: Measuring its development and outcome. *Journal of Comparative Psychology,* 1983, *97,* 327–337.

West-Eberhard, M. J. Sexual selection, social competition, and speciation. *Quarterly Review of Biology,* 1983, *58,* 155–183.

Woolfenden, G. E. Florida scrub jay helpers at the nest. *Auk,* 1975, *92,* 1–15.

Woolfenden, G. E., and Fitzpatrick, J. W. *The Florida scrub jay: Demography of a cooperatively-breeding bird.* Princeton, NJ: Princeton University Press, 1984.

Zajonc, R. B. The decline and rise of scholastic aptitude scores: A prediction derived from the confluence model. *American Psychologist,* 1986, *41,* 862–867.

Zajonc, R. B., and Markus, G. B. Birth order and intellectual development. *Psychological Review,* 1975, *82,* 74–88.

3

Cause and Function in the Development of Behavior Systems

JERRY A. HOGAN

The purpose of this chapter is to present a general framework for studying the development of behavior. Kruijt (1964) proposed that, in young animals, the motor components of behavior often function as independent units, and that only later, often after specific experience, do these motor components become integrated into more complex systems, such as hunger, aggression, and sex. The thesis to be defended here is a generalization of this proposal: The building blocks of behavior are various kinds of perceptual, motor, and central components, all of which can exist independently. The study of development is primarily the study of changes in these components themselves and in the connections among them.

The chapter itself is organized somewhat in reverse of the title. I first explain my conception of a behavior system. The basic concepts that I use are generally derived from classical ethological theory as set forth, for example, by Tinbergen (1951). There are, however, a number of differences in the way I define and use these concepts, and these differences are discussed where appropriate. The bulk of the chapter is devoted to the presentation and discussion of examples showing how behavior systems develop. Many of these examples are also "classical," but whenever possible, I include references to recent work in order to provide the reader with an entrance to the literature. At the end of the chapter, I discuss a number of general issues, including the distinction between causal and functional classification of behavior systems and the relevance of functional considerations to causal analyses.

JERRY A. HOGAN   Zoology Laboratory, University of Groningen, A.A. Haren 9750, The Netherlands, and Department of Psychology, University of Toronto, Toronto, Canada M5S 1A1.

JERRY A. HOGAN

No two occurrences of behavior are ever identical, and it is therefore necessary to sort behavior into categories in order to make scientific generalizations. These categories can be defined in different ways (e.g., structurally, causally, or functionally; cf. Hinde, 1970, Ch. 2; Hogan, 1984a,c) and at different levels of complexity (e.g., individual muscle movements, limb movements, or acts; cf. Gallistel, 1980). The concept of a behavior system is defined here structurally, and the level to be analyzed corresponds to the complexity indicated by the terms *feeding behavior, aggressive behavior, play behavior,* and so on. These terms can be considered names for behavior systems as a whole, but our analysis begins with a consideration of the parts of which these systems are constructed.

Three kinds of parts are discussed: motor parts, perceptual parts, and central parts. All of these parts are viewed as corresponding to structures within the central nervous system. For this reason, the word *mechanism* is used in the rest of this chapter in references to these parts.[1] Each motor mechanism, perceptual mechanism, or central mechanism is conceived of as consisting of some arrangement of neurons (not necessarily localized) that acts independently of other such mechanisms. These mechamisms are here called *behavior mechanisms* for two reasons. First, the actual neural connections, their location, and their neurophysiology are not of direct interest in the study of behavior. Second, the activation of a behavior mechanism results in an event of behavorial interest: a particular perception, a specific motor pattern, or an identifiable internal state.

Behavior mechanisms can be connected with one another, and the organization of these connections determines the nature of the behavior system. In order to make the discussion more specific, I shall use the feeding system of a chicken as my example, but the principles involved can be easily generalized to other animals and to other systems.

MOTOR MECHANISMS

We say a chicken is feeding when it walks about looking at the ground, when it scratches at the substrate, and when it pecks and swallows small objects. Walking, scratching, pecking, and swallowing are all easily recognizable motor patterns and can be viewed as reflecting the motor mechanisms of the feeding system. Three points here are worthy of mention.

First, although the behavior patterns of walking and so on are easily recognizable, there is considerable variation between different instances of the "same" pattern. In a practical sense, this variation does not usually interfere with the identification of a pattern, and that is sufficient for our present purpose. The second

---

[1]The word *central,* referring to a mechanism, may cause some confusion because all three types of mechanism are deemed to be structures in the central nervous system. An alternative designation would be *motivational mechanism.* I prefer the word *central* because it emphasizes the location of the structure (i.e., between perceptual and motor mechanisms). As well, later in the chapter, I use the word *motivation* to refer to the activation of all three types of mechanism.

point is essential. What we observe is only a reflection or manifestation of the motor mechanisms of the system. The motor mechanism itself is located inside the central nervous system of the animal and is responsible for coordinating the muscle movements that we actually see. Finally, the concept of a motor mechanism is clearly related to the concept *Erbkoordination* (Lorenz, 1937) or *fixed action pattern* (Hinde, 1970; Tinbergen, 1951) but is meant to be much broader in scope and to encompass all types of coordinated movements.

PERCEPTUAL MECHANISMS

Corresponding to the motor mechanisms on the output side of a behavior system are perceptual mechanisms on the input side. Perceptual mechanisms solve the problem of stimulus recognition and are often associated with particular motor mechanisms. In the feeding system of a chicken, there must be perceptual mechanisms for recognizing the objects at which the bird pecks, for what it swallows, and for the type of environment in which the bird scratches. There must also be perceptual mechanisms for recognizing changes in the chick's internal state consequent to its behavior.

Perceptual mechanisms are inherently more difficult to study than motor mechanisms because the output of a perceptual mechanism can be "seen" only after it has activated some motor mechanism. Thus, there are always more steps where variation can occur. The general method used to study perceptual mechanisms is to present stimuli that vary along different dimensions and to ascertain which combination of characteristics is most effective in bringing about certain responses. The concept *perceptual mechanism* is clearly related to concepts such as *releasing mechanism* (Baerends and Kruijt, 1973; Lorenz, 1937; Tinbergen, 1951); *Sollwert,* or *comparator mechanism* (Hinde, 1970; von Holst, 1954); *cell assembly* (Hebb, 1949); and *analyzer* (Sutherland, 1964). However, as with the term *motor mechanism, perceptual mechanism* is meant to encompass all types of stimulus recognition mechanisms.

CENTRAL MECHANISMS

The final part of a behavior system to be considered is the central mechanism, which is responsible for integrating the input from various perceptual mechanisms and coordinating the activation of various motor mechanisms. It is the central mechanism that usually corresponds to the name we give to a behavior system: a hunger mechanism, an aggression mechanism, a sexual mechanism, and so on. The concept *central mechanism* is clearly related to the neurophysiological concepts *central excitatory mechanism* (Beach, 1942); *central motive state* (Stellar, 1960), or *center* (Doty, 1976), but it will be used here in a still more general sense. Central mechanisms do not differ in any basic way from motor or perceptual mechanisms; they are distinguished separately because of their function of coordinating various motor or perceptual mechanisms.

JERRY A. HOGAN

We can now return to the concept *behavior system* and define it as an organization of perceptual, central, and motor mechanisms that act as a unit in some situations. A pictorial representation of this definition is shown in Figure 1. The first part of this definition is structural and is basically similar to Tinbergen's definition of an instinct (1951, p. 112); it is also similar to the *functional* organization of von Holst and von St. Paul (1960). Hierarchical organization is also implied in this part of the definition, and it is thus related to conceptions of Tinbergen (1951), Baerends (1976), and Gallistel (1980). See also Hogan (1981).

Further, as we shall see, there are various levels of perceptual and motor mechanisms, and the connections among them can become very complex. A diagram such as Figure 1, if expanded to encompass all the facts that are known, would soon become unmanageable. In the extreme, it would become congruent with a wiring diagram of the brain. The main function of such a diagram—and of the concept of a behavior system—is to direct our thinking into particular pathways.

The second part of the definition of a behavior system is causal: at present,

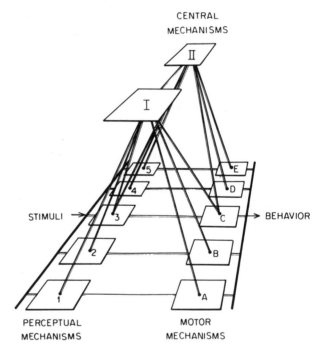

Figure 1. Conception of behavior systems. Stimuli from the external world are analyzed by perceptual mechanisms. Output from the perceptual mechanisms can be integrated by central mechanisms and/or channeled directly to motor mechanisms. The output of the motor mechanisms results in behavior. In this diagram, Central Mechanism I, Perceptual mechanisms 1, 2, and 3, and Motor mechanisms A, B, and C form one behavior system; Central Mechanism II, Perceptual Mechanisms 3, 4, and 5, and Motor Mechanisms C, D, and E form a second behavior system. 1-A, 2-B, and so on can also be considered less complex behavior systems.

the only method for determining behavioral structure is through causal (or motivational) analysis. In discussing the development of behavior systems, as we shall be interested in both structural and causal (motivational) aspects.

THE DEVELOPMENT OF BEHAVIOR SYSTEMS

In a very real sense, the development of behavior begins at conception and continues until death. Nonetheless, much can be understood about the development of behavior systems by considering only the period between birth (hatching) and maturity, and that is what I shall do here.

The thesis of this chapter is that perceptual, central, and motor mechanisms are the building blocks out of which complex behavior is formed, and that a developmental analysis requires looking for the factors causing the development of the building blocks themselves, as well as for the way connections among these building blocks become established. In some cases, these building blocks appear for the first time "prefunctionally"[2] (Schiller, 1949); that is, functional experience is not necessary for their development (though functional experience is often necessary for them to become fine-tuned). Even in such cases, developmental questions arise, and I begin with an example of such a system. I then consider a few examples of how the building blocks themselves develop and, finally, some examples of the development of more complex systems.

THE "GUSTOFACIAL REFLEX": A PREFUNCTIONALLY DEVELOPED SYSTEM

Steiner (1979) showed that newborn infants have at least three gustofacial reflexes. A sweet stimulus to the tongue elicits a "smile" reaction, a sour stimulus elicits a "pucker" reaction, and a bitter substance elicits a "disgust" reaction. The identification of these reactions by even inexperienced observers is highly reliable. In terms of the concepts discussed above, we can posit that the newborn infant has three perceptual mechanisms for particular tastes (a sweet, a sour, and a bitter mechanism) and three motor mechanisms (a smile, a pucker, and a disgust mechanism). These mechanisms and the specific connections between them are formed prefunctionally, that is, before the consequences of ingesting sweet, sour, or bitter substances have been experienced and before any social (or other) reactions to

---

[2]A building block (e.g., the pecking motor mechanism) is functional when its associated response (i.e., pecking) occurs in its adaptive context (i.e., grasping small objects). If the pecking response occurs in its normal form before the chick has ever grasped an object, the development of the pecking motor mechanism can be said to occur prefunctionally: experience grasping an object is not necessary for the development of a normal pecking response. It should be noted that saying that a behavior mechanism develops prefunctionally implies only that particular kinds of experience play no role in the development; there is no implication about the role of other kinds of experience. For example, the development of the pecking motor mechanism of the chick may well be influenced by events associated with beak movements that occur in the egg before hatching or with head and beak movements that occur during hatching. The pecking motor mechanism would nonetheless still be regarded as appearing prefunctionally. This concept is discussed in greater detail later.

these facial expressions can have been perceived. Nonetheless, there are many questions of developmental interest that can be asked about these results.

Some questions refer to changes that occur later in life. For example, how can one interpret the reaction of an adult who smiles at the taste of coffee (a bitter substance)? Presumably neither the perceptual mechanism nor the motor mechanism has changed over time: the coffee still has a bitter taste and the smile is basically the same smile. What has changed is the connection between the perceptual and the motor mechanisms. Further, the change is not simply one in which the bitter mechanism becomes attached to the smile mechanism, because other bitter substances still elicit a "disgust" expression. Identification of the changes that actually occur and the experience that is necessary requires experimental analysis (cf. Rozin, 1984; Rozin and Schiller, 1980), but this type of formulation of the problem makes that analysis easier to tackle.

A second, but closely related, question has to do with the smile mechanism. People smile not only in response to sweet tastes, but also in response to a wide range of stimuli associated with the hunger, sexual, parental, and other systems. How does the smile become attached to these various systems? This question also requires experimental analysis (cf. Blass, Ganchrow, and Steiner, 1984), and several examples of this type are considered below.

Other questions about the development of the gustofacial reflex refer to experiences of the fetus before birth. These would include possible effects of tasting and swallowing amniotic fluid or feedback from movements of facial or other muscles. We are not concerned in this chapter with such prenatal experiences, but it is important to realize that there is a complex developmental history before the emergence of even a prefunctionally developed system (see also Smotherman and Robinson, Chapter 5).

DEVELOPMENT OF PERCEPTUAL MECHANISMS

Two of the most studied examples of behavior development, song learning in birds and imprinting in various species, are both examples that involve a perceptual mechanism that develops independently of connections with central and motor mechanisms. In both cases, the development of the perceptual mechanism is inferred from tests given later in life. Several aspects of these studies seem worthwhile to mention here.

SONG RECOGNITION MECHANISMS. Some time ago, Thorpe (1958, 1961) showed that the male chaffinch, *Fringilla coelebs,* had to learn to sing its species-specific song, and that this learning occurred in two stages. First, the young bird had to hear the normal song (or, within limits, a similar song); later, it learned to adjust its vocal output to match the song it had heard when it was young. Similar results have also been found for the white-crowned sparrow, *Zonotrichia leucophrys* (Konishi, 1965; Marler, 1970), though not necessarily for other species of songbirds (e.g., Logan, 1983; Marler, 1976). The first stage of learning involves the development of a perceptual mechanism, and that is discussed here; the second stage involves the development of a motor mechanism, and that is discussed in the next section. There have been many reviews of the bird song literature (e.g., Bottjer and Arnold, 1986; Slater, 1983), and only highly selected aspects are mentioned in this chapter.

Marler (1976, 1984) proposed that the results of studies of song learning imply the existence of an auditory template, which he conceived of as a sensory mechanism that embodies species-specific information. The normal development of the template requires auditory experience of the proper sort at the proper time. In our terms, the template becomes a song-recognition (perceptual) mechanism that is partially formed at hatching.

The development of the song recognition mechanism is especially interesting because it illustrates most of the problems encountered in the development of behavior systems in general. First, the postulation of a template is equivalent to saying that a perceptual mechanism exists and, further, that it is preassigned to serve a particular function. Second, there are constraints on the kinds of experience that can affect development and on the age or stage of development at which this experience can be effective. Are the effects of experience irreversible? These constraints also vary greatly across species. The third problem relates to the process(es) by which experience has its effects on development: Are the effects of experience direct or indirect? Is mere exposure sufficient, or is some sort of reinforcement necessary? These problems are all interrelated, and aspects of them are discussed at the end of this section.

A final point about song recognition mechanisms is that the same perceptual mechanism, once it has developed, serves several different functions: in the male, it serves as a standard against which the bird's own song develops, and it also releases aggressive behavior when the male becomes territorial in the spring; in the female, it releases sexual behavior (e.g., Milligan and Verner, 1971).

SPECIES RECOGNITION MECHANISMS: IMPRINTING. Most song-recognition mechanisms serve a species recognition function, but there are many species in which song does not exist. These species apparently have analogous perceptual mechanisms that analyze visual or other sensory input. The development of such perceptual mechanisms has usually been studied in the context of imprinting. This concept, as originally elaborated by Lorenz (1935), was primarily concerned with the process by which early experience affects development. Therefore, most studies of imprinting have had a narrower focus than studies of song learning. Nonetheless, in his original discussion of imprinting, Lorenz (1935) pointed out that a newly hatched individual of some species, such as the curlew *(Numenius arquata)*, require no visual experience in order to recognize members of its own species, whereas in other species, such as the greylag goose *(Anser anser)*, a newly hatched individual apparently directs all its species-typical social behaviors to the first moving object it sees.

In our terms we would say that most, and perhaps all, species have a preassigned perceptual mechanism (a "template" again) that serves a species recognition function. In such species as the curlew, this perceptual mechanism is developed prefunctionally, whereas in such species as the greylag goose, various kinds of experience are necessary for its development. A moment's thought will make it clear that all the aspects of song recognition mechanisms mentioned above are also applicable to species recognition mechanisms, in general. In other words, song learning and imprinting are both specific examples of the general problem of the development of perceptual mechanisms. Some general principles emerging from this view will be discussed after we consider the development of food recognition mechanisms.

FOOD RECOGNITION MECHANISMS. The work of Steiner (1979), discussed above, suggests that newborn infants have well-developed perceptual mechanisms for recognizing sweet, sour, and bitter. The recognition of sweet, sour, and bitter, of course, is a rather low-level accomplishment, and a more interesting question is whether a food recognition mechanism exists and, if so, how it develops. For the moment, I will assume that a food recognition mechanism does exist, and I will review some data relevant to how it is organized (at a behavioral level) and how that organization develops.

It is perhaps wise to emphasize here that, in talking about a "food recognition mechanism" or a "song recognition mechanism," I am using these terms in a strictly (behaviorally) causal sense. That is, stimuli that activate the food recognition mechanism, for example, are those stimuli that the animal treats as food; we infer that the animal is treating a stimulus as food from the occurrence of behaviors that belong to the hunger system. Such stimuli may or may not be nutritious and could even be poisonous.

Newly hatched chicks peck at a wide variety of objects, although, even at the first opportunity, certain colors and shapes are preferred (Fantz, 1957; Hess, 1956). These preferences need not be a reflection of an undeveloped food-recognition mechanism, however, for at least two major reasons. First, pecking is a component of aggressive, sexual, and grooming behavior as well as of feeding behavior, and the stimuli that release and direct pecking in these various contexts are quite different. Second, chickens continue to peck a wide variety of objects throughout their lives, even after the objects toward which they direct their feeding, grooming, aggressive, and sexual behavior have become quite specific. Thus, it seems not unreasonable to view these early preferences as being due to a perceptual mechanism directly connected to the pecking mechanism in the same way that the various taste mechanisms are connected to specific motor mechanisms in infants. This "independent" pecking might be regarded as serving an exploratory function, and it also has many of the characteristics of play, as will be discussed later.

The putative food-recognition mechanism in newly hatched chicks must be largely unspecified because of the very wide range of stimuli that are characteristic of items that chicks will come to accept as food. Certain taste and tactile stimuli are more acceptable than others (see Hogan, 1973b, for review), but these stimuli can be effective only after the chick has the stimulus in its mouth. In some cases, taste and tactile feedback seem to be sufficient to cause an item to become recognized as food. For example, as early as 1–2 days of age, a chick that has eaten one mealworm will treat all subsequent mealworms as food. Presumably, the taste of the mealworm is sufficient for subsequent visual recognition to occur because a second mealworm will be accepted immediately after the first, and thus long before any effects of digestion could be expected to play a role (Hogan, 1966). Taste is also sufficient for a chick to develop visual recognition of a stimulus to be rejected: a 1-day-old chick will learn to reject a distasteful cinnabar caterpillar in just one trial (Morgan, 1896; see also Hale and Green, 1979). The fact that mealworms can come to be recognized as food (i.e., are avidly ingested) and other insects can come to be rejected as food before nutritive factors gain control of pecking on day 3 (see below) is evidence that the food recognition mechanism is independent of the central mechanism of the developing hunger system.

The food recognition mechanism also develops under the influence of the long-term (1–2 h) effects of ingestion. Experiments by Hogan-Warburg and Hogan (1981) provide evidence that chicks gradually learn to recognize food particles as a result of the reinforcing effects of food ingestion. In these experiments, visual stimuli from the food gained significant control over the chicks' behavior after one substantial food meal, though oral stimuli gained control of ingestion more slowly.

The development of food recognition in young kittens is similar in many ways to that of chicks (Baerends-van Roon and Baerends, 1979). Kittens begin ingesting their first solid food at about 4 weeks of age. Some items are immediately recognized as food, whereas others require various kinds of experience before being accepted (or rejected) as food. Fish odor appears to be attractive to all cats, even those with no experience of fish. Fish is ingested as early as a kitten is able to eat solid food, but the main problem for the kitten is learning how to catch a fish. This topic is discussed in the next section. Mouse odor, on the other hand, does not appear to have an inherent attractiveness for cats. Mice become recognized as food only after a kitten has eaten a mouse. This can happen if a mother cat presents a dead (and opened) mouse. It can also happen if a kitten attacks and bites a live mouse by itself. It is not yet possible to say whether the taste of the mouse is sufficient experience for its subsequent recognition as food (as in the chicks) or whether nutritional effects of digestion are necessary. The Baerendses did observe that a shrew may be caught and ingested by a naive kitten, but it is vomited within 15–20 min. Thereafter, kittens may catch and "play" with shrews, but they never ingest them. This finding suggests that the effects of digestion may be the critical experience for food recognition to develop. Such observations also indicate considerable independence of catching and eating behavior, a topic discussed later.

In a functional sense, the nutritional effects of ingestion should be the ultimate factor in determining which objects are recognized as food. But sometimes, other factors override the effects of nutrition and lead to the development of a food recognition mechanism that is maladaptive. Two observations made on chicks' food preferences are relevant here (Hogan, 1971). The first observation is that many chicks that were fed mealworms on the first few days after hatching died at about 6 or 7 days. These chicks could generally be characterized as mealworm fanatics because of their excited, positive behavior toward mealworms. These mealworm fanatics never learned to eat the regular chicken food that literally surrounded them, and they apparently died of starvation. The second observation is that many chicks that were raised on a mixture of chicken food and aquarium gravel also died at about 6 days of age, also apparently of starvation. In this case, the gravel seemed to be an exceptionally good releasing stimulus for pecking and swallowing. Both these examples suggest that factors other than the nutritional effects of ingestion can play an important role in the development of food recognition.

DISCUSSION. The results from chicks and kittens provide material for considering some of the general problems mentioned earlier in this section. First is the question of existence. The evidence suggests that perceptual mechanisms exist in at least three functional levels of organization: feature recognition, object recognition, and function recognition. Feature recognition mechanisms discriminate among various sizes, shapes, colors, smells, tastes, and so on. This is presumably the level at which the gustofacial reflex is organized in human infants. The reason for distinguishing between object recognition and function recognition is that objects with similar properties, such as food crumbs and sand, mealworms and cinnabar caterpillars, or mice and shrews, are easily recognized (after appropriate experience) as being food or nonfood, whereas other objects with greatly disparate properties, such as grain, insects, fish, and the leaves of various plants, are easily included in the food category.

Most investigators who study song or species recognition mechanisms assume that the perceptual mechanism functions only in the recognition of the "correct" song or the "ideal" mate. In these cases, the object and the function recognition mechanisms would be identical. There is reason to believe, however, that the situation is often more complex. A mockingbird, *Mimus polyglottos,* for example, mimics very accurately the songs of many different species (Baylis, 1982); therefore, it must have a number of perceptual mechanisms for recognizing each different song. Further, the various songs that the mockingbird has learned are combined into an overall song that has species-specific characteristics (Logan, 1983); therefore, there must be an additional perceptual mechanism at a higher level of organization. There are also species of birds that recognize conspecific songs individually (McGregor and Avery, 1986) or even discriminate among nonconspecific songs (Park and Dooling, 1985), findings that also imply separate object and function recognition mechanisms.

Two levels of perceptual mechanisms are also implicated in the results of some recent studies of imprinting. Ten Cate (1986) demonstrated a case of double imprinting. Young zebra finches that are exposed early in life to both zebra and Bengalese finches may later court both species. A stable preference is formed for both these species over other similar species, to which the zebra finches were not exposed when young. Further experiments investigated what kind of internal representation (perceptual mechanism) is necessary to account for this phenomenon (1987). Ten Cate concluded that a single, combined representation is sufficient to account for courtship preferences (function recognition), but that differential responding to potential mates from other species implies object recognition mechanisms as well.

The problem of constraints on what experience can be effective and at what stage of development is very general and applies to all kinds of development. This problem is addressed in the general discussion. The problem of the processes through which experience has its effects is also very general, but a few comments seem appropriate here. In particular, the development of a food recognition mechanism in chicks and kittens seems to require various kinds of reinforcement, and the objects that come to be recognized as food can change over the animal's lifetime, whereas mere exposure to an adequate song or partner is often thought to be sufficient for the development of a song or a species recognition mechanism, and subsequent changes may be difficult or impossible. Cases where mere exposure is sufficient for the development of a food recognition mechanism in various insects are known, however, and this preference is apparently irreversible (Thorpe and Jones, 1937). On the other hand, the type of interaction between (surrogate) parents and young in zebra finches seems to be important in determining to which object imprinting occurs (ten Cate, 1984), and social interaction sometimes determines which song is learned (Baptista and Petrinovich, 1984). Further, reversibility in the object to which a young bird has been imprinted (e.g., Boakes and Panter, 1985; Bolhuis and Trooster, 1988) has also been seen, as has reversibility in song learning in some species (e.g., Nottebohm, 1981). Thus, a whole range of developmental processes may be important in determining function recognition in various species.

DEVELOPMENT OF MOTOR MECHANISMS

Many motor mechanisms develop prefunctionally. For instance, young chicks show normal locomotion and pecking movements almost immediately after hatching. And within the first few days, ground scratching and various grooming movements appear. Kruijt (1964) showed that the proper functioning of these and other movements in the posthatching situation is not a necessary causal factor for their development. Of course, prehatching conditions obviously influence the development of these movements, though the processes responsible for behavioral organization remain largely unknown (Oppenheim, 1974).

It should be emphasized here that, although motor patterns are visible to an observer, motor mechanisms are not. Thus, the study of the development of motor mechanisms has many of the same inherent problems as the study of perceptual mechanisms. An example should make this difficulty clear. Kuo (1967) noted that chicks that developed with the yolk sac in an abnormal position were often crippled when they hatched. He interpreted these results to mean that the development of normal walking movements required functional experience in the egg: the legs had to push actively against the yolk sac for normal development to occur. Such experience is indeed necessary for the development of normal joints (Drachman and Sokoloff, 1966), and without properly functioning joints, a chick cannot move normally. Nonetheless, the movements of a crippled chick cannot provide evidence for whether or not the motor mechanism for walking has developed normally. Such evidence certainly does not contradict the conclusion of Hamburger (e.g., 1973) that the neural patterning underlying the walking movements of a chick develop without functional experience (cf. Lehrman, 1970).

Song Learning. Perhaps the best studied example of how a motor mechanism actually develops is the development of bird song (see Bottjer and Arnold, 1986). As we have seen above, the young bird, in many species, forms an auditory image of the song it will learn to sing. Actually, learning to sing the song does not happen until later, when the internal state (e.g., the level of testosterone) is appropriate. At this point, it appears that the bird learns to adjust its motor output to match the image it has previously formed. This adjustment must involve the bird's hearing itself because deafened birds never learn to produce any song that approaches normal song (Konishi, 1965).

There are various ways in which this auditory feedback could be effective. Experiments by Stevenson (1967) showed that hearing its species-specific song could serve as a reinforcer for an operant perching response in male chaffinches. On the basis of these results, Hinde (1970) suggested that song learning might involve matching the sounds produced by the young bird with the stored image: sounds that matched the image would be reinforced, whereas other sounds would extinguish (cf. Bottjer and Arnold, 1986; Marler and Peters, 1982). In this way, a normal song could develop in much the same way as an experimenter originally trains a rat to press a lever (Skinner, 1953).

The comparison of song learning with the process of "shaping" in an operant conditioning experiment leads one to ask a number of rather unexpected questions. For example, if song learning is the shaping of the song out of relatively undifferentiated sounds on the basis of differential reinforcement, is it possible to use any reinforcer for this purpose? Rice (1978) tried to affect the occurrence of shrill calls and twitters in young chicks by using food reinforcement but was unsuccessful. Nonetheless, these calls in young chicks are already formed when the experiment begins, and it is possible that undifferentiated sounds are amenable to shaping with a variety of reinforcers. Another question that can be asked is whether the learning of skilled movements, such as occur in some sports or in playing a musical instrument, for example, proceeds in the same way as song learning. What is the image being matched in skill learning? These questions are all aspects of the more general problem of imitation, and some of these aspects will be considered again in the next section.

Displays. A display is a behavior pattern that is adapted to serve as a signal to a conspecific. The mechanism controlling the display is thus the motor counterpart of species-recognition perceptual mechanisms discussed above. Displays are often complex, yet they typically develop prefunctionally. For example, waltzing is a courtship display in chickens that essentially involves the male's circling a female in a characteristic posture. Kruijt (1964) showed that the form of this display can be derived from components of behavior that belong to the aggression and escape systems, and that these systems are activated when waltzing first appears. Nonetheless, waltzing appears even in animals that are reared in social isolation, so social experience cannot be a necessary causal factor in its development. The occurrence of waltzing does depend in interesting ways on social experience; this topic is discussed later.

One example of a display in which social experience has been implicated as a causal factor in its development is the "oblique posture with long call" of the black-headed gull, *Larus ridibundus*. Groothuis (1985) raised gulls to the age of 1 year either in social isolation, in small groups of 2–4 individuals, or in large groups of 12. Black-headed gulls are colonial breeders, and large groups are the normal social environment for the developing young. All the birds raised in large groups, 50% of the birds raised in small groups, and 35% of the birds raised in social isolation developed the normal display. The other isolated birds and about 10% of the birds raised in small groups showed fragmentary forms of the display that were similar to some of the transitional forms that occur in normal development. Of particular interest is that about 40% of the birds raised in small groups developed an aberrant display in which the head was held in an abnormal posture. Further experience in large groups for more than a year had no effect on the form of this aberrant display. This finding contrasts with the finding that all of the isolated and other birds that showed only fragmentary forms of the display subsequently developed a normal display when placed together in a large group. A separate experiment showed that isolated birds that were injected with testosterone at 10 weeks of age all developed a normal display within a few days of injection.

One process underlying the development of this display may be the same as that suggested by Hinde for the development of bird song. There may be some sort of template sensitive to proprioceptive feedback from the display that "selects out" the correct forms from all the transitional forms that normally occur. The existence of a visual template for recognition of the display does not seem unreasonable, but it seems much less plausible that this template could also recognize proprioceptive feedback. Such a property cannot be excluded, however, and a cognitive structure that recognizes proprioceptive feedback has actually been proposed to explain the results of experiments on imitation by human infants (Field, Woodson, Greenberg, and Cohen, 1982). Nonetheless, the results from the testosterone experiments, in which essentially no transitional forms were seen, do not support such a process in the gulls. Further, the fact that many isolated birds developed a normal display means that social experience cannot be a necessary causal factor for normal development. However, the aberrant displays that developed in some birds raised in small groups lead one to suspect that social interractions can be of importance in special circumstances. A. G. G. Groothuis (personal communication, 1986) suggested that social interaction does not normally influence the development of the display, but that, during the period before the attainment of the ultimate form, abnormal social interactions (such as frequently occur in groups of 2 or 3 individuals) can distort normal development. We shall return to this idea in the discussion.

PREY CATCHING. The final example of the development of motor patterns is the prey-catching behavior of cats. This example has aspects in common with the development of individual behavior patterns just discussed, and it also provides some insight into the development of more complex behavior systems. As before, most of the material reviewed here is found in the paper by Baerends-van Roon and Baerends (1979).

Locomotion, pouncing, angling (with one paw), and biting are the basic motor patterns out of which effective prey-catching develops, and all these behaviors can be seen, prefunctionally, by the time the kitten is about 4 weeks old. The way these behaviors become integrated depends primarily on the type of prey being caught. If a mouse is the prey, locomotion and biting are sufficient to catch and kill, whereas with larger prey, pouncing is necessary in addition. If a fish is the prey, angling and biting are the necessary motor patterns. The evidence suggests that the "correct" behavior sequences are selected on the basis of the effects of the behavior. In other words, an operant shaping process can account for all the results, with the proviso that the basic elements—locomotion, pouncing, angling, and biting—are not themselves shaped. This conclusion is supported by the fact that the course of development can vary considerably among individuals even though the final result is quite stereotyped. Given the behavioral elements available, there really is only one best way to catch a mouse (or a fish), but it takes considerable experience to discover that way and to perfect it.

Two further points should be mentioned. The first is that the result, or reinforcer, that shapes the behavior is probably not related to eating (nutrition). This conclusion follows from the fact that prey catching in general is often independent of nutritional state (e.g., Polsky, 1975). It seems more likely that prey catching is an end in itself. This conclusion is also attested to by the experience of many cat owners who have fed their pets from weaning on the best cat food, but who, nonetheless, are often presented with dead birds that have been caught but not eaten.

The second point is that, unlike many cases of song learning or displays, the prey-catching sequences in cats do not "crystallize." That is, functional experience continues to be effective in shaping new sequences. For example, kittens that have developed proficient fish-catching behavior can subsequently learn to catch mice, although there is some interference from the previous learning in that such kittens take longer to learn to kill the mouse with a bite than naive kittens. Learning to catch a fish after the kitten has already developed mouse-catching behavior turns out to be considerably more difficult. The primary problem here is that older kittens have a stronger tendency to avoid getting wet than younger kittens. If the fear of water can be overcome, the fish-catching sequence can be easily acquired. This last example indicates an important problem in the study of development: It seems that certain cases of learning may be irreversible when, actually, indirect factors (such as fear of water, in this case) obscure the fact that functional experience can still have direct effects on development.

We can say that a central and a motor mechanism are connected when the occurrence of a behavior varies directly with the presence of factors known to affect the central mechanism. Consider the behavior of pecking and the central hunger mechanism in a chicken. If the amount of pecking varies directly with the amount of food deprivation, then we have evidence that hunger and pecking are connected. On the other hand, if variations in food deprivation have no effect on the amount of pecking, we have evidence that hunger and pecking are not connected, that is, are independent mechanisms. The developmental problem is how we get from the state of independence to the state of connectedness. There are actually many examples of situations in which a motor mechanism becomes connected to a particular central mechanism, including examples from the operant conditioning literature. I shall discuss some of these later, but I shall begin with some examples of the development of normal feeding behavior.

Hunger. A surprising fact about the feeding behavior of many neonatal animals is that their early feeding movements are relatively independent of motivational factors associated with food deprivation. Hinde (1970, p. 551ff.) reviewed a variety of evidence from studies on kittens, puppies, lambs, and human infants that show that the amount of suckling by a young animal is very little influenced by the amount of food it obtains. More recently, a series of studies on the development of feeding in chicks and in neonatal rats has been published, and these will be reviewed here.

A chick begins pecking within a few hours of hatching, but its nutritional state does not influence pecking until about 3 days of age (Hogan, 1971). When chicks were 1 or 2 days old, 5 h of food deprivation did not influence the subsequent rate of pecking at food, whereas, by the time the chicks were 4 or 5 days old, 5 h of food deprivation led to a large increase in pecking at food. A very similar change in the control of feeding has been found in rat pups (Blass, Hall, and Teicher, 1979; Hall and Williams, 1983). Before the age of about 2 weeks, the occurrence of behaviors such as nipple search and nipple attachment, as well as the amount of suckling itself, was not influenced by food (i.e., maternal) deprivation of as long as 22 h. After 2 weeks, however, deprived pups attached to the nipple more quickly and suckled longer than nondeprived pups. Similarly, when tested in a spatial discrimination task in a Y maze, nutritive suckling provided a greater incentive than nonnutritive suckling only after the pups were older than 2 weeks (Kenny, Stoloff, Bruno, and Blass, 1979).

The developmental question, with respect to these results, is: How do the motivational factors associated with food deprivation come to control feeding behavior? This question has not yet been answered for the rat pups, but it has for the chicks. A number of early experiments showed that some kind of pecking experience is necessary for this change in control to occur (Hogan, 1973a). Subsequent experiments (see Hogan, 1977, for a review) led to the hypothesis that it is the experience of pecking followed by swallowing that causes the connection between the central hunger mechanism and the pecking mechanism to be formed. In other words, it appears that a chick must learn that pecking is the action that leads to ingestion; once this association has been formed, nutritional factors can directly affect pecking (see Figure 2).

Subsequent experiments have shown that the association of pecking with ingestion is, indeed, the necessary and sufficient condition for pecking to become integrated into the hunger system (Hogan, 1984b). Chicks with experience of pecking followed by swallowing, whether food, sand, mealworms, or sawdust, all formed the association; whereas chicks with experience of pecking glued-down sand that they could not swallow, or with experience of swallowing liquid food or sand that was force-fed and thus not pecked at, did not form the association. Further, once the association between pecking and ingestion occurred, food deprivation influenced pecking immediately.

These data provide the best evidence available for the factors actually responsible for the formation, during normal development, of a connection between a central coordinating mechanism and a motor mechanism. Recent experiments on the development of pecking in ring doves *(Streptopelia roseogrisea)* also indicate that experience is necessary for hunger to gain control of pecking; though, in this case, the necessary experience apparently involves interaction with the parents (Graf, Balsam, and Silver, 1985).

Similar experiments with rat pups have not been done, though the problem with mammals, in general, is more complex because the suckling response drops

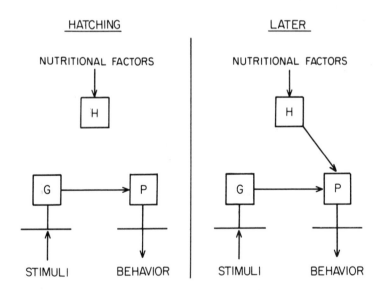

Figure 2. Interpretation of the results from Hogan (1984b). At hatching, a grain-recognition perceptual mechanism (G) and a pecking motor mechanism (P) are connected (prefunctionally) and can be viewed as forming an independent pecking system. A hunger central mechanism (H) also exists, and it may be influenced by nutritional factors, but it has no influence on the pecking system. Later, after experience of pecking followed by swallowing, the hunger mechanism becomes attached to the pecking mechanism, and the nutritional state can now influence pecking.

out altogether at weaning and is replaced by different behaviors (cf. Hall and Williams, 1983). Hall and his colleagues have shown that, under special conditions, rat pups ingest food away from the mother very soon after birth, but these experiments have not asked the same questions being asked here (also see Johanson and Terry, Chapter 7). However, there are some results from guinea pigs that are relevant (Reisbick, 1973). Guinea pigs normally begin ingesting solid food within a day of birth, and Reisbick found that experience of ingesting and swallowing was necessary before the guinea pigs showed evidence of discriminating between nutritious and nonnutritious objects. These results are very similar to the results from the chicks and have been discussed in more detail elsewhere (Hogan, 1977).

OPERANT CONDITIONING. A second source of evidence for the development of connections between central and motor mechanisms is the operant conditioning literature. The process of reinforcement, in general, can be regarded as influencing the development of connections between central and motor mechanisms. For example, the response of lever pressing is an easily recognizable motor pattern in a rat. Reinforcing lever pressing with food leads to a connection of the motor mechanism for lever pressing with the hunger system, and reinforcing with water leads to a connection with the thirst system.

Schiller (1949) reported the results of studies of problem solving by chimps. He noted that many of the behavior patterns used by his chimps to procure food that was placed out of reach were apparently the same manipulative patterns that had first appeared "spontaneously" and "prefunctionally." These patterns included "weaving," "poking and sounding," and "joining sticks." Schiller suggested that these patterns could be considered operant responses that were used to solve the problem, and that they were reinforced when the chimp was successful. In the terminology used here, we could say that the originally independent motor mechanisms responsible for the various observed behavior patterns became connected to the hunger system as a result of operant reinforcement. The test for "connection" here, as elsewhere, is to see if the occurrence of a behavior varies directly with the presence of factors known to affect the central mechanism: Do hungry chimps engage in these behaviors more than sated chimps? Schiller's results suggest that they do.

If we consider the results from the chicks discussed above, the conclusion was that a chick had to ingest and swallow some solid substance in close temporal association with pecking before pecking became attached to the hunger system. One question that follows from this conclusion is whether any movement can be attached to the hunger system in the same way.

Shettleworth (1975) looked at golden hamsters to see whether various behavior patterns could be influenced by food reinforcement. In one set of experiments, she observed animals in their home cages and in an unfamiliar environment both when deprived and when not deprived of food. In another set of experiments, she reinforced animals with food when they performed various behavior patterns, including scrabbling, digging, rearing, face washing, scratching, and scent marking. She found that food reinforcement was effective in increasing the occurrence of scratching, digging, and rearing, but that it had very little effect on the occurrence of face washing, scratching, and scent marking. The first three patterns all increased in frequency in hungry hamsters, and the latter three decreased in frequency. Thus, behavior patterns that belonged to the hamster's hunger system—when the criterion used is a positive correlation with food deprivation—could be influenced by food reinforcement, whereas behavior patterns that belonged to other systems could not.

These results indicate a considerable degree of inflexibility with respect to which motor patterns can become connected to which central mechanisms, at least in an adult hamster. It remains to be seen whether similar results would be obtained with young hamsters at the time that these behavior patterns first appear.

DEVELOPMENT OF CONNECTIONS BETWEEN PERCEPTUAL AND CENTRAL MECHANISMS

We can say that a perceptual mechanism and a central mechanism are connected when a stimulus that activates the perceptual mechanism can lead to the occurrence of the set of behaviors known to belong to the central mechanism. For instance, an egg recognition mechanism is connected to the incubation system in many birds because the presentation of an egg (or other appropriate stimulus) can lead to approach, retrieval, and settling on the nest.

HUNGER. The results with the chicks discussed above show that a mealworm recognition mechanism can become connected to the motor mechanism for pecking at least one day before nutrition (i.e., the central "hunger" mechanism) gains control of pecking. The evidence indicates that the ingestion of mealworms remains semi-independent of hunger, probably throughout life: satiated chicks avidly ingest many mealworms, and the ingestion of a substantial number of mealworms, at least in the first week after hatching, has no effect on the amount of other food subsequently ingested (Hogan, 1971). This semi-independence of mealworm ingestion and hunger is probably the same phenomenon as the semi-independence of prey catching and hunger in cats and most other predators.

The evidence necessary to show that a perceptual mechanism is, in fact, connected to a central mechanism is to show that the presentation of an adequate stimulus has the same effect on the central mechanism as a direct manipulation of the revelant internal factors, for example, by deprivation or the injection of hormones. Such evidence is most easily provided by demonstrating priming effects (Hogan and Roper, 1978, pp. 231–232). For example, the presentation of food may make an animal hungrier (the "appetizer" effect), or the presentation of a sexual stimulus may increase its sexual appetite. Such priming effects are regularly seen in adult animals, though no one seems to have asked how they develop. There is evidence in young chicks that food particles develop incentive value between 3 and 5 days posthatching (Hogan, 1971); development of incentive value probably reflects the same process involved in the development of food recognition discussed above (Hogan-Warburg and Hogan, 1981). More direct evidence of perceptual mechanisms' becoming connected to central mechanisms is provided by several examples from the learning literature.

CLASSICAL CONDITIONING. There are now numerous examples of complex, species-typical behaviors that become released by previously neutral stimuli that develop their effectiveness by means of a classical conditioning procedure. For instance, Adler and Hogan (1963) paired the presentations of a weak electric shock with a mirror to a male Siamese fighting fish and showed that full aggressive display could be conditioned to the shock. In a similar way, Farris (1967) conditioned the courtship behavior of Japanese quail to a red light. Moore (1973) showed that a small lighted key followed consistently by food elicited a food peck in a pigeon; when followed consistently by water, it elicited a drinking peck. Blass *et al.* (1984) were able to condition the ingestive behaviors of head orientation and sucking in human infants (which are unconditioned responses to the oral delivery of a sucrose solution) to gentle forehead stroking. These and many other cases exemplify the development of connection between a perceptual mechanism and a set of behaviors as a result of a classical conditioning procedure. These examples, however, do not distinguish between a connection between a perceptual mechanism and a central mechanism or directly between a perceptual mechanism and a complex motor mechanism.

There are some cases, however, where a connection between a perceptual mechanism and a central mechanism is directly implicated. Wasserman (1973) looked at the behavior of young chicks tested in a cool environment. The chicks were trained by being exposed to a lighted key for several seconds and then to presentation of heat from a heat lamp. After several pairings of the light and the heat, the chicks began to approach the key when it lighted up and showed pecking and "snuggling" movements to it. These behaviors were never shown to the heat lamp itself (which was suspended above the chicks, out of reach). Pecking and "snuggling" movements are behaviors shown by young chicks when soliciting brooding from a mother hen (Hogan, 1974). Wasserman's results imply that the recognition mechanism for the lighted key becomes connected to a thermoregulatory system in the young chick (cf. Sherry, 1981), and that the presentation of this stimulus to a cold chick elicits brooding solicitation movements.

A second example comes from the work of Hollis (1984) on aggressive behavior in the fish blue gourami *(Tricogaster tricopterus)*. She paired the presentation of a red light with a rival behind glass during the training phase of her experiment. The fish were tested by being presented the red light and then being allowed to engage in a real fight. Fish that had been conditioned responded sooner and more frequently with the aggressive behaviors of biting and tail beating than control fish that had not been conditioned. These results support the idea that the conditioned stimulus, the red light, primed the central aggression mechanism of the fish, which allowed it to respond appropriately to the rival fish.

Another example is provided by the work of Pinel and Treit (1978, 1979). These workers showed that rats that received an electric shock from a small metal rod protruding from the wall of their cage would subsequently bury the rod with whatever materials were at hand. Control rats, which had not been shocked, did not show this behavior. Presumably, the rod recognition mechanism became connected to an escape or fear system as a result of the shock, and the rat then behaved appropriately to the appearance of the rod. Finally, it is also reasonable to infer the involvement of a central mechanism in the study of human infants by Blass *et al.* (1984): 7 of 8 experimental infants cried during extinction, but only 1 of 16 control infants cried.

These examples are not exhaustive, and a number of other cases from the learning literature have been analyzed and interpreted in a somewhat similar framework by Timberlake (1983). What all these cases show is that previously neutral stimuli can, as a result of classical conditioning procedures, develop control of entire behavior systems. It is not certain that these examples provide the best model for the development of connections between perceptual mechanisms and central mechanisms under "natural" conditions and during "normal" development, but it seems likely that similar processes apply in at least some cases. We shall return to this whole issue in the discussion.

DEVELOPMENT OF CONNECTIONS AMONG PERCEPTUAL, CENTRAL, AND MOTOR MECHANISMS

The previous sections have presented evidence about the effects of various kinds of experience on the development of connections between pairs of building blocks. The principles of development that have emerged from those results are sufficient to allow us to understand much of the development of more complex systems. As we shall see, however, some new principles seem also to be involved in these more complex cases. A review of some examples of the development of hunger, aggressive, and sexual systems will illustrate how these principles operate.

HUNGER. The hunger system of an adult chicken consists of various perceptual mechanisms that serve a food recognition function, motor mechanisms that function to locate and ingest food, and a central mechanism that integrates signals from the physiological mechanisms concerned with nutrition and modulates signals from the perceptual mechanisms and to the motor mechanisms. We have seen above how the perceptual mechanisms develop and what experience is necessary for the central mechanism to develop its modulating function. With respect to motor mechanisms, the previous discussion has focused entirely on pecking. There are, however, several other motor mechanisms that are normally associated with the hunger system, such as those controlling ground scratching and locomotion. The question to be asked here is: How do these various motor mechanisms become integrated into the system?

The hypothesis of Kruijt (1964) was that motor components originally function as independent units but become integrated into a system as a result of specific experience. The development of prey catching in cats, discussed above, provides an example that is consonant with this hypothesis. Experiments on the development of feeding in chicks, however, gave results that do not conform with this schema (Hogan, 1971). In chicks, pecking is seen immediately after hatching, whereas ground scratching does not usually occur until the bird is 3 days old. Nonetheless, as soon as it appeared, ground scratching was very highly correlated with pecking, regardless of whether either movement had ever functioned to produce food (or something peckable). Locomotion was also highly correlated with pecking and ground scratching, but it occurred independently in other contexts as well. The very high intercorrelations among these three behavior patterns were seen equally under various stimulus conditions and whether the birds were hungry or sated. Under natural conditions, the correlations among these patterns remain very high, but under the conditions of the experiments, the correlation began to decrease by the end of the 1st week. One further result of interest was that the correlation between pecking and ground scratching decreased much more quickly when the chicks were deprived of food than when they were not deprived.

These results suggest that a group of motor patterns is organized, prefunctionally, into a coordinated complex, but that appropriate functional experience is necessary to maintain this organization. In the experimental rearing conditions, food was always readily available, and ground scratching, if anything, functioned to make the food less accessible. Under these conditions, the central hunger mechanism rapidly lost control of ground scratching. Pecking remained an effective behavior for procuring food and thus continued to be controlled by the central hunger mechanism. It follows that the correlation between pecking and ground scratching would decrease. The fact that the correlation remained high (for several weeks) when the chicks were not deprived of food means that the original organization of the motor mechanisms did not disintegrate; rather, it was obscured by the influence of the central hunger mechanism.

The general picture that emerges from these considerations (and from the data previously discussed) is depicted in Figure 3. A young chick has a number of feature-recognition perceptual mechanisms, an undeveloped food-recognition

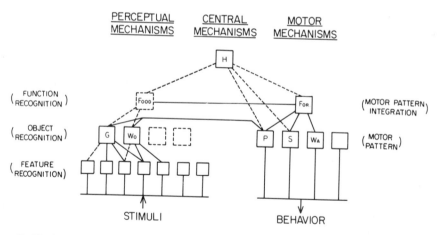

Figure 3. The hunger system of a young chick. Perceptual mechanisms include various feature-recognition mechanisms (such as of color, shape, size, and movement), object recognition mechanisms (such as of grainlike objects [G], wormlike objects [Wo], and possibly others), and a function recognition mechanism (Food). Motor mechanisms include those underlying specific behavior patterns (such as pecking [P], ground scratching [S], walking [Wᴀ], and possibly others) and an integrative motor mechanism that could be called foraging (Fᴏʀ). There is also a central hunger mechanism (H). Solid lines indicate mechanisms and connections among them that develop prefunctionally. Dashed lines indicate mechanisms and connections that develop as the result of specific functional experience.

mechanism, an independent central hunger mechanism, an integrated complex of motor mechanisms, and some connections between the perceptual and motor mechanisms; these mechanisms are available prefunctionally. The food recognition mechanism develops (perhaps simultaneously with a number of object recognition mechanisms) under the influence of experience with certain tastes or positive nutritive aftereffects of ingestion. The food recognition mechanism probably has connections to the motor mechanisms prefunctionally. A connection between the central hunger mechanism and the complex of motor mechanisms develops as a result of the experience of pecking followed by swallowing, and between the central hunger mechanism and the food recognition mechanism as a result of experience of the nutritive aftereffects of ingesting particular particles (the incentive value of food crumbs). More specific connections develop between the central hunger mechanism and particular motor mechanisms on the basis of nutritive feedback as well. These specific connections are in evidence especially when the chick is hungry, but the original prefunctional connections among perceptual mechanisms and motor mechanisms remain operative and can be seen especially when the chick is not hungry. This interpretation means that Kruijt's hypothesis is partially supported: Although the motor mechanisms are originally not independent, they can develop relatively independent connections to the central hunger mechanism.

It should be noted that the picture for the development of prey catching in kittens is not essentially different from the picture just presented for chicks. Although the individual behavior patterns used in prey catching are originally independent in the sense that the precise ordering of components is not determined, nonetheless these behavior patterns do not occur at random. A correlational analysis of the sort carried out on the chick data would undoubtedly show that the actions of pouncing, angling, and biting are highly correlated when they first appear. The specific patterns of these components that develop with respect to particular stimuli can be considered subsystems of the sort that chicks develop with respect to mealworms or to grainlike objects. These subsystems in kittens—a mouse-catching system or a fish-catching system—also have a relationship to the central hunger mechansim that is very similar to the relationship between hunger and pecking or ground scratching in chicks.

A final point is that the development of a hunger system can be greatly influenced by factors that are basically irrelevant to feeding or nutrition. The factor that has been mentioned here is fear, with respect to both the development of recognition of mealworms as food in chicks and the development of fish catching in kittens. A chick that is too afraid of a mealworm will never pick one up (Hogan, 1965), and a kitten that is too afraid of water will never learn to catch a fish. Such indirect motivational factors play an even more important role in the development of social behavior, as will be seen below.

AGGRESSION. The aggression system of an adult chicken consists of perceptual mechanisms that serve an "opponent" recognition function, various motor mechanisms that are used in fighting (including those that control threat display, leaping, wing flapping, kicking, and pecking), and a central mechanism that is sensitive to internal motivational factors (such as testosterone) and that coordinates the activation of the motor mechanisms. Kruijt (1964) showed that fighting develops from the age of about 1 week out of hopping, which is a locomotory pattern that is not initially released by or directed toward other chicks. While hopping, chicks sometimes "accidentally" bump into each other, and in the course of several days, hopping gradually becomes directed toward other chicks. Frontal threatening now occurs, and by the age of 3 weeks, pecking and kicking have been added to the interactions between chicks as well. Finally, between 2 and 3 months, normal well-coordinated adult fights are seen, which include appropriate behavior before and after the fight as well as various "irrelevant" movements that are typical of adult fights. The questions to be asked here are: First, how do the various motor mechanisms become integrated into the system, and second, what is the nature of the "opponent"?

The various behavior patterns seen in adult fighting are almost all seen to occur, independently, in the 1- to 2-week-old chick, that is, before their integration into fighting behavior. The way that normal fighting behavior develops, as just described, means that functional social experience could be a necessary factor guiding development. In fact, the results of other experiments reported by Kruijt (1964) show that this is not the case. A number of chicks were raised in social isolation for 1 week and were then confronted with each other in pairs. Many of these chicks showed aggressive behavior toward each other within minutes, or even seconds. Further, the fights that developed were characteristic of the fights of 1-month-old, socially raised chicks. Thus, social experience, rather than being a necessary factor in the development of fighting, appears to be an inhibitory factor. Such results suggest that the organization of the aggression system develops prefunctionally, and that the occurrence of aggressive behavior requires only the proper motivational state. This conclusion is also supported by the results of Evans (1968), who saw frontal threat with aggressive pecks in 2½-day-old chicks presented with an appropriate stimulus.

Whether functional social experience ever affects the organization of the motor mechanisms of the aggression system in chickens remains an open question. Males raised by Kruijt in social isolation for more than a year still showed reasonably normal aggressive patterns, and the abnormalities that were seen could be accounted for in terms of interference from other systems such as fear. Nonetheless, social experience could be necessary for fighting behavior to develop a high degree of effectiveness. One method of testing this idea is to see whether chickens can be "trained" to fight by appropriate tutors. Kuo (1967) reported that such methods are effective in training various breeds of dogs to fight.

The second question to be asked about the development of aggressive behavior in chickens is: What factors influence the development of the opponent-recognition perceptual mechanism? Here, it is clear that experience can play a role because many males raised in social isolation come to direct their aggressive behavior either to their human keepers or to their own tails. It is actually quite common to see aggressive behavior directed to humans or other species of intruders even in normally reared males, but attacking the tail seems to be peculiar to isolated males. Nonetheless, most aspects of this question remain unanswered. For example, the chicks mentioned above that were raised in social isolation for a week evidently "recognized" other chicks as "opponents" prefunctionally, because fully coordinated aggressive behavior was released by and correctly directed toward the other chick within seconds of the first encounter. But isolated chicks of the same age can also direct aggressive behavior to a light bulb hanging in the cage. Presumably, the perceptual mechanism is partially formed prefunctionally, and its further development depends on the proper experience at the proper time (just as the templates for song learning in many species), but the experiments necessary to explore this idea have not yet been done. Likewise, almost nothing is known of the relationship of the "opponent"-recognition perceptual mechanism to the "partner"-recognition perceptual mechanism, or of either of these mechanisms to the perceptual mechanism involved in "imprinting." Here, too, rather simple experiments could provide much useful information.

The results summarized above support Kruijt's hypothesis that the motor components out of which aggressive behavior develops occur independently in young chicks, but that social experience seems to be unnecessary for their integration into normal, effective aggressive behavior. The development of aggressive behavior in kittens, however, seems more nearly to conform to the hypothesis. Baerends-van Roon and Baerends (1979) described early attack behavior, which included most of the same behavior patterns previously discussed with respect to prey catching, including pouncing and biting. These patterns are apparently the same when originally directed to either a prey or another kitten, but they become modified in different ways as a result of feedback from the opponent. In particular, the force of the pounce, the extension of the claws, and the strength of the bite all become reduced after a nestmate responds in kind. The occurrence of "play" behavior, especially in the period from 4 to 8 weeks, seems to provide the kitten with essential experience for the development of normal social behavior. Two kittens that were raised in social isolation (after weaning at 7 weeks) showed either unrestrained attack or total avoidance when confronted with a normally reared cat at the age of several months. These two cats also showed abnormal maternal behavior when they later had their own litters. The Baerendses suggested that normal development requires a proper balance of attack and escape motivation.

Sex. The sex system of a normal adult rooster consists of perceptual mechanisms that serve a "partner" recognition function; motor mechanisms for locomotion, copulation (which includes mounting, sitting, treading, pecking, and tail lowering), and various displays, such as waltzing, wing flapping, tidbitting, and cornering; and a central mechanism that is sensitive to internal motivational factors such as testosterone and that coordinates the activation of the motor mechanisms. In small groups of junglefowl, Kruijt (1964) saw mounting and copulatory trampling (treading) on a model in a sitting position as early as 3–4 days, but such behavior was not common until weeks later. Full copulation with living partners did not occur before the males were 4 months old. Here, we shall ask how the motor mechanisms become integrated into the system and how partner recognition develops.

Many of the components of the copulatory sequence (mounting, sitting, pecking) are seen independently in young chicks, and there is ample opportunity for social experience to influence the occurrence and the integration of these components. Nonetheless, such experience seems irrelevant for normal development. In fact, various lines of evidence suggest that the motor mechanisms are already organized soon after hatching (if not earlier), and that their expression merely requires a sufficiently high level of motivation (internal plus external factors). For example, Andrew (1966) was able to elicit well-integrated mounting, treading, and pelvic lowering in socially isolated domestic chicks as young as 2 days old by using the stimulus of a human hand moved in a particular manner. Andrew also found that injection of testosterone greatly increased the number of chicks that responded sexually in his tests during the first 2 weeks. Further, junglefowl males that had been raised in social isolation for 6–9 months copulated successfully with females within so few encounters that it was clear that the motor mechanisms had been integrated before testing (Kruijt, 1962). The behavior of these isolated males was not completely normal, however.

The occurrence of the courtship displays presents a somewhat different picture. For example, waltzing is first seen at 2–3 months of age, when it always appears in the context of fighting. As already mentioned, the form of the display seems to develop independently of social experience. The factors controlling the occurrence of waltzing, however, seem to be largely determined by social experience. Waltzing to a female usually has the effect that the female crouches, and a crouching female is the signal for mounting and copulation. Preliminary experiments reported by Kruijt (1964) showed that the frequency of waltzing increased when mating was contingent on its occurrence and decreased when mating was not allowed. This finding suggests that, in normal development, the switch that is seen from waltzing's occurring in a fighting context to its occurring primarily in a sexual context may also require the experience of the display followed by copulation. This interpretation is also supported by the behavior of the males that were socially isolated for 6–9 months. These animals did not show waltzing (or the other displays) before mating with the female, but they did often show the displays before attacking her. Thus, copulation seems to be the reinforcer that causes the motor mechanism for waltzing to become attached to the central coordinating mechanism for sex.

Tidbitting is a display that consists of ground pecking directed to edible or inedible objects and/or ground scratching, accompanied with high, rhythmically repeated calls. It develops out of the pecking and calling that accompany "food running" (Kruijt, 1964), which can be seen in young chicks as early as 2 days. Tidbitting is especially interesting because it serves a courtship function in males but a parental function in females. In all three contexts, it serves to attract conspecifics from a distance: food running chicks attract other chicks and the mother hen, tidbitting males attract females, and food-calling (tidbitting) mother hens attract their chicks. As in waltzing, the form of the tidbitting display does not depend on social experience because it is seen in both chicks and adults that have been raised in social isolation. The causal factors controlling food running are complex and include escape, hunger, and possibly aggression (Hogan, 1966). Andrew (1966) reported that testosterone injections did *not* increase the occurrence of "juvenile tidbitting," whereas they did increase copulatory behavior. Nonetheless, in adult males, sexual factors play a primary role in the occurrence of tidbitting (Kruijt, 1964), and in adult females, parental factors play a primary role (Sherry, 1977). Here again, the switch in causal factors in the course of development implies that the motor mechanism for tidbitting develops new connections with central mechanisms. Unfortunately, there have been no experiments to determine what kind of experience is necessary for the switch in causal factors to occur.

The development of the perceptual mechanisms of the sex system seems to be much more susceptible to the effects of experience than to the development of the motor mechanisms. For example, junglefowl chicks become sexually dimorphic at about 1 month of age. By about 2 months, young males begin to show incomplete sexual behavior toward other animals, but such behavior is directed equally toward males and females. Only gradually, as a result of specifically sexual experience, does sexual behavior become directed exclusively to females (Kruijt, 1964).

It was suggested above that a preassigned perceptual mechanism exists in most species that serves a species recognition function. In chickens, such a mechanism would need to serve in at least three contexts: it should release approach and following behavior in young birds and aggressive and sexual behavior in older birds. Thus, whatever object the young chick "imprints" on, that object should be the focus of most of its subsequent social behavior.

Various studies give some support to this idea. For example, Guiton (1961) exposed male domestic chicks to either a prism-shaped or a rectangular box in the first week after hatching. He found that the chicks did preferentially follow the model to which they had been exposed, and that later they did direct various aggressive behaviors and waltzing to the model as well. In a similar study, Kruijt (1985) raised male junglefowl with a cylinder for 2 months. When the cylinder was reintroduced after sexual maturity, both aggressive and sexual behavior, including copulation attempts, were directed toward it. In both studies, however, social behavior toward the model did not continue or was directed toward other objects as well. Thus, these models did not sufficiently match whatever species-recognition mechanism had developed.

Recent results of several investigators suggest that the range of stimuli to which very strong effects of early exposure occur is more limited than was once thought. The basic finding is that young ducklings (Johnston and Gottlieb, 1981, 1985) and young chicks (Bolhuis, Johnson, and Horn, 1985; Horn, 1985; Johnson, Bolhuis, and Horn, 1985) show less permanent effects of exposure when highly artificial stimuli, such as a green ball or a red box, are used as imprinting stimuli than when more natural stimuli, such as a stuffed female mallard or a stuffed junglefowl hen, are used. Various interpretations of these results are possible, one of which is that the perceptual mechanisms for following in the young and for sexual behavior in the adult are independent. This interpretation is equivalent to saying that filial and sexual imprinting are separate processes—an idea that has been expressed before (Lorenz, 1935; Schutz, 1965).

Another possibility is that following an artificial stimulus is based on a behavior system that is different from the system responsible for following a more natural stimulus. The former may involve fear reduction by a familiar stimulus (an "exploration" system), whereas the latter may involve the whole set of responses appropriate to reacting to a mother duck or hen. The results of the Horn group show that the perceptual mechanisms for recognizing the artificial stimuli are located in a different part of the brain from the perceptual mechanisms for recognizing a junglefowl hen. Further, young chicks can recognize each other individually when only a day or 2 old (Zajonc, Wilson, and Rajecki, 1975), a finding that also means that object recognition mechanisms are independent of a partner recognition mechanism, which does not develop until much later. The fact that aggressive and sexual responses are sometimes shown to highly artificial stimuli may reflect the facts that these stimuli do have some of the characteristics of the natural stimulus and that nothing better is available. Whatever the correct explanation of these results turns out to be, it is clear that the relationship between early experience and later social behavior is more complex than was commonly thought.

It should be mentioned here that much of the work of Harlow and his students and of Hinde and his students on the development of social behavior in rhesus monkeys *(Macaca mulatta)* is also relevant to this discussion (see, for example, Harlow and Harlow, 1965; Hinde, 1974; Sackett, 1970). The parallels between the development of chicken behavior and monkey behavior are remarkable, and many of the points made in the previous discussion could have been illustrated just as easily by reference to the monkey results.

DEVELOPMENT OF INTERACTION AMONG BEHAVIOR SYSTEMS

A basic tenet of ethological theory is that various behaviors of an animal—and often the most interesting ones—are the expression of the activation of not just a single behavior system, but of the interaction of two or more behavior systems that are activated simultaneously. This is the so-called conflict hypothesis of Tinbergen (1952), which has been discussed and evaluated more recently by Baerends (1975). Although there have been many studies of how already-formed behavior systems interact, only one major study has directly addressed the development of interactions among systems—that of Kruijt (1964). His major conclusions are presented here. Baerends-van Roon and Baerends (1979) used some of Kruijt's ideas to explain aspects of their results, and these are mentioned as well.

Shortly after hatching, chicks show a surprising number of well-coordinated movements, which often occur as a response to particular stimuli. As already mentioned, these movements generally function as independent units, so that the set of factors, both external and internal, causing the occurrence of one movement is largely different from the set causing any other movement. In general, the movement with the strongest causal factors is the one that occurs, whereas movements with weaker causal factors are inhibited.

In young chicks, the interactions that occur are mostly at the level of individual motor mechanisms. In older birds, interactions are more often thought to occur between central mechanisms. At this level, the central mechanism (or the behavior system) with the strongest causal factors can also inhibit all other systems. Often, however, the causal factors for more than one behavior system are relatively strong, in which case various kinds of outcome are possible (see Hinde, 1970, for a review). The question to be asked here is whether there are any special relationships that develop among developing systems.

Kruijt's results (1964) show that the major behavior systems of escape, aggression, and sex develop in chickens in that order. Further, activation of a system already developed inhibits the expression of systems that are just beginning to develop. Thus, a young chick that shows frontal threatening and jumping to another chick may immediately stop this early aggressive behavior if it bumps into the other too hard. As the chicks grow older, and the causal factors for aggression become stronger, however, such escape stimuli no longer stop aggressive behavior. Rather, attack and escape begin to occur in rapid alternation, and various irrelevant movements start to appear during fighting. Likewise, early sexual behavior is immediately interrupted if either the attack or the escape system is activated, but later, behavior containing components of attack, escape, and sex can be seen simultaneously.

As we have seen above, there are reasons to think that the basic organization of these major systems is formed prefunctionally, and that their expression merely requires a sufficiently high level of causal factors. Insofar as this is the case, the picture described by Kruijt is the same as the picture of interacting motor mechanisms: behavior systems that are strongly activated inhibit systems that are weakly activated. The gradual appearance of more complex interactions can be interpreted as reflecting changes in the strength of causal factors (i.e., motivational changes) rather than changes in the connections among central mechanisms (i.e., developmental changes).

We can now ask whether the connections among the central mechanisms are formed prefunctionally. Here, other results of Kruijt suggest that functional experience is essential for the proper integration of behavior systems. One line of evidence comes from males raised in normal mixed sex groups. Complete male sexual behavior begins to be seen regularly in these groups at 4–5 months of age. At this stage, there are various reasons for thinking that sexual causal factors are already at "full" strength, yet sexual behavior is often mixed with overt aggression. Only gradually do overt aggressive components toward the female disappear. This change is due to specific experience with females, because males raised in male groups until 1 year of age behaved in many respects in the way that inexperienced young males do during their first encounters with females. Even in highly experienced males that show no overt aggression toward females, Kruijt's evidence suggests that agonistic tendencies (attack and/or escape) are nonetheless activated. Because these behavior systems are not expressed overtly, it follows that a particular balance between them must be struck—a balance that implies a mutual inhibition. Reaching this balance apparently requires specific experience.

This conclusion is strengthened even further by the results from experiments in which males were raised in social isolation for varying periods. Most males raised in this way for 10 months or more were never able to copulate, even after living for a year with receptive females. These males showed most of the courtship displays, but when a female crouched, they either attacked or ignored her. On the other hand, males raised in groups until they were 2½ months old and then in social isolation for 12 months copulated, when introduced to females, in the same way as inexperienced males. It is quite likely that these males never exhibited any sexual behavior during their group experience; yet when they were adults, their sexual behavior quickly became normal. Such results can be interpreted as providing evidence that this early social experience is necessary for a satisfactory integration of the aggression and escape behavior systems, and that such an integration is a prerequisite for the development of normal sexual behavior.

Results of the Baerendses, mentioned above, also support this interpretation. Their kittens that were raised in isolation from peers showed either unrestrained attack or complete avoidance when confronted with a normal kitten, and this pattern was also seen later in a sexual situation. Rhesus monkeys that were raised in isolation from peers also showed inadequate sexual behavior when adult (Harlow and Harlow, 1962). However, in both the cats and the monkeys, a particularly "good" partner was able to compensate for the behavioral deficiency in the isolation-reared animals (Harlow and Suomi, 1971; Novak and Harlow, 1975). The description of these encounters suggests that the sexual behavior system itself had not developed abnormally, but that abnormal fear or aggression interfered with the performance of sexual behavior. The conclusion that can be drawn from these studies is that well-integrated interactions among behavior systems are necessary for the normal, well-coordinated behavior we see in adult animals, and that functional experience is often necessary for such integration to occur.

DISCUSSION

SOME CAUSAL ASPECTS OF DEVELOPMENT

The process of development is extremely complex, to a large extent because so many interdependent events occur simultaneously (cf. Hogan, 1978; Kuo, 1967). Unfortunately, it is not possible to comprehend all the important variables at the same time, so that various sorts of distinctions and simplifications must be made in order to further our understanding. The basic simplification that has been made in this paper is that of describing behavior in terms of motor, central, and perceptual mechanisms and the connections among them. These mechanisms are conceived of as structural units of behavior of a particular magnitude and complexity.

Changes in behavior imply changes in the underlying behavioral mechanisms. Such changes can be of two major types: motivational and developmental. Motivational changes are viewed as being temporary and as involving the activation of particular behavioral mechanisms; developmental changes are viewed as being permanent and as involving structural changes in the mechanisms themselves or in the connections among the mechanisms. This distinction is not absolute, of course, but is useful for separating kinds of problems. It is developmental changes that have been the focus of this paper, but motivational changes often influence developmental changes.

If one accepts the thesis that the development of behavior is the result of changes in the structure of the underlying behavioral mechanisms, it is then possible to see a clear analogy between behavior development and the development of specialized cells and tissues in the embryo (e.g., Waddington, 1966). The three problems mentioned above—existence, constraints, and processes—are discussed here from this point of view, and this section concludes with a brief discussion of play.

EXISTENCE. This chapter is based on the idea that particular parts of the central nervous system subserve particular functions, and that, by the time behaviorally interesting events are occurring, these parts are preassigned. This means that, at the particular stage of development under consideration, the range of possibilities for further development of a particular behavior mechanism are so restricted that only special (i.e., already determined) kinds of experience can have a developmental effect on that mechanism. In practice, this means that, by the time of birth (or hatching), the central nervous system is already highly differentiated, with the general organization of pathways and connections already determined. By this stage of development, reversing the functions of major parts of the brain is generally impossible in the sense just discussed. Under these circumstances, it seems justified to speak of the song-recognition perceptual mechanism or the ground-scratching motor mechanism or the aggression central mechanism as prefunctionally developed units of behavioral structure subject to further (but quite restricted) differentiation on the basis of subsequent experience.

It should be realized, however, that, if we follow the development of any behavior mechanism backward in time, we can always find a stage in which the nerve cells making up the behavior mechanism could have subserved a different behavior mechanism under somewhat different conditions. If we go back still further, we will find a stage when the cells could have become something other than nerve cells, and so on. At the time of birth—an arbitrary time I have chosen for convenience—a particular set of nerve cells may have differentiated to the point where they, if they survive, will be the cells that mediate mate recognition, and in this sense, they are preassigned that function. But they are preassigned only from the point of view of future development.

CONSTRAINTS: IRREVERSIBILITY AND CRITICAL PERIODS. Insofar as behavior mechanisms can be regarded as preassigned, they illustrate the problem of the irreversibility of development. When Waddington (1966) discussed the question of whether the differentiation of cells is reversible, his answer was that "it depends." It depends on what cell, in what animal, at what stage of development, and so on. This is already an important point because similar reasoning shows that it is nonsense to ask a question such as: Is imprinting irreversible? One can only begin to answer such a question after specifying the species, the particular imprinting procedures, the stage of development, and so on.

More important, Waddington specified some of the processes that are responsible for the irreversibility of cell differentiation. For example, some or all of the genetic material may have been "used up" or may have otherwise disappeared in the course of the development of the cell; or the genetic material may still be present, but for various reasons, it cannot be accessed. The most frequent reason for irreversibility, however, seems to be that

> development involves such a complicated network of processes that it would be an extremely long and tricky process to unravel them. One could, in theory, take an automobile, dismantle it, and build the pieces up again with a little modification into two motorcycles, but it wouldn't be easy; and it is something like this that we are asking a differentiated cell to do when we try to persuade it to lose its present differentiation and develop into something else. (Waddington, 1966, pp. 54–55)

Processes with similar characteristics seem certain to underlie cases of behavioral irreversibility.

The best documented cases of total irreversibility involve motor mechanisms for bird song—as exemplified by the "crystallization" of song in the chaffinch (Thorpe, 1961) and the white-crowned sparrow (Marler, 1970). The perceptual mechanisms, or "templates," on which these songs are based are probably also fixed irreversibly once they have developed, although here the evidence is somewhat controversial (e.g., Petrinovich, 1985). It should be emphasized that not all bird songs crystallize, nor are all perceptual mechanisms underlying song recognition fixed (e.g., Baylis, 1982; Nottebohm, 1981). Many of the courtship and agonistic displays seen especially in birds, such as waltzing in chickens (Kruijt, 1964) or the oblique posture in the black-headed gull (Groothuis, 1985), are probably also fixed irreversibly once they have developed. These cases are probably all analogous to the case of cell differentiation, in which the genetic material disappears in the course of development: once these motor and perceptual mechanisms have developed, the possibility of further change no longer exists (except by formation of new nerve cells; cf. Paton and Nottebohm, 1984).

Here it is useful to emphasize the distinction between the perceptual and motor mechanisms themselves, as well as the various connections that may exist between them: even though a perceptual or motor mechanism has crystallized, there are still possibilities for alternative pathways among them. The concept of imprinting, for example, implies a change in a perceptual mechanism as a result of experience. In some species, such a change may itself be irreversible, but subsequent experience may lead to additional pathways being formed between other perceptual mechanisms and the sexual behavior system, and these new connections may mask the original imprinting. A rather difficult experimental analysis would be necessary to investigate this possibility. We have seen, however, a case such as this on the motor side in the hunger system of chickens: an original connection between pecking and ground scratching was masked, but not destroyed, by later experience.

The most common reason that behavior changes are apparently irreversible is probably the same reason that cell differentiation is irreversible: so many events would have to be undone (or compensated for) that change becomes almost impossible. A very simple case, where changes could still be made, was training a kitten to catch fish after it had already learned to catch mice (Baerends-van Roon and Baerends, 1979). Here, there were two problems. One was an indirect, motivational problem: a fear of water inhibited any attempt to catch the fish. Once the fear of water could be overcome, the kitten faced a direct, developmental problem: rearranging motor mechanisms in a different sequence. In this case, rearrangement was possible, although with some interference from the original learning.

A more complex case is the sexual behavior of male junglefowl raised in social isolation. Here, subtle aspects of the integration of the aggression and escape systems seem to be permanently missing. Because this integration plays a determining role in permitting sexual behavior to occur, these effects of social isolation are effectively irreversible, even though the copulatory motor patterns are intact. It is possible that some sort of "therapy" could be devised to cope with this problem— as was possible in the cats and monkeys raised in social isolation—but that is an empirical matter.

The fact that development is not reversible (except as discussed above) means that constraints of various sorts are inherent in developing systems. The most commonly discussed constraint is a "critical" or "sensitive" period that corresponds to the embryological concept of competence (Waddington, 1966). In essence, these concepts refer to the fact that the developing system is especially susceptible to particular external influences at particular stages of development. This topic has often been a matter of controversy, especially with respect to the factors responsible for the beginning and the end of a critical period (see Hinde, 1970). Nonetheless, the previous discussion should make clear that probably all aspects of development are associated with critical periods. At each stage of development, the animal is different from what it was; it is only to be expected that the effects of the "same" experience will be different in the different stages (cf. Schneirla, 1956; Schneirla, Rosenblatt, and Tobach, 1963). The factors that are responsible for the beginning and ending of these periods are probably different in every case.

DEVELOPMENTAL PROCESSES. A major issue that has only been hinted at in this chapter is the question: What is (are) the process(es) of behavior development? There is not yet any answer to this question, but I think several points are worth making.

First, it seems very unlikely to me that the biochemical processes responsible for altering the structure of behavioral mechanisms and their connections are different before and after a particular behavior begins to function. This line of reasoning implies that the processes responsible for learning are no different from the processes responsible for development in general. The essence of this idea is that the same structural change can be triggered by different events, for example, by genes or by the experience of "reinforcement." The important point is that the change itself cannot be classified as genetic or learned because it could have been triggered either way and it does not matter which way.

This reasoning helps us to understand more easily the various results we have discussed. For example, Groothuis (1985) found that the oblique posture in the black-headed gull developed normally when a gull was reared either in social isolation or in large social groups, but that it sometimes developed abnormally when a gull was raised with only two or three peers. This result could be interpreted as being due to a motor mechanism that, at a certain stage of its development, is competent to form particular connections. Under circumstances of social isolation, genetic information provides the trigger for the connection to form. When peers are present, certain social experience provides the trigger. If the connection requires repeated experience for completion, the probability that the average experience will be "correct" is greater in a large group than in a small group, where the effects of the behavior of one abnormal individual companion would be relatively greater. This line of reasoning suggests that social experience and genes provide alternative routes for the control of behavior system development, a suggestion that is consonant with the results for the development of the aggression system in chickens, and for the results of studies of play in several species (cf. Martin and Caro, 1985).

We can go one step further if we make another assumption. Suppose that crystallization represents the fact that structural change is no longer possible in a particular cell. It then follows that the timing of triggering events becomes crucial in determining which events will affect development. In a particular species of songbird, for example, one can imagine that, if genetically triggered events occur in the perceptual mechanism for song recognition before the young bird can hear, then the perceptual mechanism is fixed, prefunctionally, in that species, and posthatching experience can no longer have an effect. If the triggering events are delayed, however, the posthatching experience of the bird can provide the trigger. In this way, the same basic perceptual mechanism can be used for either "innate" or "learned" song recognition.

PLAY. The topic of play has been discussed extensively in the context of development. Here, I briefly present some ethological ideas about the causation of play, and I show how they complement the behavior system framework developed here. A more general treatment of play that includes a discussion of problems caused by the confusion of cause and function is given by Martin and Caro (1985) and by Burghardt (Chapter 4).

The first important idea was expressed by Lorenz (1956): "It seems to be characteristic of 'play' that instinctive movements are thus performed independently of the higher patterns into which they are integrated when functioning 'in serious'" (p. 635). In other words, the motor mechanisms are activated independently of an activation of the central mechanisms. As we have seen, insofar as Kruijt's hypothesis is correct, this is the state into which most animals are born, and of course, play is most characteristic of young animals.

As an animal grows older, the independence of motor and central mechanisms decreases, and one might expect the frequency of play to decline. That this need not be so follows from Kruijt's analysis (1964) of junglefowl ontogeny. He showed that the central mechanisms for aggression and sex only gradually develop control over the relevant motor mechanisms. Connections between the central mechanisms and the motor mechanisms may well exist at hatching or even earlier, but the causal factors activating the central mechanisms appear only gradually. Thus, "playful" motor patterns can continue to occur for some time. The analysis of the hunger system suggests that, even when particular motor patterns such as pecking and/or ground scratching become integrated into the system, these same movements can occur independently, especially when the causal factors that activate the central mechanism (i.e., the level of hunger) are weak.

Similar results are also seen in other species. Lorenz (1956) described the behavior of a young raven that showed a wide array of "playful" movements toward a strange object when not hungry, but that immediately tried to eat such an object if it was hungry. Likewise, Schiller's chimpanzees (1949) showed a playful manipulation of objects, especially when not hungry. The motor patterns of the raven and the chimps under these circumstances could be recognized as being similar to motor patterns belonging to various adult behavior systems.

Once various behavior systems have developed, it may be that play ceases. This, of course, is not true in many species. Morris (1956) suggested that play occurs when central mechanisms are switched off: "The mechanisms of mutual inhibition and sequential ordering mechanisms are not switched on and as a result there is no control over the types and sequences of motor patterns in the usual sense" (p. 643). Switching off central mechanisms would effectively return the animal to a very early stage of development, in which the appearance of play would again be expected. A more elaborate version of this idea was suggested much more recently by Baerends-van Roon and Baerends (1979) and was based on their observations of kittens. They proposed that, in cats at least, a central play mechanism exists that, when activated, actively inhibits other central mechanisms. This inhibition would have the effect of releasing the central control on motor mechanisms, and "play" could thus appear. This idea seems very attractive to me because it can explain why play seems so organized in some species: "species-typical" patterns of play can be understood as being due to a differential inhibition of central mechanisms. Further, when play occurs, its causation remains the same as Lorenz originally suggested: the independent activation of motor mechanisms. Even in species such as chickens, in which an independent central play mechanism has probably not evolved, newly hatched chicks can "play" because their motor mechanisms are relatively independent of central control, but older chickens do not play because central control cannot be inhibited.

SOME FUNCTIONAL ASPECTS OF DEVELOPMENT

An important issue, with which all the chapters in this book are concerned, is the relation of the functions of behavior to its causes. What problems must the animal solve in the particular environment it inhabits, and how can consideration of these "ecological" requirements help us to understand the development of its feeding, aggressive, sexual, and other behavior? To this point, this chapter has been concerned exclusively with a causal analysis of development, but some functional aspects are considered now.

First, however, it is necessary to make an important proviso. It is my opinion that the cause of a particular behavior and the function of that behavior are logically independent; that is, there is no necessary relation whatsoever between cause and function (Hogan, 1984a). An analogy should make this clear. The cause of a chair is the way that it is manufactured; the function of a chair is to provide a place in which to sit in comfort. Many people have studied methods of chair manufacture, and many people have studied what makes chairs comfortable. The question now becomes: Does the specification of a level of comfort tell chair manufacturers whether they should attach the arms to the frame before they attach the legs? Or if chair manufacturers use a dovetail joint rather than a butt joint, can we predict whether the chair will be more comfortable to sit in? Clearly, these are independent aspects of chair manufacture, and knowledge of one aspect does not tell us anything much about the other aspect.

Causal and functional questions are equally valid to ask, but the proviso mentioned above may make it seem that there is nothing to be gained toward understanding causal mechanisms by asking functional questions. In theory, this should be true. In practice, however, the problems that an animal must solve in order to survive provide the selection pressures that are responsible for evolution by natural selection. And it turns out that the evolutionary solutions to these problems sometimes use causal mechanisms that are related to functions that the behavior serves. We shall consider here first some examples of functional questions that do not increase our understanding of development, and then some examples that do.

IS DEVELOPMENT SELECTED? It is almost a truism that natural selection should operate at all stages of development, and not only on the adult outcome, because any developmental process that reduces the probability of reaching adulthood will be very strongly selected against—all other things being equal. Nonetheless, a genotype with advantageous consequences at a particular stage of development can be selected for only if its consequences in the adult do not reduce the fitness of the individual possessing it. What this means is that, at any particular stage of development, behavior may be far from optimal: it need only be good enough to bring the animal to adulthood.

This line of reasoning also leads to other conclusions. For example, it seems intuitively obvious that the best mechanism for regulating a particular outcome would be one that is directly sensitive to the outcome. Thus, the best mechanism for regulating nutrition, say, would be one that could directly sense the state of nutrition. This is another way of saying that an optimal mechanism should be based on a simple, direct relationship between cause and function. But as we have seen, development is an extremely complex process and one in which optimal solutions may be the exception rather than the rule. It follows that development is opportunistic in the sense that any available means will be used to produce an acceptable end. A few examples should make this point clearer.

We have seen above that pecking in newly hatched chicks is not controlled by factors related to nutrition. When it became clear that experience was necessary for nutritional control to develop, it seemed reasonable to look at the effects of various kinds of nutritional experience on the occurrence of pecking. That approach turned out not to be the key to solving the puzzle because the necessary experience was not nutritional, but an association between the act of pecking and the effects of swallowing any solid object. These results were surprising (and took a long time to discover) because of our preconceptions about the relationships between the causes and the functions of behavior. We intuitively feel that, when behavior changes in an adaptive direction, the cause of the change should be related to factors associated with the adaptation. Thus, when pecking changes in such a way that relatively more nutritive items are ingested, we infer that something about nutrition was responsible for the change. But in this case, our inference was wrong. Pecking behavior to food and sand during the test changes for reasons that are completely unrelated to nutrition.

A second example is provided by the analysis of Hall and Williams (1983) of the relationship between suckling and other ingestive behavior in rats. Suckling and eating are both behaviors that function to provide nutritive substances to rats—suckling normally for the first 3 weeks after birth and eating thereafter. In their search for the causal mechanisms underlying ingestion, Hall and his colleagues originally assumed that these mechanisms would be similar in both newborn and older animals. In fact, after many years of work, their results showed that the causal mechanisms controlling suckling are largely independent of the mechanisms controlling eating. Their analysis suggests that both systems coexist simultaneously, and that only one system is expressed at a time. Hall and Williams (1983) concluded: "Such findings for suckling illustrate the general difficulty in determining the relationship between adaptive behavior of infancy and functionally similar representations in adulthood (p. 250). More recently, Hall and Browde (1986) made similar studies of infant mice and discovered that the causal factors underlying eating are considerably different from those in rats. Thus, the study of the development of feeding behavior in chicks, rats, and mice shows that mechanisms for change have evolved that lead to an adaptive result, but that these mechanisms often bear little resemblance to our prior ideas of what they should be.

The final example makes the point of the independence of cause and function in a different way. Maynard Smith (1977) posed the question of why male mammals do not lactate—not in general, but specifically with respect to monogamous species with stable pair bonding and resulting high confidence of paternity. This question was explored by Daly (1979) from both a physiological (causal) and a fitness (functional) point of view. The complete answer to the question is complicated, but part of it relates to development:

> Functional male lactation would require changes in sexually differentiated ontogenetic processes at both prepubertal and circumpubertal stages, as well as some male analogue of lactogenic events late in pregnancy. None of these modifications seems impossible, but together they constitute a formidable barrier to the evolution of male lactation. (Daly, 1979, p. 325)

In other words, no matter how desirable a particular function might be, it cannot evolve unless the ontogenetic machinery is capable of being changed appropriately.

This is actually an example of what Waddington meant when he talked about the "complicated network of processes" in development.

ADAPTATIONS FOR DEVELOPMENT. The problems that an animal has to solve for survival put selection pressures on the causal mechanisms for the behavior that can evolve. It is for this reason that functional thinking can help us to understand causal mechanisms that we have discovered, and in some cases, it may direct our attention to seeking causal mechanisms that we would not otherwise have thought of. Here, I shall make a few functional comments about some cases we have already considered from a causal perspective.

We can first consider some aspects of nutrition acquisition. In almost all species of animal, the method of acquiring nutrition changes—willy-nilly, at least once, and often two or more times—in the course of the animal's lifetime. In mammals, for example, nutrition is provided to the embryo via the placenta and, after birth, first by suckling and later by eating. Suckling, as a motor mechanism, exists before birth and after weaning, but it is not expressed then. Thus, at some stage in development, suckling must be "switched in" to provide nutrition, and later, it must be "switched out." Similarly, in birds, the yolk sac provides nutrition in the egg and for some time after hatching; then, the young bird may receive food from its parents by gaping, and finally, it feeds itself using some sort of pecking movement. Here, too, something must regulate when gaping is used, and when pecking is used. This, then, is the problem the animal must solve. How does it do it?

The causal answer to this question is probably different for every species. We have seen at least a partial causal answer for chicks in the results we have obtained from pecking. But these results raise several obvious functional questions, two of which can be considered here. First, why should pecking not be controlled by nutritional factors at hatching? Second, why should experience be necessary for pecking to become integrated into the hunger system? One can imagine that, if pecking were originally controlled primarily by the chick's nutritional state, pecking might not occur at all until the yolk reserves were exhausted. Such a chick would not have as much experience with its world as a chick that had engaged in exploratory pecking during the first few days. Given that the control of pecking must shift sometime between hatching and the time when pecking is necessary for providing nutrients, there is no particular reason that experience should not provide the timing of the shift. On the other hand, there is one important reason that experience should provide the timing: Birds can hatch early or late with respect to their overall stage of development (and mammals can be born prematurely or past term). Endogenous timing of the switch in causal factors to or from pecking or suckling would be disastrous if, for example, a 1-week premature baby could not suckle in its first week, or if a baby could not be weaned early if its mother's milk supply were interrupted. In general, it seems certain that experiential factors provide a more reliable timing cue than endogenous factors could provide in most cases where a switch between methods of acquiring nutrition occurs.

There is at least one other set of studies that gives information about motor mechanisms being switched in or out as a result of experience: studies on the development and control of leg movements in hatching chicks. Bekoff and Kauer (1982) observed that the pattern of leg movements during hatching involved a simultaneous contraction and extension of both legs, whereas, immediately after hatching, the pattern involves the alternation pattern characteristic of walking. They then showed that it is possible to bring back the simultaneous pattern by folding the chick up in an egg-shaped container. Thus, both motor mechanisms must be present simultaneously, but particular feedback from the posture of the chick provides the information necessary for the activation of one or the other.

In this context, it is useful to return to the concept of play and to consider what function it may serve. We have seen that the essence of the concept is that motor mechanisms have a chance to be "free" of influence from central mechanisms. Such freedom may give the motor mechanisms an opportunity to become incorporated into other central mechanisms. One can imagine that such a flexible system would be useful during development, especially in cases where something may have gone wrong, and in which the so-called normal connections would not function optimally. Similar functions for play have been suggested before, but one problem with such explanations is that adult behavior develops equally well in individuals that vary greatly in the amount of play they exhibit (cf. Martin and Caro, 1985). Here, we can see a function for the developmental situation described by Groothuis (1985): Endogenous factors are sufficient to determine the development of particular behavior systems (or particular motor mechanisms), but during development, the possibility exists for experience to bring about a somewhat different outcome. Under normal conditions of development, either endogenous factors or play could provide alternative pathways to reach the same result. Only under special conditions (such as those provided the gulls by Groothuis) would the different pathways lead to different results.

THE CONCEPT OF PREFUNCTIONAL. It should be clear by now that it is quite possible to discuss the causal development of behavior without using the word *innate*. Nonetheless, it must also be clear that I have used the word *prefunctional*, defined as developing without the influence of functional experience, in many places where others would have said *innate*. In some ways, this is how Lorenz (1961, 1965) suggested the term *innate* be used, though he was not always consistent in his use (cf. Lehrman, 1970). Nonetheless, there are still some problems in a functional definition, and I shall briefly mention two of them here. But first, it may be useful to indicate why I think the concept *prefunctional* is necessary at all.

Lehrman (1970) pointed out that one important reason for the controversy between him and Lorenz was that the two were interested in different problems: Lehrman was interested in studying the effects of all types of experience on all types of behavior at all stages of development, whereas Lorenz was interested only in studying the effects of functional experience on behavior mechanisms at the stage of development at which they begin to function as modes of adaptation to the environment. In other words, Lehrman used a causal criterion to determine what was interesting to study, whereas Lorenz used a functional criterion. These two criteria are equally legitimate (cf. Hogan, 1984a), but the functional criterion used by Lorenz corresponds to the way most people think about development. In fact, it is logically consistent to talk about behavior development that is prefunctional (or innate) versus behavior development that is learned when the criterion is the absence or presence of functional experience (cf. p. 67, footnote 2). (I prefer the word *prefunctional* to the word *innate* because innate has too many additional meanings.) I think it is important to show how behavior that can be classified as prefunctional still presents interesting developmental problems that can be investigated in a causal framework. That is one of the things I have tried to do in this chapter.

It is also important to see some of the difficulties inherent in using a functional definition. Perhaps the most important of these is that the function of a behavior is not always obvious. For example, if the function of pecking is viewed as being providing nutrition, pecking becomes integrated into the hunger system prefunctionally; if the function of pecking is viewed as bringing about ingestion, then pecking becomes integrated into the hunger system through functional experience. In either case, the causal process is the same. Similar problems arise when there are alternative routes to reaching the same end, as in the development of the oblique posture in the black-headed gull.

A related problem is that the function of behavior can change over the course of time. Sometimes, this change is due to changes in the environment and sometimes to changes in the behavior mechanisms themselves. This means that, at best, the concept *prefunctional* is only relative: it can usefully be used to describe situations with respect only to the particular function that the investigator has in mind.

CONCLUSIONS

One of the remarkable things about development is how normal most individuals become in spite of large variations in the experiences to which they are exposed. Waddington (e.g., 1966) coined the term *canalization* to express this fact with respect to the morphology of the animal, and we have seen a similar picture with respect to behavior. The basic structure of the perceptual, central, and motor mechanisms, as well as the basic interconnections among these units, develops, by and large, prefunctionally. The experience of the individual is, of course, important, often in very unexpected ways, but typically, the basic structure of behavior is extraordinarily stable.

Nonetheless, development, especially of social behavior, sometimes goes seriously wrong. Such disturbed development can often be traced to peculiarities in the social experience of the young animal, especially to periods of social deprivation. In some ways, this conclusion seems to contradict earlier statements that social experience has little effect on the development of the basic structure of behavior. It is possible to reconcile this apparent contradiction by analyzing how development can produce nonfunctional results. Broadly speaking, nonfunctional outcomes of the developmental process can be due to either structural or motivational causes (or to some combination of the two).

The structural causes for abnormal behavior include the development of aberrant behavior mechanisms and the development of anomalous connections among behavior mechanisms. For example, a chick that is force-fed and is not allowed to peck in its first 2 weeks after hatching is later unable to peck at food when hungry, presumably because the motor mechanism for pecking remains independent of the central mechanism for hunger (see discussion in Hogan, 1977). Other examples include motor mechanisms, such as copulation, that get hooked up to the wrong central mechanism, such as aggression, which may then be expressed as rape. Or the partner recognition mechanism may develop with the image of the wrong species or of a member of the same sex, and interspecific courtship or homosexual behavior would be seen. Such misdevelopment (from a functional point of view) does happen, and causes for it can be studied. But in fact, structural aberrations probably account for only a small proportion of developmental problems.

Most disturbed development probably results from motivational causes such as an abnormally high activation of particular behavior systems or atypical interactions among behavior systems. For example, excessively fearful animals have general difficulties in learning new tasks (such as the older kittens learning to catch fish) and in expressing normal social behavior. And the inadequate integration of fear and aggression is probably the main reason for problems in the expression of sexual behavior, as seen in isolated roosters, cats, and monkeys. In these cases, the basic behavioral structure is present, but the more subtle interactions among behavior systems are missing. It is, of course, sometimes difficult to distinguish structural aberrations from problems of behavior system interaction. Nonetheless, the causal analysis of the development of behavior systems, as discussed in this chapter, provides a framework within which to attack these problems.

Acknowledgments

This chapter was written while I was on sabbatical leave at the Zoology Laboratory, University of Groningen, Netherlands. I thank J. P. Kruijt for providing me with facilities and a supportive environment in which to work. He and the other members of the Ethology Discussion Group—J. J. Bolhuis, I. Bossema, C. ten Cate, A. G. G. Groothuis, A. J. Hogan-Warburg, M. Hulscher-Emeis, and G. de Vos—as well as T. Piersma discussed the manuscript in detail and made many useful suggestions for improvement. Support for my travel to the Netherlands was given by the Natural Sciences and Engineering Research Council of Canada, which has also supported the research of mine reported in this chapter.

References

Adler, N. T., and Hogan, J. A. Classical conditioning and punishment of an instinctive response in *Betta splendens. Animal Behaviour*, 1963, *11*, 351–354.

Andrew, R. J. Precocious adult behaviour in the young chick. *Animal Behaviour*, 1966, *14*, 485–500.

Baerends, G. P. An evaluation of the conflict hypothesis as an explanatory principle for the evolution of displays. In G. P. Baerends, C. Beer, and A. Manning (Eds.), *Function and evolution in behaviour*. London: Oxford University Press, 1975.

Baerends, G. P. The functional organization of behaviour. *Animal Behaviour*, 1976, *24*, 726–738.

Baerends, G. P., and Kruijt, J. P. Stimulus selection. In R. A. Hinde and J. G. Stevenson-Hinde (Eds.), *Constraints on learning*. London: Academic Press, 1973.

Baerends-van Roon, J. M., and Baerends, G. P. The morphogenesis of the behaviour of the domestic cat, with a special emphasis on the development of prey-catching. *Verhandelingen der Koninklijke Nederlandse Akademie van Wetenschappen, Afd. Natuurkunde, Tweede Reeks* (Proceedings of the Royal Netherlands Academy of Sciences, Section Physics, Second Series), Part 72, 1979.

Baptista, L. F., and Petrinovich, L. Social interaction, sensitive phases and the song template hypothesis in the white-crowned sparrow. *Animal Behaviour*, 1984, *32*, 172–181.

Baylis, J. R. Avian vocal mimicry: Its function and evolution. In D. E. Kroodsma, E. H. Miller, and H. Ouellet (Eds.), *Acoustic communication in birds*, Vol. 2. New York: Academic Press, 1982.

Beach, F. A. Analysis of factors involved in the arousal, maintenance, and manifestation of sexual excitement in male animals. *Psychosomatic Medicine*, 1942, *4*, 173–198.

Bekoff, A., and Kauer, J. A. Neural control of hatching: Role of neck position in turning on hatching leg movements in post-hatching chicks. *Journal of Comparative Physiology A*, 1982, *145*, 497–504.

Blass, E. M., Hall, W. G., and Teicher, M. H. The ontogeny of suckling and ingestive behaviors. *Progress in Psychobiology and Physiological Psychology*, 1979, *8*, 243–299.

Blass, E. M., Ganchrow, J. R., and Steiner, J. E. Classical conditioning in newborn humans 2–48 hours of age. *Infant Behavior and Development*, 1984, *7*, 125–134.

Boakes, R., and Panter, D. Secondary imprinting in the domestic chick blocked by previous exposure to a live hen. *Animal Behaviour*, 1985, *33*, 353–365.

Bolhuis, J. J., and Trooster, W. J. Reversibility revisited: Stimulus-dependent stability of filial preference in the chick. *Animal Behaviour*, 1988, *36*.

Bolhuis, J. J., Johnson, M., and Horn, G. Effects of early experience on the development of filial preferences in the domestic chick. *Developmental Psychobiology*, 1985, *18*, 299–308.

Bottjer, S. W., and Arnold, A. P. The ontogeny of vocal learning in songbirds. In E. M. Blass (Ed.), *Handbook of behavioral neurobiology*, Vol. 8. New York: Plenum Press, 1986.

Daly, M. Why don't male mammals lactate? *Journal of Theoretical Biology*, 1979, *78*, 325–345.

Doty, R. W. The concept of neural centers. In J. C. Fentress (Ed.), *Simpler networks and behavior*. Sunderland, MA: Sinauer, 1976.

Drachman, D. B., and Sokoloff, L. The role of movement in embryonic joint development. *Developmental Biology*, 1966, *14*, 401–420.

Evans, R. M. Early aggressive responses in domestic chicks. *Animal Behaviour*, 1968, *16*, 24–28.

Fantz, R. L. Form preferences in newly hatched chicks. *Journal of Comparative and Physiological Psychology*, 1957, *50*, 422–430.

Farris, H. E. Classical conditioning of courting behavior in the Japanese quail *(Coturnix c. japonica)*. *Journal of the Experimental Analysis of Behavior*, 1967, *10*, 213–217.

Field, T. M., Woodson, R., Greenberg, R., and Cohen, D. Discrimination and imitation of facial expressions by neonates. *Science*, 1982, *218*, 179–181.

Gallistel, C. R. *The organization of action*. Hillsdale, NJ: Erlbaum, 1980.

Graf, J. S., Balsam, P. D., and Silver, R. Associative factors and the development of pecking in the ring dove. *Developmental Psychobiology*, 1985, *18*, 447–460.

Groothuis, A. G. G. The ontogeny of complex species-specific motor patterns, studied in gull displays. *Abstracts of the 19th International Ethological Conference*, Toulouse, 1985.

Guiton, P. The influence of imprinting on the agonistic and courtship responses of the brown leghorn cock. *Animal Behaviour*, 1961, *9*, 167–177.

Hale, C., and Green, L. Effect of initial pecking consequences on subsequent pecking in young chicks. *Journal of Comparative and Physiological Psychology*, 1979, *93*, 730–735.

Hall, W. G., and Browde, J. A. The ontogeny of independent ingestion in mice: Or, why won't infant mice feed? *Developmental Psychobiology*, 1986, *19*, 211–222.

Hall, W. G., and Williams, C. L. Suckling isn't feeding, or is it? A search for developmental continuities. *Advances in the Study of Behavior*, 1983, *13*, 219–254.

Hamburger, V. Anatomical and physiological basis of embryonic motility in birds and mammals. In G. Gottlieb (Ed.), *Behavioral embryology*, New York: Academic Press, 1973.

Harlow, H. F., and Harlow, M. K. Social deprivation in monkeys. *Scientific American*, Nov. 1962.

Harlow, H. F., and Harlow, M. K. The affectional systems. In A. M. Schrier, H. F. Harlow, and F. Stollnitz (Eds.), *Behavior of nonhuman primates*, Vol. 2. New York: Academic Press, 1965.

Harlow, H. F., and Suomi, S. J. Social recovery by isolation-reared monkeys. *Proceedings of the National Academy of Sciences*, 1971, *68*, 1534–1538.

Hebb, D. O. *The organization of behavior.* New York: Wiley, 1949.

Hess, E. H. Natural preferences of chicks and ducklings for objects of different colors. *Psychological Reports,* 1956, *2,* 477–483.

Hinde, R. A. *Animal behaviour.* New York: McGraw-Hill, 1970.

Hinde, R. A. *Biological bases of human social behaviour.* New York: McGraw-Hill, 1974.

Hogan, J. A. An experimental study of conflict and fear: An analysis of behavior of young chicks to a mealworm. Part I. The behavior of chicks which do not eat the mealworm. *Behaviour,* 1965, *25,* 45–97.

Hogan, J. A. An experimental study of conflict and fear: An analysis of behavior of young chicks to a mealworm. Part II. The behavior of chicks which eat the mealworm. *Behavior,* 1966, *27,* 273–289.

Hogan, J. A. The development of a hunger system in young chicks. *Behaviour,* 1971, *39,* 128–201.

Hogan, J. A. Development of food recognition in young chicks. I. Maturation and nutrition. *Journal of Comparative and Physiological Psychology,* 1973a, *83,* 355–366.

Hogan, J. A. How young chicks learn to recognize food. In R. A. Hinde and J. G. Stevenson-Hinde (Eds.), *Constraints on learning.* London: Academic Press, 1973b.

Hogan, J. A. Responses in Pavlovian conditioning studies. *Science,* 1974, *186,* 156–157.

Hogan, J. A. The ontogeny of food preferences in chicks and other animals. In L. M. Barker, M. Best, and M. Domjan (Eds.), *Learning mechanisms in food selection.* Waco, TX: Baylor University Press, 1977.

Hogan, J. A. An eccentric view of development: A review of *The Dynamics of Behavior Development* by Zing-Yang Kuo. *Contemporary Psychology,* 1978, *23,* 690–691.

Hogan, J. A. Hierarchy and behavior: A review of *The Organization of Action* by C. R. Gallistel. *Behavioral and Brain Sciences,* 1981, *4,* 625.

Hogan, J. A. Cause, function, and the analysis of behavior. *Mexican Journal of Behavior Analysis,* 1984a, *10,* 65–71.

Hogan, J. A. Pecking and feeding in chicks. *Learning and Motivation,* 1984b, *15,* 360–376.

Hogan, J. A. The structure versus the provenance of behavior: A comment on B. F. Skinner's "Ontogeny and phylogeny of behavior." *Behavioral and Brain Sciences,* 1984c, *7,* 690.

Hogan, J. A., and Roper, T. J. A comparison of the properties of different reinforcers. *Advances in the Study of Behavior,* 1978, *8,* 155–255.

Hogan-Warburg, A. J., and Hogan, J. A. Feeding strategies in the development of food recognition in young chicks. *Animal Behaviour,* 1981, *29,* 143–154.

Hollis, K. The biological function of Pavlovian conditioning: The best defense is a good offense. *Journal of Experimental Psychology: Animal Behavior Processes,* 1984, *10,* 413–425.

Horn, G. *Memory, imprinting, and the brain.* Oxford: Oxford University Press, 1985.

Johnson, M. H., Bolhuis, J. J., and Horn, G. Interaction between acquired preferences and developing predispositions during imprinting. *Animal Behaviour,* 1985, *33,* 1000–1006.

Johnston, T. D., and Gottlieb, G. Development of visual species identification in ducklings: What is the role of imprinting? *Animal Behaviour,* 1981, *29,* 1082–1099.

Johnston, T. D., and Gottlieb, G. Effects of social experience on visually imprinted maternal preferences in Peking ducklings. *Developmental Psychobiology,* 1985, *18,* 261–271.

Kenny, J. T., Stoloff, M. L., Bruno, J. P., and Blass, E. M. The ontogeny of preferences for nutritive over nonnutritive suckling in the albino rat. *Journal of Comparative and Physiological Psychology,* 1979, *93,* 752–759.

Konishi, M. The role of auditory feedback in the control of vocalizations in the white-crowned sparrow. *Zeitschrift für Tierpsychologie,* 1965, *22,* 770–783.

Kruijt, J. P. Imprinting in relation to drive interactions in Burmese red junglefowl. *Symposia of the Zoological Society, London,* 1962, *8,* 219–226.

Kruijt, J. P. Ontogeny of social behaviour in Burmese red junglefowl *(Gallus gallus spadiceus). Behaviour,* 1964, *Supplement 9.*

Kruijt, J. P. On the development of social attachments in birds. *Netherlands Journal of Zoology,* 1985, *35,* 45–62.

Kuo, Z. Y. *The dynamics of behavioral development.* New York: Random House, 1967.

Lehrman, D. S. Semantic and conceptual issues in the nature-nurture problem. In L. R. Aronson, E. Tobach, D. S. Lehrman, and J. S. Rosenblatt (Eds.), *Development and evolution of behavior.* San Francisco: Freeman, 1970.

Logan, C. A. Biological diversity in avian vocal learning. In M. D. Zeiler and P. Harzem (Eds.), *Advances in analysis of behavior, Vol. 3: Biological factors in learning.* Chichester, England: Wiley, 1983.

Lorenz, K. Der Kumpan in der Umwelt des Vogels. *Journal für Ornithologie*, 1935, *83*, 137–213, 289–413.

Lorenz, K. Über die Bildung des Instinktbegriffes. *Naturwissenschaften*, 1937, *25*, 289–300, 307–318, 324–331.

Lorenz, K. Plays and vacuum activities. In *L'instinct dans le comportement des animaux et de l'homme*. Paris: Masson et Cie, 1956.

Lorenz, K. Phylogenetische Anpassung und adaptive Modifikation des Verhaltens. *Zeitschrift für Tierpsychologie*, 1961, *18*, 139–187.

Lorenz, K. *Evolution and modification of behavior*. Chicago: University of Chicago Press, 1965.

Marler, P. A comparative approach to vocal learning: Song development in white-crowned sparrows. *Journal of Comparative and Physiological Psychology* (monograph supplement), 1970, *71*, 1–25.

Marler, P. Sensory templates in species-specific behavior. In J. C. Fentress (Ed.), *Simpler networks and behavior*. Sunderland, MA: Sinauer, 1976.

Marler, P. Song learning: Innate species differences in the learning process. In P. Marler and H. S. Terrace (Eds.), *The biology of learning*, Dahlem Workshop Reports—Life Sciences Research Report 29. Berlin: Springer, 1984.

Marler, P., and Peters, S. Subsong and plastic song: Their role in the vocal learning process. In D. E. Kroodsma and E. H. Miller (Eds.), *Acoustic communication in birds*, Vol. 2. New York: Academic Press, 1982.

Martin, P., and Caro, T. M. On the functions of play and its role in behavioral development. *Advances in the Study of Behavior*, 1985, *15*, 59–103.

Maynard Smith, J. Parental investment: A prospective analysis. *Animal Behaviour*, 1977, *25*, 1–9.

McGregor, P. K., and Avery, M. I. The unsung songs of great tits *(Parus major):* Learning neighbors' songs for discrimination. *Behavioural Ecology and Sociobiology*, 1986, *18*, 311–316.

Milligan, M. M., and Verner, J. Inter-populational song dialect discrimination in the white-crowned sparrow. *Condor*, 1971, *73*, 208–213.

Moore, B. R. The role of direct Pavlovian reactions in simple instrumental learning in the pigeon. In R. A. Hinde and J. G. Stevenson-Hinde (Eds.), *Constraints on learning*. London: Academic Press, 1973.

Morgan, C. L. *Habit and instinct*. London: Arnold, 1896.

Morris, D. [Discussion following Lorenz] In *L'instinct dans le comportement des animaux et de l'homme*. Paris: Masson et Cie, 1956, pp. 642–643.

Nottebohm, F. A brain for all seasons: Cyclical anatomical changes in song control nuclei of the canary brain. *Science*, 1981, *214*, 1368–1370.

Novak, M. and Harlow, H. F. Social recovery of monkeys isolated for the first year of life: I. Rehabilitation and therapy. *Developmental Psychology*, 1975, *11*, 453–465.

Oppenheim, R. The ontogeny of behavior in the chick embryo. *Advances in the Study of Behavior*, 1974, *5*, 133–172.

Park, T. J., and Dooling, R. J. Perception of species-specific contact calls by budgerigars *(Melopsittacus undulatus)*. *Journal of Comparative Psychology*, 1985, *99*, 391–402.

Paton, J. A., and Nottebohm, F. Neurons generated in the adult brain are recruited into functional circuits. *Science*, 1984, *225*, 1046–1048.

Petrinovich, L. Factors influencing song development in the white-crowned sparrow *(Zonotrichia leucophrys)*. *Journal of Comparative Psychology*, 1985, *99*, 15–29.

Pinel, J. P., and Treit, D. Burying as a defensive response in rats. *Journal of Comparative and Physiological Psychology*, 1978, *92*, 708–712.

Pinel, J. P., and Treit D. Conditioned defensive burying in rats: Availability of burying materials. *Animal Learning and Behavior*, 1979, *7*, 392–396.

Polsky, R. H. Hunger, prey feeding, and predatory aggression. *Behavioral Biology*, 1975, *13*, 81–93.

Reisbick, S. H. Development of food preferences in newborn guinea pigs. *Journal of Comparative and Physiological Psychology*, 1973, *85*, 427–442.

Rice, J. C. Effects of learning constraints and behavioural organization on the association of vocalizations and hunger in Burmese red junglefowl chicks. *Behaviour*, 1978, *67*, 259–298.

Rozin, P. The acquisition of food habits and preferences. In J. D. Matarazzo, S. M. Weiss, J. A. Herd, N. E. Miller, and S. M. Weiss (Eds.), *Behavioral health: A handbook of health enhancement and disease prevention*. New York: Wiley, 1984.

Rozin, P., and Schiller, D. The nature and acquisition of a preference for chili pepper by humans. *Motivation and Emotion*, 1980, *4*, 77–101.

Sackett, G. P. Unlearned responses, differential rearing experiences, and the development of social attachments by Rhesus monkeys. In L. A. Rosenblum (Ed.), *Primate behavior*. New York: Academic Press, 1970.

Schiller, P. H. Manipulative patterns in the chimpanzee (1949). In C. H. Schiller (Ed.), *Instinctive behavior*. New York: International Universities Press, 1957.

Schneirla, T. C. Interrelationships of the "innate" and the "acquired" in instinctive behavior. In *L'instinct dans le comportement des animaux et de l'homme*. Paris: Masson et Cie, 1956.

Schneirla, T. C., Rosenblatt, J. S., and Tobach, E. Maternal behavior in the cat. In H. Rheingold (Ed.), *Maternal behavior in mammals*. New York: Wiley, 1963.

Schutz, F. Sexuelle Prägung bei Anatiden. *Zeitschrift für Tierpsychologie*, 1965, *22*, 50–103.

Sherry, D. F. Parental food-calling and the role of the young in the Burmese red junglefowl *(Gallus g. spadiceus)*. *Animal Behaviour*, 1977, *25*, 594–601.

Sherry, D. F. Parental care and development of thermoregulation in red junglefowl. *Behaviour*, 1981, *76*, 250–279.

Shettleworth, S. J. Reinforcement and the organization of behavior in golden hamsters. *Journal of Experimental Psychology: Animal Behavior Processes*, 1975, *1*, 56–87.

Skinner, B. F. *Science and human behavior*. New York: Macmillan, 1953.

Slater, P. J. B. Bird song learning: Theme and variations. In G. A. Clark, Jr., and A. R. Brush (Eds.), *Perspectives in ornithology*. London: Cambridge University Press, 1983.

Steiner, J. E. Human facial expressions in response to taste and smell stimulation. *Advances in Child Development and Behavior*, 1979, *13*, 257–295.

Steller, E. Drive and motivation. In J. Field, H. W. Magoun, and V. E. Hall (Eds.), *Handbook of physiology*, Sec. 1, Vol. 3. Washington: American Physiological Association, 1960.

Stevenson, J. G. Reinforcing effects of chaffinch song. *Animal Behaviour*, 1967, *15*, 427–432.

Sutherland, N. S. The learning of discriminations by animals. *Endeavour*, 1964, *23*, 148–152.

ten Cate, C. The influence of social relations on the development of species recognition in zebra finch males. *Behaviour*, 1984, *91*, 263–285.

ten Cate, C. Sexual preferences in zebra finch males exposed to two species. I. A case of double imprinting. *Journal of Comparative Psychology*, 1986, *100*, 248–252.

ten Cate, C. Sexual preferences in zebra finch males exposed to two species. II. The internal representation resulting from double imprinting. *Animal Behaviour*, 1987, *35*, 321–330.

Thorpe, W. H. The learning of song patterns by birds, with especial reference to the song of the chaffinch *(Fringilla coelebs)*. *Ibis*, 1958, *100*, 535–570.

Thorpe, W. H. *Bird song*. Cambridge: Cambridge University Press, 1961.

Thorpe, W. H., and Jones, F. G. W. Olfactory conditioning and its relation to the problem of host selection. *Proceedings of the Royal Society, Series B.* 1937, *124*, 56–81.

Timberlake, W. The functional organization of appetitive behavior: Behavior systems and learning. In M. D. Zeiler and P. Harzem (Eds.), *Advances in analysis of behavior, Vol. 3. Biological factors in learning*. Chichester, England: Wiley, 1983.

Tinbergen, N. *The study of instinct*. Oxford: Oxford University Press, 1951.

Tinbergen, N. Derived activities: Their causation, biological significance, origin and emancipation during evolution. *Quarterly Review of Biology*, 1952, *27*, 1–32.

von Holst, E. Relations between the central nervous system and the peripheral organs. *British Journal of Animal Behaviour*, 1954, *2*, 89–94.

von Holst, E., and St. Paul, U. von. Vom Wirkungsgefüge der Triebe. *Naturwissenschaften*, 1960, *47*, 409–422. (Trans.: On the functional organisation of drives. *Animal Behaviour*, 1963, *11*, 1–20.)

Waddington, C. H. *Principles of development and differentiation*. New York: Macmillan, 1966.

Wasserman, E. A. Pavlovian conditioning with heat reinforcement produces stimulus-directed pecking in chicks. *Science*, 1973, *181*, 875–877.

Zajonc, R. B., Wilson, W. R., and Rajecki, D. W. Affiliation and social discrimination produced by brief exposure in day-old domestic chicks. *Animal Behaviour*, 1975, *23*, 131–138.

4

Precocity, Play, and the Ectotherm–Endotherm Transition

Profound Reorganization or Superficial Adaptation?

GORDON M. BURGHARDT

> The truth lies directly before us in the reality surrounding us. However, we can not use it as is. An unbroken description of reality would be simultaneously the truest and most useless thing in the world, and it certainly would not be science. If we want to make reality and therefore truth useful to science, we must do violence to reality. We must introduce the distinction, which does not exist in nature, between *essential* and *inessential*. By seeking out the relationships that seem essential to us, we order the material in a surveyable way at the same time. Then we are doing science.
>
> von Uexküll
> *Environment* [Umwelt] *and the inner world of animals.*
> (1909/1985, p. 227)

Reptiles have many morphological and physiological characteristics similar to those found in mammals and birds; others are seemingly only modestly modified (e.g., functional organization of the circulatory, endocrine, visual, and central nervous systems). Yet behaviorally, endotherms are often perceived to be (in effect) qualitatively different from ectotherms. This chapter explores this issue, focusing on development. Lurking in the background are questions such as: What are the phenomena that have led to the perceived distinction? If any such behavioral differences are genuine, are they profound or superficial? To what extent may any behavioral differences be due to a lack of cognitive and emotional capacities in reptiles, or may other factors be involved? Recent studies have shed light on these questions, and the answers coming in have potentially important consequences for our views of the behavior of "higher" vertebrates.

GORDON M. BURGHARDT   Departments of Psychology and Zoology, Graduate Program in Ethology (Life Sciences), University of Tennessee, Knoxville, Tennessee 37996.

Although no definitive answers can yet be given to any of the questions asked above, it appears that the relative lack of postnatal parental care, coupled with physiological differences associated with limited oxygen-consumption abilities, are responsible for the perceived behavioral differences between reptiles and endotherms. These two factors—parental care and metabolic physiology—greatly influence the behavioral development and behavioral ecology of reptiles, and they raise important theoretical issues as well as provide ample opportunities to test them. Although the emphasis here is on reptile–mammal comparisons, birds and amphibians are also discussed. After some general considerations, examples of the precocial abilities of reptiles are given, based primarily on our work with feeding, social, and defensive behaviors. Play is then discussed as one area where a difference between reptiles and mammals seems most clear. Somewhat paradoxically, play is one topic on which predictions about mammalian and avian diversity can be derived from a comparative knowledge of reptiles.

This chapter is the only one in this book that discusses vertebrates other than birds and mammals. I hope to demonstrate that, for two fundamental reasons, vertebrates other than homeotherms (homoiotherms) need to be ontogenetically and comparatively studied. The first reason is that they manifest phenomena that can be analyzed without some of the factors confounding and confusing the analysis of comparable, often homologous, phenomena in mammals and birds. Thus, some of the cantankerous theoretical controversy about whether various kinds of processes can *ever* occur may be set aside. The second reason is that the proper understanding of behavior patterns in amphibians and especially reptiles, the closest extant survivors of the stem groups of both mammal and avian evolution, is essential to the correct understanding of behavior in birds and mammals.

It is tempting to state, as is often done in the popular literature, that reptiles are born as fully blown miniatures of the adults, their precocial nature implying that they must behave just as the adults do. In fact, the two assertions do not follow. Reptiles do learn, sometimes quite rapidly (Burghardt, 1977a); their behavior is modified through experience and maturation (Burghardt, 1978); and social interactions can be complex (e.g., Greenberg, 1976). Yet it is clear that the feeding, defensive, and social behaviors of young reptiles are far more like those of adults than is true of even the most precocial of the endotherms. Amphibians, on the other hand, typically show the reverse: the larval stages are quite dissimilar from the adult stages, but the larvae can have rather complex abilities, such as kin preferences, even if reared in social isolation (Waldman, 1985). Together, reptiles and amphibians have the potential to help unravel fundamental processes in vertebrate behavioral development, such as continuity (Bateson, 1981; Sackett, Sameroff, Cairns, and Suomi, 1981) in naturalistic contexts.

Although developmental questions can be separated conceptually from those dealing with evolution, function, and proximate causation (Tinbergen, 1963), it does not follow that developmental issues are not critical in the analysis of evolution, function, and causation (Bekoff and Byers, 1985). Indeed, an understanding of development is increasingly seen as a critical neglected factor in our understanding of macroevolution (e.g., Gould, 1977). Consequently, those who study the genetic basis of behavior, especially social behavior, cannot ignore ontogenetic processes. Similarly, those studying development cannot ignore evolutionary and ecological concerns. But to say that ecological and evolutionary concerns cannot be omitted is, in fact, to say that genetic mechanisms cannot be ignored. Critics of the innate–learned, genetic–environmental, nature–nurture, or comparable dichotomies have been exercised about specific applications of the dichotomy, rather than avoiding it themselves when they get down to empirical research. Whenever one is careful to restrict one's studies to a given breed or strain or engages in a balanced cross-fostering study, one is implicitly acknowledging that the dichotomy has some validity.

Aspects of phenotypic expression are associated with genotypic and environmental (including experiential) characteristics, although interactions and mutually interdependent processes are obviously always involved in the ontogeny of any phenotypic characteristic, and nonobvious and unexpected influences and factors are always cropping up on both the genetic and the experiential fronts (Oppenheim and Haverkamp, 1985). Further, the existence within species of individual differences and plasticity in and of itself tells us nothing about the importance of either genes or experience (cf. Burghardt, 1977c). Finally, the ecological contexts in which behavioral development and behavior patterns occur are the locus of prospective effects both on natural selection (of future generations) and on the life course of the specific individual (Wiley, 1981). Developmental psychobiologists need to be continually aware of the diversity of behaviors and mechanisms and the necessary tentativeness of any theoretical framework, as well as of the limitations of the metaphors that can enrich our vision while simultaneously being blinders (e.g., parent–offspring behavior as involving symbiosis or parasitism; genetic information as a blueprint or a recipe; and phenotypes as sculptures; cf. the excellent review by Alberts, 1985).

The above approach goes counter to frequent statements that it is impossible to partition genetic and environmental sources of variation in behavioral characteristics (e.g., Mason, 1979). There is ample theoretical (e.g., Burghardt, 1977c) and practical (Plomins, DeFries, and McClearn, 1980) evidence to the contrary. A related problem is the continued ignoring of individual differences in developmental studies (e.g., Mason, 1979) and especially genetic sources of such differences in behavior. As argued below, evidence from reptiles establishes the importance of genetic variation.

Terrestrial Ecotherms and Endotherms Compared

Terrestrial Vertebrate Diversity

There are roughly 4,000 amphibian species and 6,200 reptile species living today. The former are divided into three orders: Urodela (the salamanders), Gymnophiona (the little-known burrowing wormlike caecilians), and the Salientia (frogs and toads), the largest order containing about 3,400 species. Reptiles are divided into four orders: Rhynchocephalia (one relic species, *Sphenodon*), Crocodilia (the 25 species of crocodiles, caimans, and gavials), Testudines (the turtles and tortoises, about 300 species), and the highly successful Squamata (about 3,100 lizards, 2,600 snakes, and the more than 100 species of little-known burrowing amphisbaenians ("wormlizards")). Birds are divided into 27 orders and number over 8,600 species. There are about 4,500 living mammals, which are divided into three distinctive groups: monotremes, marsupials, and the 16 orders of placentals. Eisenberg (1981) is an excellent source on mammalian diversity from the perspective of both zoology and ethology.

This catalog indicates a fact that we all "know" but continually ignore: the animals typically studied developmentally reflect only a minor sample of the diversity found within each of these four classes of terrestrial vertebrates. The comparison of related taxa was a prime concern of the early ethologists (e.g., Heinroth, 1911/1985). Yet, today, our comparative data base is still too full of blanks, our knowledge of current systematics is deficient, and we underestimate the serious difficulties attending comparisons across taxa, even those within the same genus (cf. Felsenstein, 1985; Harvey and Mace, 1982; Lauder, 1986).

Consider the program for the November 1986 annual meeting of the International Society of Developmental Psychobiology that I received while I was preparing the final draft of this chapter. Of the 106 papers (of a total of about 125) for which the species studied could be determined, fully 72 were on rodents (I include 1 paper on rabbits): 60 were on lab rats, and 7 were on mice. Primates were studied in 28 reports: 16 were on humans, 8 on rhesus monkeys, and only 4 on other primate species. A highly biased selection of mammals thus encompassed 94% of the current work. Of the 6 nonmammalian papers, 5 were on birds (all domesticated), and 1 was on bullfrogs. None were on reptiles or fish. Although it may be unfair to call this one meeting program "typical," I think the lack of species diversity in the field is both incontestable and unfortunate, regardless of the many plausible reasons—historical, practical, and otherwise—that can be given to justify the narrowness of the coverage.

The catalog also suggests some other points. In terms of numbers of both orders and species, birds can be viewed as most successful. The mammals have fewer species than reptiles, but a greater diversity of extant orders. Amphibians show the least speciation and the smallest number of extant orders, although the frogs are, next to the reptilian Squamata, the largest order in number of species. The highly successful and diverse Squamata are also the most recent reptilian order; and most of the order's radiation occurred during the teriary period, as is also true of mammals and birds. Still, there is no doubt that many of the features of squamates and probably also their behavior reflect the characteristics of early reptiles and even dinosaurs (Burghardt, 1977b). Unfortunately, some paleontologists (e.g., Ostrom, 1986) still argue from fossil evidence that dinosaurs had behavioral characteristics seeming more like those of mammals or birds than like those of the extant reptiles, although all of the behaviors discussed are found in living reptiles. Indeed, arguments have been made that birds and dinosaurs should be in the same class (review in Charig, 1976; Thomas and Olson, 1980). Endothermay is a major aspect of this debate, and in fact, endothermy plays a critical role in this chapter.

Complicating the picture is the possibility that, unlike the birds and the therian mammals (marsupials and placentals), the four reptile orders seem *not* to be a natural assemblage derived from a common ancestor; they may, in fact, be grouped together only because they lack certain traits that unambiguously set off mammals and birds, such as feathers, fur, and mammary glands. For example, Pough (1983), pointed out the large biological similarities between reptiles and amphibians, even though amphibians and the extant reptiles have been separated for a few hundred million years. Nevertheless, current reptiles "have more recent genetic continuity with mammals than they do with amphibians, and among the reptiles the crocodilian lineage separated from that of birds some 50 million years more recently than its separation from other reptilian stocks" (Pough, 1983, p. 142). Such taxonomic points may eventually prove critical in evaluating scenarios concerning the evolution of behavior and development in amniote vertebrates. In addition, the methods being used in cladistic analysis (e.g., Felsenstein, 1985; Kluge, 1985; Lauder, 1986) may prove useful in comparative developmental psychobiology. In the following discussion, lizards are emphasized both because of the large data sets available and because they appear to be the best living model for the therapsid (mammal-like) reptiles (MacLean, 1986).

A few comments on terminology are also in order. *Poikilothermy* refers to animals whose body temperature fluctuates with that of the external environment. *Homeothermy* (homoiothermy) refers to animals who maintain a constant body temperature. Reptiles and amphibians are traditionally regarded as having the former, and birds and mammals the latter. However, reptiles often have body temperatures much higher than the ambient environment because of behavioral thermoregulation, such as shuttling in and out of the sun. On the other hand, birds and mammals, especially neonates and small species, can show considerable diel variation in body temperature. The other contrast, *ectothermy* and *endothermy,* refers to the source of body heat; reptiles are typically regarded as having the former, and birds and mammals the latter. Again, a few exceptions can be cited, as in egg-brooding pythons, which can use endogenous means to raise their body temperature and hence that of their eggs, and sea turtles, which maintain a core body temperature 18°C above that of the ambient environment (Greenberg, 1980). *Heterothermy* is a useful term for endothermic animals that are not continuously homeothermic (Bartholomew, 1982). In this chapter, I use primarily the ectotherm–endotherm contrast.

PARENTAL CARE

A number of contrasts between the life history and physiological characteristics of reptiles and of endotherms are presented in Table 1. Several relate to the precocial nature of much reptile behavior. At birth, reptiles lack most (usually all) postnatal parental care and must find food, water and shelter, as well as protect themselves from adverse weather and predators, all pretty much on their own.

TABLE 1. PHYSIOLOGICAL AND LIFE HISTORY CONTRASTS BETWEEN TYPICAL
ENDOTHERMS AND REPTILES[a]

Mammals and birds	Reptiles
High basal and resting metabolic rates	Low basal and resting metabolic rates
Rich vascular system and highly oxygenated blood	Fewer capillaries and less efficient blood-transport system; blood capable of carrying far less oxygen
Capable of sustained, vigorous activity (aerobic metabolism)	Vigorous behavior sporadic and short-lived; reliance on anaerobic metabolism for sustained vigorous activity
Rapid recuperation after sustained activity and thus short period of vulnerability	Recuperation from sustained activity (to normal lactic-acid levels) measured in hours; extended period of vulnerability.
Exercise increases cardiovascular and endurance functions	No evidence of physiological benefits of exercise; exercise may even be harmful.
Endothermy provides high resting metabolism, allowing rapid onset of vigorous play. Costs of overcoming inertia increase with weight	Ectothermy allows a low-energy (conservation) lifestyle; the behaviors needed to raise body temperature to aerobic optimum are often incompatible with play.
Neonates have food, heat, shelter, and protection provided by parent	Neonates must provide most, if not all, their own resources.
Neonates have many motor and perceptual systems restricted to juvenile period (e.g., sucking)	Most neonatal behaviors show clear continuities with adult motor and perceptual systems.
Neonatal period available to develop or perfect functional social, feeding, locomotor, or antipredator skills	Most behaviors necessary for survival need to be highly functional at birth; however, skill improvement can occur.
Play research focuses on pure "delayed" benefits, vigorous motor activity	Highly likely that any "play" will also have a current benefit; play may be subtle, less obvious
"Relaxed field" common in juveniles. Play occurs most frequently when juveniles are well fed, often after feeding	"Relaxed field" rare in juveniles. Postingestion behavior in reptiles is characterized by lethargy, distended stomachs, and basking or holing up out of harm's way.
Relatively determinate juvenile growth allows for excess metabolic energy in "good times"	Relatively indeterminate juvenile growth allows most energy intake to be channelled into growth.
Neonates capable of sustained activity.	Even well-fed neonates have far less endurance than adults.
Relatively few offspring, especially in the most "playful" families	Relatively more offspring, with higher mortality, over equivalent adult lifespans.

[a]Based in part on Burghardt (1984).

The altricial–precocial dichotomy is clearly a continuum, particularly among birds and mammals. I use the dichotomy here to refer to the relative importance, amount, and duration of parental care needed for offspring to survive. The more precocial the neonate is, the more independent it is at birth or hatching regardless of its morphological aspects. This use is in contrast with the way others have used the dichotomy. For example, in referring to the state of development of the young, Calder (1984, p. 273) used *altricial* to mean "naked, blind and helpless" and *pre-*

cocial to mean "furred or feathered, eyes open, and capable of some coordinated movement on its own behalf." Harvey and Bennett (1983) used as a measure the length of the gestation period and characterized the longer periods as producing precocial young. All three, along with endothermy, are often but not always associated (Case, 1978a). Primate young, in the second two views, are highly precocial, compared to newborn rats or bears. On the basis of the usage here, primates are also highly altricial, compared to newborn lizards or snakes.

Related to the behavioral precocity of neonate reptiles is the general lack of postnatal parental care as an *essential* factor in neonate survival in the wild. All turtles deposit their eggs and abandon them. All crocodilians also lay eggs, but as far as is known, all species evidence nest guarding, hatchling release from the nest and perhaps the guiding of hatchlings to water, and maternal proximity to the young for at least the first months of life. Much individual variability in nest guarding occurs; however, this variability may relate to human or observer disturbance (personal communications, H. A. Herzog, Jr., 1975, on American alligators and A. S. Rand, 1983, on American crocodiles).

Why do crocodilians, in contrast to turtles, show this level of parental care? Most turtles are primarily aquatic, and crocodilians are always associated with water. Both groups may live and breed in the same habitats, although turtles range farther into temperate and drier areas. Even their food habits often overlap. Parental care in crocodilians may primarily provide for protection from predators. But why should this not be equally true in turtles? The shell "armor" of turtles does not seem a sufficient reason for the absence of parental care. Baby turtles typically have softer shells than the adults, and they readily and frequently fall prey to birds and other predators. Similarly, nest predation on turtle eggs is very common. Furthermore, turtle hatchlings, even of the gigantic tortoise and sea turtle species, are usually smaller and far more timid than virtually all crocodilian hatchlings. As anyone who has tried to handle hatchling crocodilians knows, they have a repertoire of defensive behaviors and a speed of response that can be painfully effective.

Adult turtles are well protected by armor, but they are typically not either fast enough on land (where all eggs are laid) or potentially dangerous enough to deter nest predators, whereas crocodilians are effective defenders against most terrestrial predators. Parental nest defense and brood care in crocodilians may also have originally arisen as a response to conspecific predation. In any event, young crocodilians emit "contact" and "distress" calls (Herzog and Burghardt, 1977), the latter when handled. Anecdotal reports suggest these calls are given when the juvenile is attached by a predator and result in the recruitment of an adult and the warding off of the predator (e.g., Gorzula, 1985). Perhaps the difference between crocodilians and turtles is related to the fact that only a few turtles vocalize at all (and then only during courtship); in juveniles, I am aware of no records of more than hisses.

But the above speculations are difficult to test, as both groups have been separated for so long and there is little variability among species or genera within each group. To some extent both groups seem "locked in" with regard to parental care.

It is in the numerically far more successful squamate groups that we observe a wide range of variability. Although most squamates seem to ignore their eggs once laid, there are lizards that brood their eggs until hatching and stay with them for at least a few days postnatally (Evans, 1959). In *Ophisaurus*, the mother may even alter the depth of her eggs in the substrate in response to temperature fluctuations (Vinegar,1968). There are oviparous and viviparous species among both lizards and snakes, and congeners use either tactic (Tinkle and Gibbons, 1977). This vivaparity may even equal advanced mammalian standards (Blackburn, Vitt, and Beuchat, 1984). And the variability in hatching times so typical of reptile eggs may relate to the differential development of the eggs as carried by the mother rather than to differences in incubation temperature after they are laid (D. Werner, personal communication, 1986). Across species, genera, and families of squamate reptiles, age at maturity and number of broods per year are related to viviparity or egg laying (Dunham and Miles, 1985).

As mentioned, some egg-brooding snakes can raise the temperature of their clutch above the ambient by physiological means (Vinegar, Hutchison, and Dowling, 1970; review in Greenberg, 1980), and recent evidence suggests that moisture regulation may also be a function of egg incubation in at least one species (York and Burghardt, 1987). Although obvious postnatal parental care in snakes has not been documented, there is some indication that newborn rattlesnakes, for example, may remain in the vicinity of their mother for several days, perhaps until the first ecdysis (Graves, Duvall, King, Lindstedt, and Gern, 1986), or follow chemical trails of adults to hibernacula (Brown and MacLean, 1983).

Frogs and salamanders are also, among the amphibians, groups in which large differences in parental care can occur, even in the same species. Duellman (1985) recognized 29 different modes of reproduction in frogs, which he derived from the familiar situation in which eggs are laid in ponds and are followed by a tadpole stage. There is even a viviparous frog, frogs that carry eggs and young on their backs, species with direct development without a larval stage, and one that broods eggs in its stomach. McDiarmid (1978) reviewed the complex and diverse modes of parental care in frogs. Among the 350 species and eight families of salamanders, parental care apparently occurs primarily in terrestrial species and largely in just one family, the Plethodontidae (lungless salamanders), a group that accounts for 61% of all salamander species (Nussbaum, 1985).

Obviously parental care was an important evolutionary step, but it may not be able to carry all the functions attributed to it in nonhuman animals (e.g., intelligence and social complexity; references in Burghardt, 1977b). Forms of parental care, often very elaborate, occur not only in fish and amphibians, as well as in a few reptiles, but also in groups as varied as coelenterates, echinoderms, mollusks, arachnids, crustacea, and insects (Grzimek, 1974). Indeed, the origins of parental care seem mostly related to ecological conditions, predation, and unknown phylogenetic factors (Gittleman, 1981). In the turtle–crocodilian comparison above conspecific aggression was postulated as a plausible origin. If we think that any functions of parental care or sociality are limited to "higher" animals, we need to address the comparative record. The diverse squamate reptiles seem to be the best group for separating out specific factors that may have been important. Data from such studies could be combined with informed paleontological theory to clarify the nature of the ectotherm-endotherm vertebrate transition (Case, 1978a; Hopson, 1973; Hotton, MacLean, Roth, and Roth, 1986; Kemp 1982; Olson, 1976; Thomas and Olson, 1980).

Physiological Adaptations

The second major suite of characteristics in which amphibians and reptiles differ from birds and mammals involves physiological energetics (see Table 1; Burghardt, 1984; Pough, 1980). No overlap in basal metabolic rate has been found for equal-sized reptiles and either mammals or birds; the difference is typically an order of magnitude, the reptile rate being 10% that of the endotherm. Most squamate reptiles are smaller than typical mammals and even birds (Pough, 1983). For example, 80% of all lizard species weight less than 20 g as adults, and 8% of all lizards weigh less than 1 g. In contrast, most rodents weight more than 20 g as adults. The situation with amphibians is even more skewed: more than half of all frogs and salamanders weigh less than 5 g as adults. The circulatory system of reptiles and amphibians is also less efficient than that of endotherms. There are typically fewer capillaries, the blood holds less oxygen, and thus, amphibians and reptiles have limited capacities for sustained aerobic metabolism, compared to endotherms (Pough, 1980).

As size decreases for endothermic vertebrates, the surface-to-volume ratio increases, and so does heat loss. Tiny endotherms have notoriously high metabolic costs and fueling requirements. Still, heat loss itself may not be the direct reason for the lower size limits (2–3 g) of mammals and birds (shrews and hummingbirds, respectively). Some insects (e.g., sphingid moths) effectively thermoregulate with a body size an order of magnitude smaller (Schmidt-Nielsen, 1984). Rather, the lower size limits for endothermic vertebrates is probably due to the "design of the oxygen supply system and the limits to the pumping capacity of the heart" (Schmidt-Nielsen, 1984; p. 208). A hummingbird or shrew heart beats 1,200–1,400 times per minute. It is clear that a like-size reptile does not have this lower limit because it does not need as much oxygenated blood. Thus, endothermy indirectly poses a minimum size constraint not applicable to reptiles and amphibians.

The evolution of endothermy in birds and mammals is an area of lively speculation. The controversy over whether dinosaurs were endothermic continues, but the advocates of dinosaur endothermy are now on the defensive. Weaver (1983), for example, has shown that giant sauropods had bodies too large, heads too small, and food too indigestible to be endothermic. Even in the therapsid reptiles that led to mammals, the evidence for endothermy is largely weak to nonexistent. Bennett and Ruben (1986) concluded that the most convincing evidence is that endothermy occurs in monotremes and therian mammals, which appear to have had a long interval of independent evolution and are most parsimoniously viewed as having independently evolved from an advanced endothermic therapsid. As for evidence from the therapsid fossils themselves, the convincing evidence is limted to complex nasal turbinals that appear only in advanced therapsids and mammals, and that serve primarily to warm inspired air and to conserve water. As for physiological theories of how endothermy arose, none seem to be tenable at the present time, particularly when individual variation within species, rather than cross-species variation, is considered (e.g., Pough and Andrews, 1984).

There are other possibilities of important differences between reptiles and endotherms (Table 1). One is that reptiles may rely on anaerobic metabolism in routine vigorous activity (in contrast to "burst" activity) more than do endotherms, and energy expenditure is thus more costly (Bennet, 1982; Burghardt, 1984; Pough and Andrews, 1985b; but see Pough and Andrews, 1985a, on cricket predation in a scincid lizard). This difference is supported by laboratory data on small rodents (Ruben and Battalia, 1979), but unfortunately, few data are available, particularly in nature (Gatten, 1985). It is definitely established, however, that reptiles have limited aerobic capacity for activity, compared to endotherms (Bennett, 1982; Pough, 1980). However, some small lizards (Cnemidophorus), although having typically low resting metabolic rates, have both high aerobic endurance capacities and oxygen consumption and thus approach mammalian levels (Garland, in press). On independent behavioral grounds, this genus of teiid lizards has been considered most mammal-like (Regal, 1978).

Also, as young, not only must reptiles locate food and feed themselves, but the energy from the food that they do ingest seems to be channeled primarily into growth, not fat, and thus healthy reptiles born the same season can differ by a factor of 5 or more in weight in late juvenile periods. For example, of a group of 12 hatchling green iguanas (Iguana iguana) from the same population in Panama that we reared in identical conditions in captivity, from June 1983 to June 1984 one male went from 19.7 g to 52.8 g, and another went from 19.2 g to 200.7 g, a ratio of 1:3.8; both were healthy and vigorous. By June of 1986, the difference had gone to 331 g and 1630 g, for a ratio of 1:4.9. Comparable data have been collected in the field (Burghardt and Rodda, unpubl., 1983). Thus, reptiles, unlike endotherms, may not have spare "fat" available for "burning off" through activity when resources are abundant. (See also discussion of play, p. 127)

Pough (1983) pointed out the physiological advantages of small size. One is that it may be better to stay small rather than simply starving if food is not plentiful enough for rapid growth. Recently, Karasov and Diamond (1985) showed that, even when kept warm, a lizard processes food 10 times more slowly than a mammal. Is this a cause, a consequence, or an adaptive correlate of the 10 times greater metabolic rate of endotherms? In the species studied, there was about a 7-fold increase in intestinal surface area in mammals, along with equal or slightly higher nutrient absorption rates. Although the mammal stayed at a higher temperature than the lizard throughout the 24-h day, this difference was found to result in only a 1.5-fold increase. Even though the data are from only a few species, these two factors combined explain the 10-fold difference (Karasov, Petrossian, Rosenberg, and Diamond, 1986).

Another unsuspected but particularly relevant ontogenetic difference may exist between reptiles and mammals. On the basis of a provocative study (on an iguanid lizard, *Scleroporus occidentalis;* Gleeson, 1979), I made the claim that reptiles may differ behaviorally from endotherms in such areas as vigorous play because physical exercise in reptiles may not lead to the enhanced or improved cardiovascular and activity functions shown to occur in mammals (Burghardt, 1984). A recent study on a lizard from another family (the agamid *Amphibolurus nuchalis;* Garland, Else, Hulbert, and Tap, in press) showed that not only did treadmill exercise for 30 min per day not lead to increased physiological function over 8 weeks, but it actually damaged the joints and skeletal muscles of the animals. Thus, what we see is the possible restriction of reptile behavior because reptiles are structurally and metabolically not built to withstand sustained activity. Furthermore, in this species (Garland and Else, in press) and in some snakes (Pough, 1977; 1978), adults, as contrasted with juveniles, have considerably greater endurance and speed capacity than simple size increase (allometry) would predict. Finally, the twelfth point, in Table 1 is supported by a study (Garland and Arnold, 1983) showing that recently fed garter snakes *(Thamnopis elegans)* had significantly decreased endurance and more awkward locomotion.

Physiological factors may intrude into social behavior in several ways. Avery (1976) studied various aspects of behavior in several species of lacertid lizards in Europe. He found that, as they ranged more northerly into cooler climes, they still had high (about 30°C) and restricted preferred body temperatures for activity, and thus, their energetic and timing (e.g., basking) needs became more acute. There was also a decrease in the time spent in nonbasking activity and annual metabolism. Avery also claimed (somewhat anecdotally) that both behavioral plasticity ("intelligence") and social complexity decreased among the more northern forms. These trends were accentuated by comparison with a well-studied but taxonomically remote African species *(Agama agama)*. Acknowledging the existence of considerable diversity, Avery nonetheless concluded that "complex social behaviour is only possible in environments in which thermoregulation is not paramount" (p. 256). And in fact, the best examples of complex social behavior in amphibians and reptiles are found in tropical species, which can more easily approach homeothermy. Additionally, Werner (1982) noted that the lack of predation on Galapagos land iguanas *(Conolophus)* may have allowed the evolution of prolonged and conspicuous male–male combat not seen in mainland iguanas.

REPTILES AND THEORIES OF DEVELOPMENT

Are these differences in parental care and physiology between reptiles and endothermic amniotes constraints on the behavioral repertoires of these groups, or are they just reflections of selective pressures that could easily have pushed the animals in other directions? This question is of crucial importance in our theoretical picture of vertebrate behavioral development. As pointed out above, many workers in developmental psychobiology work with and cite data primarily from only a few species of birds and mammals, and some explicitly limit their comparative analyzes to mammals and birds (e.g., Bekoff and Byers, 1985; Wittenberger,

1979). Yet, without an evolutionary anchor point, any similarities are mere analogies or convergences (homoplasy), or comparisons at the grade level, be they comparisons of song learning in birds with language learning in humans, parental care in birds and mammals, imprinting in ducks and sheep, the determinants of neonatal sucking in rats and humans, or the hormonal determinants of sexual behavior in rats and quail.

An additional factor from the adult reptiles' vantage point is that they, as parents, are not encumbered with the costs in time, energy, and various risks that go along with protecting, provisioning, and generally taking care of their young, which are found in even the most precocial birds and mammals. If the neonate mammal and bird is essentially a parasite on its parents, as evocatively argued by Galef (1981; see also Trivers, 1972), then these costs are transferred to the parents. Are there any factors intrinsic to the reptilian level that preclude extensive homeothermlike parental care? Two possibilities stand out. One involves the aforementioned energetic factors. Extensive provisioning of young in the manner of songbirds, say, may be inconceivable, given reptilian energetic constraints in term of endurance and aerobic metabolism.

Lactation in mammals is a clear difference from reptiles that has imposed a series of physiological and behavioral adaptations in both parents and young. Duvall (1986) and Guillette and Hotton (1986) have speculated on the evolution of lactation and viviparity in therapsid reptiles and the early mammals. Although it is generally held that the primitive state of neonate mammals is altricial (as in monotremes and marsupials), this condition clearly did not arise overnight, and the shift from precocial to altricial young is viewed here as a gradual process in both the reptile–mammal and the reptile–bird transitions.

Although neonate reptiles do not need the amount of nutrients that neonate endotherms typically do, they can use a relatively large amount because of their indeterminate juvenile growth rates (i.e., growth rates can vary widely, depending on food intake, as contrasted with the less variable or determinate growth seen in endotherms). Growth rates in reptiles are typically an order of magnitude less than those in mammals at all body sizes (Calder, 1984; Case, 1978b). Thus, rapid growth rates should be selected for, especially because reptile neonates are typically smaller than endotherms and, by growing quickly, can outgrow possible predators and competitors. The importance of this factor is magnified by the lack of parental care. Of course, life history traits, such as age to sexual maturity and typical growth rates, also differ among reptiles as a function of foraging mode, oviparity, and clutch size (e.g., Dunham and Miles, 1985; Huey and Pianka, 1981).

Our field data on green iguanas recaptured throughout the first months of life in Panama and Venezuela indicate that 4-fold weight differences among yearlings in the same habitat are not unusual. In our captive colony of same-age animals from Panama reared in our laboratory from a few weeks of age, we found that both males and females that were offered ad lib food showed different growth rates, the rates in males being more variable; yet all were healthy. As we have not lost a single animal (of 12) in 4½ years, differential mortality is not a confound. Gordon Rodda (unpubl.) has argued that female mate choice in iguanas may be influenced by the male's contribution to heritable growth rate variation in hatch-lings. Hatchling iguanas are highly vulnerable to predation, so outpacing predators quickly is a good strategy if food is available. For folivores such as green iguanas, food is usually plentiful. Thus, the point here is that, not only are neonate reptiles more precocial, but there are consequences for the parents in providing care to relatively precocial young, as well as to the more altricial young typical of most endotherms.

The second possibility involves the role that endotherm parents play in the thermoregulation of their offspring. Neonate birds and mammals are often effec-tively poikilothermic and develop reliable homeothermy only after days or weeks, especially if born or hatched without fur or feathers. Hot-blooded birds and mam-mals can warm their offspring with their own heat; reptile parents, however, even if shuttling in and out of the sun, may find this difficult. And because neonate endotherms are capable of producing at least some body heat, insulated nests, sib-ling huddling (Alberta and May, 1984), and other features can markedly increase the value of parental behavior. Although some snakes do raise the temperature of their eggs by physiological means (Greenberg, 1980), the overall costs are unknown. The rarity of such temperature regulation indicates that although rep-tiles are not precluded from evolving endothermy, a suite of associated character-istics would be needed for its spread and development.

Crews and Moore (1986) argued that, in studies of reproduction in terrestrial vertebrates, we need increased use of comparative studies of diverse species under ecologically appropriate conditions, or "natural experiments." Studies of devel-opment, just as of reproduction, need this perspective in combining studies of proximate mechanisms and evolutionary and ecological factors. Identification of trajectories of behavioral ontogeny are enchanced when the role of parental care can be evaluated without the disruptive effects on numerous behavior systems that hand rearing or isolation rearing can impose on species normally reared by their parents. Consider Harlow's experiments (Harlow and Harlow, 1965) on mother-deprived monkeys, for example, or the difficulty until recent years of raising a rat or a mouse from birth without a rodent parent. The mere fact that critical parental care is absent in reptiles may lead some to dismiss the relevance of the reptile grade to gaining insights into behavioral development. This is a shortsighted view. Study-ing a phenomenon where it is questionably present or even absent may give us more insights into the evolutionary and developmental origins of behavior than studying it in its more elaborated and derived forms (Burghardt, 1984). Thus, care-ful selection of reptiles—especially related groups, such as the skinks, where dif-ferent levels of viviparity, egg brooding, and postantal parental care occur (Black-burn *et al.*, 1984)—can be of potential value.

Rearing mammals or birds in the absence of typical parental care can lead to conclusions on the role of specific kinds of experience in the ontogeny of behavior (cf. Lorenz, 1965). Such conclusions are, however, often suspect because of the very deprivation involved. The recent demonstrations that rat pups raised without mothers have a basic core repertoire of feeding behaviors have been critical (e.g., Hall and Williams, 1983). But because normal species-typical experience is lacking, one cannot rule out the equifinality possibility so nicely applied to ontogeny by

Bateson (1976). In other words, the same outcome may result from more than one "path," and thus, deprivation experiments may not be conclusive, no matter how elegant. In this equifinality, we see something akin to the phenomenon of vicarious function established by physiological psychologists: a part of the brain may be principally involved in a given function, but if it is destroyed, its job can be taken over by another part of the brain that normally would not be at all involved. Although not obviating the role that ablation studies can play, such findings encourage judicious interpretation.

Another issue relevant to reptile–endotherm comparisons is the question of rate of development, not just of the animal as a whole but of the various sensory, nervous system, and effector mechanisms. One form of such heterochrony is the differential sequencing of such systems. For example, in rat pups, the chemical senses develop first, the auditory system second, and vision (eye opening) last. Heterochrony clearly has implications for behavioral development and opens up the possibility of selective deprivation experiments in neonatal mammals. By studying animals whose virtually entire sensory, nervous system, and motor development has taken place in the relatively closed environment of egg or womb, we can evaluate the theoretical essentiality of putative processes.

SPECIFICITY AND DIVERSITY IN NEONATE REPTILE BEHAVIOR

Having laid out some of the basic but stereotyped differences in the biology and natural history of reptiles and mammals as classes, I will now consider several kinds of precocial neonatal behavior to which these differences may have relevance, among them food recognition and ingestion, antipredator behavior, social structure and organization, and communication.

FOOD SELECTION

The remarkable abilities of many mammals to find and recognize diverse food types may be based on some form of training by the parents. In fact, studies such as those by Galef (1977) have shown the subtle ways in which parental diet as well as imitationlike processes may be at work. But again, one potent proof against the necessity of such processes is the presence of specific abilities in reptiles with no parental care.

For example, our lab has studied the prey choice of newborn and newly hatched snakes for many years. What we have found is that ingestively naive neonate snakes can recognize, by chemical cues alone, the prey items typically captured and eaten by the species. These differences can often be dramatic (see review in Burghardt, 1970); rat snakes *(Elaphe)* respond to rodent and chick chemical cues; eastern and plains garter snakes *(Thamnophis* sp.) to earthworm, leech, frog, salamander, and fish cues; green snakes *(Opheodrys)* to insect cues; vine snakes *(Uromacer)* to lizard cues (Henderson, Binder, and Burghardt, 1983); queen snakes *(Regina)* to freshly molted crayfish cues; and so on. Maternal prenatal feeding experience during gestation does not seem to affect the neonatal preferences (Burghardt, 1971), nor even lifelong diets (Burghardt, 1978). Arnold (1981) demonstrated substantial heritabilities in *T. elegans* via breeding studies and sibling comparisons within and between litters. Neonates born to females from different populations of the same species may show different preferences (Arnold, 1981; Burghardt, 1970); and considerable variation within litters also occurs (Burghardt, 1975b). The poststrike increase in tongue flicking and the onset of prey trailing in viperine snakes when striking live prey has been shown to occur in adult zoo-born and zoo-reared snakes that had never been exposed to or fed live prey (O'Connell, Greenlee, Bacon, Chiszar, 1982).

But such specificity does not rule out the possibility that other cues (e.g., vision; Drummond, 1985) may play important roles. Nor does it preclude the modifiability of preferences because of postnatal feeding experience (Arnold, 1978; Burghardt, Wilcoxon, and Czaplicki, 1973; Fuchs and Burghardt, 1971) nor even because of exposure to stimulating chemicals in the absence of ingestion (Burghardt, 1970). On the other hand, all postnatal changes are not due to experience, for Mushinsky and Lotz (1980) showed that some species of water snakes *(Nerodia)* alter their chemical prey preference as they grow in spite of being fed exclusively on one type of prey. The preference shift seems to track changes in prey choice with snake size in the field. Thus, congenital, experiential, and maturational factors all play varying roles that differ across species, and it is not possible to state that specificity in one species precludes specificity in others, a common implicit assumption in development and evolution (Burghardt, 1977c).

Simply because these processes can be demonstrated in reptiles is no proof that they occur in mammals and birds. But in light of the similarities in other aspects of their biology and the demonstration that such complex innate processes can occur, it seem parsimonious to postulate that they can take place, even although, as in reptiles, experiential processes of some subtlety can be superimposed. However, more recently, comparable chemosensory food-related responses *have* been demonstrated in rat pups (Ganchrow, Steiner, and Csnetto, 1986) and human infants (Steiner, 1979).

ANTIPREDATOR BEHAVIOR

Some aspects of intraspecific communication and affect in reptiles and amphibians may be limited or, rather, may be different from those in birds and mammals because of the lack of intensive parent–offspring bonds. But in another area, defense, this very lack of parental care and bonding has led to an extraordinary richness of neonatal behaviors that are meant to startle, injure, deceive, or in other ways prevent being attacked or eaten. Such precocious defensive displays are more marked in neonatal reptiles than in amphibians, of course, as most of the latter go through an aquatic larval stage in which active defense is rare. But in those amphibians that have direct development, or in newly metamorphosed animals, diverse defensive tactics are also seen, including poisonous skin and glands and aposematic coloration.

A reptile's initial response to another organism is often flight, biting, threatening, and so on (review in Greene, 1987). Survival made such responses necessary, whereas neonate birds or mammals, being protected, could afford more exploratory or endearing behaviors. In precocious mammals and birds, we do see examples of well-developed defensive responses (Harvey and Greenwood, 1978), although they are often limited to freezing and reliance on protective cryptic coloration, as in white-tailed deer and many ungulates. When actually picked up, however, many mammals and birds may bite, claw, and squirm.

We have recently begun an extensive comparative study of defensive responses in natricine snakes and their development. I noticed in my studies on feeding behavior in newborn snakes that, at birth or hatching, some species strike out on any disturbance (such as black rat snakes, *Elaphe obsoleta;* northern banded water snakes, *Nerodia sipedon;* and aquatic water snakes, *Thamnophis couchii aquaticus,* whereas others, such as queen snakes *(Regina septemvittata)* and Butler's garter snakes *(T. butleri),* did not threaten or try to bite even when handled (also see Burghardt, 1978). On the face of it, such differences are quite perplexing, as we are dealing with often similar-sized and appearing sympatric species apparently subject to comparable predators. Careful systematic comparative work in the laboratory was lacking until recently.

Scudder and Burghardt (1983) tested laboratory-reared water snakes *(Nerodia)* from three species. The snakes were all offspring born to captive females from the same area in western Tennessee. Although the repertoire of defensive reactions to being approached and picked up by a human were similar, the relative frequency of such actions differed among the three species. One species *(N. cyclopion)* was most prone to use the most intense defensive response (striking), and one *(N. fasciata)* was by far the least likely to strike. Females in all three species were more likely to flatten and less likely to strike than males, but only in *N. fasciata* was this a significant difference. Because the animals had been reared in the laboratory in similar cages, had been isolated most of the time, and had been fed the same diet, the species and sex differences did not seem to be experiential in origin. Still, why the differences existed is not at all clear. And as the animals were 14 months of age when tested, the neonatal responses were undocumented.

Arnold and Bennett (1984) carried out a careful study of antipredator responses in many individuals roughly 2 weeks old born to 15 female plains garter snakes *(Thamnophis radix).* These authors found a characteristic but variable set of responses to a tail-touching stimulus that they could sum and use as a score of defensive arousal. They showed that littermates were more similar to each other than they were to offspring of other litters, on the average, and that substantial heritabilities (about 0.43) occurred.

Building on the preceding studies, Hal Herzog and I (Herzog and Burghardt, 1986) set out to look at species differences more thoroughly than in my incidental observations in the past. This study was stimulated by the birth in our lab of litters of a garter snake species restricted to Mexico, *T. melanogaster,* in which both the adults and the newborns were highly prone to strike any intruding stimulus.

Neonate snakes respond to approach and contact by humans and other animals with a variety of behaviors, depending on the species. These may include "defensive" tongue flicks (Gove, 1979; Gove and Burghardt, 1983), coiling, writhing, tail vibration, hissing, neck expansion, cloacal discharge, head hiding, flight, and striking. The last two behaviors were of especial interest, as they were clear opposites and, unlike some others, would occur even when the snake was only approached by a "threatening" object, but not touched or handled. Our method was to individually test snakes isolated at birth in individual plastic boxes. Testing was within the first 24 h after birth in an 59 × 54 cm arena. The experimenter introduced the snake into the arena and brought his forefinger to the front of the snake's snout at about 2 cm away and kept it as close as possible to that distance for 60 s. After a 30-s interval, the finger was reintroduced but, this time, was moved back and forth at the rate of about 4 cps. These are referred to as moving and nonmoving tests, respectively.

Our first study (Herzog and Burghardt, 1986), based on at least 70 newborn snakes from each species tested within 24 h after birth, showed that neonate *T. melanogaster* were most prone to strike and that neonate *T. sirtalis* and *T. butleri* were far less likely to do so. Concurrent open-field tests showed no pattern of relationship between such defensive responses and latency to locomote in the open-field or ambulation time. We found considerable similarity in the pattern of response by the neonates and adult females from the same populations when tested under comparable conditions.

A second study on habituation showed that, although daily tests led to rapid suppression of the response, recovery was rapid, and groups soon once again sorted themselves out as they had been sorted originally. Correlations across trials remained quite high and consistent. However, *T. melanogaster* habituated more than *T. butleri,* even considering the higher baseline of the former. More important is the fact that litter differences were great in both species, and so were individual differences within litters, not only in the readiness to strike, but also in the rate and extent of habituation. Such individual variability in both feeding and antipredatory behavior in neonate snakes from the same population and even within the same litter cannot be easily explained by calling on some postnatal experience difference or the effects of sex.

SOCIAL ORGANIZATION

Crocodilians have not only extended postnatal parental care but complex hierarchies and territorial systems (Garrick, Lang, and Herzog, 1978), vocalization and postural communication systems, and perhaps one of the most sophisticated magnetic orientation systems yet demonstrated in vertebrates (Rodda, 1985). In caimans, group coordinated capture of fish also occurs (Schaller and Crawshaw, 1982).

Snakes and turtles also show some remarkable social behavior, but their social organization is poorly understood. A fair amount is known about lizards, however.

The two radiations involving the largest sized individuals, the monitors and iguanas, seem to have really rather remarkable social structures (e.g., Auffenberg, 1981; Burghardt, 1977b; Burghardt and Rand, 1982). I will limit dicussion here to iguanas.

Green iguanas *(Iguana iguana)* are large herbivorous lizards found throughout much of Central and South America. Their ecology and behavior have been extensively studied in Panama since the mid-1960s, and other major studies have taken place in Honduras, Curaçao, Colombia, Costa Rica, and Venezuela. Although other iguana species have also been studied (references in Burghardt and Rand, 1982), the social behavior of green iguanas has been most thoroughly explored. Green iguanas have a polygynous mating system in which males defend an elevated spatial territory typically devoid of food or resources other than sleeping perches and basking sites. Females select from among these territories and may compete among themselves and set up dominance hierarchies (Burghardt, unpublished observations, 1982; Rodda, personal communication, 1982). Males and females display with head and dewlap bobs, and male displays, at least, are individually discriminable (Dugan, 1982a, b).

Ontogenetically, we have found that neonate iguanas emerging from communal nest sites in Panama are highly gregarious and engage in numerous obvious social behaviors, such as tongue touching and synchronizing movements (Burghardt, 1977b; Burghardt, Greene, and Rand, 1977). Hatchlings emigrate from their nest sites in groups and tend to remain in proximity to each other for many months. This is shown in sleeping-group size; an adaptive reason for such grouping may lay in our observations that those in larger groups have faster growth rates (Burghardt and Rand, 1985).

The role that thermoregulation may play in sociality in green iguanas is suggested by Boersma's study (1982) of marine iguanas *(Amblyrhynchus)* in the Galapagos. She found that they form large sleeping piles (huddles) at night. These serve to retard body cooling, especially of the innermost animals, to the extent that food digestion is greatly speeded up; the "lucky" animals are also ready to "go" earlier in the morning than their cooler conspecifics, which need more time to warm up.

Although the neonate sociality of iguanas may be related to their subsequent adult behavior, agonism also occurs. In our lab colony of 12 wild-caught hatchlings, now 4½ years old, aggression between males became damaging when they reached sexual maturity, and the second, third, and fourth largest males had to be removed. Interestingly, the smallest male, only about 20% the weight of the dominant, was never attacked, even though he gave assertion displays frequently and, on one occasion, bit the dewlap of the large male rather vigorously, with no response from the latter (V. Cobb, personal communication, 1985). He has not been observed to copulate with females or even to attempt to.

There are other reasons for viewing neonate iguanas as having ecological and social adaptations different from those of the adult. Hatchling iguanas have an eye spot on their upper eyelid that gives the impression that their eyes are open when, in fact, they are closed (photo in Burghardt, 1977b). This eyespot may be used in social communication among basking or sleeping iguanas, especially the latter, as basking iguanas almost always have their eyes open and are alert. On the other hand, the eyespot could fool a predator by falsely signalling alertness.

Another difference from adults is that, after observing the emergence from nest sites of iguanas during complete daylight monitoring on Slothia, a tiny islet used for communal nesting in Panama, we discovered, (through the use of fencing surrounding the nest site), that as many or more hatchlings emerge during the night than during the day (Drummond and Burghardt, 1983). This observation was of considerable interest because iguanas are otherwise completely diurnal in their activities, generally becoming active only after warming up in the morning sun, not even moving until well after dawn, and moving to sleeping perches or burrows shortly before sunset and well before dark. Indeed, iguanas are highly visual lizards with good color and form perception (Rensch and Adrian-Hinsberg, 1964). The hatchlings appear to visually monitor each other as well as predator and landscape features when migrating from the nest site, as well as from the islet itself (Burghardt, 1977b; Drummond and Burghardt, 1982). Many hatchlings, in contrast, left the nest holes in complete darkness when the air temperature was (24–26°C), well below their normally preferred activity body temperature. After nest emergence, no further nocturnal behavior has been recorded.

Why this nocturnal activity? Perhaps it is a means of avoiding predators, such as birds and basilisk lizards, which begin to gather at communal nest sites during hatch times and have been observed capturing hatchlings (Greene, Burghardt, Dugan, and Rand, 1978). During diurnal emergence, the iguanas may peer out of the holes repeatedly and may wait for hours before making their move, lending support to the predation hypothesis (Burghardt *et al.*, 1977; Drummond and Burghardt, 1982). We have observations and films of successful and unsuccessful dive-bomb attacks by birds *(Anis)* on iguanas at the entrance to their nest holes.

The young often emerge in groups and leave the nest site together in the same direction (Drummond and Burghardt, 1982). Groups seem to make better "decisions" than do singletons. Iguanas hatching from different holes may approach one another and lick or tongue-touch each other (Burghardt *et al.*, 1977). The grouping behavior seems to be related to several factors that can not yet be totally partitioned. Avoiding predation is an obvious one, of course, but enhanced decision-making for orientation and movements, the location of food and sleeping resources, the social stimulation of feeding, and the mutual transmittal of the hindgut fermentation microbes (Troyer, 1982) that aid in processing a high-cellulose diet are all possibilities.

In summary, a careful consideration of the behavioral ecology of the neonates is necessary to even postulate evolutionary as well as proximate explanations. Animals without parental care often allow the uncovering of relations between ecological and behavioral parameters in neonates because the buffering effects of parental care are absent.

GORDON M.
BURGHARDT

The sensory channels and the perceptual cues used by reptiles to communicate are diverse and involve chemicals, visual cues, tactile stimuli, and sounds (especially diverse in crocodilians and geckonid lizards). Whereas sounds are generally less salient in most reptiles, vision may be superior to that of many mammals, but inferior to that of most birds, although diurnal-nocturnal habits are undoubtedly influential. Many lizards seem to have excellent form and color vision. Chemical cues, especially those perceived through the olfactory and vomeronasal organs, may be typically more salient, at least in snakes, than in many mammals and birds.

The early ontogeny of displays in lizards poses a number of interesting questions. A study by Roggenbuck and Jenssen (1986) established that the performance of head bobs in newly hatched eastern fence lizards *(Sceloporus undulatus)* is basically complete and in the adult form shortly after birth. In a study of filmed displays by 36 laboratory-born animals from 8 clutches, the authors found that duration measures of the first 12 units in each display (which were of two major types) were remarkably consistent over time. Further, of the approximate 60% of the variance explained between lizards for both A and B displays, about 24% was attributable to that between clutches and about 28% to that among clutchmates. Only 7% was due to age (up to adulthood). Furthermore, the stereotypy of the displays neither increased nor decreased over time. But such stereotypy, rather than making this behavior developmentally uninteresting, poses some intriguing questions. For example, the context in which the behavior occurred or the message being conveyed is not at all clear in the hatchlings and juveniles. The authors suggested that their failure to discern a function for hatchling displays, as well as for the apparently haphazard stimulation of display performance by the lizards, may indicate that the lizards were playing, or that hormones or conditioning may significantly affect "the function of reptilian communication behavior" (p. 164).

Such ideas lead to the question of the role of experience in reptiles. Although reptiles do have much more specific "instinctive" (genetically programmed) knowledge for getting started in the world, this does not mean that learning is unimportant. Reptiles can learn rather complex things, but we must deal with their world, not a mammalian one. Thus, body temperature, food habits and eating schedule, and seasonality, among other factors, must be considered.

Emotional expressions are even less easy to study in reptiles. Their general lack of the whines, cries, screams, and whimpers when hurt or suffering that mammals and sometimes birds express makes it difficult to infer affective state. Lack of vocal communication is undoubtedly related to the lack of parental care and the diminished need for such signals to communicate neonatal needs to parents and other protective adults, and vice versa. Such factors mean that our usual methods of analysis can not suffice and makes even Griffin's "communication window" approach (1981) to the mind of animals less useful when dealing with animals that have different, or perhaps limited, intraspecific communicatory needs. Nonetheless, careful study is needed of communication mechanisms in reptiles, both ontogenetic and comparative. Recent speculation on the role of pheromones in therapsid (mammal-like) reptiles (Duvall, 1986; Duvall, Emg, and Graves, 1983); can also help us to frame evolutionary hypotheses testable on extant reptiles and mammals.

REPTILES, PRECOCITY, AND THE EVOLUTION OF PLAY

Definitions of play have been repeatedly discussed (see listings in Baldwin and Baldwin, 1981; Fagen, 1981), but the influential definition of play used by Bekoff and Byers (1981) captures the "objective" features:

> *Play* is all motor activity performed postnatally that appears to be purposeless in which motor patterns from other contexts may often be used in modified form and altered temporal sequencing. (p. 300)

The critical word here is *purposeless*. But the other major issue is that we have not been able to eliminate subjective elements. Indeed, Martin and Bateson (1985) stated that terms such as *enjoyable, rewarding,* and *spontaneous,* as anthropomorphically seen by humans, are essential components of locomotor play in cats. Martin and Caro (1985) combined the two ideas and wrote that "the distinguishing feature of play seems to be the subjective sense on the part of the observer that the behavior lacks any obvious prupose or immediate benefit" (p. 64). This is essentially the conclusion reached by Smith, Takhvar, Gore, and Vollstedt (1985, p. 39) in a review on play in children (play is "enjoyable" and "characterised by pretence"). Thus, by default, most students of play have assumed that its benefits *must* be delayed. Martin and Caro (1985) advanced a useful revision of the above definition:

> Play is all locomotor activity performed postnatally that *appears* to an observer to have no obvious immediate benefits for the player, in which motor patterns resembling those used in serious functional contexts may be used in modified forms. The motor acts constituting play have some or all of the following structural characteristics: exaggeration of movements, repetition of motor acts, and fragmentation or disordering of sequences of motor acts. Social play refers to play directed at conspecifics; object play refers to play directed at inanimate objects; locomotor play refers to apparently spontaneous movements which carry the individual about its environment; and predatory play refers to play directed towards living or dead prey. (p. 65)

The application of a defintion also needs to be addressed with empirical studies. Smith and Vollstedt (1985) tested five play criteria (intrinsic motivation, positive affect, nonliterality, dominated by means not ends, and flexibility) with observers of children and found that all but intrinsic motivation were associated with play ratings, and that higher ratings ocurred when two or more criteria were met simultaneously.

A serious problem, as pointed out by Martin (1984) and persuasively documented in Martin and Caro (1985), is the fact that no clear functions of play have been established in either animals or humans, although many plausible hypotheses and circumstantial evidence have been put forth (e.g., Bekoff and Byers, 1981; Byers, 1984; Fagen, 1981; Poirier, 1978; Smith, 1978, 1982). The proposed functions of play can be grouped into five major areas: the benefits accruing by way of physical exercise, perfection of nonsocial skills, perfection of social skills (including competitive relationships related to social roles), cognitive CNS development, and behavioral innovation. Chiszar (1985) added the interesting idea that play may inform parents about the competence of offspring. Not being able to establish *why* animals play has hindered research greatly.

Besides the issue of function, the other three basic ethological queries are those addressing causation, ontogeny, and evolution. All four need to be addressed in the field of play. It is my reading of the literature that our understanding of these areas of play research are also rather primitive. The issue of evolution, particularly of the transition from nonplaying animals to those that play, has been neglected. Most previous models of play, including the mathematical ones (Fagen, 1981), suffer from this neglect.

OVERVIEW OF THE SURPLUS RESOURCE MODEL

Recently (Burghardt, 1982, 1984), I considered the evolution of play from nonplay by comparing reptiles, in which there is no good evidence of play, with mammals and birds. All orders of mammals seem to have at least some representatives that play. Play in birds is more restricted both taxonomically and topographically (Fagen, 1981; Ficken, 1977). No clear evidence of play appears in fishes, amphibians, or invertebrates. MacLean (1986) also argued that play is a primary behavioral distinction between reptiles and mammals that must be addressed. My treatment of play took its cue from the surplus energy theory as put forth by Spencer (1872), which has rarely received attention since the attack by Groos (1898), and which apparently was never explicitly applied to the reptile/mammal-bird transitions. Smith (1978) provided a balanced overview of the history of various play theories, including the surplus energy theory.

Surplus resource theory was originally formulated as a qualitiative model that outlined a different way of looking at play. Two underlying premises of this approach are (a) that the benefits of play may often be minor, adventitious, and of value only under limited conditions, and (b) that play has its origin in behavior that has proximal causes and benefits, any delayed benefits being a derived phenomenon of generally less importance than is currently supposed. Critical transition activities may be difficult to recognize as play. Thus, the dilemmas of definition and function are more inherent in the phenomena than in the researchers' lack of experimental and observational precision. Highly organized vigorous play could thus be an exaptation, not an adaptation, in the terminology of Gould and Vrba (1982).

Basically, the theory is based on three concepts: energy, boredom, and deterioration. Supporting evidence for these three notions is given in Burghardt (1984). Only a brief synopsis is provided here, preparatory to the presentation and evaluation of some predictions deriving from the theory. The main, but not exclusive, focus is on comparisons and contrasts (Table 1) that, taken together, largely underlie the *discontinuity* in play between reptiles and endotherms.

ENERGY. As discussed above, reptiles are limited in their ability to engage in sustained vigorous behavior because of their low maximal rates of oxygen consumption and their reliance on anaerobic metabolism. Mammals generally have more effective means of turning stored energy into active behavior that has fewer detrimental effects, such as exhaustion. This is true even if the costs of endothermy are added in. Thus, a most important point to keep in mind is that physiological metabolic limitations deter reptiles from engaging in mammalian-style vigorous play. Reptiles do engage in exploration and curiosity, however (see below). Motivational energy or drives are a different use of the term *energy* that should not be confused with its meaning here. I earlier treated four usages of *energy* and *surplus* as applied to play (Burghardt, 1984). Given that mammalian physiology is more conducive to play, how did the evolution from the reptile to the mammal levels occur?

DETERIORATION. The evolution of parental care removed some of the selective pressures maintaining the precise precocial abilities that neonate reptiles needed for survival in the absence of parental nurturance, guidance, and protection. Thus, neonatal endotherms underwent a certain amount of "degeneration" of systems of innate response mechanisms because of relaxed natural selection as well as selection for behavior more adaptive in a parental care system. Threshold changes, stereotypy, and stimulus control may all have been affected, as well as the underlying physiological and motivational conditions. The neonate endotherm had to adapt to a rather different environment. Play in primates seems to be positively correlated with the degree of immaturity and the length of dependency (Poirier, 1978). The view of Groos (1898) that infancy in mammals exists because of play is still favorably quoted today. I think he had it reversed. Today, we recognize that neonates are not merely incomplete, poorly adapted versions of the adult.

Consider the implications of the Hall and Williams (1983) research showing that, when carefully teased apart, neonatal feeding in rats (sucking) shares few or no developmental continuities with adult feeding. Further, neonatal feeding experience or maternal care plays virtually no role in the topography of rat feeding. That is, mammals with evolved behavior patterns specifically adapted to the parental care niche have retained the species-typical behavior that reptiles have always displayed precocially. To some extent, then, the term *deterioration* may be misleading. What may have happened in the transition between reptiles and mammals was a parentally induced domesticationlike process, paralleling the changes seen in species domesticated by humans (cf. Price, 1984) in which animals are removed from the selection presssures that keep certain skills honed. Here, a form of heterochrony (neoteny) often occurs, as in dog breeds that retain juvenile morphology and behavior (see also Gould, 1977, especially his discussion of progenesis; Coppinger, Glendinning, Torop, Malthay, Sutherland, and Smith, 1987; Fagen, 1981).

BOREDOM. Along with parental care came a less stimulating, as well as less demanding, environment. There is some evidence, reviewed by Baldwin and Baldwin (1977), that optimal arousal is a factor in play. Certainly, we know that neonate mammals often need sensory stimulation for proper development and even enhanced learning (Hofer, 1981; Poirier, 1978). In an archaic cretaceous mammal, with its motivational, sensory, neurological, and response systems for serious precocial behavior still largely intact *and* necessary for adult behavior, the thresholds for such responses neonatally may have been lowered at the same time that the stimuli evoking the responses were being broadened and the resulting behavior became more disorganized. But these response systems were still important as early precursors of counterpart activities performed by the adult (such as foraging, prey killing and handling, defense and escape, and finding and using shelter). *Boredom,* although not a scientific term, seems to capture the idea I am trying to convey here, perhaps better than any other (it was also used by Lancy 1980). Suboptimal afference (suggested by N. Greenberg, personal communication, 1986), stimulus seeking, drives leading to stimulus change or novelty, and optimal arousal also convey aspects involved.

IMPLICATIONS. The chief difference of this approach from previous ones is that the initial advantages of incipient playlike behavior did not involve any particular functions (such as perfecting later behavior, increasing endurance, and incorporating flexibility). "Play" was a disparate constellation of *ad hoc* mechanisms used to maintain the continuity of the endothermal and behaviorial systems bridging the periods of juvenile dependence and adult responsibilities. The deterioration of certain neonatal response systems through parental care, the lowering of thresholds and the broadening of effective stimuli, and the increased aerobic metabolic capacities resulting from endothermy led to a reorganization of developmental processes so that play, as well as other experiential avenues, was not only available to homeotherms but may very well have had to be exploited by them for continued survival, by replacing lost, suppressed, or maturationally delayed "instincts."

An independent drive or motivation for play, which does seem to occur (e.g., Kortlandt, 1955; Rasa, 1984), would be a subsequent evolutionary development that takes us further from the origins of play itself. Such motivation may have some connection with Piaget's earliest stage of play in children (1962): mastery or practice play. There appears to be no firm evidence for an animal analogue of Piaget's second stage (symbolic play) unless we force interpretations of cats playing with balls of yarn, although his third stage (games with rules) may superficially resemble social play in both animals and human toddlers.

Ultimately, the difficulties in defining play or in adequately distinguishing it from other developmental processes seem to be due to the diffuse nature of play itself, not to a failure of our ability to delimit and define. In any event, play may have been a major factor in the eventual "improved" ability of endotherms, compared to that of reptiles, to have an enlarged repertoire of highly skilled response systems, as modeled by means of a topographic landscape (Figure 1). It should be noted that the ordinate represents a measure of behavioral complexity, not fitness. To reach this new level of behavioral complexity, endotherms had to dip into an ontogenetic valley of less precocial and independent behavior and to forgo the neonatal precocial complexity found in reptiles. Kortlandt (1955) argued independently that the function of play is to allow animals to have more complex abilities and to adapt precisely as adults to changing environmental conditions in ways that innate skills could not provide for. Thus, the animal has an innate drive to learn via play, rather than being provided with innate skills, My view is compatible with this idea and offers a broad evolutionary scenario for the transition. But it should be emphasized that any function of play is almost certainly a polishing and not a formative one, and also that other pathways may exist to the same end.

Increased brain size is, by this approach, not a causal correlate of play, but more an additional setting factor, perhaps a consequence of increased metabolic rates (cf. Armstrong, 1983; Harvey and Bennett, 1983; Martin, 1981). Regardless, recent experiments (Renner and Rosenzweig, 1986) do not support the view (Fagen, 1981) that *social* play differs in rats raised in environmentally enriched or impoverished conditions and is responsible for the increased brain weights found in the former condition.

A new formulation of a problem that allows us to look at phenomena in a

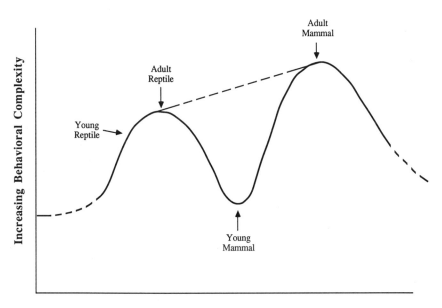

Figure 1. A topographic landscape illustrating the argument that the complexity of behavior in endotherms, especially mammals, resulted from a reorganization of the ontogeny of some response systems. Changes in neonatal behavior and its experiential basis are derived from a more effective metabolism, the evolution of parental care and the consequential deterioration of precocial response systems, and the motivational and stimulus needs of the young animal.

different light and that brings together scattered data and insights has its value even if the overall framework cannot be easily proved or tested. But clearly such "retrospective validity" is of limited use if it does not also lead to asking specific questions and predicting outcomes. Such hypothesis testing is difficult in comparative ethology and psychology when one is dealing with diverse animals with a host of adaptations and phylogenetic histories that reflect a constellation of selective pressures and their ensuing costs and benefits. Nonetheless, I will now play the game of making ontogenetic and comparative predictions, with an "all things being equal" proviso. Although there are traps in this game, they are of the same sort found in all comparative analyses, although often unrecognized (see Jarman, 1982, and Clutton-Brock and Harvey, 1984, for recent reviews of interspecific comparisons in ethology and sociobiology).

A major problem in comparing the quality and quantity of play engaged in by different species is the range of variability one finds within a species, especially among different populations (see below). This variability is compounded by the different methods used to record and classify behavior; by the necessary reliance on field, captive, and even home-reared animals; and by the lack of any information at all for most species of mammals and birds. Still, a series of predictions resutling from the surplus resource view outlined here, made as strong as feasible, may, at the very least, encourage observations that will lead to more effective comaprative integrative formulations. I have relied heavily on Fagen's (1981) thorough review of play in my evaluation of existing data. These predictions should be evaluated quantitatively and probabilistically.

The main reason for presenting these ideas is to demonstrate that considerations of ectotherm–endotherm differences can provide some ideas for looking at the comparative diversity of behavior within birds and mammals.

COMPARATIVE EVIDENCE AND PREDICTIONS

Let us now consider some predictions about play in mammals and birds, beginning with those related to metabolism. These are a combination of comparative questions and experimentally and descriptively addressable developmental aspects. Body size plays an important role in these predictions, which were derived initially without benefit of the recent allometric and comparative physiology reviews, which, however, are germane and will be essential for their adequate testing once sufficient data are in place (e.g., Calder, 1984; Peters, 1983; Schmidt-Nielsen, 1984). The first nine predictions stem from metabolic considerations, and predictions 10–19 from developmental considerations:

1. *Very small endotherms should play rarely, simply, or not at all.* The smallest birds and mammals are larger than the smallest reptiles and amphibians. They are not as small as reptiles and amphibians because of the enormous costs of endothermy as the volume-to-surface-area ratio decreases (Tracy, 1977; also see p. 115). Indeed, some small endotherms, such as hummingbirds, have body temperatures that fluctuate widely, even in adults, and neonates of many species cannot adequately thermoregulate by themselves. In situations where energy is so limiting, surplus

resource theory holds that play would not occur unless the benefits were very great. Tiny hummingbirds, rodents, and other high-metabolic-rate animals have rarely, if ever, been reported to play. Prediction 1 thus states that small endotherms are less likely to play because they are in an energy-limiting situation unlikely to provide for an accumulation of an expendable resource. Furthermore, their energy needs often must be satisfied by a huge expenditure of time. A 10-g warbler must capture almost two prey per minute of a 12-h active day (Peters, 1983).

2. *Within the smallest body-size lineages (e.g., a family) the smaller species should be less playful than moderate-size or large members.* This is a corollary of Prediction 1 and may explain why house mice, for example, play far less, and less complexly (i.e., no social play), than do rats (Poole and Fish, 1975). Fagen (1981, pp. 81–82) gave a beautiful example of the relationship between body size and the complexity of play in dasyurid marsupials, where the small "mouselike" species have the simplest play. As the taxa become larger in body size range, as in mustelids, the relationship apparently does not hold (Gittleman, pers. comm, 1986). But social complexity also varies greatly, the larger being more solitary and more omnivorous.

3. *Animals larger than the typical mammal should often play in less metabolically costly ways.* Although, below a certain size within a lineage, play should be less evident, large and bulky mammals should show less whole-body vigorous play involving rapid rolling over, jumping, and so on. Play should instead involve more head and limb movements than involvement of the entire body. Garland (1983a) showed that, over all mammals, the optimal size with regard to maximal running speed is about 119 kg. We also know that the per kilogram cost of locomotion goes down as animal size increases, although the total costs do go up. But the picture apparently changes if rapid locomotion is involved. Thus, for a 10-g mammal to run at minimum gallop speed, the metabolic rate would only have to double from the zero-speed rate, whereas for a 450-kg mammal the rate would be 11.8 times faster (Calder, 1984).

It has been shown that the cost of moving vertically up slopes or of carrying loads is independent of body size (Schmidt-Nielsen, 1984). This means that the relative increased aerobic cost for small endotherms of climbing, jumping, and otherwise engaging in the vigorous behavior characteristic of play is far less than for large mammals (Taylor, Caldwell, and Rowntree, 1972). Huey and Hertz (1982, 1984) made a similar finding for sprint speed in different sizes of an agamid lizard; they even found that maximum speed in a small lizard running up a 60° slope was about the same as on the level. Interestingly, acceleration seemed largely independent of both body size and slope. Clearly, the predatory and defensive maneuvers of a large animal can be quick. But a size should be reached at which "turning on" full-body vigorous activity, as will as the frequent starts, stops, jumps, and turns of vigorous play, should have increasing costs for a heavy mammal and thus is best done only for behavior with a current function, one less likely to be called play. Some variance may be related to the degree of physical activity normally engaged in by the adult—ungulates, perhaps, because they have evolved mechanisms for turning on and off flight rapidly in their open environment habitats. Careful assessment of play in rhino, buffalo, elephant, whale, bear, gorilla, and other large species is needed. In any event, Peters (1983) concluded that larger animals may be generally less active than small ones. The increased possibility of serious injury during rapid locomotion in large animals may also contribute to this difference.

4. *Play should be very sensitive to nutritional and thermal needs.* Like small endotherms, animals of any size that have evolved with severe and continuing constraints on nutrition and thermoregulation should be less likely to play than related species in more benign environments. Also, species that rely on toxic or nutrient-poor food (e.g., anteaters and folivores) should, *as species,* play little, for their metabolic rates are lower (McNab, 1980), and they are generally less active than related species with more nutritious diets (cf. frugivorous and folivorous monkeys). In species where play is prominent, play should be readily dispensed with in times of even mild thermal and nutritional stress. This prediction has been confirmed in squirrel monkeys, bighorn sheep, caribou, and vervet monkeys in wild populations (Baldwin and Baldwin, 1974; Berger, 1979; Lee, 1984; Müller-Schwarze and Müller-Schwarze, 1982) and in experimental manipulations of captive groups of monkeys and deer (Baldwin and Baldwin, 1976; Müller-Schwarze, Stagge, and Müller-Schwarze, 1982). Other evidence supports this proposition (Lancy, 1980) and suggests additional characteristics of benign environments.

Geist (1983) argued that the evolution of Ice Age mammals derived from a proximal mechanism by which the developing zygote in a well-fed mother received signals that prepared it to behave differently from offspring of poorly fed mothers; in particular, the latter indicates the presence of intense competition for limited available resources. The offspring of a female on a high-protein diet is "always on the go! It explores, runs, plays, and is much on the move" (p. 126). Along with other traits, this one leads to a dispersal phenotype that is the source of new species. In contrast, an offspring of a restricted-diet mother is physically smaller, more lethargic, and more aggressive, seeking to reduce maintenance costs to a minimum, and thus is termed a *maintenance phenotype.*

5. *Well-cared-for captive animals should play more than their wild counterparts.* Young mammals, besides having food, thermal, and defensive needs supplied in part by parents, have the time and metabolic capacities for play. Adults not only need to provide for themselves and any offspring but also are confronted with demands for territorial establishment and defense, maintaining social position, finding and courting mates, building and maintaining shelters, and so on. In captivity, these demands are reduced, and boredom, among other factors, may lead to increased adult play (see also above paragraph). In fact, this is what has been often noted: greater play frequency by both juveniles and adults in captivity, with a proportionally greater increase among adults (Fagen, 1981). Observations on pet and hand-reared animals certainly point out the possibility and form of play behaviors. They tell us little about the ubiquity and importance of play in natural environments.

6. *Birds and mammals with very low rates of metabolism should play less than those with higher metabolic rates.* Folivores might be predicted to be particularly low in play, along with other animals eating low-energy or potentially toxic food (e.g., ant specialists). Their metabolic rates are relatively low (McNab, 1980). Indeed, play in sloths, anteaters, and so on is rare and/or very subtle and in slow motion. Even a primate, the slow loris, was thought not to play until recently (Ehrlich and Musicant, 1977). The problem in testing this prediction (which is a rearrangement of Prediction 4) within a group such as primates is that, even for this most well-studied family, the time budget data are limited, and the observation conditions are diverse and really not comparable (see Table 5-1 in Fagen, 1981).

7. *As a group, birds should be less playful than mammals.* Factually, the data support this prediction (Fagen, 1981), which follows from the metabolic data indicating that birds are more likely to operate at their physiological limits than are mammals, to be more continuously active, and to have higher body temperatures and energy requirements to boot. Birds are also smaller, on the average, than mammals, the majority of species being in the songbird range, or weighing less than a small rodent such as *Peromyscus*. In addition, postnatal growth in birds is much faster than in mammals: the time required to double in weight is roughly one-third as long in birds, and growth to adulthood is even more pronounced in favor of birds. Likewise, oviparity among homeotherms is faster than viviparity in terms of both embryological and postnatal growth (Calder, 1984; Case, 1978b). Together, these points suggest that birds have used endothermy to maximize rapid growth, continuing the reptilian growth pattern, but much more effectively; thus, the surplus energetic and temporal resources are less available for play, as it is typically recognized.

Adultlike "serious" behavior, although not as precocial as in reptiles, could have been developmentally delayed in even very altricial songbirds, and more "hard-wired" maturation could take place without the deterioration of response systems because development is so rapid. On the other hand, it is possible that birds merely began hatching out their young at less developed stages than did reptiles. Such premature hatching could have been a consequence of several factors, one of which is that postnatal growth is always relatively faster than prenatal growth, a fact leading Calder (1984) to argue that, all things being equal, selection should favor an early altricial birth. As Fagen (1981) suggested, avian play needs much more study; some species, such as the raven, are apparently among the most playful animals known. Study of the ethology, the life history, and the physiology of such species would add greatly to theoretical developments in play research.

8. *Species that engage in sporadic vigorous behavior (e.g., foraging excursions) should play more than species that are active near the limits of their physiology.* This prediction may seem somewhat contradictory in comparison to reptiles because many reptiles are indeed capable of intermittent rapid behavior. But growing endotherms (Table 1) are more able to store energy (fat) in "good times," to engage in

aerobic activity, and to recuperate quickly, activities especially important for less-than-life-sustaining (capturing prey or outrunning predators) responses. Again, this phenomenon also applies to Prediction 4 and may be applied both to species (as here) and to populations living under different conditions.

This view predicts that more play should occur in animals (e.g., carnivores, ungulates, and primates) when they do not have to devote a substantial amount of their time or energy budget to essential activities. In lizards, the percentage of daily energy expenditure devoted to locomotion is generally much higher than in mammals (Garland, personal communication, 1986). Garland's (1983b) analysis suggests that small mammals should have small percentages ($<$ 1%) of their daily energy expenditure devoted to transport (locomotion) costs. In contrast, for large mammals, this percentage can reach 5%–15% or more. For large sedentary mammals, this cost is of little energetic significance. But for large mammals that need to be prepared to move long distances rapidly, and that thus have evolved the ingestion and the energetic budgets to do so, periods of rich resources provide them with available, expendable resources. Expending these resources through play may be a way of maintaining cardiovascular and muscular tone through exercise, perhaps derived from appetitive behavior. The frequent comments that play is pleasurable may be a reflection of the self-reinforcing nature of such activities. The classical ethological view that the goal of appetitive behavior was the attainment of releasing stimuli, and that performance of the resulting consummatory acts was the source of reinforcement, not the biological need served (Craig, 1918), can be amended to accommodate many of the features of play in surplus resource theory.

9. *Animals in an energy-efficient medium for locomotion (e.g., water) should be more playful than others. Additionally, animals both terrestrial and either aerial or aquatic should be most playful in the more energy-efficient medium.* Aquatic mammals, *as a group,* are probably the most playful (Fagen, 1981). Is this fact unrelated to the energy-efficient medium they locomote in and the large surpluses of fat accumulated for insulation purposes that can be expended in favorable conditions? Birds also perform their most vigorous play when flying or soaring. Otters are a good example of a play "champion" (Fagen, 1981) whose terrestrial play often involves sliding down snow and mud banks into water. I have recently found this prediction derived from energetics independently proposed in Peters (1983, p. 98). If play is to be found in a reptile, well-fed sea turtles in warm oceans may be the ones.

10. *Early in ontogeny, exploration and play should be difficult to distinguish, becoming more clear-cut later.* Deriving play from the exploratory and curiosity motives unquestionably present in reptiles (e.g., Burghardt, Allen, and Frank, 1986; Chiszar, Carter, Knight, Simonsen, and Taylor, 1976; Greenberg, 1985) would mean that, in reptiles, any play, defined as nonfunctional responses, would be hard to identify if it did exist, and also that, in the neonatal bird and mammal, such responses also would be hard to recognize. This difficulty has been well accepted even by those asserting that, later in ontogeny, a clear functional and topographic distinction appears (e.g., Hutt, 1966; West, 1977). Adang (1985) pointed out that

exploration can apply to social as well as physical environments. Note that the definition of play by Martin and Caro above does not allow for any distinction between exploration and (especially) locomotor and object play.

11. *Play should peak after neonates are less dependent on parents for food, warmth, and so on. Thus, precocial birds and mammals show play earlier than altricial species.* The evidence for this prediction seems quite straightforward. Ungulates and precocial rodents engage in locomotor play earlier than altricial relatives. Comparative data on deer show that caribou have less extended care till weaning, and that they begin playing earlier, compared to black-tailed or white-tailed deer (Müller-Schwarze and Müller-Schwarze, 1982).

Precocial locomotor behavior obviously makes possible the vigorous activities characteristic of play. But note that exploration is also not only possible but necessary to survival in precocial neonates. Certainly, newly hatched snakes and green iguanas engage in investigatory tongue-flicking behavior (Chiszar *et al.*, 1976) within seconds on exposure to the "light of day" (Burghardt, 1977b, and personal observation, 1965).

12. *Precocial species should be less playful than altricial species.* The more precocial the species, and thus the more reptilelike in a way that the theory views as critical, the less playlike behavior should be seen. Perhaps the best evidence for this prediction comes from birds. Those species most playful have extended periods of parental care of an intimate nature. Thus, in birds, one finds play in parrots and corvids, but it is rare or absent in waterfowl (Fagen, 1981). One should be cautious in comparing animals with different levels of precocity across major phylogenetic chasms, however, because of the large number of life history and physiological factors I postulate as influencing the nature and extent of play. Holding these relatively constant, as in comparing within a family, or order, at best, is called for. Thus, in the Pelecaniformes, there is evidence that the extent of play is correlated with the degree of altricial behavior (Fagen, 1981). Similarly, caribou, which begin play earlier than white-tailed deer, seem to be largely limited to locomotor and rotational play, whereas black-tailed and white-tailed deer engage in more social play and spend more time playing in general (Müller-Schwarze, 1984).

13. *Ontogenetically, there should be a trend from more energetically costly to more subtle play as animals mature.* Once play is liberated from the energetic costs early in ontogeny (for altricial animals), vigorous play should peak and then decline. For example, black bears that we observed (Burghardt, 1975a) showed a definite transition from wrestling and chasing games to those involving jaw wrestling and head jockeying. That is, play should begin to involve more head and limb movements than movements of the entire body insofar as morphologically possible. Orangutans also show this trend (Zucker, Dennon, Puteo, and Maple, 1986), as do primates in general (Symons, 1978).

This trend is due to several factors. One is the relation between body size and activity (Prediction 3), which also appears to hold ontogenetically (although the power function may be lower; Andrews and Pough, 1985). Another is the simple allocation of time; as animals mature, "serious" behaviors, such as finding food and mates and avoiding predators, must be performed by weaned and matured endotherms (see also Zucker *et al.*, 1986).

Of course, many have noted that the frequency of play is much lower in adult animals. An explanation for this shift was offered by Baldwin and Baldwin (1977), who postulated that the ontogenetic decline is due to a learning process in which older animals have reached a point where "there is little more novelty reinforcement to be had" (p. 368), and play thus extinguishes. One would think that a simple test would be to look at animals with limited play experience as juveniles. But this approach, too, would lead to little adult play, for "exploration and play behavior cannot gain much habit strength in deprived environments where there is little sensory stimulation reinforcement and, thus, these behaviors would be likely to extinguish quickly" (p. 368). Thus, this alternative explanation is untestable as stated.

14. *Juvenile animals may play in ways that presage important adult activities because of the presence of neurological, hormonal, motivational, and sensory mechanisms. These may also be sexually dimorphic.* Certainly, we know that precocial adultlike behavior of a sexual and aggressive nature can be stimulated in neonates by hormonal treatment in early life (e.g., Noble and Zitrin, 1942, for chicks; Crews, 1985, for garter snakes). However, sex differences in play and exploration may also be hormonally influenced (Baldwin and Baldwin, 1977; Poirier, 1978). They also may be environmentally stable. Coelho and Bramblett (1982) found that sex differences in baboon play were unaffected by major differences in rearing conditions.

Although it might be expected that females that are smaller than males as adults have more energy available for play, selection may have favored a more conservative expenditure of physical energy because of the need for more metabolic resources for reproduction. In those reptiles where male–male combat is absent, females are usually the larger sex, as number of offspring in most reptiles is associated with body size. In mammals and birds, clutch and litter size is far less dependent on female body size. In canids, were sex differences in adult roles are slight, sex differences are not found in play in spite of marked differences in levels of adult sociality (Biben, 1983).

15. *Sex differences in the frequency and type of play should be most pronounced in species in which adults are behaviorally dimorphic and in which experience is important in the ontogeny of social, locomotor, feeding, and defensive skills.* Insofar as the social roles and the behavioral repertoires differ between juveniles and adults and depend on experience, one would expect to find differences in the nature and extent of play between the sexes in juveniles. This expectation seems to be fulfilled in the literature, particularly in primates (e.g., Symons, 1978), where the more active and agonistic play of males early in ontogeny has been well documented. Because juveniles are more behaviorally monomorphic than adults, play provides one source of raw material for the elaboration and perfection of such differences. But note that this is a relatively weak prediction because there is nothing orthogenetic about the evolutionary paths that should result from the archaic play phe-

notypes postulated here. But, combining the ontogeny of sex differences with the different needs of adult males in different kinds of societies, Byers (1984) predicted the the more polygynous the society, the more diverse should be the play styles of male and female juveniles.

16. *Interindividual differences in the amount of play in various contexts (e.g., predatory and social) may reflect motivational level and maturation rather than correlating with later skill level.* Attempts to show relationships among different levels of play between individuals within litters and later behavior have been relatively unconvincing (Bekoff and Byers, 1981; Martin and Caro, 1985). But the search for such relationships is based on the assumption that skills are being learned or practiced. It is equally tenable to begin with the view that the timing and intensity of play differences is due to individual differences in motivational, metabolic, and sensory thresholds. In this view, precocity is an anticipation of adult proficiency and propensity, rather than being causally involved in shaping proficiency in those activities. This point can also apply to species differences in play that seem to covary with adult social responses (e.g., the hyrax; Caro and Alawi, 1985).

17. *Solitary locomotor-rotational play should be more common—and more representative of ancestral species—than social or object play.* If play is, in the first instance, derived from endogenous processes set in motion only by a lack of environmental stimulation, than it would follow that, in the absence of further development, "play" would most likely involve simple locomotor acts. Such activity is also common to most kinds of more complex play. In fact, locomotor-rotational play is by far the most common type. Byers (1984) surveyed the ungulates, where a reasonably complete data set exists, and documented that only about half of the species showing locomotor-rotational play exhibit social play. If a species has only one kind of play in its repertoire, it is most likely to be this one. (See also Prediction 2.)

18. *Behavior patterns necessarily performed in early neonatal life in birds and mammals should be rarely found elaborated in play.* One of the problems in defining and recognizing play in animals seems to be the perceived necessity that play be nonfunctional. This requirement seems overly restrictive (cf. Burghardt, 1982, and Smith, 1982). In any event, the surplus resource view suggests that highly functional ("serious") neonatal behaviors would not present the setting and motivational circumstances conducive to play. The elaboration and use of such behaviors in later life in different contexts is termed *ritualization*, which is defined by many of the characteristics of play, with the exception that it is deemed *more* stereotyped than its source behavior (see also Kortmulder, 1983). For example, many birds feed one another during courtship in a manner reminiscent of parent–offspring interactions.

19. *Behavior patterns largely evolved by neonatal endotherms (sucking, gaping, and thermoregulation) should rarely be found in play, although they may be found in adults in ritualized forms, particularly in courtship.* The absence of these behaviors in play puzzled Fagen (1981), but it is a corollary of Prediction 18. The fact that behaviors can occur later in courtship indicates that there is nothing intrinsic in them that

precludes their use in other contexts. And it has been noted that much animal "play" can itself appear to be formalized and even stereotyped in its repetitive nature.

FINAL THOUGHTS

I have argued here for a look at play from the reptile up, as it were, rather than, as is usual, from the human down. I have indicated a number of predictions compatible with, if not directly derivable from, the surplus resource view. Clearly, much more comparative work, particularly of a quantitative nature, is needed before even the correlational evidence can be marshaled one way or the other. The predictions listed here are clearly not independent of one another, nor are they presented in the most parsimonious way. The points about body size, metabolic rates, and play incidence could be reduced to one statement about an "optimal" size for play resulting from the constraints of energy budgets in very small endotherms and the large incremental costs of activity in large endotherms. Also, the 19 predictions are not either the only or the most well-phrased ones possible.

To experimentally test the surplus resource theory in the areas of ontogeny, physiology, and function will be difficult. I have not incorporated here studies on physiological and other proximate mechanisms that may also relate to play, such as those on "warm-up" effects (Golani, Bronchti, Moualem, and Teitelbaum, 1981) and on drug and nervous system interventions. Prenatal nutrition and motility, the temporal course of weaning, litter size, and hormonal variation may become future areas of proximal investigation. The areas covered by Predictions 14 and 16 seem particularly important in relation to developmental psychobiology. But experimental studies of very playful advanced animals are unlikely to give us much information on the question of origins, (Burghardt, 1977c), whereas studies on animals that play rarely, ambiguously, or in a less than vigorous manner are hard to plan, control, and interpet. Thus, correlational studies remain useful, as in the evidence that longevity in mammals can be explained by body size, metabolic rate, brain size, and preferred activity temperature, with the higher values being correlated with longevity (Hofman, 1983; Sacher, 1976, 1978; Sacher and Staffelt, 1974), or McNab's (1980) relation of basal metabolism rate to reproductive rate and food habits. It must be remembered, however, that comparative physiology is just beginning to provide data relevant to the comparative issues discussed here, and that the trends noted here may not stand up when more complete and well-controlled data are available (e.g., Hayssen and Lacy, 1985).

The larger goals of this and other efforts, however, should be to broaden our comparative approaches, to consider the ecology and pacing of behavioral development, to look for and evaluate the possible constraints underlying species differences, and to try to integrate, without confounding, proximal and evolutionary analyzes. Greene's distinction (1986) between pattern and process in evolutionary comparisons needs to be applied as solid comparative data appear. More analyses of within-species variation in animals from the same population living in comparable circumstances are needed to test the functional aspects of play, as well as the presumptive factors in the evolution of differences within reptiles and endotherms and in the transition between reptiles and both mammals and birds. If we are to speak to a larger audience, we need to present, through informed synthesis and speculation, a picture of where we are that allows some patterns to be detected from the many isolated data points so painstakingly and elegantly gathered. This book represents a step toward this end.

Acknowledgments

This chapter is based in part on talks given to the Winter Animal Behavior Conference, Park City, Utah in January 1984 and to the Animal Behavior Society, Raleigh, North Carolina, in June 1985. Preparation was supported in part by NSF Research Grant BNS 82-17569. The following provided valuable comments on early drafts: Elliot Blass, Ted Garland, Valerius Geist, John Gittleman, Neil Greenberg, Harry Greene, and Gordon Rodda.

REFERENCES

Adang, O. M. J. Exploratory aggression in chimpanzees. *Behaviour,* 1985, *95,* 138–163.
Alberts, J. R. Ontogeny of social recognition: An essay on mechanism and metaphor in behavioral development, In E. S. Gollin (Ed.), *The comparative development of adaptive skills: Evolutionary implications.* Hillsdale, NJ: Erlbaum, 1985.
Alberts, J. R., and May, B. Non-nutritive, thermotactile induction of filial huddling in rat pups. *Developmental Psychobiology,* 1984, *17,* 161–181.
Andrews, R. M., and Pough, F. H. Metabolism of squamate reptiles: Allometric and ecological relationships. *Physiological Zoology,* 1985, *58,* 214–231.
Armstrong, E. Relative brain size and metabolism in mammals. *Science,* 1983, *220,* 1302–1304.
Arnold, S. J. Some effects of early experience on feeding responses in the common garter snake, *Thamnophis sirtalis. Animal Behaviour,* 1978, *26,* 455–462.
Arnold, S. J. The microevolution of feeding behavior. In A. C. Kamil and T. D. Sargent (Eds.), *Foraging behavior: Ecological, ethological, and psychological approaches.* New York: Garland STPM, 1981.
Arnold, S. J., and Bennett, A. F. Behavioral variation in natural populations. III. Antipredator displays in the garter snake *Thamnophis radix. Animal Behaviour,* 1984, *32,* 1109–1118.
Auffenberg, W. *The behavioral ecology of the Komodo monitor.* Gainsville: University of Florida Press, 1981.
Avery, R. A. Thermoregulation, metabolism and social behaviour, In A. d'A. Bellairs and C. B. Cox (Eds.), *Morphology and biology of reptiles.* London: Acedemic Press, 1976.
Baldwin, J. D., and Baldwin, J. I. Exploration and social play in squirrel monkeys *(Saimiri). American Zoologist,* 1974, *14,* 303–315.
Baldwin, J. D., and Baldwin, J. I. Effects of food ecology on social play: A laboratory simulation. *Zeitschrift für Tierpsychologie,* 1976, *40,* 1–14.
Baldwin, J. D., and Baldwin, J. I. The role of learning phenomena in the ontogeny of exploration and play. In S. Chevalier-Skolnikoff and F. E. Poirier (Eds.), *Primate biosocial development: Biological, social, and ecological determinants.* New York: Garland, 1977.
Baldwin, J. D., and Baldwin, J. I. *Beyond sociobology.* New York: Elsevier, 1981.
Bartholomew, G. A. Energy metabolism. In M. S. Gordon (Ed.), *Animal physiology: Principles and adaptations.* New York: Macmillan, 1982.
Bateson, P. Rules and reciprocity in behavioural development. In P. Bateson and R. A. Hinde (Eds.), *Growing points in ethology.* London: Cambridge University Press, 1976.
Bateson, P. Discontinuities in development and changes in the organization of play in cats. In K. Immelmann, G. W. Barlow, L. Petrinovich, and M. Main (Eds.), *Behavioral development: The Bielefeld interdisciplinary project.* Cambridge: Cambridge University Press, 1981.
Bekoff, M., and Byers, J. A. A critical reanalysis of the ontogeny and phylogeny of mammalian social and locomotor play: An ethological hornet's nest. In K. Immelmann, G. W. Barlow, L. Petrinovich, and M. Main (Eds.), *Behavioral development: The Bielefeld interdisciplinary project.* Cambridge: Cambridge University Press, 1981.

Bekoff, M., and Byers, J. A. The development of behavior from evolutionary and ecological perspectives in mammals and birds. *Evolutionary Biology,* 1985, *19,* 215–286.

Bennett, A. F. The energetics of reptilian activity. In C. Gans and F. H. Pough (Eds.), *Biology of the reptilia,* (Vol. 13) London: Academic Press, 1982, pp. 155–199.

Bennett, A. F., and Ruben, J. A. The metabolic and thermoregulatory status of therapsids. In N. Hotton III, P. D. MacLean, J. J. Roth, and E. C. Roth (Eds.), *The ecology and biology of mammal-like reptiles.* Washington, D.C.: Smithsonian Institution, 1986.

Berger, J. Social ontogeny and behavioural diversity: Consequences for Bighorn sheep *Ovis canadensis* inhabiting desert and mountain environments. *Journal of Zoology (London),* 1979, *188,* 251–266.

Biben, M. Comparative ontogeny of social behaviour in three South American canids: the maned wolf, crab-eating fox and bush dog: Implications for sociality. *Animal Behaviour,* 1983, *31,* 814–826.

Blackburn, D. G., Vitt, L. J., and Beuchat, C. A. Eutherian-like reproductive specializations in a viviparous reptile. *Proceedings of the National Academy of Sciences,* 1984, *81,* 4860–4863.

Boersma, P. D. The benefits of sleeping aggregations in marine iguanas, *Amblyrhynchus cristatus.* In G. M. Burghardt and A. S. Rand (Eds.), *Iguanas of the world: Their behavior, ecology, and conservation.* Park Ridge, NJ: Noyes, 1982.

Brown, W. S., and MacLean, F. M. Conspecific scent-trailing by newborn timber rattlesnakes, *Crotalus horridus. Herpetologica,* 1983, *39,* 430–436.

Burghardt, G. M. Chemical perception in reptiles. In J. W. Johnston, Jr., D. G. Moulton, and A. Turk (Eds.), *Communication by chemical signals.* New York: Appleton-Century-Crofts, 1970.

Burghardt, G. M. Chemical cue preferences of newborn snakes: Influence of prenatal maternal experience. *Science,* 1971, *171,* 921–923.

Burghardt, G. M. Behavioral research on common animals in small zoos. In National Academy of Sciences (Eds.), *Research in zoos and aquariums.* Washington, DC: National Academy of Sciences, 1975a.

Burghardt, G. M. Chemical prey preference polymorphism in newborn garter snakes *Thamnopis sirtalis. Behaviour,* 1975b, *52,* 202–225.

Burghardt, G. M. Learning processes in reptiles. In C. Gans and D. Tinkle (Eds.), *The biology of the reptilia.* Vol. 7. *Ecology and behavior.* New York: Academic Press, 1977a.

Burghardt, G. M. Of iguanas and dinosaurs: social behavior and communication in neonate reptiles. *American Zoologist,* 1977b, *17,* 177–190.

Burghardt, G. M. Ontogeny of communication. In T. Sebeok (Ed.), *How animals communicate.* Bloomington: University of Indiana Press, 1977c.

Burghardt, G. M. Behavioral ontogeny in reptiles: whence, whither, and why. In G. M. Burghardt and M. Bekoff (Eds.), *The development of behavior: Comparative and evolutionary aspects.* New York: Garland STPM, 1978.

Burghardt, G. M. Comparison matters: Curiosity, bears, surplus energy, and why reptiles do not play. *Behavioral and Brain Sciences,* 1982, *5,* 159–160.

Burghardt, G. M. On the origins of play. In P. K. Smith (Ed.), *Play in animals and humans.* London: Basil Blackwell, 1984.

Burghardt, G. M., Wilcoxon, H. C., and Czaplicki, J. A. Conditioning in garter snakes: Aversion to palatable prey induced by delayed illness. *Animal Learning and Behavior,* 1973, *1,* 317–320.

Burghardt, G. M., Greene, H. W., and Rand, A. S. Social behavior in hatchling green iguanas: Life at a reptile rookery. *Science,* 1977, *195,* 681–691.

Burghardt, G. M., and Rand, A. S. (Eds.). *Iguanas of the world: Their behavior, ecology, and conservation.* Park Ridge, NJ: Noyes, 1982.

Burghardt, G. M., and Rand, A. S. Group size and growth rate in hatchling green iguanas *(Iguana iguana). Behavioral Ecology and Sociobiology,* 1985 *18,* 101–104.

Burghardt, G. M., Allen, B. A., and Frank, H. Exploratory tongue flicking by green iguanas in laboratory and field. In D. Duvall, D. Müller-Schwarze, and R. M. Silverstein (Eds.), *Chemical signals in vertebrates,* Vol. 4. New York: Plenum Press, 1986.

Byers, J. Play in ungulates. In P. K. Smith (Ed.), *Play in animals and humans.* London: Basil Blackwell, 1984.

Calder, W. A., III. *Size, function, and life history,* Cambridge: Harvard University Press, 1984.

Caro, T. M., and Alawi, R. M. Comparative aspects of behavioural development in two species of free-living hyrax. *Behaviour,* 1985, *95,* 87–109.

Case, T. J. Endothermy and parental care in the terrestrial vertebrates. *Amercian Naturalist,* 1978a, *112,* 861–874.

Case, T. J. On the evolution and adaptive significance of postnatal growth rates in the terrestrial vertebrates. *Quarterly Review of Biology*, 1978b, *53*, 243–282.

Charig, A. J. "Dinosaur monophyly and a new class of vertebrates": A critical review. In A. d'A. Bellairs and C. B. Cox (Eds.), *Morphology and biology of reptiles*. London: Academic Press, 1976.

Chiszar, D. Ontogeny of communicative behaviors. In E. S. Gollin (Ed.), *The comparative development of adaptive skills: Evolutionary implications*. Hillsdale, NJ: Lawrence Erlbaum, 1985.

Chiszar, D., Carter, T.; Knight, L., Simonsen, L., and Taylor, S. Investigatory behavior in the plains garter snake *(Thamnophis radix)* and several additional species. *Animal Learning and Behavior*, 1976, *4*, 273–278.

Clutton-Brock, T. H., and Harvey, P. Comparative approaches to investigating adaptation. In J. R. Krebs and N. B. Davies (Eds.), *Behavioural ecology*, 2nd ed. Sunderland, MA: Sinauer, 1984.

Coelho, A. M. Jr., and Bramblett, C. A. Social play in differentially reared infant and juvenile baboons *(Papio* sp.) *American Journal of Primatology*, 1982, *3*, 153–160.

Coppinger, R., Glendinning, J., Torop, E., Matthay, C., Sutherland, M., and Smith, C. Degree of behavioral neoteny differentiates canid polymorphs. *Ethology*, 1987, *75*, 89–108.

Craig, W. Appetites and aversions as constituents of instinct. *Biological Bulletin*, 1918, *34*, 91–107.

Crews, D. Effects of early sex steroid hormone treatment on courtship behavior and sexual attractivity in the red-sided garter snake, *Thamnophis sirtalis parietalis. Physiology and Behavior*, 1985, *35*, 569–575.

Crews, D., and Moore, M. C. Evolution of mechanisms controlling mating behavior. *Science*, 1986, *231*, 121–125.

Drummond, H. The role of vision in the predatory behavior of natricine snakes. *Animal Behavior*, 1985, *33*, 206–215.

Drummond, H., and Burghardt, G. M. Orientation in dispersing hatchling green iguanas, *Iguana Iguana*. In G. M. Burghardt and A. S. Rand (Eds.), *Iguanas of the world: Their behavior, ecology, and conservation*. Park Ridge, NJ: Noyes, 1982.

Drummond, H. D., and Burghardt, G. M. Nocturnal and diurnal nest emergence in green iguanas. *Journal of Herpetology*, 1983, *17*, 290–292.

Duellman, W. E. Reproductive modes in anuran amphibians: Phylogenetic significance of adaptive strategies. *South African Journal of Science*, 1985, *81*, 174–178.

Dugan, B. A. A field study of the headbob displays of male green iguanas *(Iguana iguana):* Variation in form and context. *Animal Behaviour*, 1982a, *30*, 327–338.

Dugan, B. A. The mating behavior of the green iguana, *Iguana iguana*. In G. M. Burghardt and A. S. Rand (Eds.), *Iguanas of the world: Their behavior, ecology, and conservation*. Park Ridge, NJ: Noyes, 1982b.

Dunham, A. E., and Miles, D. B. Patterns of covariation in life history traits of squamate reptiles: The effects of size and phylogeny reconsidered. *American Naturalist*, 185, *126*, 231–257.

Duvall, D. A new question of pheromones: Aspects of possible chemical signaling and reception in the mammal-like reptiles. In N. Hotton III, P. D. MacLean, J. J. Roth, and E. C. Roth (Eds.), *The ecology and biology of mammal-like reptiles*. Washington, DC: Smithsonian Institution, 1986.

Duvall, D., King, M. B., and Graves, B. M. Fossil and comparative evidence for possible chemical signaling in the mammal-like reptiles. In D. Müller-Schwarze and R. M. Silverstein (Eds.), *Chemical signals in vertebrates*, Vol. 3. New York: Plenum Press, 1983.

Ehrlich, A., and Musicant, A. Social and individual behaviors in captive slow lorises. *Behaviour*, 1977, *60*, 195–220.

Eisenberg, J. F. *The mammalian radiations*. Chicago: University of Chicago Press, 1981.

Evans, L. T. A motion picture study of maternal behavior of the lizard, *Eumeces obsoletus* Baird and Girard. *Copeia*, 1959, 103–110.

Fagen, R. *Animal play behavior*. New York: Oxford University Press, 1981.

Felsenstein, J. Phylogenies and the comparative method. *American Naturalist*, 1985, *125*, 1–15.

Ficken, M. S. Avian play. *Auk*, 1977, *94*, 573–582.

Fuchs, J. L., and Burghardt, G. M. Effects of early feeding experience on the responses of garter snakes to food chemicals. *Learning and Motivation*, 1971, *2*, 271–279.

Galef, B. J., Jr. The social transmission of food preferences: An adaptation for weaning in rats. *Journal of Comparative and Physiological Psychology*. 1977, *91*, 1136–1140.

Galef, B. J., Jr. The ecology of weaning: Parasitism and the achievement of independence by altricial animals. In D. J. Gubernick and P. H. Klopfer (Eds.), *Parental care in mammals*. New York: Plenum Press, 1981.

Ganchrow, J. R., Steiner, J. E., and Csnetto, S. Behavioral displays to gustatory stimuli in newborn rat pups. *Developmental Psychobiology*, 1986, *19*, 163–174.

Garland, T., Jr. The relation between maximal running speed and body mass in terrestrial mammals. *Journal of Zoology*, 1983a, *199*, 157–170.

Garland, T., Jr. Scaling the ecological cost of transport to body mass in terrestrial mammals. *American Naturalist*, 1983b, *121*, 571–587.

Garland, T., Jr. Locomotor performance and activity metabolism of *Cnemidophorus tigris* in relation to natural behaviors. In J. Wright (Ed.), *Biology of* Cnemidophorus, Seattle: University of Washington, in press.

Garland, T., Jr., and Arnold, S. J. Effects of a full stomach on locomotory performance of juvenile garter snakes. *Copeia*, 1983, *1983*, 1092–1096.

Garland, T., Jr., and Else, P. L. Seasonal, sexual, and individual variation in endurance and activity metabolism in a lizard. *American Journal of Physiology (Regulatory, Integrative and Comparative Physiology)*, in press.

Garland, T., Jr., Else, P. L., Hulbert, A. J., and Tap, P. Effects of endurance training and captivity on activity metabolism of a lizard. *American Journal of Physiology (Regulatory, Integrative and Comparative Physiology.)*, in press.

Garrick, L. D., Lang, J. F., and Herzog, H. A., Jr. Social signals of adult American alligators. *Bulletin of the American Museum of Natural History*, 1978, *160*, 157–192.

Gatten, R. E., Jr. The use of anaerobiosis by amphibians and reptiles. *American Zoologist*, 1985, *25*, 945–954.

Geist, V. On the evolution of ice age mammals and its significance to an understanding of speciations. *The ASB Bulletin*, 1983, *30*, 109–133.

Gittleman, J. L. The phylogeny of parental care in fishes. *Animal Behaviour*, 1981, *29*, 936–941.

Gleeson, T. T. The effects of training and captivity on the metabolic capacity of the lizard *Sceloporus occidentalis*. *Journal of Comparative Physiology*, 1979, *129*, 123–128.

Golani, I., Bronchti, G., Moualem, D., and Teitelbaum, P. "Warm-up" along dimensions of movement in the ontogeny of exploration in rats and other infant mammals. *Proceedings of the National Academy of Sciences USA*, 1981, *78*, 7226–7229.

Gorzula, S. Are caimans always in distress. *Biotropica*, 1985, *17*, 343–344.

Gould, S. J. *Ontogeny and phylogeny*. Cambridge: Harvard University Press, 1977.

Gould S. J., and Vrba, E. S. Exaptation—A missing term in the science of form. *Paleobiology*, 1982, *8*, 4–15.

Gove, D. A comparative study of snake and lizard tongue-flicking with an evolutionary hypothesis. *Zeitschrift für Tierpsychologie*, 1979, *51*, 58–76.

Gove, D., and Burghardt, G. M. Context correlated parameters of snake and lizard tongue-flicking. *Animal Behaviour*, 1983, *31*, 718–723.

Graves, B. M., Duvall, D., King, M. B., Lindstedt, S. L., and Gern, W. A. Initial den location by neonatal prairie rattlesnakes: functions, causes, and natural history in chemical ecology. In D. Duvall, D. Müller-Schwarze, and R. M. Silverstein (Eds.), *Chemical signals in vertebrates*, Vol. 4. New York: Plenum Press, 1986.

Greenberg, N. Observations on social feeding in lizards. *Herpetologica*, 1976, *32*, 348–352.

Greenberg, N. Physiological and behavioral thermoregulation in living reptiles. In R. D. K. Thomas and E. C. Olson (Eds.), *A cold look at the warm-blooded dinosaurs*. Boulder, CO: Westview Press, 1980.

Greenberg, N. Exploratory behavior and stress in the lizard, *Anolis carolinensis*. *Zeitschrift für Tierpsychologie*, 1985, *70*, 89–102.

Greene, H. W. Diet and arboreality in the emerald monitor, *Varanus prasinus*, with comments on the study of adaptation. *Fieldiana (Zoology)*, 1986, New Series 31 (1370), 1–12.

Greene, H. W. Antipredator responses in reptiles. In R. Huey and C. Gans (Eds.), *Biology of the reptilia*, Vol. 16, New York: Wiley, 1987.

Greene, H. W., Burghardt, G. M., Dugan, B. A., and Rand, A. S. Predation and the defensive behavior of green iguanas (*Reptilia, Lacertilia, Iguanidae*). *Journal of Herpetology*, 1978, *12*, 169–176.

Griffin, D. R. *The question of animal awareness: Evolutionary continuity of mental experience*. (2nd ed.). New York: Rockefeller University Press, 1981.

Groos, K. *The play of animals*. New York: D. Appleton, 1898.

Grzimek, B. *Animal life encyclopedia*, 13 vols. New York: Van Nostrand, 1974.

Guillette, L. J., Jr., and Hotton, N., III. The evolution of mammalian reproductive characteristics in therapsid reptiles. In N. Hotton III, P. D. MacLean, J. J. Roth, and E. C. Roth (Eds.), *The ecology and biology of mammal-like reptiles*. Washington, DC: Smithsonian Institution, 1986.

Hall, W. G., and Williams, C. L. Suckling isn't feeding, or is it? A search for developmental continuities. *Advances in the Study of Behavior; 13,* 219–254.

Harlow, H. F., and Harlow, M. K. Effects of various mother-infant relationships on rhesus monkey behaviors. In B. M. Foss (Ed.), *Determinants of infant behaviour,* Vol. 4. London: Methuen, 1965.

Harvey, P. H., and Bennett, P. M. Brain size, energetics, ecology and life history patterns. *Nature,* 1983, *306,* 314–315.

Harvey, P. H., and Greenwood, P. J. Anti-predator defence strategies: some evolutionary problems. In J. R. Krebs and N. B. Davies (Eds.), *Behavioral ecology: An evolutionary approach,* Oxford: Blackwell, 1978.

Harvey, P. H., and Mace, C. M. Comparisons between taxa and adaptive trends: problems of methodology. In King's college Sociobiology Group (Eds.)., *Current problems in sociobiology.* Cambridge: Cambridge University Press, 1982.

Hayssen, V., and Lacy, R. C. Basal metabolic rates in mammals: Taxonomic differences in the allometry of BMR and body mass. *Comparative Biochemistry and Physiology,* 1985, *81A,* 741–754.

Heinroth, O. Contributions on the biology, especially the ethology and psychology of the Anatidae. (D. Gove and C. J. Mellor, trans.,). In G. M. Burghardt (Ed.), *The foundations of comparative ethology.* New York: Van Nostrand Reinhold, 1911/1985.

Henderson, R. W., Binder, M. H., and Burghardt, G. M. Responses of neonate Hispaniolan vine snakes *(Uromacer frenatus)* to prey extracts. *Herpetologica,* 1983, *39,* 75–77.

Herzog, H. A., and Burghardt, G. M. Vocalization in juvenile crocodilians. *Zeitschrift für Tierpsychologie,* 1977, *44,* 294–304.

Herzog, H. A. Jr., and Burghardt, G. M. Development of anti-predator responses in snakes. I. Defensive and open-field behaviors in newborns and adults of three species of garter snakes. *Journal of Comparative Psychology,* 1986, *100,* 372–379.

Hofer, M. A. Parental contributions to the development of their offspring. In D. J. Gubernick and P. H. Klopfer (Eds.), *Parental care in mammals.* New York: Plenum Press, 1981.

Hofman, M. A. Energy metabolism, brain size and longevity in mammals. *Quarterly Review of Biology,* 1983, *58,* 495–512.

Hopson, J. A. Endothermy, small size, and the origin of mammalian reproduction. *American Naturalist,* 1973, *107,* 446–451.

Hotton, N., III, MacLean, P. D., Roth, J. J., and Roth, E. C. (Eds.) *The ecology and biology of mammal-like reptiles.* Washington, DC: Smithsonian Institution, 1986.

Huey, R. B., and Hertz, P. E. Effects of body size and slope on sprint speed of a lizard *(Stellio (Agama) stellio). Journal of Experimental Biology,* 1982, *97,* 401–409.

Huey, R. B., and Hertz, P. E. Effects of body size and slope on acceleration of a lizard *(Stellio stellio). Journal of Experimental Biology,* 1984, *110,* 113–123.

Huey, R. B., and Pianka, E. R. Ecological consequences of foraging mode. *Ecology,* 1981, *62,* 991–999.

Hutt, C. Exploration and play in children. In P. A. Jewell and C. Loizo (Eds.), *Play, exploration and territory in mammals.* London: Symposium Zoological Society, 1966.

Jarman, P. Prospects for interspecific comparison in sociobiology. In King's College Sociobiology Group (Eds.), *Current problems in sociobiology.* Cambridge: Cambridge University Press, 1982.

Karasov, W. H., and Diamond, J. M. Digestive adaptations for fueling the cost of endothermy. *Science,* 1985, *228,* 202–204.

Karasov, W. H. Petrossian, E., Rosenberg, L., and Diamond, J. M. How do food passage rate and assimilation differ between herbivorous lizards and nonruminant mammals? *Journal of Comparative Physiology B,* 1986, *156,* 599–609.

Kemp, T. S. *Mammal-like reptiles and the origin of mammals.* New York: Academic Press, 1982.

Kluge, A. G. Ontogeny and phylogenetic systematics. *Cladistics,* 1985, *1,* 13–27.

Kortlandt, A. Aspects and prospects of the concept of instinct (vicissitudes of the hierarchy theory). *Archives Néerlandaises de Zoologie,* 1955, *11,* 155–284.

Kortmulder, K. Play-like behaviour: An essay in speculative ethology. *Acta Biotheoretica,* 1983, *32,* 145–166.

Lancy, D. F. Play in species adaptation. *Annual Review of Anthropology,* 1980, *9,* 471–495.

Lauder, G. V. Homology, analogy, and the evolution of behavior. In M. H. Nitecki and J. A. Kitchell (Eds.), *Evolution of animal behavior: Paleontological and field approaches.* New York: Oxford University Press, 1986.

Lee, P. C. Ecological constraints on the social development of vervet monkeys. *Behaviour,* 1984, *91,* 245–262.

Lorenz, K. *Evolution and modification of behavior.* Chicago: University of Chicago Press, 1965.

MacLean, P. D. Neurobehavioral significance of the mammal-like reptiles (therapsids). In N. Hotton III, P. D. MacLean, J. J. Roth, and E. C. Roth (Eds.), *The ecology and biology of mammal-like reptiles.* Washington, DC: Smithsonian Institution, 1986.

Martin, P. The time and energy costs of play behaviour in the cat. *Zeitschrift für Tierpsychologie,* 1984, *64,* 298–312.

Martin, P., and Bateson, P. The ontogeny of locomotor play behaviour in the domestic cat. *Animal Behaviour,* 1985, *33,* 502–510.

Martin, P., and Caro, T. M. On the functions of play and its role in behavioral development. *Advances in the Study of Behavior,* 1985, *15,* 59–103.

Martin, R. D. Relative brain size and basal metabolic rate in terrestrial vertebrates. *Nature,* 1981, *293,* 57–60.

Mason, W. Ontogeny of social behavior. In P. Marler and J. G. Vandenbergh (Eds.), *Handbook of behavioral neurobiology.* Vol. 3. *Social behavior and communication.* New York: Plenum Press, 1979.

McDiarmid, R. W. Evolution of parental care in frogs. In G. M. Burghardt and M. Bekoff (Eds.), *The development of behavior: Comparative and evolutionary aspects.* New York: Garland STPM, 1978.

McNab, B. Food habits, energetics, and the population biology of mammals. *American Naturalist,* 1980, *116,* 106–124.

Müller-Schwarze, D. Analysis of play behaviour: What do we measure and when? In P. K. Smith (Ed.), *Play in animals and humans.* London: Basil Blackwell, 1984.

Müller-Schwarze, D., and Müller-Schwarze, C. Play behaviour in free-ranging caribou, *Rangifer tarandus. Acta Zoologica Fennica,* 1982, *175,* 121–124.

Müller-Schwarze, D., and Müller-Schwarze, C., Play behavior in mammals: persistence, decrease and energetic compensation after play deprivation in deer fawns. *Science,* 1982, *215,* 85–87.

Mushinsky, H. R., and Lotz, K. H. Responses of two sympatric water snakes to the extracts of commonly ingested prey species: ontogenetic and ecological considerations. *Journal of Chemical Ecology,* 1980, *6,* 1624–1629.

Noble, G. K., and Zitrin, A. Induction of mating behavior in male and female chicks following injection of sex hormones. *Endocrinology,* 1942, *30,* 327–334.

Nussbaum, R. A. The evolution of parental care in salamanders. *Miscellaneous Publications Museum of Zoology, University of Michigan,* 1985, *169,* 1–50.

O'Connell, B., Greenlee, R., Bacon, J., and Chiszar, D. Strike-induced chemosensory searching in old world vipers and new world pit vipers at the San Diego Zoo. *Zoo Biology,* 1982, *1,* 287–294.

Olson, E. C. The exploitation of land by early tetrapods. In A. d'A. Bellairs and C. B. Cox (Eds.), *Morphology and biology of reptiles.* London: Academic Press, 1976.

Oppenheim, R. W., and Haverkamp, L. Early development of behavior and the nervous system: An embryological perspective. In E. M. Blass (Ed.), *Handbook of behavioral neurobiology,* Vol. 8. New York: Plenum Press, 1985.

Ostrom, J. H. Social and unsocial behavior in dinosaurs. In M. H. Nitecki and J. A. Kitchell (eds.), *Evolution of animal behavior: Paleontological and field approaches.* New York: Oxford University Press, 1986.

Peters, R. H. *The ecological implications of body size.* Cambridge: Cambridge University Press, 1983.

Piaget, J. *Play, dreams and imitation in childhood.* New York: Norton, 1962.

Plomin, R., DeFries, J. C., and McClearn, G. E. *Behavioral genetics: A primer.* San Francisco: W. H. Freeman, 1980.

Poirier, F. E. Functions of primate play behavior. In E. O. Smith (Ed.), *Social play in primates.* New York: Academic Press, 1978.

Poole, T. B., and Fish, J. An investigation of playful behaviour in *Rattus norvegicus* and *Mus musculus* (Mammalia). *Journal of Zoology (London),* 1975, *175,* 61–71.

Pough, H. Ontogenetic change in blood oxygen capacity and maximum activity in garter snakes *(Thamnophis sirtalis). Journal of Comparative Physiology B,* 1977, *116,* 337–345.

Pough, H. Ontogenetic changes in endurance in water snakes *(Natrix sipedon):* Physiological correlates and ecological consequences. *Copeia,* 1978, 69–75.

Pough, H. The advantages of ectothermy for tetrapods. *American Naturalist,* 1980, *115,* 92–112.

Pough, H. Amphibians and reptiles as low energy systems. In W. P. Aspey and S. I. Lustick (Eds.), *Behavioral energetics: The cost of survival in vertebrates.* Columbus: Ohio State University Press, 1983.

Pough, F. H., and Andrews, R. M. Individual and sibling-group variation in metabolism of lizards: The aerobic capacity model for the origin of ectothermy. *Comparative Biochemistry and Physiology,* 1984, *79A,* 415–419.

Pough, F. H., and Andrews, R. M. Energy costs of subduing and swallowing prey for a lizard. *Ecology,* 1985a, *66,* 1525–1533.

Pough, F. H., and Andrews, R. M. Use of anaerobic metabolism by free-ranging lizards. *Physiological Zoology,* 1985b, *58,* 205–213.

Price, E. O. Behavioral aspects of animal domestication. *Quarterly Review of Biology,* 1984, *59,* 1–32.

Rasa, O. A. E. A motivational analysis of object play in juvenile dwarf mongooses *(Hologale undulata rufula). Animal Behaviour,* 1984, *32,* 579–589.

Regal, P. Behavioral differences between reptiles and mammals: An analysis of activity and mental abilities. In N. Greenberg and P. D. MacLean (Eds.), *Behavior and neurology of lizards.* Rockville, MD: DHEW Publ. No. (ADM) 77-491, 1978.

Renner, M. J., and Rosenzweig, M. R. Social interactions among rats housed in grouped and enriched conditions. *Developmental Psychobiology,* 1986, *19,* 303–313.

Rensch, B., and Adrian-Hinsberg, C. Die visuelle Lernkapazität von Leguanen. *Zeitscrhrift für Tierpsychologie,* 1964, *20,* 34–42.

Rodda, G. H. Navigation in juvenile alligators. *Zeitschrift für Tierpsychologie,* 1985, *68,* 65–77.

Roggenbuck, M. E., and Jenssen, T. A. The ontogeny of display behavior in *Sceloporus undulatus* (Sauria: Iguanidae). *Ethology,* 1986, *71,* 153–165.

Ruben, J. A., and Battalia, D. E. Aerobic and anaerobic metabolism during activity in small rodents. *Journal of Experimental Zoology,* 1979, *208,* 73–76.

Sacher, G. A. Evaluation of the entropy and information terms governing mammalian longevity. *Interdisciplinary Topics in Gerontology,* 1976, *9,* 69–82.

Sacher, G. A. Evolution of longevity and survival characteristics in mammals. In E. L. Schneider (Ed.), *The genetics of aging.* New York: Plenum Press, 1978.

Sacher, G. A., and Staffeldt, E. F. Relation of gestation time to brain weight for placental mammals: implications for the theory of vertebrate growth. *American Naturalist,* 1974, *108,* 593–615.

Sackett, G. P., Sameroff, A. J., Cairns, R. B., and Suomi, S. J. Continuity in behavioral development: theoretical and empirical issues. In K. Immelmann, Barlow, G. W., Petrinovich, L., and Main, M. (Eds.), *Behavioral development: The Bielefeld interdisciplinary project.* Cambridge: Cambridge University Press, 1981.

Schaller, G. B. and Crawshaw, P. G. Fishing behavior of Paraguayan caiman. *Copeia,* 66–72.

Schmidt-Nielsen, K. *Scaling: Why is animal size so important.* Cambridge: Cambridge University Press, 1984.

Scudder, R. M., and Burghardt, G. M. A comparative study of defensive behavior in three sympatric species of water snakes *(Nerodia). Zeitschrift für Tierpsychologie,* 1983, *63,* 17–26.

Smith, E. O. A historical view on the study of play: statement of the problem. In E. O. Smith (Ed.), *Social play in primates.* New York: Academic Press, 1978.

Smith, P. K. Does play matter? Functional and evolutionary aspects of animal and human play. *Behavioral and Brain Sciences,* 1982, *5,* 139–155.

Smith, P. K. and Vollstedt, R. On defining play: An empirical study of the relationship between play and various play criteria. *Child Development,* 1985, *56,* 1042–1050.

Smith, P. K., Takhvar, M., Gore, N., and Vollstedt, R. Play in young children: problems of definition, categorization and measurement. *Early Child Development and Care,* 1985, *19,* 25–41.

Spencer, H. *The principles of psychology* (2nd ed), Vol. 2. London: Williams and Norgate, 1872.

Steiner, J. E. Human facial expressions in response to taste and smell stimulation. *Advances in Child Development and Behavior,* 1979, *13,* 257–295.

Symons, D. *Play and aggression: A study of rhesus monkeys.* New York: Columbia University Press, 1978.

Taylor, C. R., Caldwell, S. L., and Rowntree, V. J. Running up and down hills: Some consequences of size. *Science,* 1972, *178,* 1096–1097.

Thomas, R. D. K., and Olson, E. C. (Eds.) *A cold look at the warm-blooded dinosaurs.* Boulder, CO: Westview Press, 1980.

Tinbergen, N. On the aims and methods of ethology. *Zeitschrift für Tierpsychologie,* 1963, *20,* 410–433.

Tinkle, D., and Gibbons, J. W. The distribution and evolution of viviparity in reptiles. *Miscellaneous Publications; Museum of Zoology, University of Michigan,* No. 154, 1977.

Tracy, C. R. Minimum size of mammalian homeotherms: Role of the thermal environment. *Science,* 1977, *198,* 1034–1035.

Trivers, R. L. Parental investment and sexual selection. In B. Campbell (Ed.), *Sexual selection and the descent of man.* Chicago: Aldine-Atherton, 1972.

Troyer, K. Transfer of fermentation microbes between generations in a herbivorous lizard. *Science,* 1982, *216,* 540–542.

Vinegar, A. Brooding of the eastern glass lizard, *Ophisaurus ventralis. Bulletin of the southern California academy of sciences,* 1968, *67,* 65–68.

Vinegar, A., Hutchinson, V. H., and Dowling, H. G. Metabolism, energetics, and thermoregulation during brooding of snakes of the genus *Python* (Reptilia, Boidae). *Zoologica,* 1970, *55,* 19–50.

von Uexküll, J. Environment [Umwelt] and inner world of animals. (C. J. Mellor and D. Gove, trans.). In G. M. Burghardt (Ed.), *The foundations of ethology.* New York: Van Nostrand Reinhold, 1909/ 1985.

Waldman, B. Sibling recognition in toad tadpoles: Are kinship labels transferred among individuals? *Zeitschrift für Tierpsychologie,* 1985, *68,* 41–57.

Weaver, J. C. The improbable endotherm: the energetics of the sauropod dinosaur *Brachiosaurus. Paleobiology,* 1983, *9,* 173–182.

Werner, D. Social organization and ecology of land iguanas, *Conolophus subcristatus,* on Isla Fernandina, Galapagos. In G. M. Burghardt and A. S. Rand (Eds.), *Iguanas of the world: Their behavior, ecology, and conservation.* Park Ridge, NJ: Noyes, 1982.

West, M. J. Exploration and play with objects in domestic kittens. *Developmental Psychobiology,* 1977, *10,* 53–57.

Wiley, R. H. Social structure and individual ontogenies: Problems of description, mechanism, and evolution. *Perspectives in Ethology,* 1981, *4,* 105–133.

Wittenberger, J. F. The evolution of mating systems in birds and mammals. In P. Marler and J. G. Vandenbergh (Eds.), *Handbook of behavioral neurobiology,* Vol. 3. New York: Plenum Press, 1979.

York, D. S., and Burghardt, G. M. Nesting and brooding in the Malayan pit viper, *Calloselasma thodostoma:* Temperature, relative humidity, and defensive behavior. *Herpetological Journal,* in press.

Zucker, E. L., Dennon, M. B., Puleo, S. G., and Maple, T. L. Play profiles of captive adult orangutans: A developmental perspective. *Developmental Psychobiology,* 1986, *19,* 315–326.

5

The Uterus as Environment
The Ecology of Fetal Behavior

WILLIAM P. SMOTHERMAN AND SCOTT R. ROBINSON

INTRODUCTION

Speculation about the importance of experience before birth dates to the origins of science itself. The belief that knowledge, habits, and personality traits could be imparted to the unborn child through experiences of the mother was widespread in classical and medieval society. Aristotle himself speculated on the importance of prenatal life:

> As soon then as the offspring of all animals are born, especially those born imperfect, they are in the habit of sleeping, because they continue sleeping also within the mother when they first acquire sensation. . . . But nevertheless they are found to wake even in the womb (this is clear in dissections and ovipara), and then they immediately fall into a sleep again. This is why after birth also they spend most of their time in sleep. (*De generatione animalium*, p. 321)

Empirical understanding of the world of the fetus began to unfold only in the last century through the pioneering efforts of Preyer (1885), Swenson (1926), Angulo (1932), and others, who initiated the development of techniques for observing the fetus *in utero*. An interest in the origins of reflexes and neuromuscular development was the impetus behind these early studies of fetal movement (see Gottlieb, 1976; Hamburger, 1963; Hooker, 1952, for reviews). This emphasis promoted the general view that early fetal movements originate in simple reflex arcs and lack intrinsic organization or coordination (Windle, 1940). The focus on evoked activity also diverted attention from spontaneous fetal movement.

WILLIAM P. SMOTHERMAN AND SCOTT R. ROBINSON   Laboratory for Psychobiological Research, Departments of Psychology and Zoology, Oregon State University, Corvallis, Oregon 97331.

Although these now classic studies documented that mammalian fetuses are active before birth, little was learned about why fetuses move (rat—Angulo, 1932; Swenson, 1926; guinea pig—Avery, 1928; Carmichael, 1934; rabbit—Pankratz, 1931; cat—Coronios, 1933; Tilney and Kubie, 1931; Windle and Griffin, 1931; sheep—Barcroft and Barron, 1939; Barcroft, Barron and Windle, 1936; humans—Hooker, 1936; Minkowski, 1928).

Understanding why particular behavioral patterns occur entails analysis at four distinct levels (Hailman, 1976; Tinbergen, 1963). Research can focus on (a) proximal causal mechanisms and neuromuscular regulation involved in the dynamic control of movement; (b) ontogenetic development of behavior in the individual; (c) phylogenetic history of behavior in the population; or (d) ultimate biological functions responsible for maintaining or preserving behavior in the population. The last of these categories of explanation—biological function—is often referred to as the *selective value* or *adaptive significance* of behavior (Hinde, 1970), terms that presume that the behavioral attributes confer advantages in terms of survival or reproductive success.

With specific regard to fetal behavior, three kinds of explanation have been proposed to account for the function of fetal movement (Oppenheim, 1981). One hypothesis, the epiphenomenal view, presumes no adaptive significance at all for fetal behavior. Movement by the fetus before birth may simply represent an accidental or incidental epiphenomenon of structural development, a manifestation of neural maturation that lacks biological significance during the prenatal period. Support for the epiphenomenon view has varied historically but was especially strong during the early days of fetal reflexology (1920s–1930s), when fetal motility was widely used as an index of neuromuscular development (Coghill, 1940; Windle and Becker, 1940). Because the prevailing presumption was that fetal movements lack organization and adaptive significance, prenatal "motility" has repeatedly been viewed as qualitatively different from postnatal "behavior" (Hamburger, 1963, 1973; Windle, 1944).

Two competing explanations contradict the epiphenomenon view. They maintain that fetal movements have beneficial consequences, either for the fetus itself (functional) or for its subsequent behavioral and morphological development (preparatory). The preparatory hypothesis holds that fetal movements represent incipient stages that foreshadow the development of mature postnatal patterns of adaptive behavior. By this view, fetal behavior may provide practice or experience that is crucial for the development of motor coordination and its expression in organized postnatal behavior (Bekoff, Byers, and Bekoff, 1980). Further, prenatal activity and the course of behavioral development may be influenced by information obtained *in utero*. Although notions of prenatal experience have existed in vague and imprecise forms for centuries (e.g., Aristotle—see above quote; Erasmus Darwin, 1796; Lamarck, 1809), it has more recently been conceptually linked with the epigenetic viewpoint, as elaborated by Kuo (1967).

The functional hypothesis, which is complementary to the preparatory view, asserts that fetal behavior may be functional and adaptive during the prenatal period (Oppenheim, 1981). Amniote embryos (reptiles, birds, and mammals) develop in environments wholly different from the external world of their postnatal life, a fact suggesting that anatomical and behavioral attributes may be functional during prenatal development to promote the survival and well-being of the embryo. Transient anatomical structures, such as the placenta and the umbilical cord, have certainly been recognized as ontogenetic adaptations that function only *in utero* (Gould 1977), but relatively little attention has been directed toward behavioral adaptations in higher vertebrate embryos (cf. Oppenheim, 1981, 1982). Some patterns of fetal behavior may represent just such ontogenetic adaptations.

Although largely ignored during the early period of fetal research, the underlying basis of fetal movement is receiving renewed interest in fields as diverse as developmental psychobiology, neuroembryology, obstetrics and pediatrics, fetal medicine and surgery, and teratology. Empirical study of fetal behavior has long been hindered, of course, by the necessity of intervening in the developmental process to observe fetuses. For example, fetuses cannot survive after removal from the uterus, yet general maternal anesthesia suppresses and distorts normal fetal activity *in utero,* thereby prohibiting direct fetal observation. Only recently have new technologies and improvements of older methods begun to circumvent these long-standing difficulties to bring a fresh, experimental approach to the study of fetal behavior, prenatal development, and adaptation *in utero.*

Innovations such as real-time ultrasonography and fetal monitoring have provided useful insights into general fetal activity (Birnholz, 1984; de Vries, Visser, and Prechtl, 1982; Rayburn, 1982), but a detailed understanding of fetal capabilities and interactions with the prenatal environment will continue to depend on directly observing fetal behavior *in utero.* Three alternative procedures have recently been developed to surgically prepare pregnant rats while circumventing the suppressive effects of general anesthesia. These include two irreversible techniques for chemical and physical transection of the spinal cord (Basmajian and Ranney, 1961; Kirby, 1979; Kodama and Sekiguchi, 1984; Narayanan, Fox, and Hamburger, 1971; Narayanan, Narayanan, and Browne, 1982) and reversible spinal anesthesia produced by lidocaine injection (Smotherman, Robinson, and Miller, 1986a). Whereas the irreversible techniques allow for the observation of fetuses over an extended period of time (2 h or longer), the reversible preparation now provides a tool for repeated prenatal study of the same fetus and a comparison of prenatal and postnatal behavior.

By these methods, it is now possible to advance understanding of the biological significance of fetal movement. Because behavior reflects the interaction between an organism and its environment, this chapter first describes some of the environmental circumstances in which the fetus behaves. Although the uterus reduces contact between the fetus and the outside world, many external stimuli still impinge directly on the fetus (by transmission through the body wall and the uterus) or indirectly through the mother (transported by maternal circulation and transplacental diffusion). Further, the uterus itself undergoes change. Several parameters in the uterine environment vary among mothers, successive pregnancies, and over the course of gestation. To understand the influence of these environmental factors, it will be useful both to exploit natural variation within the uterus and to induce exaggerated variation through the experimental manipulation of laboratory animals.

After characterizing the fetal environment, the focus of this discussion shifts to fetal behavior itself. Most of this overview relies on data collected from rat *(Rattus norvegicus)* and human fetuses, simply because more is known about fetal behavior in these two species than in any other mammals. In particular, we describe the behavioral repertoire for rat and human fetuses from the origins of movement through parturition. This base of descriptive information provides a starting point for measuring the degree of organization of spontaneous fetal activity and assessing the responsiveness of fetal behavior to environmental change. Together, these investigations of the organization and responsiveness of fetal behavior converge toward the ultimate goal of understanding the importance of behavior during the prenatal period.

Evolutionary Roots of Fetal Development

Mammalian reproduction is the culmination of an evolutionary trend among terrestrial vertebrates toward greater parental investment in the early development of the embryo. The origin of the amniote egg, a necessity for reproduction on land, brought about a transition from the external to the internal fertilization of ova, with the early stages of embryonic development promoted by the protected, aqueous envelope of the egg. Crocodilians and virtually all birds invest additional energy into the incubation of eggs and the parental care of hatchlings. The importance of parental investment to the young in mammalian evolution is preserved in the few extant species of monotremes (platypus and echidna), which exhibit lactation and extended parental care. In all other mammals, fertilization and early embryonic development is internalized and further buffered from unpredictable perturbations in the external environment (Lillegraven, 1979).

In marsupials, a diverse group of mammals ranging from South American opossums to Australian kangaroos, internal development is incomplete. Embryos emerge from the urogenital sinus at a primitive stage of development and migrate to the mother's teats, which generally are located within a protected marsupium. Offspring remain inside the pouch for an extended time and, toward the end of this period, may partially exit or leave the pouch for brief excursions, eventually returning to the protected maternal environment. Some investigators have emphasized that this pattern of marsupial reproduction, rather than being primitive, is, in fact, an adaptive strategy that permits a high reproductive potential while preserving flexibility in the face of fluctuating environmental conditions (Parker, 1977). Some marsupials exercise considerable facultative control over reproduction, including delayed implantation of fertilized ova, simultaneous development of different-age offspring (on different teats), and premature termination of a reproductive effort under harsh conditions (Sharman and Calaby, 1964).

Eutherian mammals have further extended the period of intrauterine embryonic development through the evolutionary innovation of the chorioallantoic placenta, the principal organ of prenatal life support. Prolonged interface of maternal and embryonic tissues has necessitated sophisticated physiological adaptations for suppressing the immunological rejection of the embryo. Vertebrates exhibit an efficient system of defense that can distinguish between "self" and "nonself" to enable the recognition and destruction of invading organisms. Yet, developing embryos of virtually all higher vertebrates (excepting only a few parthenogenetic lizards) are composed of cells and tissues that derive from both maternal and paternal genes. For prolonged internal development to be possible, immunological defenses must be disarmed to prevent rejection of the embryo.

To accomplish this end, eutherian mammals have evolved an unprecedented level of biochemical and physiological cooperation between the embryo and the mother (Lillegraven, 1975). The result is a system of viviparous reproduction in which the embryo is isolated during early life and emerges into the external environment at a relatively advanced stage of physical and nervous development (Hamburger, 1963; Parker, 1977). This strategy finds extreme expression in precocial species, which bear young that are furred, remarkably coordinated, responsive to environmental stimuli, and nearly independent. In a traditional frame of reference, the early appearance of sensory responsiveness and locomotor independence has been viewed as the point of origin of behavioral development. Yet the behavioral competencies of newborn placental mammals are at the same time the end products of prenatal development. An understanding of the process of behavioral development will benefit from a more thorough investigation of fetal behavior and the intrauterine environment in which the fetus develops.

FEATURES OF THE PRENATAL ENVIRONMENT

Adult behavior under natural conditions, by definition, represents a continuous and changing interaction between the animal and its environment. As ethologists and behavioral ecologists have long maintained, it is imperative to recognize the relevant features of an animal's environment if the animal's behavior is to be fully understood. We believe that recognition of the salient characteristics of the prenatal environment is equally important for the correct interpretation of fetal behavior. Although current methodologies require that fetuses be brought into the laboratory for study, the fetus itself remains within its natural intrauterine environment. This presents an unusual situation in behavioral research: fetal subjects can be observed in the analogue of their native habitat without sacrificing the experimental control that is possible only in a laboratory setting.

LIFE SUPPORT SYSTEM OF THE FETUS

In albino rats, multiple embryos (Days 1–14 of gestation, before the onset of motility) and fetuses (Days 15–22, after the onset of motility) develop within a duplex uterus; the two uterine horns are physically separate (each having its own cervix), and fetuses in the left horn are completely isolated from those in the right (Ramsey, 1982). Although the uterus itself is loosely suspended within the peritoneum, the smooth muscles that comprise the uterus form an elastic tube that limits the space available for fetal movement. As each conceptus grows during gestation, the uterus undergoes distension and thinning, gradually changing in shape from spheroidal (resembling a string of pearls) to cylindrical (Bradin, 1948). The rate of shape change, which is indicative of the tension in the uterine wall, varies with the number of fetuses in the horn: when fewer than four fetuses are present, the spheroidal shape may persist until term. As long as the shape of the uterus remains spheroidal, the area of contact between adjacent fetuses is small or absent. Only as the uterus takes on a cylindrical shape does the area of contact expand (up to the full diameter of the uterus), thereby increasing the potential for direct physical or chemical interaction between fetuses.

Within the uterus, embryonic tissues differentiate early in gestation to give rise to the fetus itself and to the anatomical structures that constitute the fetal life-support system. The principal components of this system are the placenta, the umbilical cord, the extraembryonic membranes, and the amniotic fluid. Although this life support system provides for the physiological needs of the fetus and buffers it from fluctuating environmental conditions in the external world, each component of the system is subject to variation and undergoes systematic change during gestation. Recognizing how these components vary is central to understanding the possible influences of the intrauterine environment on fetal behavior. Figure 1 summarizes some of the developmental milestones and sources of environmental variation experienced by the rat fetus during gestation.

The placenta is the vital interface between the developing fetus and the mother. It provides both a point of physical attachment to the wall of the uterus and a means of chemical exchange between maternal and fetal blood supplies. Nutrients, oxygen, and biologically important chemicals are transported to the

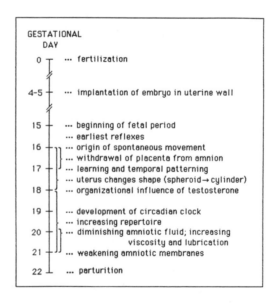

Figure 1. Chronology of important environmental changes within the uterus during gestation in the rat.

fetus by simple diffusion, facilitated diffusion, and active transport across the placenta, and fetal wastes are returned for removal by maternal circulation (Finnegan, 1979). Early in gestation, the rat embryo is supported entirely by an inverted yolk-sac placenta, which does not intergrow with maternal tissues (Ramsey, 1982). By Day 12, however, the true chorioallantoic placenta, formed from a fusion of embryonic and maternal tissues, becomes functional. At this time, compounds of molecular weight less than 600 are readily transported to the fetus, whereas compounds with weights in excess of 1,000 cross the placenta with difficulty (Beaconsfield, Birdwood, and Beaconsfield, 1980; Mirkin, 1973). Thus, substances ranging from amino acids and simple sugars to hormones and small peptides can circulate to the fetus (Finnegan, 1979).

Through Day 15, the placenta is hemispheric in shape and wraps around the sphere of concentric extraembryonic membranes that surround the fetus. This placental envelope withdraws from the fetus and flattens against the wall of the uterus over the next 2 days, assuming its mature discoid shape (Ramsey, 1982). Like the changes in shape of the uterus during gestation, the flattening of the placenta removes a physical buffer between adjacent fetuses, increasing the potential for intersibling contact. At the same time, thinning of the trophoblastic epithelium, where the placenta joins the uterus, facilitates the transport of slow-diffusing substances to the fetus (Mirkin, 1973). Thus, placental maturation markedly alters the physical and chemical environment of the fetus during the last few days of gestation.

Each fetus is joined to its placenta by arterial and venous circulation through the umbilical cord, the only specialized conduit between mother and fetus. Although the cord is flexible and allows considerable freedom of movement for the fetus within the amnion, it nevertheless tethers the fetus and limits the range of fetal movement. The length of the umbilical cord increases steadily over the fetal period (Days 15–21), apparently in response to tensile forces, but it exhibits considerable variation among individual fetuses (Moessinger, Blanc, Marone, and Polsen, 1982). Because the umbilical cord is responsible for oxygen transport from the placenta, obstruction of the cord can induce hypoxia, with detrimental consequences for fetal health and movement (McCullough and Blackman, 1976; Meier, Bunch, Nolan, and Scheidler, 1960).

A series of extraembryonic membranes, especially the chorion and the amnion, envelops the fetus and physically segregates it from the placenta, the uterus, and the other fetuses. The primary function of these flexible, transparent membranes is to contain and to help regulate the aqueous medium surrounding the fetus (Adolph, 1967). The presence of fluid-filled sacs around the fetus provides physical protection, a relatively stable osmotic environment, and the space necessary for fetal movement. Because each fetus is enveloped by its own membranes and fluids, the adjacent fetuses are relatively isolated and never directly touch. Amniotic fluid, which serves as a reservoir for fetal waste products (Jeffcoate and Scott, 1959) and contains important nutritional and immunological factors that are ingested by the fetus (Abbas and Tovey, 1960; Lev and Orlic, 1972), provides odor cues to the fetus that help coordinate early postnatal mother–infant interaction (Pedersen and Blass, 1981, 1982). Near term, when fluid volume is greatly diminished, the lubricant qualities of amniotic fluid may continue to help prevent adhesions and to facilitate movement (Moessinger *et al.*, 1982).

The two principal fluid pools contained by the extraembryonic membranes include exocoel fluid, which occupies the smaller space between the chorion and the amnion, and amniotic fluid, which fills a larger volume within the amnion, where it directly bathes the fetus. During the early stages of development, before the fetal tissues exhibit any secretory activity, fluid is produced by the placenta and the amnion (Jeffcoate and Scott, 1959). Later, after the maturation of the embryonic organs, the fetal pulmonary, alimentary, and renal systems contribute to amniotic fluid production and composition (Adolph, 1967). Amniotic fluid is also regularly ingested and irregularly aspirated by the fetus soon after the onset of fetal movement (Marsh, King, and Becker, 1963). In the rat fetus, the opposing processes of fluid production and elimination lead to a complete turnover of water content every 3 h (Wirtschafter and Williams, 1957a,b) and a steady increase in fluid volume through Day 19 of gestation. However, amniotic fluid begins to decline in volume on Day 20, and by Day 21, it is virtually absent (Marsh *et al.*, 1963; Tam and Chan, 1977). Coincident with the reduction in amniotic fluid volume near term is a marked increase in fluid viscosity (increasing 5- to 16-fold from Day 19 to Day 21; Marsh *et al.*, 1963), an alteration in the protein and urea content of the fluid (Wirtschafter and Williams, 1957a,b; Tam and Chan, 1977), and an increase in the lubricant quality of the fluid (Smotherman, unpublished data, 1986). In part, these changes may be facilitated by a more rapid rate of fluid ingestion by the fetus during the last 2 days of gestation (Marsh *et al.*, 1963).

THE FETUS

Physical growth of the fetus is exponential from shortly after conception through parturition (fetal body mass doubles every 1.2 days; Knox and Lister-Rosenoer, 1978). In contrast, the growth of the placenta, the umbilical cord, and the amniotic fluid (through Day 19) is linear (Plentl, 1959; Tam and Chan, 1977). Consequently, as development proceeds, the fetus occupies an ever larger fraction of the total volume within the amnion and is faced with a continually shrinking space in which to move (Figure 2). Near term, the fetus essentially occupies the entire volume within the amniotic sac. In species bearing multiple offspring, such as the rat, the problem of intrauterine space is compounded by crowding within each uterine horn (Barr, Jensh, and Brent, 1970). In our laboratory, rats bear an average of 13.4 pups in their first pregnancy, but actual uterine density varies from 0 to 14 fetuses in each uterine horn, often creating highly discrepant distributions of fetuses (a discrepancy of four or more is evident in 34% of all litters; Figure 3). The intrinsic variability of uterine density and interhorn distribution promotes variation in other features of the prenatal environment, such as uterine shape (affecting intersibling contact), intrauterine crowding (affecting the space available for movement), and uterine position (the location of each fetus within the uterus relative to other fetuses).

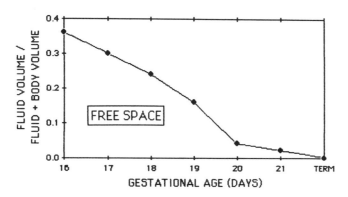

Figure 2. The amount of free space available for movement *in utero* by fetal rats during gestation. The index of free space is derived from the ratio of amniotic fluid volume to the total volume within the extraembryonic membranes (estimated from fluid volume + fetal body mass). The sharp decline in free space on Day 20 coincides with the sharp reduction in amniotic fluid and the rapid growth of the fetus.

Uterine position may be an especially important example of natural variation within the prenatal environment. The uterus is narrower at the ovarian and the caudal ends, perhaps exacerbating fetal restraint for fetuses in terminal positions. Rat fetuses growing at the ovarian or the caudal ends of the uterus are 5–10% smaller (Barr *et al.,* 1970) and are bounded by only a single sibling, whereas fetuses in central positions are larger and are sandwiched between siblings. Moreover, the availability of blood-borne factors (oxygen, amino acids, and neuroregulators, including hormones) may vary with uterine position (Wigglesworth, 1964). Although incompletely understood, the maternal blood supply to the uterus appears to flow from the caudal toward the ovarian ends of each horn (Del Campo and Ginther, 1972). As a consequence, fetuses at the caudal end of the uterus experience higher concentrations of nutrients and lower concentrations of wastes in the maternal blood than fetuses at the ovarian end. High uterine density accentuates this difference by expanding the number of fetuses linked in series, creating

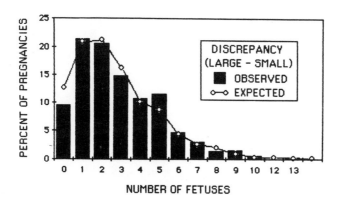

Figure 3. Variability in the distribution of fetuses between horns of the rat uterus. The observed discrepancy between uterine horns and the expected distribution based on a model of random assortment are depicted.

the potential for marked variation in the chemical microenvironments of fetuses at different uterine positions.

Male and female fetuses are distributed throughout the uterine horn, but in any particular pregnancy, the relative positions of males and females may produce unique environments for fetuses within the horn. On Days 16–18, male fetuses begin to produce testosterone (Baum, 1979), which is responsible for organizing brain areas that control adult sexually dimorphic behavior. Morphological sexual differentiation (anogenital distance) becomes evident by Day 18. Owing to the proximity of arterial and venous blood vessels supplying the uterus, it has been suggested that testosterone produced by male fetuses may diffuse into the blood supply of other fetuses in the horn (Babine and Smotherman, 1984; Del Campo and Ginther, 1972; Meisel and Ward, 1981). Similarly, testosterone may diffuse directly across the amniotic membranes of adjacent fetuses (Richmond and Sachs, 1984). However mediated, differential exposure to testosterone during prenatal development can contribute to the masculinization of the anatomical and behavioral attributes of females, particularly those female fetuses in positions adjacent to males or on the ovarian side of males in the same uterine horn. Uterine position, and consequent prenatal testosterone exposure, has been demonstrated to affect the reproductive behavior of adult female rats (Tobet, Dunlap, and Gerall, 1982), avoidance responding in female mice (Hauser and Gandelman, 1983), and responsiveness to exogenous testosterone administration (Babine and Smotherman, 1984). Predictions about the effects of prenatal exposure to testosterone are complicated by uterine density (which may dilute or concentrate the exposure), the sex ratio within the horn, and the possibility that the blood flow may reverse direction in portions of the uterine circulation (Del Campo and Ginther, 1972).

In most mammals, the sex ratio at birth is approximately 1:1, although a slight but important bias favors males. This nearly equal sex ratio is also characteristic of rats bred in our laboratory. However, male and female fetuses may not be distributed randomly within a uterine horn. At the ovarian end of the uterus, no sex bias is evident, but approximately twice as many males as females are present at term at the caudal end (Smotherman, unpublished data, 1986). This unequal distribution of the sexes may be mediated by differential mortality of embryos in the ovarian and caudal positions (Barr *et al.,* 1970; Beck, 1967). The relevance of male–female distribution within the uterus may extend beyond prenatal hormone exposure. During parturition and the immediate postnatal period, mother rats provide male offspring with more anogenital licking than females (Moore, 1982; Moore and Morelli, 1979; Smotherman, unpublished data, 1983). Factors that may influence the order of delivery of fetuses during parturition—including presentation (vertex vs. breech), uterine density, uterine laterality, and sex—are poorly understood (Fuller, McGee, Nelson, Willis, and Culpepper, 1976; Taverne, van der Weyden, Fontijne, Ellendorff, Naaktgeboren, and Smidt, 1977). Regardless of the exact order of delivery, it appears unavoidable that mothers will be exposed to male offspring before females in the majority of births. In this way, uterine position, sex, and birth order may interact to influence the onset of maternal behavior and the discrimination of different-sex pups (Moore, 1984).

Clearly, the intrauterine habitat of the fetus varies. Different-age fetuses do not occupy exactly the same environment, so changes in fetal behavior with advancing age (described below) cannot be presumed to be the result of maturation without environmental influence. Similarly, same-age fetuses are faced with varying conditions, depending on uterine density, uterine position, sex of wombmates, maternal age, diet and physiological condition, and the effects of their own behavior on morphology (e.g., umbilical cord length and amniotic fluid volume). Because the variable elements of the fetal environment constitute components of a highly integrated system, perturbations in any one component are likely to result in cascading effects throughout the fetal life-support system. Yet, we are only beginning to glimpse the importance of intrauterine variation in behavioral and morphological development.

Techniques for Investigating Fetal Behavior

Experimental analysis of behavioral development in mammalian fetuses is complicated by two general methodological problems: how to manipulate uterine features and how to assess the effects of these environmental manipulations on fetal behavior. Until recently, indirect inference has been the most common approach to solving these problems. In teratological research, for example, pregnant females are exposed to various experimental conditions (e.g., drugs, toxins, or other chemical substances) and the consequences of this prenatal exposure are inferred from postnatal anatomy (e.g., the loss, reduction, or malformation of body parts). When applied to questions of fetal behavior, however, this method of indirect inference ignores the essential intervening variable: the fetus *in utero*.

A more direct approach to the study of prenatal influences on behavior has involved the controlled manipulation of the immediate uterine environment and postnatal assessment of its behavioral consequences. An experiment used to investigate the influence of prenatal sensory experience on postnatal taste preferences exemplifies this approach (Smotherman, 1982b). Day-20 rat fetuses were exposed *in utero* to a chemosensory stimulus (apple juice) or to its saline control by intra-amniotic injection (Blass and Pedersen, 1980; Stickrod, 1981). This exposure was achieved by briefly externalizing the distended, transparent uterus, injecting apple juice into each amniotic sac, and returning the uterus to the peritoneal cavity. The animals were delivered at term by cesarean section, were reared by foster mothers, and were allowed to grow to adulthood. As adults, when presented with a choice between apple juice and tap water, the rats prenatally exposed to apple juice consumed significantly more apple juice than control rats lacking prenatal experience with apple juice. Moreover, the preference for apple juice was specific; no corresponding preference for a novel maple solution was apparent. This experiment clearly demonstrates how postnatal behavior, such as taste preference and fluid consumption, can be manipulated by a novel taste or odor cue present *in utero* late in gestation.

This "second-generation" approach to the study of fetal behavior—direct manipulation of the intrauterine environment with postnatal assessment of behavior—has proved successful in identifying behaviorally active substances and a capacity to learn *in utero* (Smotherman, 1982a; Stickrod, Kimble, and Smotherman, 1982a,b). Nevertheless, the approach is limited by having to assess the effects of prenatal manipulations postnatally. The delay between the manipulation and the testing prohibits a direct measurement of the responses of fetuses to environmental stimuli. In general terms, restriction to postnatal testing severely limits what we can learn about the fetus itself, its sensory capabilities, the existence of behavioral continuities between prenatal and postnatal life, and the importance of the interaction between the fetus and its environment in subsequent behavioral development. These issues call for a "third-generation" methodology: the direct observation of fetal behavior.

One strategy that has grown out of the technological breakthroughs of the 1970s and 1980s has been to replace invasive surgery with remote sensing techniques. Fetal monitoring and real-time ultrasonography have proved especially valuable in research concerned with human fetal movement. External fetal monitors can detect heart rate, uterine contraction, fetal respiratory movements, and gross fetal body movements (McLeod, Brien, Loomis, Carmichael, Probert, and Patrick, 1983; Robertson, Dierker, Sorokin, and Rosen, 1982; Sterman and Hoppenbrouwers, 1971); but cannot make finer distinctions among fetal behaviors. Real-time ultrasonography provides greater resolution, enabling researchers to describe an extensive repertoire of movements by the human fetus (Birnholz, 1984; de Vries *et al.*, 1982; Rayburn, 1982). The principal difficulty with ultrasonography, however, is that high resolution is difficult to maintain throughout a period of observation; therefore, any attempt to conduct a continuous, systematic observation of the fetuses becomes complicated.

With the aim of overcoming these limitations, our laboratory has adapted and currently uses several alternative surgical methodologies (on animal subjects) that enable direct, high-quality observation of fetal behavior. Under ether anesthesia, the spinal cord of a pregnant rat is surgically or chemically transected (Smotherman, Richards, and Robinson, 1984) or reversibly blocked with lidocaine (Smotherman *et al.*, 1986a) to eliminate the transmission of afferent stimuli posterior to the site of intervention. The female is then placed in a holding apparatus, her uterus is externalized through a midventral laparotomy, her hindquarters and uterus are immersed in a constant-temperature (37.5°C) bath of isotonic saline (Locke's solution) (Galigher and Kozloff, 1971), and the uterus is allowed to float freely within the fluid medium.

After a delay of 20 min, during which the effects of ether administration completely dissipate (Kirby, 1979), two fetuses are selected as subjects, one from the ovarian end of each uterine horn. The subject fetuses are observed under one of three environmental conditions: in uterus, in amnion, or in bath. When the subject fetus is studied in uterus, it remains within the unmanipulated uterus, and behavior is viewed through the semitransparent uterine wall of the uterus. The in-amnion preparation involves delivery of the subject fetus through a 10- to 15-mm incision in the uterine wall into the water bath, with care taken to preserve the connection between placenta and uterus; behavior is viewed through the transparent extraem-bryonic membranes. The in-bath preparation also involves the delivery of the sub-ject fetus through a uterine incision, maintaining the placental-uterine attachment intact, and additionally involves the removal of the extraembryonic membranes that surround the fetus. The behavior of each subject fetus is recorded during a 10-min observation session.

Although invasive, like all methods for investigating fetal behavior, these "third-generation" techniques enable high-quality behavioral observations not oth-erwise obtainable. These procedures are also demonstrably benign. Fetuses observed in uterus with the mother under reversible spinal anesthesia can be replaced in the mother's body cavity and delivered normally at term. Such pups are morphologically and behaviorally indistinguishable from unmanipulated pups (Smotherman *et al.*, 1986a).

Observation of fetuses in uterus provides the closest approximation to the nat-ural prenatal environment, and preparation of fetuses in amnion and in bath per-mits a detailed analysis of fetal movements and precise control over chemosensory and tactile stimulation. These techniques have been successfully applied to the analysis of age-related change in fetal behavior (Smotherman and Robinson, 1986); the emergence of behavioral organization (Smotherman and Robinson, 1986); fetal sensory capabilities (Smotherman and Robinson, 1985a); fetal learning and responsiveness to conditioned stimuli *in utero* (Smotherman and Robinson, 1985b); and the effect of experimentally induced behavioral suppression *in utero* on the development of subsequent physical anomalies (Barron, Riley, and Smotherman, 1986; Smotherman, Woodruff, Robinson, del Real, Barron, and Riley, 1986b). Each of these areas of inquiry is discussed below.

Fetal Movements: Motility or Behavior?

Spontaneous fetal activity is remarkably dissimilar to adult patterns of behav-ior. Individual limbs, the head, and the body trunk exhibit movements ranging from barely perceptible flexion of digits to vigorous wriggling and twisting of the whole body. Verbal descriptions of these movements in diverse species are striking in their similarity. Spontaneous fetal activity has been variously characterized as "the usual spontaneous, purposeless, squirming trunk, head and leg movements" (Windle and Griffin, 1931, p. 165) and "unintegrated, aimless movements" (Naray-anan *et al.*, 1971, p. 121). Superficially, fetal activity appears to lack orientation and coordination. Movements of individual body parts seem dissociated from one another and appear to occur without temporal or spatial organization.

Because recognizable action patterns are rare or absent during the prenatal period, most researchers have used arbitrary categories to summarize fetal activity (e.g., "local," "regional," and "total" movements; Narayanan *et al.*, 1971) or have quantified the discrete movements of individual body parts (Narayanan *et al.*, 1982; Smotherman *et al.*, 1984). In our laboratory, seven basic categories of movement by the rat fetus are distinguished: foreleg, hindleg, head, mouth, curl, stretch, and twitch. These patterns are described in Table 1 and Figure 4. These exclusive movement categories are scored by entry into a real-time event recorder (with interrater reliability in excess of .90), creating a continuous record of spontaneous fetal activity in timed sequence during an observation period. To facilitate more inclusive levels of analysis, several summary categories are derived from the basic categories of fetal behavior to reflect the total amount of movement (whole activity and component activity) and simultaneous movement of two or more body parts (complex movement; Table 1). We have used this protocol in the observation of more than 1,000 rat fetuses under different experimental conditions. Fetuses have been observed at all ages from Day 16 (when spontaneous movement first appears) through Day 21 (just hours before parturition), thereby providing information on developmental changes in fetal behavior.

The first signs of movement are evident in the rat fetus late on Day 15 of gestation (Angulo, 1932). Spontaneous activity, consisting of simple movements of the forelegs and lateral flexions of the body trunk (curls), becomes apparent within 12 h (Day 16) (Figure 5; Smotherman and Robinson, 1986). Foreleg movements continue to dominate fetal activity throughout gestation (comprising 45% of all fetal behavior), although their relative abundance declines during gestation. With the subject fetus observed in uterus, foreleg and curl movements reach their highest

---

TABLE 1. CATEGORIES OF FETAL BEHAVIOR

INDIVIDUAL CATEGORIES OF MOVEMENT

Head: Any discernible movement of the head, involving flexion and/or rotation of the head and neck.

Mouth: One cycle of opening and closing the mouth, exclusive of movements of the tongue.

Foreleg: Flexion or extension of one or both forelimbs originating at the shoulder, elbow, wrist, or digits.

Hindleg: Flexion or extension of one or both hindlimbs originating at or distal to the pelvis.

Twitch: A momentary, spasmodic contraction of muscles of the lateral and ventral portions of the trunk in the general vicinity of the diaphragm.

Curl: Ventral or lateral flexion or torsion of the entire body trunk, causing the posterior end of the body to move to one side of the median sagittal plane.

Stretch: Dorsal extension of the body trunk, causing the body to straighten or curve backward with the pelvic region moving above the horizontal plane of the body.

SUMMARY CATEGORIES OF FETAL ACTIVITY

Complex movement: Two or more individual movement patterns that occur simultaneously (e.g., foreleg and mouth).

Whole activity: The total number of times a fetus is recorded as active. Each complex movement is scored as a single whole act.

Component activity: The total number of individual body-part movements of a fetus. Each behavioral component of a complex movement is scored as a separate component act.

ADDITIONAL CONTEXTUAL CATEGORY

Mother active: Any movement of the upper body or forelegs of the restrained female rat that causes the free-floating uterus and fetuses under observation to be passively moved.

frequencies of occurrence on Day 17 of gestation, coincidentally with the first appearance of several other categories of movement (hindleg, head, mouth, twitch, and complex movement). By Day 18, head and hindleg movements also reach their developmental peak, as do complex movement and overall activity. These categories exhibit a plateau or a slow decline in frequency through Day 21. The three remaining types of fetal movement exhibit their developmental peak *in utero* later in gestation: stretch peaks on Day 19, mouth on Day 20, and twitch on Day 21. In addition, several new and rare movements, such as eye blinking (a brief contraction of the muscles surrounding the eye) and ear wiggling (a movement of one or both ears and the loose skin adjacent to the ears), and patterned combinations of simpler movements, such as wiping (synchronous movement of the forepaws along the side of the head) and chewing the paws (placement of the forepaws in the mouth), appear during the last few days of gestation.

Few comparable data are available for the emergence of spontaneous fetal behavior in other mammals. In species that bear precocial young, such as guinea pigs (*Cavia porcellus*—Carmichael, 1934) and sheep (*Ovis aries*—Barcroft and Barron, 1939), fetal movement originates at a relatively earlier point in gestation than in the rat or cat (*Felis catus*—Windle and Griffin, 1931). The earliest spontaneous movements generally involve flexion of the forelimbs and lateral bending of the trunk, with hindlimb movement appearing later. The first movements of the human fetus are discernible at 7.5 weeks postmenstrual age (de Vries *et al.*, 1982). Movement of arms appears earlier in gestation (at about 12 weeks) than movement of legs (after 14 weeks). Overall activity increases rapidly during Weeks 10–15, continues to increase gradually and plateaus over the next 15–20 weeks, and begins to decline during the 2–3 weeks before birth (Edwards and Edwards, 1970).

For rats and humans, the two species for which comparative data are available, the emergence of spontaneous movement closely parallels the responsiveness of the fetuses to tactile stimulation. Local cutaneous stimulation of rat fetuses (using

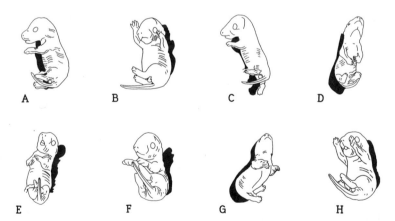

Figure 4. Line drawings depicting typical patterns of movement in basic categories of fetal behavior: (A) resting posture; (B) foreleg; (C) hindleg; (D) head; (E) mouth; (F) curl; (G) stretch and head (a complex movement); and (H) mouth and foreleg (wiping, also a complex movement).

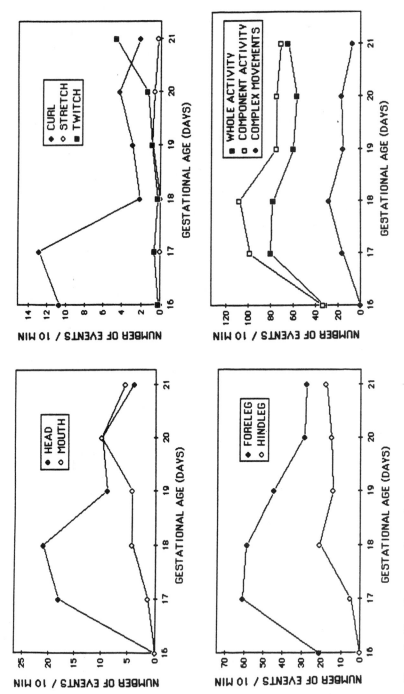

Figure 5. Mean frequency of seven basic patterns of fetal behavior and three summary categories over 10-min periods plotted as a function of gestational age: head and mouth (upper left); curl, stretch, and twitch (lower left); foreleg and hindleg (upper right); and whole activity, component activity, and complex movement (lower right). Data are for fetuses observed in utero. Please note that the ordinates of the four graphs use different scales.

164

a probe, bristle, or brush) can elicit movements from the forelimbs on Day 16, coincidentally with the earliest spontaneous movements (Angulo, 1932; Narayanan *et al.*, 1971). The vibrissae in the perioral region are also sensitive on Day 16, but stimulation typically evokes generalized trunk flexion. By Day 17, trunk movement can be elicited by direct stimulation of the flanks. Local stimulation on Day 18 generally evokes responses from multiple regions of the body ("diffuse mass action"; Narayanan *et al.*, 1971). These generalized responses of rat fetuses gradually give way to more localized movements on Days 19–20. Behavioral data for human fetuses observed from aborted pregnancies are similar (Hooker, 1952). The timing of the earliest evoked responses corresponds closely to the first spontaneous movements at 7.5 weeks. Close correspondences also have been identified between the earliest ages of evoked and spontaneous movements of the arms and legs, head, mouth, and trunk of the human fetus (de Vries *et al.*, 1982).

The principal conclusion to be drawn from these studies is that mammalian embryos exhibit a clear dichotomy between an early nonmotile period of development and a later motile period. Reflexogenic and apparently spontaneous movements appear at virtually the same point in gestation, although the precise timing varies among different species. Further, the onset of motility appears to correspond to significant changes in the developing nervous system. Fetal muscular activity is not myogenic and hence must arise from nervous stimulation (Straus and Weddell, 1940). Reflex transmission has been detected within isolated spinal cords of fetal rats on Day 15.5 (Saito, 1979), when fetal motility is first evident. Similarly, synapse formation in the cervical spinal cord of human fetuses occurs at 8 weeks of gestation (Okado, 1980, 1981), coincidentally with the origin of human fetal motility. Expansion of the behavioral repertoire of rat fetuses on Day 17 occurs at about the same time that intersegmental spinal reflexes appear, and neuronal inhibition of spinal discharge does not develop until Day 19.5 (Saito, 1979). These observations suggest that fetal activity may be organized at the spinal level, a view that fits well with findings that spontaneous activity in fetal rats is not eliminated following spinal cord section (Hooker, 1930) or decapitation (Narayanan *et al.*, 1971).

Further parallels have been identified between fetal behavior and the maturing chemistry of the central nervous system. In rats, neuronal maturation and synaptogenesis occur as early as Day 13 and proceed at an increasing rate throughout the last third of gestation, encompassing the period of origin and the expansion of fetal behavior (Coyle, 1977). This neural maturation is illustrated by the emergence of specialized receptor sites for various centrally active neuroregulators, many of which become functional in a patterned sequence within the CNS. Benzodiazepine binding sites, for example, are first evident on Day 14 in the spinal cord and the lower brain stem, and they subsequently emerge in a caudal-to-rostral pattern in the diencephalon (Day 15) and the telencephalon and the neocortex (Day 18; Schlumpf, Richards, Lichtensteiger, and Mohler, 1983). Other specific receptors identified during the fetal period include neurotensin (Pazos, Palacios, Schlumpf, and Lichtensteiger, 1985); opiate (Coyle and Pert, 1976); beta-adrenergic (Bruinink, Lichtensteiger, and Schlumpf, 1982); oxytocin and vasopressin (Whitnall, Key,

Ben-Barak, Ozato, and Gainer, 1985); and muscarinic cholinergic binding sites (Schlumpf, Palacios, Cortes, Pazos, Bruinink, and Lichtensteiger, 1985). In general, these binding sites undergo the most rapid period of expansion during gestational Days 16–18, coincidentally with rising levels of fetal activity.

Several parallels may be identified between these patterns of fetal development and the behavior of chick embryos *(Gallus domesticus)*, which have been the subject of intensive experimental investigation (Hamburger, 1963; Hamburger and Oppenheim, 1967; Provine, 1973). In chicks, motility begins at about Day 4 of incubation with slight head movements, followed by movement of other body parts over the next 3 days. During this period, spontaneous activity is clearly nonreflexogenic; chick embryos are not responsive to tactile stimulation until Day 7 (Provine, 1973). From the onset of motor activity to Day 13, movement by the chick embryo is spontaneous and rhythmic and appears jerky and uncoordinated. These periodic movements are controlled at the spinal level, as evidenced by their lack of response to spinal transection (Hamburger, 1973; Hamburger and Balaban, 1963) and the correlation of movement with the patterning of burst discharges in the spinal cord (Provine, 1973). Following Day 13, the periodicity of spontaneous movement slowly disappears, and overall activity declines. By Day 17, coordinated prehatching movements can be identified, which gradually increase in relative abundance up to the time of hatching on Day 21. In contrast to early periodic movements, coordinated hatching movements (such as tucking the head and pipping) and shifts of body position (rotation, mediated by leg movement) are governed by central processes in the brain and disappear following spinal transection (Oppenheim and Narayanan, 1968) or forebrain ablation (Bekoff, 1981; Oppenheim, 1972). These differences in the underlying neural control of chick activity have substantiated the qualitative distinction between early periodic motility (Types I and II movement) and later prehatching behavior (Type III movement; Hamburger and Oppenheim, 1967).

Although it is tempting to draw attention to the similarities in motor development between avian embryos and mammalian fetuses, several striking dissimilarities also exist. Most important, the onset of movement occurs at a much more advanced stage of development in mammals than in birds. The first movements by a chick embryo occur when the limbs are little more than buds, the nervous system is rudimentary, and the sensory apparatus is almost nonexistent (Hamburger, 1963). In contrast, the first movements by a fetus occur when the limbs are well formed, complete with motor and sensory innervation. For this reason, fetuses do not exhibit spontaneous motility before tactile responsiveness (Narayanan *et al.*, 1971). Fetuses also do not exhibit the jerky, periodic movements characteristic of Type I chick motility.

Two salient points may be concluded from these basic descriptions of behavioral development. First, movement patterns originate and peak at varying points during gestation. Heterochronous patterning of motor development has been interpreted as evidence that different body regions mature earlier than others (Kodama and Sekiguchi, 1984; Narayanan *et al.*, 1971). In some instances, the appearance of new movements follows a cephalocaudal pattern of development (e.g., forelegs move before hindlegs). But numerous exceptions to this pattern (e.g., oral movements appear and peak much later than limb movements) refute any simple head-to-tail explanation of behavioral ontogeny. Moreover, the maturation of the central nervous system, which governs fetal movement, appears to follow exactly the reverse pattern of development (caudal to rostral).

Second, at this qualitative level of analysis, there is little indication of coordination or integration of fetal behavior, particularly at earlier ages. The fact that various movement categories originate and peak at different points during gestation highlights the apparent independence of fetal movements. The unstructured aspect of prenatal activity has long been recognized for chick embryos (Kuo, 1932) and has been emphasized by use of the term *motility* in place of *behavior* (e.g., Angulo, 1932; Bekoff *et al.*, 1980; Hamburger, 1963). Whereas behavior is characterized by structure, coordination, and responsiveness to sensory stimuli, movements by mammalian fetuses and avian embryos lack apparent organization and neural influence above the spinal level. These observations have led to the conclusion that the "unstructured performance of the chick embryo up to 17 days, and similar performances of reptilian and mammalian embryos, hardly deserve the designation of 'behavior'" (Hamburger, 1973, p. 53).

Organization of Fetal Behavior

Since the early 1980s, fetal movement has been subjected to new methods of analysis. These studies question the long-standing conclusion that prenatal motility is qualitatively different from postnatal behavior. Basic descriptions of fetal development (summarized in the previous section) clearly indicate that fetal behavior is not coextensive with mature adult behavior. Nevertheless, evidence from many sources indicates that fetal movements exhibit subtle organization and incipient coordination. In rat fetuses, behavioral organization is evident in the diversity of fetal movements, the synchronous movement of different body parts, and the nonrandom temporal patterning of activity. Many of these features have been identified in the behavior of human fetuses as well.

The behavioral repertoire of rat fetuses continually expands from its origins on Day 16 through parturition. With each day, the gross appearance of individual movements and the emergence of rare but coordinated acts (e.g., wiping) increase the resemblance of the fetus to the newborn. Subjectively, older fetuses exhibit a larger repertoire of behavioral patterns and distribute their activity more evenly among different behaviors than do younger fetuses. This impression is confirmed by a quantitative measure of behavioral diversity derived from the standard information theory index of entropy (Shannon and Weaver, 1949):

$$H = \sum_{i=1}^{n} (p_i - \log_2 p_i) \tag{1}$$

where n is the number of behavioral categories, p is the probability that behavior i will occur in a given 1-s interval, and H is the overall entropy or diversity of behavior expressed in bits per act. *H* will vary from a value of 0 (when one category has a probability of 1.0) to a maximum of $\log_2 n$ (when all categories are equally probable). When fetuses are observed in uterus, this measure of diversity increases sharply over Days 16–18, plateaus on Days 18–20, and declines on Day 21 (Figure 6), a progression reflecting changes in the repertoire of fetal movements over the course of gestation (Smotherman and Robinson, 1986). In fact, this information index underestimates diversity late in gestation, when the seven basic movement categories become more variable in their expression (i.e., subcategories of behavior become recognizable), several new patterns of movement appear (eye blink and ear wiggle), and coordinated movements become evident (wiping and chewing the paws). When this additional variability is considered, behavioral diversity exhibits a monotonic increase from Day 16 through term even though overall activity peaks on Day 18.

Although the data are incomplete, this picture of a continuously expanding behavioral repertoire is also apparent in human fetal development. Ultrasonographic imaging during the first half of gestation has revealed that only one behavioral category ("just discernible movement") can be recognized at the onset of fetal movement (7.5 weeks; de Vries, *et al.*, 1982). Within 3 weeks, the number of distinguishable categories increases to 9, and by 13 weeks, 16 behavioral categories are recognizable. Comparable descriptions of repertoire changes during the last half of gestation are unavailable, although fetuses do continue to exhibit new patterns of movement (Birnholz, 1981; Birnholz and Benacerraf, 1983).

Behavioral organization can also be indicated by the integration of separate body parts into a single pattern of behavior. This kind of organization is exemplified by interlimb synchronization in chick embryos (Provine, 1980). Early during incubation, the simultaneous movement of both wings occurs about as often as of one wing and the ipsilateral leg (about 11% of wing movements are synchronous on Day 7). Beginning on Day 13, however, synchronous movement of two wings increases in frequency, whereas wing–leg synchrony decreases. By Day 19, 85% of

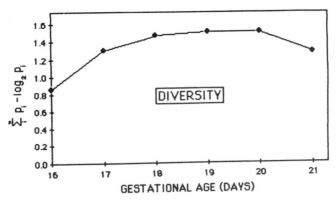

Figure 6. Mean values of behavioral diversity plotted as a function of gestational age for rat fetuses observed in uterus. Diversity is calculated from the Shannon–Weaver index of entropy; for seven categories of behavior, the maximum diversity = 2.81 bits/act.

all wing activity involves synchronized movement of both wings even though the level of overall wing activity is reduced (70% fewer movements on Day 19 than on Day 13). Because the steady increase in interwing synchronization cannot be accounted for by the chance association of independent parts (overall activity declines, reducing the probability of chance association) or by generalized movement (diffuse mass action cannot explain the reduction in wing–leg synchronization), it must be interpreted as evidence of early coordination of embryonic movement.

In the rat fetus, the simultaneous movement of two or more parts (complex movement) may be a comparable example of behavioral organization. The principal difficulty in using complex movement as an indication of early organization is distinguishing between chance coincidence and true synchronization of movement. Even if different body parts move independently of each other, as has been claimed repeatedly (Angulo, 1932; Narayanan *et al.*, 1971), one should expect that two body parts will occasionally move at the same instant by chance association. The probability of chance synchrony is directly proportional to overall activity; thus, the higher frequency of complex movements by rat fetuses on Days 17–20 may simply reflect greater activity at these ages. To investigate this possibility, we used an index of synchronicity (complex movement/whole activity) to provide a direct measure of synchronous movement as a function of overall activity (Smotherman and Robinson, 1986). This measure reveals that complex movements generally constitute a small percentage of total activity on Days 16 and 17, become relatively more common on Days 18–20, and decline in proportion to simple movements on Day 21 (subject fetuses are observed in uterus). These fluctuations in synchronicity during the course of gestation suggest that simultaneous movements are not necessarily the consequence of chance association.

A stochastic model can more accurately describe complex movement as a function of whole activity. The probability (p) of any fetal movement's occurring in a given 1-s interval can be estimated for each fetus by dividing total whole activity by the number of intervals during an observation (10 min $\times$ 60 s = 600 intervals). Based on this estimator, the chance association of two simultaneous movements (i.e., a complex movement consisting of two component acts) is equal to the joint probability of two movements (p^2), the chance association of three acts is equal to the joint probability of three movements (p^3), and so on. Thus, the expected frequency of complex movement is given by the equation:

$$ f = 600 \times \sum_{i=2}^{n} p^i \qquad (2) $$

where p^i is the joint probability of i simultaneous movements, n is the number of behavioral categories, and f is the expected frequency of complex movements.

Figure 7 depicts the goodness of fit with the random model by summarizing the mean difference between observed and expected frequencies of complex movement at various gestational ages (Smotherman and Robinson, 1986). The occurrence of synchronous movement is well described by the stochastic model on Days 16 and 17 of gestation, but it deviates from predicted frequencies thereafter. Specifically, complex movements are more abundant than expected on Days 18–20, indicating that fetuses are beginning to synchronize the movement of different body parts. Near term, however, the situation is reversed, and complex movements become less frequent than expected, a finding suggesting that movements are dispersed to prevent temporal overlap. The initial synchronization and later dispersal of fetal movements are indicative of central organization and may represent an incipient form of motor coordination.

Another striking example of synchronously organized motor activity is interlimb coordination, as described for Day 20 rat fetuses by Bekoff and Lau (1980). In addition to synchronous occurrence, truly coordinated movements are linked spatially and rhythmically, sharing a common direction, orientation, and duration. Close inspection of videotaped movement sequences revealed that contralateral limbs (within the same girdle) exhibit similar stroke durations, and the phases of left and right strokes are offset by 0.5. (A phase value of 0 or 1.0 occurs when two limbs are moved simultaneously in the same direction.) The observed phase relationship, which is apparent for both forelimbs and hindlimbs, indicates that Day 20 fetuses are capable of coordinated alternation in limb movement. Further, fetal interlimb coordination resembles the timing and pattern of normal postnatal swimming movements (Bekoff and Trainer, 1979). The duration of stroke cycles and phase relationships of forelimb–forelimb and hindlimb–hindlimb alternation observed in rat fetuses is within the normal range for 1-day-old rat pups.

An additional source of evidence for prenatal behavioral organization is the temporal patterning of spontaneous fetal behavior. Temporal patterning can assume many forms, ranging from highly stereotyped periodicity to circadian rhythms to aperiodic clustering of behavioral acts. Examples of all three kinds of temporal patterning have been described for human and rat fetuses. Simple periodicity is well illustrated by the spasmodic Type I movements of the chick embryo

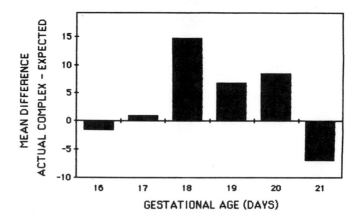

Figure 7. Direction and magnitude of discrepancies between observed and expected frequencies of complex movement plotted as a function of gestational age. Expected frequencies are based on a model of chance association of simple movements. Observed and expected frequencies do not differ significantly on Days 16 and 17, but do thereafter.

(Hamburger and Balaban, 1963), which exhibit a period (the average time between peaks in the cycle) on the order of a few seconds. Although rhythmic, the underlying organization of periodic movements has been demonstrated to derive from patterned bioelectric activity in the chick spinal cord (Ripley and Provine, 1972). Periodic movement by the chick embryo disappears by about Day 13 of incubation and is replaced by intermittent movements and later coordinated prehatching behavior (Hamburger and Oppenheim, 1967).

As mentioned earlier, the highly stereotyped, periodic movements described for avian embryos are not characteristic of mammalian fetuses. However, rhythmic activity involving gross body movements has been described for the human fetus by means of external monitoring and ultrasonographic techniques. As part of a larger study of the ontogeny of rest–activity patterns in neonates, Sterman and Hoppenbrouwers (1971) recorded human fetal body movements during Weeks 21–39 of gestation. Spectral analysis of the polygraphic activity records revealed two distinct rhythms in fetal movement that are maintained throughout the last half of gestation. The period of the faster rhythm is 40 min, which approximates the normal rest–activity cycle of newborn infants (period = 47 min) and is nearly identical to the normal REM cycle of the neonate (period = 39 min) (Stern, Parmelee, Akiyama, Schultz, and Wenner, 1969). The period of the slower rhythm is 96 min, which corresponds to no known behavioral cycle in the human neonate (Sterman, 1972) but is suggestively similar to the normal REM cycle of adults (Globus, 1970). The existence of long-period activity cycles in the human fetus has recently been corroborated by independent studies (Dierker, Pillay, Sorokin, and Rosen, 1982; Granat, Lavie, Adar, and Sharf, 1979).

Human fetal movements also exhibit shorter period oscillations (Robertson, 1985; Robertson *et al.*, 1982). Fourier analysis of external monitoring data collected during Weeks 21–35 of gestation has revealed two more rhythms in gross body movements. The dominant rhythm exhibits a period of about 2.5 min, which corresponds to a similar short-period rhythm in general activity of newborn infants (Robertson, 1982). This dominant rhythm is superimposed on a weaker, secondary rhythm with a period of only 1.0 min. The secondary rhythm is expressed in the tendency for body and limb movements to occur in short bursts.

The behavior of many adult mammals is tied to the normal day–night cycle of the environment. The "biological clock" responsible for circadian rhythmicity has been identified within the suprachiasmatic nucleus (SCN) of the hypothalamus (Moore, 1981). By means of deoxyglucose metabolic neural mapping techniques, the SCN has been shown to be functional on gestational Day 19 in rat fetuses (Reppert and Schwartz, 1984b) and in late-gestation fetuses of squirrel monkeys (*Saimiri sciureus;* Reppert and Schwartz, 1984a). In both rats and primates, the pattern of activity in the SCN was in phase with the maternal circadian cycle, a finding suggesting that the fetal clock is entrained by maternal coordination (Reppert and Schwartz, 1983). These findings are especially remarkable because most circadian rhythms of rodents are not overtly expressed until 2–3 weeks after birth (Aschoff, 1981). Thus, the metabolic activity of the fetal SCN is the earliest indication of circadian rhythmicity in rats.

External monitoring has provided evidence of circadian rhythms in human fetal motor activity. Ultrasound scanning has been used to measure changes in the frequency of fetal breathing and gross body movements over 24-h periods at 35 weeks' gestation (Patrick, Natale, and Richardson, 1978). First, it was found that fetal breathing and body movements exhibited a period of increased activity at intervals of about 1.5 h, in approximate agreement with the slower rhythm reported by Sterman and Hoppenbrouwers (1971). Second, fetal activity increased significantly between 0100 and 0700, with the percentage of time spent active rising from the daily average of 32% to an early morning average of 44%. The period of increased fetal activity corresponded to the times when the mothers were asleep. To date, these findings are the only evidence of circadian rhythmicity in fetal behavior.

Rhythmic activity is an important manifestation of behavioral organization in time, but temporal dependencies can also be evident in nonrhythmic behavior. For instance, events that are randomly generated with respect to time exhibit a broad range of time lags between events (interevent intervals). Truly random acts occur independently of the time lag since the preceding event, and patterned events show temporal dependencies reflected in the distribution of interevent intervals. By plotting the cumulative number of interevent intervals as a function of interval length, information regarding bout structure (whether individual events are clustered, randomly distributed, or evenly spread in time) can be obtained. This cumulative distribution should approximate an exponential decay function if the probability of an additional event's occurring in a given interval is constant and independent of the time lapse since the preceding event (Hailman 1974; Smotherman et al., 1984).

This analytic technique has recently been applied to the question of the temporal patterning of behavior in rat fetuses (Smotherman and Robinson, 1986). Figure 8 (top) presents two representative distributions for fetuses observed in uterus on Day 16 and Day 21 of gestation. Although both distributions appear to fit the exponential decay function quite well, systematic deviation is apparent in the Day 21 plot, indicating a greater frequency of short-duration intervals (0–5 s) than would be predicted by a random model. When the plots are compared at all gestational ages (Days 16–21), it is apparent that the frequency of short-duration intervals between acts exceeds expected values by only 18% on Day 16 but increases to a discrepancy of 103% by Day 21 (Figure 8, bottom). The fact that short intervals are more prevalent than expected indicates that the probability of a behavioral act's occurring in a given interval is higher if immediately preceded by another act. What these graphs reveal is a developmental change from independence of behavioral movements to a clustering of behavioral acts in time. A lack of temporal organization is characteristic of young fetuses (which also exhibit few complex movements) but is strongly evident among older fetuses (in spite of the decrease in synchronicity on Day 21).

To date, this quantitative approach has been applied to the temporal patterning of behavior only in rat fetuses. Representative graphs of human fetal activity obtained by ultrasonography, however, appear to conform to the general pattern of temporal independence at early ages (8–9 weeks), followed by the emergence of short-interval clustering over the next 5–10 weeks of gestation (de Vries *et al.*, 1982). These data further suggest that different patterns of movement vary in their temporal patterning, ranging from apparently random temporal distribution (startle movements) to highly clustered activities (head flexion and arm movements). This finding is consistent with our own observations of rat fetuses (Smotherman and Robinson, 1986), in which some categories of behavior can occur with stereotyped periodicity (bouts of mouth opening) or at varying intervals (head and limb movements).

The behavioral sophistication implied by these studies of repertoire diversity, movement synchronization, and temporal patterning is evidence that motor activity by the fetus, especially late in gestation, exhibits structure and incipient coordi-

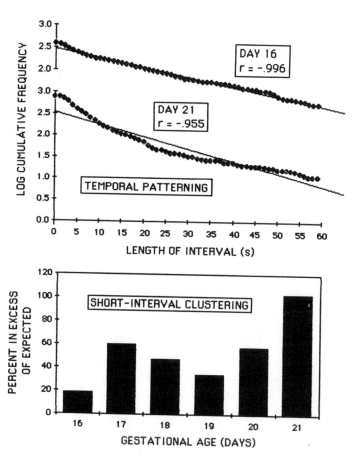

Figure 8. *(Top)* The cumulative distributions of intervals between successive behavioral acts by rat fetuses plotted on a logarithmic axis as a function of length of interval. Points are superimposed on the least-squares regression lines for each plot. The two graphs depict the characteristic lack of temporal patterning on Day 16 and deviation from random patterning on Day 21 for fetuses observed in utero. *(Bottom)* Abundance of short-duration inter-event intervals (0–5 s) in excess of expected frequencies for all six gestational ages. The difference between the observed and the expected frequency (based on a model of random patterning) is expressed as a percentage of the expected frequency.

nation. In the rat fetus, stochastic models are adequate to account for the organization of movement at the earliest gestational ages (Days 16 and 17), but they
break down thereafter. In the human fetus, the existence of up to five superimposed activity rhythms, some of which relate to REM cycles in the neonate and the
adult, suggests a degree of behavioral control above the spinal level. All of these
points of evidence argue that behavioral organization in the mammalian fetus
begins to emerge shortly after the origin of movement and is well developed before
parturition.

FETAL RESPONSIVENESS TO ENVIRONMENTAL CONDITIONS

RESPONSIVENESS TO SENSORY STIMULI

Although general descriptions of fetal behavior in the rat are available and an
understanding of the features of the prenatal environment is developing, relatively
little is known about fetal responsiveness to variable conditions *in utero*. We know
from indirect anatomical and physiological evidence that many of the sense organs
of mammalian fetuses are structurally developed before birth (Bradley and Mistretta, 1975; Mistretta and Bradley, 1986). We also have direct behavioral evidence
that the senses of tactoreception, chemoreception (olfaction and/or taste), and
audition are functional in the prenatal period among at least some species. In contrast, prenatal visual sensitivity appears to be poorly developed or absent in most
mammals (Bradley and Mistretta, 1975; Geubelle, 1984; Mistretta and Bradley,
1986).

Sensitivity of rat, guinea pig, sheep, cat, and human fetuses to cutaneous tactile stimulation has been recognized since the classic studies of fetal reflexology in
the 1920s and 1930s. Tactoreceptors become functional coincidentally with or
slightly before the onset of spontaneous fetal behavior. In fact, this concurrent
development has prompted some critics to doubt true behavioral spontaneity and
to interpret fetal activity as "movements of reflex nature for which the stimulus is
unknown" (Humphrey, 1953). This extreme position is defended less often today
(Oppenheim, 1981), in part because of experiments that have demonstrated continued spontaneous fetal activity, although altered in form and patterning, following sensory deafferentation (Dawes, Fox, LeDuc, Liggins, and Richards, 1972).
Our own research with rat fetuses has shown that repeated tactile stimulation activates fetuses above basal spontaneous levels (Smotherman and Robinson, in press).

Perception of other mechanical stimuli, as in audition, exhibits variable
expression among different species. Rats probably lack auditory sensation at birth,
but guinea pig fetuses can detect and respond to external sounds as early as 15
days before birth (Romand, 1971), and humans can respond by Week 28 of gestation (Birnholz and Benecerraf, 1983; Geubelle, 1984). The acoustic environment
of the fetus is rich, comprising an assortment of sounds generated within the
mother (by her eating, drinking, breathing, gastrointestinal activity, and cardiovascular activity) and attenuated sounds transmitted (vocalizations) or originating out-

side the mother (environmental noise; Armitage, Baldwin, and Vince, 1980; Walker, Grimwade, and Wood, 1971).

The receptors and CNS structures associated with chemoreception develop relatively early in gestation in most mammals (Bradley and Mistretta, 1975; Mistretta and Bradley, 1986), perhaps because many potentially important chemical cues readily cross the placenta, and the fetus develops within a rich chemical environment. Deoxyglucose metabolic neural mapping techniques have demonstrated in rats that the accessory olfactory bulb of the brain is active before birth, a finding indicating that rat fetuses are sensitive to olfactory cues normally present in amniotic fluid (Pedersen, Stewart, Greer, and Shepherd, 1983). Fetal behavior can be measurably activated on Day 19 by intra-amniotic presentation of a mint solution and can be greatly activated by repeated intraoral infusions of mint, lemon, orange, or sucrose solutions (Smotherman and Robinson, 1985a, in press). Conversely, fetal movements are suppressed following acute exposure to ethanol *in utero* (McLeod *et al.*, 1983; Smotherman *et al.*, 1986b). These findings suggest that novel chemosensory stimuli derived from the maternal diet and transported to the fetus across the placenta may play a role in the control and development of normal fetal behavior.

MATERNAL INFLUENCES

Although mammalian embryos can now be grown *in vitro* through advanced stages of development (Austin, 1973), the study of viable fetuses isolated from maternal influence is not yet possible. Yet, we know that the mother's diet, physical condition, and habits can have a profound influence on fetal well-being. The teratological literature is replete with examples of chemical substances that can be transported across the placenta to alter fetal development (e.g., fetal alcohol syndrome—Abel, 1984; and opiate-abstinence syndrome—Umans and Szeto, 1985). Similarly, prolonged maternal stress during pregnancy can affect the reproductive physiology and behavior of offspring (Ward, 1984). Most recently, physical exercise by pregnant mothers has been reported to reduce the birth weight of offspring (Lotgering, Gilbert, and Longo, 1985). The multiplicity of maternal influences on long-term fetal development suggests that fluctuations in maternal activity or physiological state can similarly affect short-term fetal behavior.

Currently, only indirect evidence is available for a maternal influence on fetal behavior. In adult animals, circadian activity rhythms are governed by an endogenous biological clock (believed to exist in the SCN of the hypothalamus), which is entrained to the exogenous light cycle of the outside world. In rodent and primate fetuses, the SCN is functional before birth but is isolated from external photic entrainment. Reppert and Schwartz (1983) demonstrated that the phase of the circadian cycle in the fetal SCN coincides with the maternal cycle, and that an induced phase shift in the maternal cycle results in a corresponding shift in the fetal cycle. This finding provides evidence that circadian rhythmicity during the prenatal period is coordinated by the mother.

Maternal coordination of fetal activity is indicated by external monitoring data on human infants (Sterman, 1972). The slower of two fetal activity cycles (period = 96 min) disappears after birth, a finding implying that it is regulated by some feature of the prenatal environment. In fact, the peaks of fetal activity generally correspond to periods of REM activity by the mother (Sterman and Hoppenbrouwers, 1971; Figure 9). This observation has led to the speculation that human fetal activity is partly related to periodic fluctuations in maternal physiology. Supporting evidence for this idea is provided by ultrasonic measurements of human fetal activity (Patrick *et al.*, 1978), which showed an inverse relationship between periods of fetal and maternal activity. Moreover, fetal breathing and body movements increase in occurrence during the second and third hour following the ingestion of food by the mother. The timing of activity peaks corresponds to the period of peak and decline in the concentration of glucose in maternal plasma.

In rats, maternal state has been implicated as an influence on fetal behavior by the demonstration that different methods of preparing the mother for the observation of fetuses are associated with different patterns of fetal activity (Smotherman *et al.*, 1984). The three techniques currently available—spinal transection, chemomyelotomy, and reversible lidocaine anesthesia—were developed to eliminate the need for general maternal anesthesia, which passes to the fetus and virtually extinguishes fetal movement. The outward effects of all three procedures on maternal behavior are identical and are well suited to the direct study of fetuses (Basmajian and Ranney, 1961; Kirby, 1979; Smotherman *et al.*, 1986a). However, a close analysis of fetal behavior reveals that overall activity is least when the mothers are prepared by chemomyelotomy and greatest when reversible lidocaine anesthesia is used. More important, individual categories of fetal movement are differentially affected, and patterns of developmental change are altered. Differences among preparations in overall fetal activity, individual patterns of movement, and temporal patterning of fetal behavior must be mediated through altered behavior

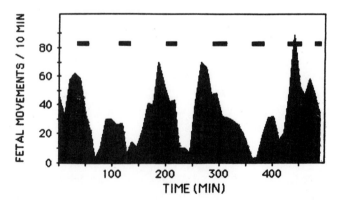

Figure 9. Comparison of the long-period activity cycle of a representative human fetus with its mother's REM cycle (indicated by solid bars). The correspondence between peaks of fetal activity and periods of maternal REM sleep seen here was observed in approximately 65% of the paired comparisons, a finding indicating a degree of relationship between these events. (Redrawn from Sterman and Hoppenbrouwers, 1971.)

or physiology of the mother. However, the actual mechanisms of this maternal influence remain unknown.

FETAL HYPOXIA

Windle (1944) and Humphrey (1953) criticized many of the original studies of fetal behavior by pointing out that fetuses are extremely sensitive to reduced oxygen availability when observed *in utero*. Although more recent studies have attempted to eliminate the effects of fetal hypoxia (e.g., Kirby, 1979; Narayanan *et al.*, 1971; Smotherman *et al.*, 1984), the role of oxygen availability in the dynamic control of spontaneous fetal behavior remains at issue. Classic experiments with cat, sheep, and human fetuses (Barcroft and Barron, 1939; Humphrey, 1953; Windle and Becker, 1940) identified several behavioral changes that accompany hypoxia. Initially, fetuses are hypersensitive to tactile stimulation and exhibit an increase in jerky movements of individual parts, especially forelimbs. Continued oxygen deprivation depresses irritability and slows spontaneous activity. Fetal movements become more generalized and sustained, comprising synchronous movements of head, limbs, and body trunk. Total asphyxia eventually eliminates spontaneous movement completely, with rhythmic respiratory movements (mouth opening and thoracic spasms) disappearing last.

In a more recent program of research with dog fetuses *(Canis domesticus)*, Arshavsky and his co-workers have extended these findings by documenting a battery of motor and physiological responses associated with transient hypoxia (Arshavsky, Arshavskaya, and Praznikov, 1976). Fetuses respond to the onset of hypoxia in a predictable sequence, beginning with jerky movements of individual body parts, followed by slower, sustained movements involving multiple parts of the body ("generalized motor reactions"). At the same time, the heart rate and the arterial blood pressure of the fetus are elevated. The initial increase in fetal heart rate and activity is apparently not a side effect of hypoxia; rather, it is a behavioral response controlled by the stimulation of sinocarotid chemoreceptors, which have been identified in the fetus (Biscoe, Bradley, and Purves, 1969).

Transient episodes of hypoxia may be induced by subtle changes within the intrauterine environment even under normal circumstances. For example, after the onset of motility on Day 16, the relative orientation of fetuses within the uterus—and thus, the region of body contact between adjacent fetuses—is constantly shifting. Late in gestation, with reduction in amniotic fluid volume, the physical buffer between fetuses disappears. At this time, a shift in the body position of one fetus can cause it to press against the umbilical cord of an adjacent sibling, thereby inducing a transient impairment of oxygen flow to the second fetus. In an analogous fashion, other changes in the fetal environment, such as postural changes by the mother, torsion of the uterus, or postural changes by the fetus itself, could result in a temporary restriction of umbilical circulation and a reduced availability of oxygen to the fetus. Impairment of umbilical circulation is a common source of complication during parturition in humans. Any of these short-term

WILLIAM P.
SMOTHERMAN AND
SCOTT R.
ROBINSON

changes in umbilical circulation, and the consequent temporary hypoxia, may play a role in the normal control of spontaneous fetal behavior.

FETAL RESTRAINT

Advancing fetal development is accompanied by a progressive diminution in free space within the uterus. At least three environmental factors, which are confounded during normal development, contribute to growing restraint: continuously increasing fetal body size, decreasing amniotic fluid volume, and increasing amniotic fluid viscosity. Uterine density (the number of fetuses in the same horn of the uterus) also contributes to intrauterine crowding by multiplying the effects of fetal growth. Greater fetal restraint should necessitate additional energy expenditure for fetal movement. Therefore, it is reasonable to expect some behavioral adjustments by the fetus in response to increased restraint late in gestation.

Comparing the behavior of rat fetuses in different physical environments provides the best evidence for an effect of intrauterine restraint on fetal movement. In most observational studies of animal fetuses, the subjects are not viewed through the wall of the uterus (in contrast to the behavioral summary above). Rather, fetuses are surgically externalized from the uterus—the placental-uterine connection being maintained—and are observed in amnion (through the transparent extraembryonic membranes) or in bath (with membranes removed; Bekoff and Lau, 1980; Kirby, 1979; Kodama and Sekiguchi, 1984; Narayanan *et al.*, 1971, 1982; Smotherman *et al.*, 1984; Smotherman and Robinson, 1985a). Because the three fetal preparations differ primarily in the freedom of movement they permit, they provide a means of assessing fetal restraint in same-age fetuses (Smotherman and Robinson, 1986).

In bath observation, which minimizes restraint, reveals the highest levels of activity in virtually all categories of rat fetal behavior (Figure 10). Conversely, fetuses studied in uterus, where restraint is greatest, exhibit the least activity.

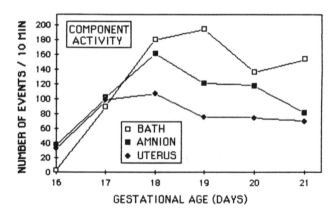

Figure 10. Total component activity of the rat fetuses observed in one of three environmental conditions—in uterus, in amnion, or in bath—plotted against gestational age. The lower activity of fetuses in uterus suggests a suppressive influence of fetal restraint on fetal behavior after Day 17.

Restraint not only affects overall activity but alters the distribution of behavior among categories as well; behavioral diversity is least in uterus and greatest in bath. As expected, restraint exhibits its most pronounced effect late in gestation. Movements of the body trunk, including curl and stretch, are especially sensitive to the effects of restraint: these behaviors are relatively frequent on Day 21 among fetuses in amnion or in bath but are rare among fetuses in uterus. Complex movements show a similar pattern of developmental change under different environmental conditions. Synchronicity does not vary with fetal environment except on Day 21, when the occurrence of complex movements increases over Day 20 levels in bath but decreases slightly in amnion and sharply in uterus. Because overall activity and behavioral diversity do not exhibit corresponding declines on Day 21, the decrease in synchronous movement in amnion and in uterus argues that fetuses perform the same number and kinds of actions but distribute these actions with less temporal overlap. Thus, fetal restraint influences the temporal patterning of fetal activity as well.

INTERSIBLING INFLUENCE

There are two general ways that fetuses can influence the behavior of their intrauterine cohabitants: indirectly, by collectively modifying the prenatal environment, or directly, by physical or chemical interaction among siblings. The principal example of indirect influence is the effect of uterine density on fetal development. In rats, the number of fetuses within the uterus is inversely correlated with body weight at birth (Barr *et al.*, 1970), a difference that is retained at least until early adulthood (Milkovic, Paunovic, and Joffe, 1976). Retarded fetal and placental growth in crowded uteri has also been reported in guinea pigs (Eckstein, McKeown, and Record, 1955; Ibsen, 1928), mice (McLaren, 1965), and humans (McKeown and Record, 1953). Singleton mouse fetuses, created by the surgical removal of all other fetuses from the uterus, are heavier at birth and mature earlier than fetuses that develop with siblings. Moreover, singletons are more active *in utero* than same-age fetuses exposed to the influence of siblings (Gandelman and Graham, 1986). More data are needed to extend these findings and to determine the scope of influence of uterine density on normal behavioral development.

There is still no direct evidence that fetal behavior is influenced by direct interaction among siblings. However, we know that rat fetuses are responsive to tactile stimulation (Angulo, 1932; Narayanan *et al.*, 1971; Smotherman and Robinson, 1985a), and therefore, that siblings in adjacent uterine positions may physically interact, providing a direct intersibling influence on behavior. Physical interaction becomes possible with the change in uterine shape on Day 18, and this possibility is accentuated by the reduction of amniotic fluid volume on Days 20–21. Direct intersibling influence may also be mediated by exchanged chemical cues. If the behavior of one fetus is altered because of local environmental conditions (e.g., transient hypoxia or tactile stimulation), chemical substances may be produced that diffuse directly across extraembryonic membranes or circulate in the maternal blood supply to affect the behavior of other fetuses in the uterus. Fetal stress, for instance, often results in raised cortisol levels or meconium staining of amniotic fluid. Although substances produced by the fetus have not yet been demonstrated to alter the behavior of siblings, chemical interaction between fetuses has been implicated in altered morphological and behavioral development. The best example of such an interaction is the effect of the prenatal exposure of female fetuses to testosterone produced by male siblings, described earlier (Babine and Smotherman, 1984; Hauser and Gandelman, 1983; Meisel and Ward, 1981; Richmond and Sachs, 1984).

UTERINE POSITION

Fetuses necessarily develop in different locations within the uterus, and microenvironmental conditions may vary systematically among different uterine positions. This possibility is supported by the finding that fetal body weight in rats varies significantly with uterine position (Barr *et al.*, 1970; Smotherman, unpublished data, 1986). However, the discrepancy in body weight is abrupt, smaller fetuses developing only in the terminal uterine positions at the ovarian and caudal ends of each horn. Embryonic mortality also varies with uterine position, ranging from 2.6 resorptions per 100 implants at the ovarian end to 14.5 resorptions per 100 implants at the caudal end (Barr *et al.*, 1970; Beck, 1967). Differential mortality may partly explain the observed discrepancy in the ratio of male to female fetuses. Rats in our laboratory exhibit an approximate 1:1 sex ratio at the ovarian end and intermediate positions within the uterus. However, at the caudal position nearest the cervix, the number of male fetuses exceeds the number of females by nearly 2:1 (Smotherman, unpublished data, 1986). The discontinuities in fetal body weight, mortality, and sex ratio suggest that development is altered by environmental conditions that vary continuously within the uterus (such as gradients of nutrients, oxygen, or waste disposal) or are unique to terminal positions (such as uterine constriction). Data on the direct behavioral influence of uterine position are unavailable. However, fetuses in terminal positions (ovarian and caudal) may be more susceptible to transient hypoxia or less subject to physical interaction between siblings than fetuses in intermediate positions. At the least, it is reasonable to expect that environmental stimuli that vary with uterine position may play a role in the control of spontaneous fetal behavior.

THE BIOLOGICAL FUNCTION OF FETAL BEHAVIOR

Sufficient data are now available to allow us to begin to evaluate the relative merits of the epiphenomenal, preparatory, and functional views of fetal behavior. The epiphenomenal hypothesis—in effect, the null—is rapidly becoming untenable. We have attempted to document how fetal behavior exhibits subtle organization, incipient coordination, and responsiveness to environmental conditions *in utero*. Such behavioral sophistication is unexplained as a mere side effect of development. Fetal behavior also has effects on both the immediate prenatal environment and the subsequent behavioral and morphological development. In the face of these discoveries, the assertion that fetal movement is a nonfunctional manifestation of neural maturation probably should be rejected.

CONTINUITY

Evidence for continuity between prenatal and postnatal behavior is growing. As we have discussed, fetal behavior in the rat becomes diverse, synchronized, and temporally organized during the last 4–5 days of gestation (Smotherman and Robinson, 1986), increasing its resemblance to postnatal pup behavior. Certain features of fetal behavior, such as the coordinated alternation of forelimbs and hindlimbs in Day 20 rat fetuses, bear a striking similarity in form and timing (stroke duration and phase relationship) to the limb movements of 1-day-old rat pups (Bekoff and Lau, 1980; Bekoff and Trainer, 1979). Movements of the mouth, the diaphragm, and the intercostal muscles of rat fetuses can circulate amniotic fluid to the lungs (Marsh *et al.,* 1963) and are virtually identical to the first functional respiratory movements after birth (Smotherman and Robinson, 1986). Prenatal breathing movements are also recognizable in human fetuses (de Vries *et al.,* 1982; Nijhuis, Martin, Gommers, Bouws, Bots, and Jongsma, 1983). Temporal rhythmicity is expressed by human fetuses, which show several behavioral cycles that appear to be coextensive with neonatal sleep–wake and activity rhythms (Dierker *et al.,* 1982; Robertson, 1985; Sterman and Hoppenbrouwers, 1971).

The sensory responsiveness of fetuses to experimental stimulation further emphasizes the continuity between prenatal and postnatal behavior. Recent experiments concerning fetal responsiveness to chemosensory stimulation have used a technique in which a fine polyethylene cannula is implanted in the mouth of a rat fetus. With the cannula in place, controlled volumes and concentrations of various chemosensory solutions can be infused without interrupting ongoing fetal behavior. These experiments have demonstrated that rat fetal behavior is activated by various novel chemosensory cues (e.g., mint, lemon, orange, and sucrose). Close examination of the response of fetuses relative to the moment of infusion has revealed that fetal activity is actually suppressed during the first 5-s interval following stimulus presentation but rebounds to a net increase in activity during the second and subsequent 5-s intervals after infusion (Smotherman and Robinson, in press). The transient suppression is not seen, however, in fetuses that had prior prenatal experience (exposure 2 days earlier) with the chemosensory stimulus (Figure 11). This pattern of initial suppression and delayed activation in response to a novel stimulus, but not to a familiar stimulus, resembles the well-known orienting reflex (OR) described for a variety of mammalian species (Hinde, 1970). The OR is characterized by a transient inhibition of ongoing activity, a reorientation of the head and the sensory organs toward the source of stimulation, an adjustment of posture, and various physiological changes, such as heart rate deceleration, peripheral vasoconstriction, and an increase in skin conductance (Rohrbaugh, 1984).

Rat fetuses are also activated by prenatal infusions of milk (commercial light cream, which is similar in composition to rat milk). On infusion of milk into the mouth, fetuses exhibit extensor responses that resemble the stereotyped "stretch reflex" of newborn pups on the receipt of milk ejection while suckling (Drewett, Statham, and Wakerley, 1974; Hall and Rosenblatt, 1977; Smotherman and Robinson, 1987). Although only suggestive, these findings illustrate how adaptive postnatal behavior may be foreshadowed by fetal responsiveness during the prenatal period.

Most recently, investigators have concluded that human fetuses exhibit behavioral states that may correspond to the four recognized sleep–wake states of the human neonate (Nijhuis *et al.*, 1983; Timor-Tritsch, Dierker, Hertz, Deagan, and Rosen, 1978). After 36 weeks of gestation, correlated patterns of fetal heart rate, body movement, and eye movement satisfy three defining criteria of behavioral states: central coordination, stable association over an extended period, and expression in more than one behavioral variable (Nijhuis, Prechtl, Martin, and Bots, 1982). Fetal behavioral states also recur cyclically, a finding that probably reflects an underlying connection between periodic wakefulness and the long-period activity rhythms described earlier (e.g., Sterman and Hoppenbrouwers, 1971).

Prenatal sensory experience can influence the course of behavioral development, determining the range of effective stimuli and the form of response. For instance, the importance of prenatal auditory experience has been the subject of intensive study in birds. In gull chicks *(Larus atricilla),* for example, some species-typical vocalizations by adults activate movements by the embryo within the egg; other calls suppress activity (Impekoven and Gold, 1973). Experience with parental vocalizations is important in posthatching individual recognition in guillemot chicks *(Uria aalge)* and species identification in domestic mallard ducklings *(Anas*

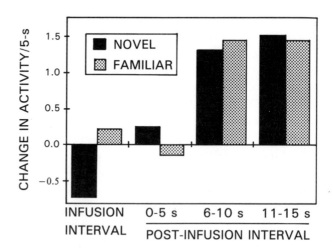

Figure 11. Differential response of rat fetuses to oral infusions (20 μl) of novel or familiar mint solution. Responses are plotted relative to baseline activity, which is the mean number of component acts during the 1-min interval preceding infusion. Response scores reflect the mean change from baseline in component activity during four 5-s intervals following infusion. Although both mint solutions have the net effect of activating behavior, novel mint suppresses activity at the moment of infusion.

mammalian fetuses has received comparatively little attention. However, Vince (1979) exposed guinea pigs fetuses to alien vocalizations (chicken clucking) *in utero* and measured their response to various sounds after birth. Neonatal guinea pigs exposed to the calls showed a differential heart-rate response as a function of pre- natal experience. Naive guinea pigs (lacking prenatal exposure) were startled by the novel sounds, as evidenced by a rapid increase in heart rate. In contrast, expe- rienced guinea pigs (with prenatal exposure) exhibited a more stable heart rate and were not startled. Yet, both groups showed a normal response to species-typical guinea pig vocalizations. The biological significance of this mechanism in guinea pigs is not known.

The importance of prenatal auditory experience under more natural circum- stances has been dramatically demonstrated by the work of DeCasper and his coworkers with human infants. They initially discovered that human newborns alter their rate of nonnutritive sucking to gain access to tape recordings of the mother's voice, and that the mother's voice is preferred over the voice of an unfamiliar female (DeCasper and Fifer, 1980). This technique was subsequently used to trace the sensitive period, during which maternal voice acquires its reinforcement value, to the prenatal period. Pregnant women were asked to read aloud passages from a children's story (Dr. Seuss's *The Cat in the Hat*). Within three days of birth, new- borns preferred to hear their mothers read from the familiar story over an unfa- miliar passage (*The King, The Mice, and the Cheese*; DeCasper and Spence, 1986). In an analogous way, recorded sounds of maternal heartbeat are reinforcing to the neonate (DeCasper and Sigafoos, 1983), and heartbeat sounds are preferred by infants over unfamiliar voices (Panneton and DeCasper, 1984). These findings sug- gest that some form of auditory perceptual learning occurs when fetuses are exposed to the normal acoustic environment *in utero*. These experiences have implications not only for the behavior of the neonate, but also for the nature of the parent–infant interaction (Bell and Harper, 1977).

Prenatal experience with chemosensory stimuli can also guide postnatal inter- actions between mother and offspring. Suckling, for example, is an early vital post- natal behavioral pattern that consists of a complex sequence of activities initiated by the location of and attachment to the nipple. Initial nipple attachment is facil- itated by the olfactory characteristics of amniotic fluid placed on the nipples during parturition by the mother (Blass and Teicher, 1980; Teicher and Blass, 1976). Sub- sequent experiments have documented how manipulation of the prenatal experi- ence with amniotic fluid can alter normal nipple attachment (Pedersen and Blass, 1982). On Day 20 of gestation, citral, a tasteless lemon scent, was injected into the amniotic fluid of fetuses *in utero* (Blass and Pedersen, 1980; Stickrod, 1981) and was presented again immediately after birth. Pups that received both prenatal and postnatal exposure to citral attached to washed nipples painted with citral, but pups that received only prenatal or postnatal exposure, or neither, failed to attach to citral-painted washed nipples. Further, citral-exposed pups did not attach to nipples bearing amniotic fluid. These data clearly illustrate the continuity in pre- natal and postnatal olfactory experience.

The ability to precisely manipulate chemosensory experience *in utero* has yielded clear evidence of prenatal learning in the rat fetus. With the mother under ether anesthesia, the uterus is externalized through a midventral incision, and individual rat fetuses are exposed by intra-amniotic injection to a novel chemosensory stimulus (mint solution) on Day 17 of gestation. Immediately after stimulus presentation, each fetus receives an intraperitoneal (ip) injection of lithium chloride (LiCl), an agent that induces an illness reaction in adult rats and that generally suppresses spontaneous fetal activity. Following treatment, the uterus is replaced in the mother, and the incision sutured closed. Two days later, on Day 19, the mother and the fetuses are prepared for direct observation of fetal behavior, and each subject fetus is reexposed to the conditioned mint stimulus (without associated LiCl). On reexperiencing the taste and odor of mint, the fetuses exhibit a marked suppression in fetal activity that resembles the normal response to LiCl injection (Smotherman and Robinson, 1985b). This response, which now has been replicated several times in our laboratory, demonstrates that fetuses can acquire and express a conditioned aversion to a chemosensory stimulus *in utero*.

In subsequent experiments, this conditioning technique has provided new information concerning the sensory and learning capabilities of the rat fetus. The form and magnitude of the conditioned response varies with the concentration of the mint solution presented on Day 19, a finding indicating the existence of either a sensory threshold or an ability of the fetus to discriminate among different stimulus concentrations (Smotherman and Robinson, 1985a). Fetuses also do not generalize the conditioned response to other novel chemosensory cues—lemon, for example. Although aversive conditioning does not alter fetal responsiveness to novel tastes and odors, it may modify the central processes responsible for regulating responsiveness in other sensory modalities. This possible effect is documented by an experiment in which fetuses were aversively conditioned to mint in the normal way and were then exposed to both the conditioned olfactory cue and tactile stimulation two days later (Smotherman and Robinson, in press). Unconditioned fetuses responded to repeated tactile stroking (with a camel hair brush) with increased activity. Conditioned fetuses, exposed to a control saline solution before testing, also exhibited greater activity when stroked. However, conditioned fetuses pretreated with the conditioned mint stimulus were not activated by stroking. In fact, with repeated application of the tactile stimulus, responsiveness diminished (Figure 12). The discovery of this contingent response to tactile stimuli as a function of prior experience with a contextual odor satisfies many of the criteria for the alteration of a behavioral state in the fetus (Nijhuis *et al.*, 1982).

Fetuses conditioned *in utero* can retain the learned association until well after birth. Pups treated prenatally, but tested before weaning, (1) avoided mothers' nipples painted with the aversive odor stimulus (Stickrod *et al.*, 1982a); (2) avoided wood shavings scented with the aversive odor (Stickrod *et al.*, 1982b), and (3) exhibited longer latencies to attach to a nipple in the presence of the conditioned odor (Smotherman, 1982b). Prenatal experience with a novel, unconditioned chemosensory cue (apple juice) can be retained into adulthood to influence drinking preferences; apple juice is preferred over tap water by prenatally exposed rats

(Smotherman, 1982a). Experiences and associations formed *in utero* reflect more than the emerging capabilities of the fetus; they can shape and direct important postnatal patterns of behavior. Such continuity across the transition from prenatal to postnatal life may be more important than was once thought in the normal ontogeny of mammalian behavior.

ONTOGENETIC ADAPTATION

In addition to preparing the fetus for postnatal life, it has been suggested that some fetal behaviors may be ontogenetic adaptations (Oppenheim, 1981). Certain anatomical structures, such as the placenta and the umbilical cord, function solely to maintain the fetus until parturition. Likewise, certain features of fetal behavior may be functional during gestation and serve to improve the ability of the fetus to survive and develop normally within the changing environment of the uterus. Although the idea of ontogenetic adaptation has been current since the turn of the century (Baldwin 1902), investigators are still faced with a paucity of data. Nevertheless, a few lines of evidence suggest that fetal behavior is indeed adaptive during the prenatal period.

Behavioral adaptations of more primitive amniote embryos have long been recognized. The prehatching and hatching behavior of avian embryos provides a case in point. In chick embryos, the last few days of incubation are characterized by a predictable sequence of activities, beginning with a shift of body position within the egg and soon followed by tucking (coordinated head movements that culminate in the placement of the head under one wing), draping (pushing the bill toward the air space at the top of the shell), penetration of the membranes with

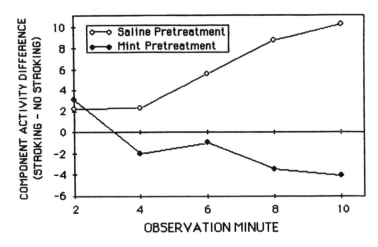

Figure 12. Differential response of rat fetuses to stroking following exposure to saline or mint. Each point represents the mean activity difference between stroked and control (unstroked) fetuses. Tactile stroking was administered immediately before the second, fourth, sixth, eighth, and tenth minute of each observation session. Activity scores are the number of component acts during the 60-s interval after stroking. The responses of saline- and mint-pretreated fetuses did not differ during Minute 2, but did thereafter.

the beak (associated with the onset of lung respiration), pipping (breaking through the egg shell with the aid of a specialized egg tooth on the beak), climax rotation (extending the crack in a circle around the top of the shell), and thrusting (removing the shell cap and emerging; Oppenheim, 1973). The adaptive value of these movements is obvious, yet they occur only during a short period in the life of the bird.

Analagous behavioral adaptations are recognized in the embryos of marsupial mammals. Following a relatively short gestation, marsupials give birth to very immature offspring; at birth, the 12-day-old embryos of the American opossum *(Didelphis virginiana)* are comparable in development to the rat embryo on Day 10. The newborn marsupial must move under its own power, without maternal aid, from the orifice of the urogenital sinus to the teats within the pouch. Locomotion in marsupial embryos is facilitated by deciduous claws that aid forepaw grasping, well-developed foreleg muscles (in contrast to the mere buds of the hindlimbs), and motor innervation sufficient to control coordinated locomotor activity (Sharman, 1973). The visual and auditory senses are still in embryonic stages of development at birth, but olfaction is functional and probably helps guide the embryo to the pouch (Sharman and Calaby, 1964). After reaching the pouch, the embryo attaches to a teat with the aid of a flattened oral shield, which functions somewhat like an air-tight washer (Sharman, 1973). Thus, newborn marsupials, which by most criteria are less mature than the fetuses of placental mammals, exhibit anatomical and behavioral adaptations that are vital to their survival and development.

In spite of the performances of other amniote embryos, the possibility of ontogenetic behavioral adaptations in placental fetuses has only recently come under consideration (Oppenheim, 1981). One form of behavioral adaptation, whether prenatal or postnatal, involves the active modification of environmental conditions. In rats, the aqueous medium in which the fetus develops provides space for growth and movement, and the volume of this space appears to be regulated, in part, by active ingestion and elimination by the fetus (Lev and Orlic, 1972; Marsh *et al.,* 1963). The marked decrease in amniotic fluid volume that occurs on Days 20–21 is probably brought about by increased rates of fluid ingestion (Marsh *et al.,* 1963; Tam and Chan, 1977). In contrast to other causes of oligohydramnios (e.g., premature rupture of the amnion), this decrease in fluid volume is accompanied by an increase in fluid viscosity and protein content (Wirtschafter and Williams, 1957a, b). Thus, the restraining influence of oligohydramnios may be compensated late in gestation by the improved lubricant qualities of the fluid.

The umbilical cord also contributes to confinement *in utero.* The position and activity of the fetus is limited by the length of the cord. Tensile forces produced by fetal movement are thought to be responsible for umbilical cord growth, with greater activity stimulating cord growth and providing greater freedom of movement (Moessinger *et al.,* 1982). Thus, it appears that fetuses have some measure of control over their own immediate environment through the regulation of conditions that facilitate or restrict movement.

A second form of adaptation involves behavioral adjustments to compensate for less than optimal environmental conditions. The behavior of rat fetuses under varying conditions of intrauterine restraint may be an example of such compensation. Late in gestation, rat fetuses perform fewer complex movements even though overall activity remains high (refer to Figure 7). Similarly, synchronous movements decline in frequency, whereas individual movements become strongly clustered (refer to Figure 8). The effect of these behavioral adjustments is to slightly disperse fetal movements, thereby reducing temporal overlap under conditions of high fetal restraint (Smotherman and Robinson, 1986).

Fetal behavior in response to oxygen deprivation may provide an additional example of ontogenetic adaptation. In the early studies of reflexogenic activity in the fetus, several investigators noted an increased sensitivity of the fetus to tactile stimulation during the early phases of hypoxia (Angulo, 1932; Windle and Becker, 1940). Among these heightened reflexes are stretch responses of the limbs and body bending (Humphrey, 1953). If, as seems likely, the fetus is naturally exposed to transient episodes of hypoxia *in utero,* whether induced by physical contact with adjacent fetuses or entanglement of the umbilical cord, these reflex patterns may be functional in altering the position of the fetus and relieving the cause of oxygen deprivation. Interestingly, body curls (bending) are among the most vigorous movements exhibited by rat fetuses and are commonly elicited by aversive stimulation (Smotherman and Robinson, 1985b). In human fetuses, complete change in body position can be brought about by alternating leg movement and twisting of the trunk (de Vries *et al.,* 1982). In addition, increased motor activity by the fetus during hypoxic episodes appears to facilitate a rise in heart rate, arterial blood pressure, and rate of blood flow through the placenta, which also helps compensate for reduced oxygen availability (Arshavsky *et al.,* 1976). The characteristic behavioral response to hypoxia by fetuses apparently disappears at birth. Newborn rat pups subjected to hypoxia perform rhythmic breathing movements (lip smacking) and wiping movements, in which the forepaws are drawn along the side of the head (R. Almli, personal communication, 1985). These movements may be functional in removing obstructions from the head and in facilitating breathing, but they are wholly different in form and effect from the generalized body movements of the hypoxic fetus observed *in utero.*

Another set of ontogenetic adaptations may be evident in the environmental and behavioral changes that occur immediately before parturition. In humans, most fetuses move into the vertex (head-down) presentation before birth. Throughout gestation, changes in body position are accompanied by fetal activity, especially coordinated leg and body movements (de Vries *et al.,* 1982). Similar movements are exhibited by fetuses during cephalic version (Suzuki and Yamamuro, 1985). The highest frequency of cephalic version occurs between Weeks 28 and 32 of gestation, at about the same time that the uterus changes shape and begins to restrain fetal movement (Suzuki and Yamamuro, 1985). Conditions associated with suppressed fetal movement *in utero,* such as fetal alcohol syndrome, congenital paralysis, or uterine malformation, are also correlated with a significant increase in breech births (Braun, Jones, and Smith, 1975; Suzuki and Yamamuro, 1985). In addition, the behavior and reflexes of breech fetuses are often qualitatively and quantitatively different from vertex fetuses (Luterkort and Marsal,

1985). From these lines of evidence, it appears that cephalic version is due to an adaptive behavioral response by the fetus to altered environmental conditions *in utero*. Thus, vertex presentation in humans—and behavior-induced changes in amniotic fluid volume, viscosity, and lubrication in the rat—illustrates how fetal behavior may facilitate the process of parturition.

In each case, the patterns of fetal behavior responsible for these effects are retrogressive structures; they either disappear at the time of parturition (fetal responses to restraint and hypoxia) or are transformed as postnatal patterns of behavior (breathing and locomotor movements). Just as temporary physical structures, such as the placenta, the umbilical cord, and the extraembryonic membranes, are clear examples of anatomical adaptation to the prenatal environment, retrogressive movement patterns provide the most compelling evidence for ontogenetic behavioral adaptation (Gould, 1977; Oppenheim, 1982). It therefore appears that many features of fetal behavior are functional at the time of their expression *in utero*.

Fetal behavior also has long-term consequences for the health and viability of the organism. Prenatal movement plays a necessary role in the fetus's normal physical and behavioral development (Hofer, 1981; Moessinger, 1983). There exists a reciprocal causal relationship between physical structure and fetal behavior during ontogeny. For example, the rhythmic intake and expulsion of amniotic fluid is important in normal pulmonary development (Vyas, Milner, and Hopkins, 1982). Prolonged inactivity, resulting from congenital myopathy, neural dysfunction, oligohydramnios, or experimental curare administration, causes fetuses to develop physical anomalies, such as joint contractures, facial and skin deformation, pulmonary hypoplasia, and growth deficiency (Mease, Yeatman, Pettett, and Merenstein, 1976; Moessinger, Bassi, Ballantyne, Collins, James, and Blanc, 1983; Moessinger *et al.*, 1982). Some of the same outcomes can occur among rat fetuses that remain in the uterus beyond their normal gestation (Smotherman, unpublished data, 1986).

Behavior is not a trivial aspect of fetal life. Normal muscular, skeletal, neural, and behavioral development is probably facilitated by fetal activity. Conversely, altered morphological and behavioral development is a likely consequence of grossly modified fetal behavior. A corollary of this conclusion is that any substance or external influence that alters fetal activity or characteristics of the fetal environment should be viewed as a potential teratogen (Smotherman *et al.*, 1986b).

CONCLUDING REMARKS

Behavior and its underlying functional neurology does not suddenly appear at the moment of birth. It is manifested soon after the fetus develops the neural and motor structures necessary for movement. Prenatal behavioral processes occur within an environment that shares certain features with the postnatal world. The intrauterine environment exhibits systematic and random variation, it is modifiable by fetal growth and activity, and it is both vital and, occasionally, suboptimal for fetal survival. Since the mid-1970s, revitalized interest in mammalian behavioral development has interfaced with technological improvements in methods for studying the fetus *in utero,* creating a vigorous new field that is beginning to change our view of life during the prenatal period. Our optimism is admittedly biased, but we believe that the current renaissance in fetal research will provide fundamental new insights into long-standing questions about the nature of the relationship between mind and body and the epigenetic interplay between inheritance and experience in behavioral ontogeny (Kuo, 1967). This sentiment is expressed in a passage by Samuel Coleridge (1885), which, coincidentally, was published in the same year as Preyer's original study of the fetus:

> Yes—the history of a man for the nine months preceding his birth would probably be far more interesting and contain events of greater moment, than all the three score and ten years that follow it!

Acknowledgments

We thank Patricia LaVallee and Ted Trask for their diligent archival work in the preparation of this chapter. William P. Smotherman is supported by Grant HD 16102-06 and Research Career Development Award HD 00719-02 (NIH).

References

Abbas, T. M., and Tovey, J. E. Proteins of the liquor amnii. *British Medical Journal,* 1960, *2,* 476–479.

Abel, E. L. Prenatal effects of alcohol. *Drug and Alcohol Dependence,* 1984, *14,* 1–10.

Adolph, E. F. Ontogeny of volume regulations in embryonic extracellular fluids. *Quarterly Review of Biology,* 1967, *42,* 1–39.

Angulo y Gonzalez, A. W. The prenatal development of behavior in the albino rat. *Journal of Comparative Neurology,* 1932, *55,* 395–442.

Aristotle. *De generatione animalium* ("On the generation of animals," trans. by A. Platt). Chicago: Encyclopaedia Britannica, 1952.

Armitage, S. E., Baldwin, B. A., and Vince, M. A. The fetal sound environment of sheep. *Science,* 1980, *208,* 1173–1174.

Arshavsky, I. A., Arshavskaya, E. I., and Praznikov, V. P. Motor reactions during the antenatal period correlated with the periodic change in the activity of the cardiovascular system. *Developmental Psychobiology,* 1976, *9,* 343–352.

Aschoff, J. (Ed.). *Handbook of behavioral neurobiology.* Vol. 4. *Biological rhythms.* New York: Plenum Press, 1981.

Austin, C. R. (Ed.). *The mammalian fetus in vitro.* London: Chapman & Hall, 1973.

Avery, G. T. Responses of foetal guinea pigs prematurely delivered. *Genetic Psychology Monographs,* 1928, *3,* 245–331.

Babine, A. M., and Smotherman, W. P. Uterine position and conditioned taste aversion. *Behavioral Neuroscience,* 1984, *98,* 461–466.

Baldwin, J. M. *Development and evolution.* New York: Macmillan, 1902.

Barcroft, J., and Barron, D. H. The development of behavior in foetal sheep. *Journal of Comparative Neurology,* 1939, *70,* 477–502.

Barcroft, J., Barron, D. H., and Windle, W. F. Some observations on genesis of somatic movements in sheep embryos. *Journal of Physiology,* 1936, *87,* 73–78.

Barr, M., Jr., Jensh, R. P., and Brent, R. L. Prenatal growth in the albino rat: Effects of number, intra-uterine position and resorptions. *American Journal of Anatomy,* 1970, *128,* 413–428.

Barron, S., Riley, E. P., and Smotherman, W. P. The effects of prenatal alcohol exposure on umbilical cord length in fetal rats. *Alcoholism: Clinical and Experimental Research*, 1986, *10*, 493–495.

Basmajian, J. V., and Ranney, D. A. Chemomyelotomy: Substitute for general anesthesia in experimental surgery. *Journal of Applied Physiology*, 1961, *16*, 386.

Baum, M. J. Differentiation of coital behavior in mammals: A comparative analysis. *Neuroscience and Biobehavioral Reviews*, 1979, *3*, 1–20.

Beaconsfield, P., Birdwood, G., and Beaconsfield, R. The placenta. *Scientific American*, 1980, *243*, 94–102.

Beck, S. L. Effects of position in the uterus on fetal mortality and on response to trypan blue. *Journal of Embryology and Experimental Morphology*, 1967, *17*, 607–624.

Bekoff, A. Embryonic development of the neural circuitry underlying motor coordination. In W. M. Cowan (Ed.), *Studies in developmental neurobiology: Essays in honor of Viktor Hamburger*. New York: Oxford University Press, 1981.

Bekoff, A., and Lau, B. Interlimb coordination in 20-day-old rat fetuses. *Journal of Experimental Zoology*, 1980, *214*, 173–175.

Bekoff, A., and Trainer, W. The development of interlimb coordination during swimming in postnatal rats. *Journal of Experimental Biology*, 1979, *83*, 1–11.

Bekoff, M., Byers, J. A., and Bekoff, A. Prenatal motility and postnatal play: Functional continuity? *Developmental Psychobiology*, 1980, *13*, 225–228.

Bell, R. Q., and Harper, L. V. *Child effects on adults*. Hillsdale, NJ: Erlbaum, 1977.

Birnholz, J. C. The development of human fetal eye movement patterns. *Science*, 1981, *213*, 679–681.

Birnholz, J. C. Fetal neurology. In R. C. Sanders and M. Hill (Eds.), *Ultrasound annual 1984*. New York: Raven Press, 1984.

Birnholz, J. C., and Benecerraf, B. R. The development of human fetal hearing. *Science*, 1983, *222*, 516–518.

Biscoe, T. S., Bradley, G. W., and Purves, J. J. The relations between carotid body chemoreceptor activity and carotid sinus pressure in the cat. *Journal of Physiology* (London), 1969, *203*, 40P.

Blass, E. M., and Pedersen, P. E. Surgical manipulation of the uterine environment of rat fetuses. *Physiology and Behavior*, 1980, *25*, 993–995.

Blass, E. M., and Teicher, M. H. Suckling. *Science*, 1980, *210*, 15–22.

Bradin, L. T. An analysis of the growth of the products of conception in relation to uterine accommodation in the Norway rat. *Anatomical Record*, 1948, *100*, 643.

Bradley, R. M., and Mistretta, C. M. Fetal sensory receptors. *Physiological Reviews*, 1975, *55*, 352–382.

Braun, F. H. T., Jones, K. L., and Smith, D. W. Breech presentation as an indicator of fetal abnormality. *Journal of Pediatrics*, 1975, *86*, 419–421.

Bruinink, A., Lichtensteiger, W., and Schlumpf, M. Characterization and ontogeny of monoaminergic- and spirodecanone-binding sites. In A. M. G. Stella, G. Gombos, G. Benzi, and H. S. Bachelard (Eds.), *Proceedings of the Fourth Meeting of the European Society for Neurochemistry, Catania: Basic and clinical aspects of molecular neurobiology*. Catania, Italy: European Society for Neurochemistry, 1982.

Carmichael, L. An experimental study in the prenatal guinea pig of the origin and development of reflexes and patterns of behavior in relation to the stimulation of specific receptor areas during the period of active fetal life. *Genetic Psychology Monograph*, 1934, *16*, 337–491.

Coghill, G. E. Early embryonic somatic movements in birds and in mammals other than man. *Monographs of the Society for Research in Child Development*, 1940, *5*, 1–48.

Coleridge, S. T. *Miscellanies, aesthetic and literary*. London: Bell & Sons, 1885.

Coronios, J. D. Development of behavior in the fetal cat. *Genetic Psychology Monograph*, 1933, *14*, 283–386.

Coyle, J. T. Biochemical aspects of neurotransmission in the developing brain. *International Review of Neurobiology*, 1977, *20*, 65–103.

Coyle, J. T., and Pert, C. B. Ontogenetic development of 3H-naloxone binding in rat brain. *Neuropharmacology*, 1976, *15*, 555–560.

Darwin, E. *Zoonomia: Or the law of organic growth*, Vol. 2. Philadelphia: E. Earle, 1796.

Dawes, G. S., Fox, H. E., LeDuc, B. M., Liggins, G. D., and Richards, R. T. Respiratory movements and rapid eye movement sleep in the foetal lamb. *Journal of Physiology* (London), 1972, *220*, 119–143.

DeCasper, A. J., and W. P. Fifer. Of human bonding: Newborns prefer their mothers' voices. *Science*, 1980, *208*, 1174–1176.

DeCasper, A. J., and Sigafoos, A. D. The intrauterine heartbeat: A potent reinforcer for newborns. *Infant Behavior and Development*, 1983, *6*, 19–25.

DeCasper, A. J., and Spence, M. J. Prenatal maternal speech influences newborns' perception of speech sounds. *Infant Behavior and Development*, 1986, *9*, 133–150.

Del Campo, C. H., and Ginther, O. J. Vascular anatomy of the uterus and ovaries and the unilateral luteolytic effect of the uterus: Guinea pigs, rats, hamsters, and rabbits. *American Journal of Veterinary Research*, 1972, *33*, 2561–2578.

de Vries, J. I. P., Visser, G. H. A., and Prechtl, H. F. R. The emergence of fetal behavior. I. Qualitative aspects. *Early Human Development*, 1982, *7*, 301–322.

Dierker, L. J., Pillay, S. K., Sorokin, Y., and Rosen, M. G. Active and quiet periods in the preterm and term fetus. *Obstetrics and Gynecology*, 1982, *60*, 65–70.

Drewett, R. F., Statham, C., and Wakerley, J. B. A quantitative analysis of the feeding behaviour of suckling rats. *Animal Behaviour*, 1974, *22*, 907–913.

Eckstein, P., McKeown, T., and Record, R. G. Variation in placental weight according to litter size in the guinea pig. *Journal of Endocrinology*, 1955, *12*, 108–114.

Edwards, D. D., and Edwards, J. S. Fetal movement: Development and time course. *Science*, 1970, *169*, 95–97.

Finnegan, L. P. Pathophysiological and behavioural effects of the transplacental transfer of narcotic drugs to the foetuses and neonates of narcotic-dependent mothers. *Bulletin on Narcotics*, 1979, *31*, 1–58.

Fuller, G. B., McGee, G. E., Nelson, J. C., Willis, D. C., and Culpepper, R. D. Birth sequence in mice. *Laboratory Animal Science*, 1976, *26*, 198–200.

Galigher, A. E., and Kozloff, E. N. *Essentials of practical microtechnique* (2nd ed.). Philadelphia: Lea & Febiger, 1971.

Gandelman, R., and Graham, S. Development of the surgically produced singleton mouse fetus. *Developmental Psychobiology*, 1986, *19*, 343–350.

Geubelle, F. Perception of environmental conditions by the fetus in utero. In P. O. Hubinont (Ed.), *Progress in reproductive biology and medicine*. Basel: S. Karger, 1984.

Globus, G. G. Quantification of the REM sleep cycle as a rhythm. *Psychophysiology*, 1970, *7*, 248–253.

Gottlieb, G. Conceptions of prenatal development: Behavioral embryology. *Psychological Review*, 1976, *83*, 215–234.

Gottlieb, G. Roles of early experience in species-specific perceptual development. In R. N. Aslin, J. R. Alberts, and M. R. Petersen (Eds.), *Development of perception*, Vol. 1. New York: Academic Press, 1981.

Gould, S. *Ontogeny and phylogeny*. Cambridge, MA: Belknap Press, 1977.

Granat, M., Lavie, P., Adar, D., and Sharf, M. Short-term cycles in human fetal activity. I. Normal pregnancies. *American Journal of Obstetrics and Gynecology*, 1979, *134*, 696–701.

Hailman, J. P. A stochastic model of leaf-scratching bouts in two emberizine species. *Wilson Bulletin*, 1974, *86*, 296–298.

Hailman, J. P. Uses of the comparative study of behavior. In R. B. Masterson, W. Hodos, and H. Jerison (Eds.), *Evolution, brain, and behavior: Persistent problems*. Hillsdale, NJ: Erlbaum, 1976.

Hall, W. G., and Rosenblatt, J. S. Suckling behavior and intake control in the developing rat pup. *Journal of Comparative and Physiological Psychology*, 1977, *91*, 1232–1247.

Hamburger, V. Some aspects of the embryology of behavior. *Quarterly Review of Biology*, 1963, *38*, 342–365.

Hamburger, V. Anatomical and physiological basis of embryonic motility in birds and mammals. In G. Gottlieb (Ed.), *Studies on the Development of Behavior and the Nervous System*. Vol. 1. *Behavioral embryology*. New York: Academic Press, 1973.

Hamburger, V., and Balaban, M. Observations and experiments on spontaneous rhythmical behavior in the chick embryo. *Developmental Biology*, 1963, *7*, 533–545.

Hamburger, V., and Oppenheim, R. Prehatching motility and hatching behavior in the chick. *Journal of Experimental Zoology*, 1967, *166*, 171–204.

Hauser, H., and Gandelman, R. Contiguity to males in utero affects avoidance responding in adult female mice. *Science*, 1983, *220*, 437–438.

Hinde, R. A. *Animal behaviour: A synthesis of ethology and comparative psychology*. New York: McGraw-Hill, 1970.

Hofer, M. A. *The roots of human behavior*. San Francisco: Freeman, 1981.

Hooker, D. Early fetal activity in mammals. *Yale Journal of Biology and Medicine*, 1936, *8*, 579–602.

Hooker, D. *The prenatal origin of behavior*, 18th Porter Lecture Series. Lawrence: University of Kansas Press, 1952.

Humphrey, T. The relation of oxygen deprivation to fetal reflex arcs and the development of fetal behavior. *Journal of Psychology*, 1953, *35*, 3–43.

Ibsen, H. L. Prenatal growth in guinea pigs with special reference to environmental factors affecting weight at birth. *Journal of Experimental Zoology*, 1928, *51*, 51–91.

Impekoven, M., and Gold, P. S. Prenatal origins of parent-young interactions in birds: A naturalistic approach. In G. Gottlieb (Ed.), *Studies on the development of behavior and the nervous system.* Vol. 1. *Behavioral embryology.* New York: Academic Press, 1973.

Jeffcoate, T. N. A., and Scott, J. S. Polyhydramnios and oligohydramnios. *The Canadian Medical Association Journal*, 1959, *80*, 77–86.

Kirby, M. L. A quantitative method for determining the effect of opiates on fetal rats in utero. *Problems of Drug Dependence, NIDA Research Monograph*, 1979, *27*, 191–197.

Knox, W. E., and Lister-Rosenoer, L. M. Timing of gestation in rats by fetal and maternal weights. *Growth*, 1978, *42*, 43–53.

Kodama, N., and Sekiguchi, S. The development of spontaneous body movement in prenatal and perinatal mice. *Developmental Psychobiology*, 1984, *17*, 139–150.

Kuo, Z. Y. *The dynamics of behavior development: An epigenetic view.* New York: Random House, 1967.

Lamarck, J. B. *Philosophie zoologique*, 1809. ("Zoological philosophy," trans. by H. Elliot). New York: Hafner, 1963.

Lev, R., and Orlic, D. Protein absorption by the intestine of the fetal rat in utero. *Science*, 1972, *177*, 522–524.

Lillegraven, J. A. Biological considerations of the marsupial-placental dichotomy. *Evolution*, 1975, *29*, 707–722.

Lillegraven, J. A. Reproduction in Mesozoic mammals. In J. A. Lillegraven, Z. Kielan-Jaworowska, and W. A. Clemens (Eds.), *Mesozoic mammals: The first two-thirds of mammalian history.* Berkeley: University of California Press, 1979.

Lotgering, F. K., Gilbert, R. D., and Longo, L. D. Maternal and fetal responses to exercise during pregnancy. *Physiological Reviews*, 1985, *65*, 1–36.

Luterkort, M., and Marsal, K. Fetal motor activity in breech presentation. *Early Human Development*, 1985, *10*, 193–200.

Marsh, R. H., King, J. E., and Becker, R. F. Volume and viscosity of amniotic fluid in rat and guinea pig fetuses near term. *American Journal of Obstetrics and Gynecology*, 1963, *85*, 487–492.

McCullough, M. L., and Blackman, D. E. The behavioral effects of prenatal hypoxia in the rat. *Developmental Psychobiology*, 1976, *9*, 335–342.

McKeown, T., and Record, R. G. The influence of placental size on foetal growth in man, with special reference to multiple pregnancy. *Journal of Endocrinology*, 1953, *9*, 418–426.

McLaren, A. Genetic and environmental effects on foetal and placental growth in mice. *Journal of Reproduction and Fertility*, 1965, *9*, 79–98.

McLeod, W., Brien, J., Loomis, C., Carmichael, L., Probert, C., and Patrick, J. Effect of maternal ethanol ingestion on fetal breathing movements, gross body movements and heart rate at 37 to 40 weeks gestational age. *American Journal of Obstetrics and Gynecology*, 1983, *145*, 251–257.

Mease, A. D., Yeatman, G. W., Pettett, G., and Merenstein, G. B. A syndrome of ankylosis, facial anomalies and pulmonary hypoplasia secondary to fetal neuromuscular dysfunction. *Birth Defects*, 1976, *12*, 193–200.

Meier, G. W., Bunch, M. E., Nolan, C. Y., and Scheidler, C. H. Anoxia, behavioral development, and learning ability: a comparative-experimental approach. *Psychology Monograph*, 1960, *74*(1), 1–48.

Meisel, R. L., and Ward, I. L. Fetal female rats are masculinized by male littermates located caudally in the uterus. *Science*, 1981, *220*, 437–438.

Milkovic, K., Paunovic, J., and Joffe, J. M. Effects of pre- and postnatal litter size reduction on development and behavior of rat offspring. *Developmental Psychobiology*, 1976, *9*, 365–375.

Minkowski, M. Neurobiologische Studien am menschlichen Foetus. *Handbuch die biologische Arbeitsmethoden*, 1928, Abt. V, Teil 5B, Heft 5, Ser. Nr. 253, 511–618.

Mirkin, B. L. Maternal and fetal distribution of drugs in pregnancy. *Clinical Pharmacology and Therapeutics*, 1973, *14*, 643–647.

Mistretta, C. M., and Bradley, R. M. Development of the sense of taste. In E. M. Blass (Ed.), *Handbook of behavioral neurobiology.* Vol. 8. *Developmental psychobiology and developmental neurobiology.* New York: Plenum Press, 1986.

Moessinger, A. C. Fetal akinesia deformation sequence: An animal model. *Pediatrics*, 1983, *72*, 857–863.

Moessinger, A. C., Blanc, W. A., Marone, P. A., and Polsen, D. C. Umbilical cord length as an index of fetal activity: Experimental study and clinical implications. *Pediatric Research,* 1982, *16,* 109–112.

Moessinger, A. C., Bassi, G. A., Ballantyne, G., Collins, M. H., James, L. S., and Blanc, W. A. Experimental production of pulmonary hypoplasia following amniocentesis and oligohydramnios. *Early Human Development,* 1983, *8,* 343–350.

Moore, C. L. An olfactory basis for maternal discrimination of sex of offspring in rats *(Rattus norvegicus). Animal Behaviour,* 1981, *29,* 383–386.

Moore, C. L. Maternal Behavior of rats is affected by hormonal condition of pups. *Journal of Comparative and Physiological Psychology,* 1982, *96,* 123–129.

Moore, C. L. Maternal contributions to the development of masculine sexual behavior in laboratory rats. *Developmental Psychobiology,* 1984, *17,* 347–356.

Moore, C. L., and Morelli, G. A. Mother rats interact differently with male and female offspring. *Journal of Comparative and Physiological Psychology,* 1979, *93,* 677–684.

Narayanan, C. H., Fox, M. W., and Hamburger, V. Prenatal development of spontaneous and evoked activity in the rat. *Behaviour,* 1971, *40,* 100–134.

Narayanan, C. H., Narayanan, Y., and Browne, R. C. Effects of induced thyroid deficiency on the development of suckling behavior in rats. *Physiology and Behavior,* 1982, *29,* 361–370.

Nijhuis, J. G., Prechtl, H. F. R., Martin, C. B., Jr., and Bots, R. S. G. M. Are there behavioural states in the human fetus? *Early Human Development,* 1982, *6,* 177–195.

Nijhuis, J. G., Martin, C. B., Jr., Gommers, S., Bouws, P., Bots, R. S. G. M., and Jongsma, H. W. The rhythmicity of fetal breathing varies with behavioural state in the human fetus. *Early Human Development,* 1983, *9,* 1–7.

Okado, N. Development of the human cervical spinal cord with reference to synapse formation in the motor nucleus. *Journal of Comparative Neurology,* 1980, *191,* 495–513.

Okado, N. Onset of synapse formation in the human spinal cord. *Journal of Comparative Neurology,* 1981, *201,* 211–219.

Oppenheim, R. W. Experimental studies on hatching behavior in the chick. III. The role of the midbrain and forebrain. *Journal of Comparative Neurology,* 1972, *146,* 479–505.

Oppenheim, R. W. Prehatching and hatching behavior: A comparative and physiological consideration. In G. Gottlieb (Ed.), *Studies on the development of behavior and the nervous system.* Vol. 1. *Behavioral embryology.* New York: Academic Press, 1973.

Oppenheim, R. W. Ontogenetic adaptations and retrogressive processes in the development of the nervous system and behaviour: A neuroembryological perspective. In K. J. Connolly and H. F. R. Prechtl (Eds.), *Maturation and development: Biological and psychological perspectives.* Philadelphia: Lippincott, 1981.

Oppenheim, R. W. The neuroembryological study of behavior: Progress, problems, perspectives. In R. K. Hunt (Ed.), *Current topics in developmental biology.* Vol. 17. *Neural development, Part 3.* New York: Academic Press, 1982.

Pankratz, D. S. A preliminary report on the fetal movements in the rabbit. *Anatomical Record,* 1931, *48,* 58–59.

Panneton, R. K., and DeCasper, A. J. *Newborns prefer intrauterine heartbeat sounds to male voices.* Paper presented at the International Conference on Infant Studies, New York, April 1984.

Parker, P. An ecological comparison of marsupial and placental patterns of reproduction. In B. Stonehouse and D. Gilmore (Eds.), *The biology of marsupials.* Baltimore: University Park Press, 1977.

Patrick, J., Natale, R., and Richardson, B. Patterns of human fetal breathing activity at 34 to 35 weeks' gestational age. *American Journal of Obstetrics and Gynecology,* 1978, *132,* 507–513.

Pazos, A., Palacios, J. M., Schlumpf, M., and Lichtensteiger, W. Pre- and postnatal ontogeny of brain neurotensin receptors: an autoradiographic study. *Society for Neuroscience Abstracts,* 1985, *15,* 602.

Pedersen, P. E., and Blass, E. M. Olfactory control over suckling in albino rats. In R. N. Aslin, J. R. Alberts, and M. R. Peterson (Eds.), *The development of perception: Psychobiological processes.* Hillsdale, NJ: Erlbaum, 1981.

Pedersen, P. E., and Blass, E. M. Prenatal and postnatal determinants of the 1st suckling episode in albino rats. *Developmental Psychobiology,* 1982, *15,* 349–355.

Pedersen, P. E., Stewart, W. B., Greer, C. A., and Shepherd, G. M. Evidence for olfactory function in utero. *Science,* 1983, *221,* 478–480.

Plentl, A. A. The dynamics of the amniotic fluid. *Annals of the New York Academy of Science,* 1959, *75,* 746–761.

Preyer, W. *Specielle Physiologie des Embryo. Untersuchungen über die Lebenserscheinungen vor der Geburt.* Grieben: Leipzig, 1885.

Provine, R. R. Neurophysiological aspects of behavior development in the chick embryo. In G. Gottlieb (Ed.), *Studies on the Development of Behavior and the Nervous System.* Vol. 1. *Behavioral embryology.* New York: Academic Press, 1973.

Provine, R. R. Development of between-limb movement synchronization in the chick embryo. *Developmental Psychobiology,* 1980, *13,* 151–163.

Ramsey, E. M. *The placenta: Human and animal.* New York: Praeger, 1982.

Rayburn, W. F. Clinical implications from monitoring fetal activity. *American Journal of Obstetrics and Gynecology,* 1982, *144,* 967–980.

Reppert, S. M., and Schwartz, W. J. Maternal coordination of the fetal biological clock in utero. *Science,* 1983, *220,* 969–971.

Reppert, S. M., and Schwartz, W. J. Functional activity of the suprachiasmatic nuclei in the fetal primate. *Neuroscience Letters,* 1984a, *46,* 145–149.

Reppert, S. M., and Schwartz, W. J. The suprachiasmatic nuclei of the fetal rat: Characterization of a functional circadian clock using 14C-labeled deoxyglucose. *Journal of Neuroscience,* 1984b, *4,* 1677–1682.

Richmond, G., and Sachs, B. D. Further evidence for masculinization of female by males located caudally in utero. *Hormones and Behavior,* 1984, *18,* 484–490.

Ripley, K. L., and Provine, R. R. Neural correlates of embryonic motility in the chick. *Brain Research,* 1972, *45,* 127–134.

Robertson, S. S. Intrinsic temporal patterning in the spontaneous movement of awake neonates. *Child Development,* 1982, *53,* 1016–1021.

Robertson, S. S. Cyclic motor activity in the human fetus after midgestation. *Developmental Psychobiology,* 1985, *18,* 411–419.

Robertson, S. S., Dierker, L. J., Sorokin, Y., and Rosen, M. G. Human fetal movement: Spontaneous oscillations near one cycle per minute. *Science,* 1982, *218,* 1327–1330.

Rohrbaugh, J. W. The orienting reflex: performance and central nervous system manifestations. In R. Pavasuramam and D. R. Davies (Eds.), *Varieties of attention.* New York: Academic Press, 1984.

Romand, R. Maturation des potentiels cochléaires dans la période périnatale chez le Chat et chez le Cobaye. *Journal de Physiologie* (Paris), 1971, *63,* 763–782.

Saito, K. Development of spinal reflexes in the rat fetus studied in vitro. *Journal of Physiology,* 1979, *294,* 581–594.

Schlumpf, M., Richards, J. G., Lichtensteiger, W., and Mohler, H. An autoradiographic study of the prenatal development of benzodiazepine-binding sites in rat brain. *Journal of Neuroscience,* 1983, *3,* 1478–1487.

Schlumpf, M., Palacios, J. M., Cortes, R., Pazos, A., Bruinink, A., and Lichtensteiger, W. Development of drug and neurotransmitter binding sites in fetal rat brain. *Society for Neuroscience Abstracts,* 1985, *15,* 602.

Shannon, C. E., and Weaver, W. *The mathematical theory of communication.* Urbana: University of Illinois Press, 1949.

Sharman, G. B. Adaptations of marsupial pouch young for extra-uterine existence. In C. R. Austin (Ed.), *The mammalian fetus in vitro.* London: Chapman & Hall, 1973.

Sharman, G. B., and Calaby, J. H. 1964. Reproductive behaviour in the red kangaroo, Megaleia rufa, in captivity. *C.S.I.R.O. Wildlife Research,* 1964, *9,* 58–85.

Smotherman, W. P. In utero chemosensory experience alters taste preferences and corticosterone responsiveness. *Behavioral and Neural Biology,* 1982a, *36,* 61–68.

Smotherman, W. P. Odor aversion learning by the rat fetus. *Physiology and Behavior,* 1982b, *29,* 769–771.

Smotherman, W. P., and Robinson, S. R. Novel and aversive chemosensory stimuli: Discrimination by the rat fetus in utero. *Society for Neuroscience Abstracts,* 1985a, *11,* 837.

Smotherman, W. P., and Robinson, S. R. The rat fetus in its environment: Behavioral adjustments to novel, familiar, aversive and conditioned stimuli presented in utero. *Behavioral Neuroscience,* 1985b, *99,* 521–530.

Smotherman, W. P., and Robinson, S. R. Environmental determinants of behaviour in the rat fetus. *Animal Behaviour,* 1986, *34,* 1859–1873.

Smotherman, W. P., and Robinson, S. R. Prenatal expression of species-typical action patterns in the rat fetus (*Rattus norvegicus*). *Journal of Comparative Psychology,* 1987, *101,* 190–196.

Smotherman, W. P., and Robinson, S. R. Behavior of rat fetuses following chemical or tactile stimulation. *Behavioral Neuroscience,* in press.

Smotherman, W. P., Richards, L. S., and Robinson, S. R. Techniques for observing fetal behavior in utero: a comparison of chemomyelotomy and spinal transection. *Developmental Psychobiology*, 1984, *17*, 661–674.

Smotherman, W. P., Robinson, S. R., and Miller, B. J. A reversible preparation for observing the behavior of fetal rats in utero: Spinal anesthesia with lidocaine. *Physiology and Behavior*, 1986a, *37*, 57–60.

Smotherman, W. P., Woodruff, K. S., Robinson, S. R., del Real, C., Barron, S., and Riley, E. P. Spontaneous fetal behavior after maternal exposure to ethanol. *Pharmacology Biochemistry and Behavior*, 1986b, *24*, 165–170.

Sterman, M. B. The basic rest-activity cycle and sleep: developmental considerations in man and cats. In C. P. Clemente, D. P. Purpura, and F. E. Mayer (Eds.), *Sleep and the maturing nervous system*. New York: Academic Press, 1972.

Sterman, M. B., and Hoppenbrouwers, T. The development of sleep-waking and rest-activity patterns from fetus to adult in man. In D. J. McGinty and A. M. Adinolfi (Eds.), *Brain development and behavior*. New York: Academic Press, 1971.

Stern, E., Parmelee, A. H., Akiyama, Y., Schultz, M. A., and Wenner, W. H. Sleep cycle characteristics in infants. *Pediatrics*, 1969, *43*, 65–70.

Stickrod, G. In utero injection of rat fetuses. *Physiology and Behavior*, 1981, *27*, 557–558.

Stickrod, G., Kimble, D. P., and Smotherman, W. P. In utero taste/odor aversion conditioning in the rat. *Physiology and Behavior*, 1982a, *28*, 5–7.

Stickrod, G., Kimble, D. P., and Smotherman, W. P. Met-5-enkephalin effects on associations formed in-utero. *Peptides*, 1982b, *3*, 881–883.

Straus, W. L., and Weddell, G. Nature of the first visible contractions of the forelimb musculature in rat fetuses. *Journal of Neurophysiology*, 1940, *3*, 358–369.

Suzuki, S., and Yamamuro, T. Fetal movement and fetal presentation. *Early Human Development*, 1985, *11*, 255–263.

Swenson, E. A. *The development of movement of the albino rat before birth*. Ph.D. Thesis, University of Kansas, 1926.

Tam, P. P. L., and Chan, S. T. H. Changes in the composition of maternal plasma, fetal plasma and fetal extraembryonic fluid during gestation in the rat. *Journal of Reproduction and Fertility*, 1977, *51*, 41–51.

Taverne, M. A. M., van der Weyden, G. C., Fontijne, P., Ellendorff, F., Naaktgeboren, C., and Smidt, D. Uterine position and presentation of minipig-fetuses and their order and presentation at birth. *American Journal of Veterinary Research*, 1977, *38*, 1761–1764.

Tilney, F., and Kubie, L. S. Behavior in its relation to the development of the brain. I. *Bulletin of Neurology Instutute, New York*, 1931, *1*, 229–313.

Timor-Tritsch, I. E., Dierker, L. J., Hertz, R. H., Deagan, N. C., and Rosen, M. G. Studies of antepartum behavioral state in the human fetus at term. *American Journal of Obstetrics and Gynecology*, 1978, *132*, 524–528.

Tinbergen, N. On aims and methods of ethology. *Zeitschrift für Tierpsychologie*, 1963, *20*, 410–429.

Tobet, S. A., Dunlap, J. L., and Gerall, A. A. Influence of fetal position on neonatal androgen-induced sterility and sexual behavior in female rats. *Hormones and Behavior*, 1982, *16*, 251–258.

Tschanz, B. Trottellummen: Die Entstehung der personlichen Beziehungen zwischen Jungvogel und Eltern. *Zeitschrift für Tierpsychologie*, 1968, *4*, 1–103.

Umans, J. G., and Szeto, H. H. Precipitated opiate abstinence in utero. *American Journal of Obstetrics and Gynecology*, 1985, *151*, 441–444.

Vince, M. A. Postnatal effects of prenatal sound stimulation in the guinea pig. *Animal Behaviour*, 1979, *27*, 908–918.

Vyas, H., Milner, A. D., and Hopkins, I. E. Amniocentesis and fetal lung development. *Archives of the Diseases of Children*, 1982, *57*, 617–618.

Walker, D., Grimwade, J., and Wood, C. Intrauterine noise: A component of the fetal environment. *American Journal of Obstetrics and Gynecology*, 1971, *109*, 91–95.

Ward, I. L. The prenatal stress syndrome: Current status. *Psychoneuroendocrinology*, 1984, *9*, 3–11.

Whitnall, M. H., Key, S., Ben-Barak, Y., Ozato, K., and Gainer, H. Neurophysin in the hypothalamo-neurohypophysial system. *Journal of Neuroscience*, 1985, *5*, 98–109.

Wigglesworth, J. S. Experimental growth retardation in the foetal rat. *Journal of Pathology and Bacteriology*, 1964, *88*, 1–13.

Windle, W. F. *Physiology of the fetus*. Philadelphia: W. B. Saunders, 1940.

Windle, W. F. Genesis of somatic motor function in mammalian embryos: A synthesizing article. *Physiological Zoology*, 1944, *17*, 247–261.

Windle, W. F., and Becker, R. F. Relation of anoxemia to early activity in the fetal nervous system. *Archives of Neurology and Psychiatry,* 1940, *43,* 90–101.

Windle, W. F., and Griffin, A. M. 1931. Observations on embryonic and fetal movements of the cat. *Journal of Comparative Neurology,* 1931, *52,* 149–188.

Wirtschafter, Z. T., and Williams, D. W. The dynamics of protein changes in the amniotic fluid of normal and abnormal rat embryos. *American Journal of Obstetrics and Gynecology,* 1957a, *74,* 1022–1028.

Wirtschafter, Z. T., and Williams, D. W. Dynamics of the amniotic fluid as measured by changes in protein patterns. *American Journal of Obstetrics and Gynecology,* 1957b, *74,* 309–313.

6

Sexual Differentiation of Behavior in the Context of Developmental Psychobiology

PAULINE YAHR

INTRODUCTION

Sexual differentiation refers to processes of biological development by which tissues and cells become committed to masculine or feminine phenotypes. Even among mammals and birds, in which chromosomes determine sex, most tissues and cells that become sexually dimorphic are sexually indifferent initially. They have the potential to produce either a male or a female version of the adult form. In most cases, the sexual phenotype that they develop depends not on their own genotype but on factors in their environment. Thus, sexual differentiation resembles, and presumably reflects, the same processes by which all specialized cells differentiate from a common precursor, the fertilized egg. Granted, some embryonic tissues can produce structures of only one sex. Yet, even in these cases, the sexual indifference of early development is apparent because tissues that can produce the structures of the other sex are present as well.

The environmental factors that induce sexual differentiation are usually chemicals, such as hormones, that originate elsewhere in the organism, but they can arise externally. In some reptiles, sex is determined by the temperature at which eggs hatch (Bull, 1980). In at least one mammalian species, parental care also differs according to the sex of the offspring (Moore, 1984; Moore and Morelli, 1979;

PAULINE YAHR   Department of Psychobiology, University of California, Irvine, California 92717.

197

Richmond and Sachs, 1984b), and it has been suggested that this difference can intensify the development of sex differences in behavior. Yet, in this case, young males are treated differently from young females because the males emit a hormonally controlled odor that evokes parental attention. Thus, the sensory stimulation can be seen as a mechanism that mediates the effects of sex-related hormones. Enhanced hormone secretion may, in turn, mediate the effects of the sensory stimulation (Moore and Rogers, 1984).

Because behavior is not a tissue, it does not undergo sexual differentiation directly. Nonetheless, it responds as if it did because it reflects activities of sexually differentiated tissues and cells, including parts of the brain and the spinal cord. The purpose of this chapter is to review research on sexual differentiation of behavior as a product of the histogenesis, the morphogenesis, and the cellular differentiation of the nervous system. To prepare for this discussion, we will review basic principles of developmental biology as revealed in the sexual differentiation of the reproductive system.

SEXUAL DIFFERENTIATION OF THE REPRODUCTIVE SYSTEM

Sexes are defined by the kinds of gametes that can or would be produced. Individuals with the type of gonad (ovary) that makes large, sessile gametes (ova) are females. Those with the type of gonad (testis) that makes small, mobile gametes (sperm) are males.

The sexually indifferent embryonic gonads of mammals—or at least, those of placental mammals (Burns, 1955; Fadem and Tesoriero, 1986)—differentiate as testes or ovaries depending on the presence or absence of a segment of the Y chromosome that contains a testis-organizing gene (Gordon and Ruddle, 1981), but the particular gene involved is not known. Since the mid-1970s, research on this issue has tested the hypothesis that the testis-organizing gene is the gene for H-Y antigen (Haseltine and Ohno, 1981; Wachtel, 1983), a plasma membrane protein coded on the long arm of the Y. Regardless of their sex chromosome karyotype, somatic cells of embryonic gonads make membrane receptors for H-Y antigen. If the individual carries the H-Y gene, most, if not all, of its cells secrete H-Y antigen. According to the H-Y hypothesis, it is the exposure of the cell surface receptors to H-Y antigen that induces the somatic cells of the gonads to differentiate as Sertoli cells, which then aggregate to form seminiferous tubules (Jost and Magre, 1984). These events commit the gonad to becoming a testis. The germ cells, which do not have receptors for H-Y, differentiate as spermatogonia in response to stimuli provided by the cords. The Leydig cells, which are the steroidogenic cells of the testes, differentiate later and may also be responding to stimuli from the seminiferous cords.

The H-Y hypothesis was supported by the observation that many individuals whose sex chromosome karyotype and gonadal phenotype are discordant show concordance between gonadal phenotype and the presence of H-Y antigen. Most XY females lack H-Y antigen, apparently because that segment of the Y was deleted during gamete formation. Most XX males have H-Y antigen, apparently because the H-Y segment of the Y translocated to another chromosome, usually the X. However, some individuals with testes do not have H-Y antigen, and some individuals with ovaries do (McLaren, Simpson, Tomonari, Chandler, and Hogg, 1984; Savikurki and de la Chapelle, 1984). These discrepancies between H-Y antigen phenotype and gonadal phenotype raised the possibility that a segment of the Y other than the one coding for H-Y antigen causes testis formation. Recently, deoxyribonucleic acid (DNA) hybridization analyses showed that the genes for H-Y antigen and for the formation of testes are located on different parts of the Y chromosome in humans (Simpson, Chandler, Goulmy, Disteche, Ferguson-Smith, and Page, 1987). The testis-determining gene is on the short, not the long, arm of the Y (Vergnaud, Page, Simmler, Brown, Rouyer, Noel, Botstein, de la Chapelle, and Weissenbach, 1986). It will be interesting to learn whether it codes for a protein that acts within cells of the embryonic gonad or whether it, like H-Y, codes for a protein produced by many cell types but for which only gonadal cells have receptors.

If the testis-organizing gene is absent, the embryonic gonads differentiate sexually as ovaries, but their histological differentiation is delayed relative to the histological differentiation of testes (Gordon and Ruddle, 1981; Jost, 1972; Wilson, George, and Griffin, 1981). The inductive relationship between somatic and germ cells is also different when ovaries rather than testes form. Ovarian differentiation begins when germ cells near the surface of the gonad start meiosis. These meiotic cells differentiate as oogonia and induce surrounding somatic cells to form follicles. Finally, the relationship between steroid biosynthesis and histological differentiation is different for the two types of gonads. The ovary begins to secrete estradiol (E_2) even before its histological differentiation has clearly begun (Wilson *et al.*, 1981). This developmental sequence raises the possibility that E_2 promotes histological differentiation of the ovary.

One feature of gonadal differentiation that recurs repeatedly in the sexual differentiation of mammals is that specific signals are needed to differentiate phenotypes typical of males. Sometimes, as in the case of the gonads, the signal actively promotes the development of masculine traits (traits that are usually more prominent in males). In these cases, we say that the signal masculinizes development. In other cases, the signal actively suppresses the development of feminine traits (traits that are usually more prominent in females). In these cases, we say that it defeminizes development. Yet, whether they require masculinization or defeminization, the phenotypes typical of mammalian males develop only when their specific signal is present. Without it, mammalian tissues and cells differentiate sexually as female.

Of course, sexual differentiation is only one aspect of gonadal development and does not ensure that the gonads produced will be fully functional. For example, whereas Sertoli and Leydig cells can form from cells with two X chromosomes, sperm apparently cannot (Gordon and Ruddle, 1981; Haseltine and Ohno, 1981). Thus, XX males, like males with two X's and a Y, are sterile. In the case of XY females, fertility varies with the species. In some species, such as voles, XY females produce ova, but in others, such as humans, they do not. Because women with only one X are also sterile, it appears that human oogenesis requires two X chromosomes. For every tissue undergoing sexual differentiation, and in the case of behavior, the same principle emerges; that is, sexual differentiation is only one component of sexual development.

Sexual differentiation is not even the only differentiating step that the gonads and the other sexually dimorphic tissues undergo. Both before and after sexual differentiation, these tissues go through the same histogenic processes that all other tissues undergo, including differentiation of specific cell types. In studying developmental biology, it is important to distinguish how a tissue or cell progresses along a pathway from how that pathway is chosen. In studying sexual development, it seems equally important to distinguish sexually differentiating events from the differentiating events that produce the sexually indifferent precursor or that transform the sexually committed tissue into its mature form, even though the mechanisms of differentiation are probably the same in each case.

Given the premium on coordinating sexual differentiation of the various body parts, it is not surprising that all other tissues that sexually differentiate do so after the gonads have formed and take their cues from the gonads. Both the genitalia and the reproductive tract provide examples of this phenomenon, yet reveal interesting differences in how sexual differentiation can be accomplished. In mammals, individual genital tissues can follow either a masculine or a feminine path, depending on whether testosterone (T), a steroid hormone from the testes, is present or absent (Wilson *et al.*, 1981). Regardless of their genetic sex, tissues that form a penis if T is present form a clitoris if it is not. The tissue that forms labia in the absence of T forms a scrotum when exposed to T. If, as a result of a genetic mutation, an individual with testes can not respond to T, the effect on the sexual differentiation of the genitalia is the same as if T were absent (Hauser, 1963; Perez-Palacios, Ulloa-Aguirre, and Kofman-Alfaro, 1984). With a developmental system like this one, in which a single primordium follows one or the other path, it is not possible to obtain both masculine and feminine versions of the adult form, although intermediate forms can develop, depending, for example, on the amount of T available during sexual differentiation.

In contrast, it is possible for both masculine and feminine reproductive tracts to develop in the same individual because they are derived from separate primordia. Both male and female fetuses form Müllerian ducts, which can produce a female reproductive tract. In addition, both sexes form Wolffian ducts, which can produce a masculine reproductive tract. Wolffian ducts produce their derivatives if T is present (Wilson *et al.*, 1981). Otherwise, they regress. Müllerian ducts produce their derivatives unless they are exposed to Müllerian inhibiting substance, a glycoprotein made by Sertoli cells (Jost and Magre, 1984). Thus, testicular secretions independently masculinize and defeminize the development of the mammalian reproductive tract.

Like Wolffian ducts and genitalia, many other tissues differentiate sexually depending on whether T is present or absent during a restricted stage of their development. The brain and the spinal cord are among them. For example, brains of female mammals contain cells—sometimes in the preoptic area (POA), sometimes in the medial basal hypothalamus (MBH)—that enable the anterior pituitary to secrete the surge of luteinizing hormone (LH) necessary for ovulation (Feder, 1981a; Goodman, 1978; Knobil and Plant, 1978; Shander and Barraclough, 1980; Terasawa and Weigand, 1978; Weigand and Terasawa, 1982). Except in primates, the ability to show an LH surge is sexually dimorphic in mammals (Barbarino, DeMarinis, and Mancini, 1983; Buhl, Norman, and Resko, 1978; Elsaesser and Parvizi, 1979; Hodges, 1980; Karsch and Foster, 1975; Karsch, Dierschke, and Knobil, 1973; Neill, 1972; Steiner, Schiller, Barber, and Gale, 1978). These sex differences can be reversed by reversing the sex difference in early exposure to T. For example, male rats (Gorski and Wagner, 1965; Harris and Levin, 1965) and gerbils (Ulibarri and Yahr, 1988) cannot make transplanted ovaries ovulate unless the males are gonadectomized shortly after birth (see Figure 1). Conversely, female rats (Barraclough, 1961; Gorski, 1968; Gorski and Wagner, 1965) and gerbils (Ulibarri and Yahr, 1988) that are injected with T propionate (TP) shortly after birth often lose the ability to ovulate. In fact, early exposure to T causes anovulatory sterility in all mammals studied to date, with the exception of primates (Feder, 1981b; Plapinger and McEwen, 1978; Resko and Ellinwood, 1984). Applying T or E_2, which is a metabolite of T, directly to the POA or the MBH of newborn female rats also induces anovulatory sterility (Christensen and Gorski, 1978; Döcke and Dörner, 1975; Hayashi, 1976; Hayashi and Gorski, 1974; Nadler, 1973; Nordeen and Yahr, 1982).

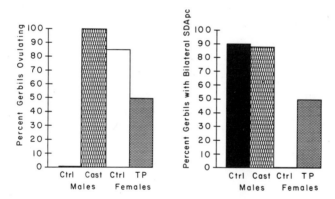

Figure 1. The effects of reversing the normal sex difference in perinatal exposure to T on the sexual differentiation of gonadotropin secretion and brain structure in gerbils. The graph on the left shows the normal sex difference in the ability to make ovaries ovulate among control (Ctrl) males and females. Such sex differences in ovulation indicate a sex difference in LH secretion. Male gerbils castrated (Cast) on the day of birth can secrete the LH surge required for ovulation. In contrast, half of the females given 100 μg TP on the day after birth were sterile as adults because they could not secrete the LH surge. The graph on the right shows the normal sex difference in the presence or absence of the SDApc, a small, dense cell group in the HPOA of adult male gerbils (see the section titled "Which Neural Tissues Contribute to Sexual Differentiation of Behavior?"). Although normal females rarely, if ever, have an SDApc in adulthood, and never have it bilaterally, half of the adult females given TP neonatally had bilateral SDApcs. Although postnatal exposure to T can masculinize this brain structure, removing T from the circulation shortly after birth does not prevent SDApc development in males. Thus, sexual differentiation of the SDApc apparently begins before birth (Adapted from Ulibarri and Yahr, 1988).

Other cells in the nervous system that differentiate sexually contribute to sex differences in behavior. In some cases, the neural systems that produce masculine and feminine responses develop from separate primordia, analogous to the reproductive tract. Hypothalamic areas controlling masculine and feminine copulatory behaviors provide examples (Christensen and Gorski, 1978; Davis and Barfield, 1979a,b; Davis, McEwen, and Pfaff, 1979b; Nordeen and Yahr, 1982). In other cases, sex differences in behavior reflect a continuum of development by one cell group, analogous to the genitalia. The forebrain areas controlling singing in songbirds provide examples here (Nottebohm and Arnold, 1976; Nottebohm, Kasparian, and Pandazis, 1981).

CELLULAR MECHANISMS UNDERLYING SEXUAL DIFFERENTIATION: BASIC ISSUES

The sexually differentiating effects of T may be mediated by one of its locally formed metabolites, E_2 or dihydrotestosterone (DHT), by a combination of the two, or by unmetabolized T. This varies with the tissue and the phenotype. E_2 mediates defeminization of the brain regions controlling LH secretion (MacLusky and Naftolin, 1981). DHT induces the early growth of the penis. Unmetabolized T induces the formation of Wolffian duct derivatives and sensitizes the penis so that it will enlarge at puberty when reexposed to T (Imperato-McGinley et al., 1974, 1980; Wilson et al., 1981). When a metabolite is involved in the actions of T, it is generally assumed that the cells that contain the metabolizing enzyme(s) are the same cells that contain receptors for the metabolite(s). Although this must often be true, it is possible that some tissues pass a metabolite from one cell type, where it was made, to another, where it is used.

Whether T is metabolized or not, there is no reason to believe that the cellular mechanisms by which the active steroid effects sexual differentiation differ in any fundamental way from the mechanisms by which steroids alter cellular activities in adulthood (Gorski and Gannon, 1976; Liao, Tymoczko, Castaneda, and Liang, 1975; O'Malley and Means, 1974). In most cases, steroids act in adults by binding to intracellular receptors. Steroid hormones freely enter all cells because they are lipid-soluble; however, only cells with specific receptors for the hormone can accumulate and respond to it directly. The receptors are proteins loosely associated with the nucleus (King and Green, 1984; Welshons, Lieberman, and Gorski, 1984). After binding the steroid, they become more tightly associated with the nucleus and attach to acceptor sites on the chromatin. This attachment alters the transcription of DNA to ribonucleic acid (RNA). Any and all forms of RNA may be affected, including ribosomal RNA (rRNA), transfer RNA (tRNA) and heterogeneous nuclear RNA (hnRNA), from which messenger RNA (mRNA) is eventually formed (Anderson, 1982; Hamilton, 1968; Luck and Hamilton, 1975; Maenpaa, 1972; Wicks, Greenman, and Kenney, 1965). The changes in transcription may be qualitative or quantitative. Some hormone-sensitive genes, particularly those coding for hnRNA, may be transcribed only when the hormone is present or only when it is absent. Others may be transcribed more or less often under hormonal control. These transcriptional changes, in turn, effect changes in mRNA translation into protein. Depending on the target cells involved, the affected proteins may be proteins that become incorporated into the cell membrane, synthetic or degradative enzymes, or secreted proteins or peptides that can affect other cells (for examples from brain, see Bigeon and McEwen, 1982; DeVries *et al.,* 1984b; Dohanich, Witcher, Weaver, and Clemens, 1982; Luine and McEwen, 1977; Luine and Rhodes, 1983; Luine, McEwen, and Black, 1977; Rainbow, DeGroff, Luine, and McEwen, 1980; Shivers, Harlan, Morrell, and Pfaff, 1983; Vacas and Cardinali, 1980; Wallis and Luttge, 1980).

Although these basic features of steroid hormone action are the same at all stages of development, their consequences can change. For example, the chromatin acceptor sites may be associated with different genetic loci at different developmental stages, as they apparently are for different cell types of the adult, leading to the synthesis of different mRNAs (Anderson, 1982; Spelsberg, Littlefield, Seelke, Dani, Torjodo, Boyd-Leiner, Throll, and Kon, 1983). The intra- and extracellular environments, which certainly change developmentally, also limit the ability of the cell and its neighbors to respond to any changes in protein synthesis that may occur.

In addition to interacting with intracellular receptors that regulate transcription, it appears that steroid hormones sometimes interact with cell surface receptors or alter membrane permeability (McEwen, Krey, and Luine, 1978; Moss and Dudley, 1984). Yet, for our purposes, the point is the same, namely, that there is no reason to believe that the fundamental mechanisms by which hormones effect sexual differentiation differ from the mechanisms by which they alter cellular activity in adulthood, although the details and consequences of those actions may change.

As noted above, there is also no reason to believe that the basic mechanisms by which tissues sexually differentiate are different from the mechanisms responsible for histogenesis and morphogenesis in general. Similarly, the mechanisms by which gonadal secretions and testis-organizing genes specify the sexual phenotypes of cells are presumably the same mechanisms by which local tissue-organizing factors and other genes specify other cellular phenotypes. In each case, differentiation commits cells to display only some of the genetically possible phenotypes. In each case, specialization is achieved at the expense of pluripotency. Once development has proceeded along a path, or has failed to proceed, the cells and tissues are no longer as capable as they previously were (or as their precursors were) of following alternative routes. Although the fertilized egg contains the same genome that the somatic cells of the adult do, each adult cell performs metabolic feats that the egg cannot. Yet, none of the adult cells can produce a complete organism, as the egg can. Similarly, during the stage of development when the embryonic gonads of mammals can form either testes or ovaries, they can not produce steroids or gametes (Wilson *et al.*, 1981). By the time they acquire these capacities, they can no longer form gonads of the opposite sex.

As the genotype remains the same (with the exception of certain cells in the immune system), restrictions on the phenotypes that cells can express must involve changes in the environment. The intracellular environment may be responsible, as the cytoplasm can determine which genes are transcribed (Gurdon, 1970; Gurdon and Woodland, 1968) and the composition and distribution of chromatin proteins can determine which genes are accessible for transcription (Davidson and Britten, 1973; Rosenfeld, Amaro, and Evans, 1984; Sutcliffe, Milner, Gottesfeld, and Reynolds, 1984). The external environment of precursor cells can also play a role in determining which restrictions will be imposed on the daughter cells. This influence is illustrated by the variety of neural and endocrine cells that form from specific populations of neural crest cells if they are transplanted to different parts of the body before they migrate (LeDouarin, 1984). Left *in situ*, each population would produce only a few cell types. However, the mechanism involved here is unclear. Each transplanted population may be a heterogeneous group of highly committed cells, many of which are normally weeded out by the selective effects of the environment. Alternatively, individual neural crest cells may have the capacity to produce daughters with a variety of phenotypes (Weston, Girdlestone, and Ciment, 1984). Differentiation can also occur after a terminal division, as exemplified by the formation of mature neurons from immature ones, or neuroblasts. Although many aspects of a neuron's phenotype have already been determined by the time it is born, others depend on its environment. Elongation and branching of the axon, elaboration of the dendritic arbor, and even the neurotransmitters and neuromodulators produced can depend on the availability of trophic factors, on the arrangement of other cell groups, or on the synaptic connections formed (Berg, 1984; Black, Adler, Dreyfus, Jonakait, Katz, La Gamma, and Markey, 1984; Jacobson, 1978; Levi-Montalchini, 1982). Once a neuron's shape and transmitter phenotype are established, though, they are usually permanent, showing us again that differentiation involves phenotypic commitment.

Yet, *differentiation* and *phenotypic commitment* are relative terms. The cells of the embryonic gonads, for example, represent one point in the continuum of differentiation that characterizes development. From one perspective, they are highly differentiated, having lost their ability to form other organs, much less a complete individual. They are committed to forming gonads or to failing to develop at all. However, they are not yet committed to forming one type of gonad. Even in the adult, differentiation and phenotypic commitment are not absolute. Particularly when exposed to unusual circumstances, such as when transplanted into embryos or into other parts of the body, when exposed to pharmacological agents, or when deprived of normal inputs (Black *et al.*, 1984; Coulombe and Bronner-Fraser, 1986; Cotman and Nieto-Sampedro, 1984), some mature cells lose their old phenotypes and acquire new ones. But the ability of differentiated cells to change their phenotypes varies from one cell type to another and from species to species. We all know that amphibians regenerate lost limbs, whereas mammals do not, although it may someday be possible to induce this process therapeutically. Similarly, some fish can change sex in adulthood (Robertson, 1972; Shapiro, 1980), whereas mammals cannot, although, having changed, the fish cannot necessarily revert to its earlier sexual phenotype. Understanding the relative nature of differentiation will be helpful when we discuss the sexual differentiation of behavior, particularly when we consider when a hormone may or must act to masculinize or defeminize a response.

As noted above, differentiation determines which phenotypes a cell displays, including the degree to which it displays them in response to various stimuli. In the case of sexual differentiation, one of the phenotypes most often affected by T (or a metabolite) is the later ability to respond to gonadal steroids. In some cases, T decreases sensitivity to a steroid. Defeminization of gonadotropin secretion in rats illustrates this phenomenon. In rats, as in various other mammals, the LH surge needed for ovulation is secreted in response to rising E_2 levels. Because E_2 secretion by the ovary is itself stimulated by LH, this is an example of positive feedback. Acting perinatally in male rats, T decreases the ability of the POA to respond to the positive feedback effects of E_2 in adulthood. In other cases, T increases sensitivity to a steroid. Here, the human penis/clitoris provides an example. Although adult women show some clitoral enlargement if given T (Money and Ehrhardt, 1972), the growth is not comparable to the penile growth that occurs at puberty in normal men or in men with the "penis at 12" syndrome (Imperato-McGinley, Guerrero, Gautier, and Peterson, 1974; Imperato-McGinley, Peterson, Lishin, Griffin, Cooper, Draghi, Berenyi, and Wilson, 1980), even though the latter men show little penile development before puberty. In discussing behavior, we will see more examples of increases and decreases in sensitivity to gonadal steroids as a result of earlier exposure to T.

SEXUAL DIFFERENTIATION AS A MECHANISM FOR PRODUCING SEX DIFFERENCES IN BEHAVIOR

Sexual differentiation is the most important, but not the only, biological process producing sex differences in behavior. Some differences between the sexes simply reflect differences in the hormones circulating in adulthood. The ovaries of an adult female, for example, secrete more E_2 than the testes of an adult male. As a result, some behaviors that are sensitive to E_2 are shown more by females than by males. In rats, running in a running wheel is sensitive to E_2. Female rats run more than male rats do, but reversing their hormonal environments in adulthood readily reverses the sex difference in their behavior (Gentry and Wade, 1976). Giving males the same amount of E_2 benzoate (EB), relative to body weight, that stimulates wheel running in females elicits the heterotypical level of running (i.e., the level typical of the opposite sex). Ovariectomizing females, thereby depriving them of E_2, makes them as inactive as castrated males.

The feminine copulatory behavior of ferrets provides another example of this phenomenon. Under the influence of their own gonadal hormones, and when tested with a partner of the opposite sex, male and female ferrets display the typical sex differences in copulatory behaviors. However, when gonadectomized and given EB, male and female ferrets are equally receptive to males that establish a neck grip as a prelude to mounting (Baum and Gallagher, 1981; Baum, 1976). To determine if the high levels of feminine copulatory behavior shown by the male ferrets were due to the use of large hormone doses that could mask sex differences in responsiveness to E_2, Baum and Gallagher tested each sex with several EB doses. The dose–response curves for the two sexes were the same. Thus, there do not appear to be any sex differences in sensitivity to E_2 in regard to feminine copulatory behavior in this species.

Many other sexually dimorphic behaviors that are controlled by gonadal steroids in adulthood can not be sex-reversed in adulthood. Most move in the heterotypical direction, but few show complete reversal. Moreover, one usually needs more hormone to elicit the behavior heterotypically than homotypically. In other words, the ability to respond behaviorally to gonadal steroids differs in adult males and adult females. These sex differences are often established through the actions of gonadal hormones during early development.

Masculine and feminine copulatory behaviors of rats provide good examples of such sexual differentiation of behavior. The feminine copulatory behavior of rats involves a distinctive posture, called *lordosis*, in which the animal's back is concavely arched, its head and rump are elevated, and its tail is held to one side. If female rats have been exposed to E_2 followed by progesterone (P), they adopt this posture reflexively in response to tactile stimulation of their flanks and perineum, as occurs when they are mounted by males. In large doses, EB alone can stimulate lordosis, but at physiological levels, E_2 and P synergize (Davidson, Rodgers, Smith, and Block, 1968; Edwards, Whalen, and Nadler, 1968; Hardy and DeBold, 1971). Male rats, in contrast, rarely show lordosis when mounted, even when given ovarian hormones (Clemens, Shryne, and Gorski, 1970; Edwards and Thompson, 1970; Gerall and Kenney, 1970; Pfaff, 1970; Pfaff and Zigmond, 1971; Whalen and Edwards, 1967; Whalen, Luttge, and Gorzalka, 1971). The males are less receptive than the females when EB is used alone but are particularly insensitive to the synergistic effects of P. These sex differences in responsiveness to E_2 and P differentiate under the control of T shortly after birth. Neonatally androgenized female rats are as unreceptive as normal males when given EB and P in adulthood. Neonatally castrated males resemble normal females. If the number of lordotic responses is expressed as a percentage of the mounts received (this is known as the *lordosis quotient*, or LQ), we see that normal females and neonatally castrated males both obtain high LQ scores with EB and P. The extent to which sexual behavior is defeminized by testicular androgens seems to vary, though, with the strain. In some strains, sex differences in sensitivity to E_2 are seen only at some stages of the daily light–dark cycle (Södersten, 1984) or disappear completely if the hormone is given as frequent pulses (Södersten, Pettersson, and Eneroth, 1983). In other strains, the sex difference in sensitivity to E_2 persists when pulses are used (Moreines, McEwen, and Pfaff, 1986).

In addition to copulatory behaviors *per se*, the sexual behavior of female rats includes a variety of proceptive behaviors, such as ear wiggling and a hopping-and-darting locomotory pattern, with which the female solicits sexual attention (Beach, 1976). Like lordosis, these aspects of feminine sexual behavior are stimulated by E_2 and P in adulthood (Fadem, Barfield, and Whalen, 1979; Tennent, Smith, and

Davidson, 1980) and show sex differences in sensitivity to E_2 and P that differentiate under the control of T through metabolism to E_2 (Davis *et al.*, 1979a; Fadem and Barfield, 1981; Whalen and Olsen, 1981).

The masculine copulatory behavior of rats consists of a series of mounts, intromissions, and ejaculations. During a mount, the male approaches the female from the rear, clasps her flanks, and thrusts several times with his pelvis before dismounting. If he detects the female's vaginal opening with his penis during one of these thrusts, he performs a deeper thrust and dismounts abruptly. This behavioral pattern characterizes an intromission. After several intromissions, the male displays an ejaculatory pattern of behavior that involves an even deeper and more prolonged thrust and a slower dismount. These behavioral patterns are all stimulated in adult males by the presence of T. Female rats also show more masculine copulatory responses, particularly mounts, when given T than when deprived of gonadal steroids; however, the females are not as responsive to T as the males are, particularly in regard to the display of intromission and ejaculatory patterns (Beach, 1971; Gerall and Ward, 1966; Gerall, Hendricks, Johnson, and Bounds, 1967; Grady, Phoenix, and Young, 1965; Hart, 1968; Larsson, 1966; Pfaff, 1970; Pfaff and Zigmond, 1971; Thomas *et al.*, 1980, 1982, 1983; Whalen and Edwards, 1967). Like the sexual differentiation of feminine sexual behavior, the sexual differentiation of masculine sexual behavior occurs perinatally in rats under the influence of T. If female rats are exposed to TP shortly after birth, the masculine sexual behavior that they show in adulthood when reexposed to T is much more complete. If male rats are deprived of T or its metabolites perinatally, they display much less masculine sexual behavior, particularly intromissions and ejaculations, than normal males do, even when the adult hormone titers of the two groups are equated.

Behaviors Susceptible to Sexual Differentiation

Copulatory behaviors are the most thoroughly studied behaviors that undergo sexual differentiation, but they are by no means the only ones. Several other social behaviors become sexually dimorphic as a result of gonadal steroids acting developmentally to establish sex differences in adult sensitivity to gonadal steroids. One of the patterns of aggression shown by mice is a good example (Bronson and Desjardins, 1968, 1970; Edwards, 1968, 1969; Peters, Bronson, and Whitsett, 1972). In mice, as in most species, males are more aggressive toward conspecific males than females are. This intermale aggression is stimulated by T circulating in adulthood. Castrated male mice seldom fight unless T is exogenously replaced. Giving adult females T increases the probability that they will attack males and fight back when attacked; however, T-treated females rarely display as much aggression toward males as males do when given the same amount of hormone. This residual sex difference can be eliminated by first exposing females to T perinatally and then reexposing them to T as adults. Castrating males as neonates makes them less sensitive to T in adulthood, as females normally are. Behaviors used as threats or as courtship or territorial displays often fit the same pattern, including singing by songbirds (Arnold, 1975; Gurney, 1982; Gurney and Konishi, 1980) and scent marking by gerbils (Thiessen, Friend, and Lindzey, 1969; Turner, 1975).

Still other social and nonsocial behaviors are sexually dimorphic and respond to gonadal steroids acting developmentally and/or in adulthood (Beatty, 1979; Goldman, 1978). However, among the cases in which a developmental effect of gonadal steroids has been demonstrated, the need for hormonal stimulation later in development varies. Some sexually differentiated behavior patterns do not appear until puberty, such as the preference that female rats show for sweets, but do not require continued exposure to ovarian steroids once they have fully developed. In other cases, the sexually differentiated behavior develops without further exposure to gonadal hormones. Play behaviors of primates are an example of a behavior that sexually differentiates under the control of T but that does not require gonadal hormones for its later expression (Goy, 1978; Goy and Phoenix, 1971; Joslyn, 1973). Primate play is sexually dimorphic in that males show a good deal more rough-and-tumble play than females do. The role of T in the sexual differentiation of this behavior is demonstrated by the fact that female rhesus that are exposed to T during gestation show as much rough play as males do. Sexual differentiation of play is apparently complete before birth, as males castrated at birth also play as roughly as normal males. Because the play patterns in question are shown by juveniles (i.e., well before gonadal hormone secretion increases at puberty), it appears that gonadal hormones are not necessary for their display. The fact that prenatally androgenized females, neonatally castrated males, and gonadally intact males all show more rough-and-tumble play than females do, despite their differing gonadal states, reinforces this conclusion. The play behavior of rats seems to follow the same pattern (Meaney and Stewart, 1981a,b). The sexually dimorphic postures that dogs assume for urination also differentiate sexually under the control of T but do not require hormonal stimulation for their later display (Beach, 1974; Ranson and Beach, 1985). When male dogs are castrated as adults, they do not abandon the leg-lift urination style, even though they do less scent marking (i.e., they urinate less often and/or distribute the urine over fewer signposts). Thus, although we often detect sexual differentiation of behavior as a change in sensitivity to gonadal steroids, it can clearly alter other parameters instead or as well.

Different Behaviors Undergo Sexual Differentiation Independently

In discussing the reproductive system, we noted that reliance on a few signals produced by the gonads, primarily T, increases the probability that the various tissues that undergo sexual differentiation do so in a complementary fashion. The same applies to the sexual differentiation of behavior. Nonetheless, different target tissues—or more accurately, different phenotypes—can differentiate independently. The exceptions are cases in which the differentiation of one tissue or phenotype limits the developmental options of others, which then sexually differentiate secondarily. By manipulating development experimentally and by studying individuals with specific genetic mutations, we can attempt to determine which behavioral effects of T reflect independent events of sexual differentiation and which ones are interdependent. This type of analysis also provides clues about whether the masculine and feminine forms of a behavior are the products of a single tissue, which can differentiate in one direction or another, or the products of different tissues, which can differentiate separately.

Independent differentiation is seen in the development of masculine and feminine copulatory behaviors. These two patterns of copulatory behavior have different neural substrates (Davis and Barfield, 1979a,b; Davis *et al.*, 1979b), and neither differentiates at the expense of the other. If female hamsters are injected with a low dose of TP after birth, they display high levels of mounting when reexposed to TP in adulthood and tested with a receptive female (DeBold and Whalen, 1975). These same females display high levels of lordosis when given EB and P and tested with a male that will mount them. Similarly, male rats injected as neonates with 1,4,6,-androstatriene-3,17-dione (ATD), which prevents the metabolism of T to E_2, display both masculine and feminine sexual responses as adults, depending on the consorts provided (Davis *et al.*, 1979a). Their feminine responses are more complete (i.e., they were more likely to show proceptive behavior) if they are castrated and given EB and P than if they are tested under the influence of their testes, but in either case, they show lordosis when mounted. Both of these examples show that the masculinization of copulatory behavior is not necessarily accompanied by defeminization.

The defeminization of sexual behavior can also occur without masculinization. To obtain clues about the functional correlates of E_2 binding in the hypothalamus-preoptic area (HPOA), Ernie Nordeen and I needed to obtain precisely such separations in the display of copulatory behavior (Nordeen and Yahr, 1983). By giving newborn female rats TP systemically or E_2 in the HPOA, and then screening them for responsiveness to gonadal steroids in adulthood, we obtained defeminized females that showed no signs of masculinzation. As illustrated in Figure 2, these females had LQ scores of 0–10 when given EB and P, yet virtually never mounted when given EB and DHT. Because most females to which we gave TP neonatally were at least partially masculinized as well as being defeminized, we assume that our ability to dissociate these processes in some individuals was due to individual differences in sensitivity to T on the day after birth. Such individual differences may reflect differences in the length of gestation, the rate of maturation, and/or the prior exposure to T *in utero*. An example of complete defeminization accompanied by partial masculinization is also available in the behavior of male rats carrying the *tfm* (testicular feminization) mutation. These males are deficient in androgen receptors but have a normal complement of estrogen receptors in the HPOA (Olsen and Whalen, 1982). Although *tfm* males do not normally display lordosis when given EB and P, they do if they are castrated shortly after birth (Olsen, 1979a; Olsen and Whalen, 1981). They are also less likely than their littermate controls to show intromissive and ejaculatory patterns in adulthood when given estrogen and/or androgen (Olsen, 1979b; Shapiro, Levine, and Adler, 1980).

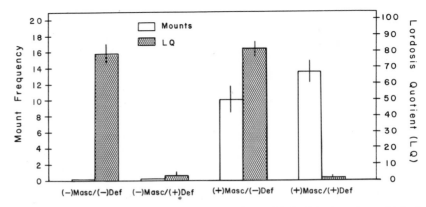

Figure 2. An illustration of the fact that the masculinization and defeminization of sexual behavior are independent processes in rats. The data shown are for female rats that received subcutaneous injections of TP, HPOA implants of E_2, or no exogenous hormone neonatally. As adults, these females were tested for lordosis after receiving EB and P and for mounting after receiving EB and DHT. Some groups, designated (−)Masc, showed no sign of masculinization in that they almost never mounted other females. Other groups, designated (+)Masc, mounted regularly. Each of these groups consisted of two subsets. One, designated (−)Def, showed no sign of defeminization in that they obtained high LQ scores. The other subset, designated (+)Def, was clearly defeminized. These females almost never showed lordosis when mounted. (Adapted from Nordeen and Yahr, 1983.)

Different components of masculine or feminine sexual behavior can also differentiate independently. In ferrets, for example, the receptive component of feminine sexual behavior is not defeminized by T, but the proceptive component is. Whereas male ferrets treated with EB as adults adopt a receptive stance when another male grips them by the scruff of the neck, they do not approach other males as readily as female ferrets do (Baum, Stockman, and Lundell, 1985). The tendency to be attracted to males is suppressed by early exposure to T. Male ferrets castrated 5 or 20 days after birth display approach patterns similar, but not identical, to those of females. In rats, the intromissive component of masculine sexual behavior is masculinized by the artificial androgen R1881, but the ejaculatory component is not (Olsen, 1985).

SPECIES, STRAIN, AND INDIVIDUAL DIFFERENCES RELATED TO SEXUAL DIFFERENTIATION

Ferrets and rats illustrate the principle that a sexually dimorphic behavior may be sexually differentiated to different degrees in different species. When given ovarian steroids, male ferrets become as receptive as conspecific females, but male rats do not. Thus, male rats are more defeminized than male ferrets in regard to this behavior. Sometimes, such cross-species comparisons are helpful in the testing of hypotheses about development. For example, as noted earlier, the defeminization of sexual behavior in male rats is largely due to a decreased sensitivity to P. In ferrets, P does not synergize with E_2 to elicit feminine copulatory behavior. Baum

(1979) therefore suggested that the defeminization of copulatory behavior occurs only in species in which the adult expression of the behavior involves a synergism between E_2 and P. Yet, among species in which E_2 and P do synergize, quantitative differences in sexual differentiation remain. Relative to conspecific females, male hamsters show more lordosis behavior than male rats do (Tiefer, 1970), although both species show synergistic effects of E_2 and P. Thus, male rats are more defeminized than male hamsters. Such comparisons raise interesting questions, though, about what baseline(s) should be used for quantifying sexual differentiation.

If we view sexual differentiation as a process that produces sex differences in a population or species of mammals, the expression of a phenotype by females provides a reasonable baseline from which to measure sexual differentiation in males from the same population. For both masculinization and defeminization, the phenotypic distribution of the females is the best available index of how males would have developed if the sexually differentiating signal(s) had been absent. For feminine functions, females also provide an index of functionally complete development. For masculine functions, the phenotypic distribution of the males serves this purpose. Yet, when studying sexual differentiation as a process of individual development, the argument for using the phenotypic distribution of the females to define the baseline from which to assess masculinization and defeminization, and for using the phenotypic distribution of the males to define complete masculinization, is less clear because the same factors that create differences between the sexes can contribute to the variation seen within each sex.

It has been hypothesized, for example, that some female rats are exposed to more T than others because they gestate between two male sibs, because they gestate rostrally to a male sib (downstream in terms of blood flow), or simply because of the number of males in the litter (Clemens, 1974; Clemens, Gladue, and Coniglio, 1978; Meisel and Ward, 1981). Such females have been reported to have longer anogenital distances, to display more mounting behavior in adulthood when given T, and to develop anovulatory sterility sooner after receiving TP postnatally than other females do (Clemens, 1974; Clemens *et al.*, 1978; Meisel and Ward, 1981; Richmond and Sachs, 1984a; Tobet, Dunlap, and Gerall, 1982), although the changes in mounting are not always seen (Slob and Van der Schoot, 1982). In other words, the development of some normal females may involve a mild version of the same processes that masculinize genital, behavioral, and neuroendocrine development in males. Similarly, in guinea pigs, females that develop immediately rostrally to males are more sensitive than other normal females to TP in adulthood in terms of its ability to stimulate mounting, but not in terms of its ability to stimulate genital sniffing or hip swaying (Gandelman, 1986). However, the amniotic fluid that surrounded these masculinized females did not contain a greater amount of T. In mice, females that gestate between two males are exposed to more T than females that gestate between two females and differ from them reproductively in ways that may reflect mild masculinization and defeminization (vom Saal and Bronson, 1978, 1980a,b). They are more aggressive toward conspecifics and display more urinary scent marking. They also have longer and more irregular estrous cycles and are less sexually attractive to males. However, these two subsets of the normal female population do not differ in their overall reproductive capacity and are equally sensitive to E_2 as assessed by induction of lordosis and negative feedback control of LH secretion. Moreover, they do not differ in their adult levels of T; thus, the increased aggressiveness and tendency to scent-mark suggest that females that develop between two males are more sensitive to T as adults. This suggestion is directly supported by the observation that they begin attacking males after about 16 daily injections of TP, whereas females that gestate between two females require about 25 (Gandelman, vom Saal, and Reinisch, 1977). However, even females that gestate some distance from males may be affected by their brothers' T, as female mice born as singletons almost never attack even after 60 days' exposure to T (Gandelman and Graham, 1976).

Male mice that gestate between two females are exposed to more E_2 than males that gestate between two males (vom Saal, Grant, McMullen, and Laves, 1983). Because E_2 mediates some of T's effects on sexual differentiation, this exposure could enhance masculinization and/or defeminization. On the other hand, the E_2 could antagonize the interaction of T or DHT with the androgen receptors. Then, masculinization and/or defeminization would be retarded. Indeed, there is evidence that both situations obtain (vom Saal *et al.*, 1983). The male mice that gestate between two females mount and intromit more readily than males that gestate between two males. In contrast, males exposed to more E_2 prenatally are less sensitive to the aggression-inducing effects of T. They are more sensitive to at least some adult effects of EB and P. When given these steroids, they are more sexually attractive to males than are males that gestate between two males. In short, the masculinizing and defeminizing processes of sexual differentiation seem to occur to varying degrees during the development of each sex. The extent to which they occur is just much greater in males.

Because mammals gestate internally, they are exposed to androgens and estrogens formed by the placenta, by the mother's ovaries, and by the maternal and fetal adrenals, whether or not the fetus's own gonads or those of their sibs are secretory (Gibori and Sridaran, 1981; Slob and Vreeburg, 1985; Sridaran, Basuray, and Gibori, 1981). Thus, variations in steroid secretion from one mother or pregnancy to another may also contribute to individual differences in the display of sexually differentiated phenotypes within each sex. The level of stress to which a pregnant female rat is exposed is an example of a situation that alters both the hormonal milieu of the gestating young, particularly the males, and their adult behavior (Ward and Ward, 1985). If a mother rat is stressed during the last week of gestation, her male fetuses have higher than normal levels of T on Day 17 of gestation, which is the day before T levels normally peak. However, this elevated level of T does not persist. In fact, on Days 18–19 of gestation, when male rats normally show a surge of T secretion, T levels are depressed. So is the activity of aromatase, the enzyme that converts T to E_2, in the brain. Behaviorally, these males are less defeminized and less masculinized than normal males. When given EB and P and tested with male consorts, they show more feminine sexual behavior than normal males, but less than normal females. When given TP and a female consort, the prenatally stressed males show some masculine sexual responses, but they either fail to ejaculate or do so only after receiving prolonged hormonal or social stimulation. Granted, males that are reproductively incompetent (e.g., males that do not ejaculate) represent an extreme point on the normal male continuum. Nonetheless, the prenatal stress syndrome reinforces the suggestion that masculinization and defeminization can be viewed as processes that occur to different degrees in normal males as well as in normal females.

This possibility is further supported by the observation that female rats are slightly defeminized by normal exposure to estrogen from their mother's ovaries. Female rats born to mothers that were ovariectomized midway through pregnancy (P was given exogenously to maintain the pregnancy) obtained higher LQ scores as adults when given EB, with or without P, than control females did (Witcher and Clemens, 1987). Injecting the mother with the aromatase inhibitor ATD intensified this effect. Even if the mother remains gonadally intact, ATD injections can enhance the display of feminine (sexual) behavior among the young (Clemens and Gladue, 1978), although this effect varies with strain (Whalen and Olsen, 1981; Whalen, Gladue, and Olsen, 1986). Thus, during normal development, the baseline level of exposure to steroids that results from internal gestation may affect sexual development, even though it could not, by definition, produce differences between the sexes.

WHEN ARE BEHAVIORS SUSCEPTIBLE TO SEXUAL DIFFERENTIATION?

Pushing sexual differentiation in a signaled direction (e.g., masculinizing and defeminizing mammals) requires two things—that the signal be available and that the sexually indifferent tissue have the capacity to respond. Either of these factors can vary with the animal's age. Histochemical analyses of fetal and neonatal testes and assays of T in blood indicate that mammalian testes begin secreting T when or before the reproductive tract sexually differentiates and before behavioral sexual differentiation begins, where this age is known (Resko, 1985). The fetal-neonatal testes remain active for days or weeks, depending on the species, before entering the quiescent phase that persists until puberty. Yet, within this early period of T secretion, one must empirically determine when any particular tissue or phenotype can respond. There is no theoretical basis for predicting when this should be, with one exception. Defeminization should not occur prenatally unless a mechanism exists for protecting females from becoming reproductively incompetent as a result of exposure to their brothers', their mother's, or placental hormones. Mechanisms for providing such protection include a high threshold for defeminization, a blood protein that sequesters circulating steroid, or an enzyme system that rapidly inactivates the hormone. Delaying sensitivity to the defeminizing effects of T until after birth prevents the problem.

The ages at which a sexually indifferent tissue can respond to a masculinizing or defeminizing signal are often restricted, in some cases because the tissue embarks on a feminine plan of development. In some other cases, the sexually indifferent precursor may regress. In studying sexual differentiation of behavior, we often do not know the precise tissues or cells involved. Nonetheless, we sometimes see the same phenomenon of age-related changes in the capacity of the phenotype to respond to a sexually differentiating signal. When this occurs, the interval during which the sexual differentiation of a phenotype can be pushed in the signaled direction is called the *critical period*. At this point, though, we should recall our earlier discussion about the relative nature of differentiation and phenotypic commitment. These critical periods are *operationally* defined by changes in the dose of hormone needed to effect sexual differentiation at different ages or by age-related changes in the effectiveness of a given hormone dose.

In some cases, the critical period for sexual differentiation is different from the period during which the hormone elicits the adult response. The ability of TP to defeminize LH secretion in female rats is already declining by 5 days of age and is largely gone by 10 days (Gorski, 1968), whereas the ability to show postive feedback does not develop until 22–24 days of age (Andrews, Mizcjewski, and Ojeda, 1981; Ronneklein, Ojeda, and McCann, 1978). In other cases, the critical period overlaps the ages at which hormones can evoke an adultlike response. The lordosis behavior of female rats is still susceptible to defeminization 6 days after birth, but it can also be elicited by EB and P at this age (Clemens *et al.*, 1970; Williams, 1987).

For any particular phenotype, the critical period for sexual differentiation can vary from species to species. In guinea pigs, which have a long gestation for rodents (63–70 days), prenatal exposure to T defeminizes copulatory behavior, but postnatal exposure does not (Goy, Bridson, and Young, 1964; Phoenix, Goy, Gerall, and Young, 1959). In rats, which have a shorter gestation (20–22 days), susceptibility to the defeminizing effects of T on lordosis is clearly present after birth (Whalen and Edwards, 1967). These differences may simply reflect differences in neural maturation at birth. Indeed, among rodents, the age at which copulatory behavior undergoes sexual differentiation seems relatively constant when calculated from fertilization, but this relationship does not seem to hold for other groups of mammals (Feder, 1981c; Ford, 1982, 1983).

Within a species, critical periods vary from one phenotype to another, although they often overlap. To the extent that male rats are more sensitive to T or its metabolites in terms of mounting, the data discussed above suggest that the masculinization of sexual behavior is well under way prenatally, whereas the defeminization of sexual behavior occurs primarily after birth. Ferrets show the opposite pattern: the defeminization of sexual behavior begins before masculinization. To fully defeminize proceptivity in male ferrets, the testes must be present throughout the first 3 weeks after birth; however, the first 5 days constitute a critical period that determines whether or not young ferrets can respond to the defeminizing effects of T over the next 2 weeks (Baum *et al.*, 1985). Giving female ferrets T prenatally defeminizes their proceptive behavior in that it eliminates the dose-dependent effects of EB on attraction to males in adulthood (Baum and Tobet, 1986). Delaying T treatment until 6 days after birth eliminates this effect, although the hormone can still partially masculinize females at this age. It increases their tendency to mount other females and to grip them by the nape of the neck (Baum and Erskine, 1984; Baum *et al.*, 1985). Similarly, male ferrets that are castrated 6 days after birth show no signs of masculinization but have already been partially defeminized in terms of their social preferences.

Critical periods also vary with the methods used to measure them. As noted above, it is most useful to view critical periods as curves describing, for example, the effects of a given dose of T, administered to females at different ages, on the later expression of the behavior. The curve may broaden if we use a larger dose of T, a longer acting form of T (e.g., TP), or a more active metabolite, or if we make the hormone available for more than 1 day (e.g., by using Silastic implants or daily injections). Still a different impression of the critical period may be gained by attempting to stop masculinization or defeminization in males instead of by attempting to induce it in females. Similarly, the critical period varies with the testing conditions used in adulthood, including the dose of hormone given to elicit the behavior, how often the animals are tested, the criterion set for the display of the behavior, and whether one records the percentage of subjects displaying it or how often each of them responds.

In terms of cellular mechanisms, the beginning and end of a critical period may depend on very different things. Hence, one end of the critical period may be more flexible than the other. The critical period for a neuron involved in the sexual differentiation of behavior may begin, for example, when the neuron begins producing intracellular receptors for T or its metabolites, or when the neuron begins synthesizing the metabolizing enzyme(s). The period may end when the cell dies, when it makes synaptic contact with other cells, or when biochemical events occur that determine which genes will be available for transcription. The ease with which one can push the animal's phenotype in the signaled direction after the critical period depends on how the critical period is terminated. Clearly, it will be difficult, if not impossible, to masculinize or defeminize a phenotype if the pertinent cells no longer exist (i.e., if they die unless exposed to T during the critical period), if they no longer produce steroid receptors, if they would have to migrate to a new location, or if they would have to receive inputs from or project to cells that no longer exist. Alternatively, if masculinization or defeminization involves killing the cells (i.e., if they die when exposed to T), or if reversing sexual differentiation requires changing the biochemical or morphological phenotypes of cells (e.g., extending or retracting processes, or synthesizing a new neurotransmitter, a new neurotransmitter receptor, or a new hormone-metabolizing enzyme), then it may be achievable at any age, although it may require pharmacological levels of hormone.

THE ROLE OF T METABOLISM IN SEXUAL DIFFERENTIATION OF BEHAVIOR

One of the most intriguing discoveries about the sexual differentiation of the brain and behavior is that aromatization to E_2 mediates many effects of T. Among mammals, E_2 seems particularly important for defeminizing the HPOA, but it contributes to masculinization as well. Several lines of evidence led to these conclusions (for detailed reviews, see MacLusky and Naftolin, 1981; Naftolin and MacLusky, 1984; Whalen, Yahr, and Luttge, 1985). First, fetal and neonatal brains contain both the aromatase enzyme and estrogen receptors. Aromatase activity and E_2 binding are especially high in the HPOA. Second, androgens that can be aromatized (e.g., T) often have more potent effects on sexual differentiation than androgens that cannot (e.g, DHT). Third, aromatase inhibitors and antiestrogens can counteract the defeminizing effects of T on copulatory behavior. Fourth, the sexual behavior of *tfm* males, which have estrogen but not androgen receptors, is defeminized and partially masculinized by T. Fifth, under conditions in which estrogens have easy access to the developing brain, they defeminize and/or masculinize copulatory behavior in much lower doses than T does.

The discovery that circulating E_2 does not necessarily enter the nuclei of fetal or neonatal brain cells undergoing sexual differentiation allowed the last piece of the aromatization puzzle to fit into place. For some time after other evidence pointed to a role for aromatization, questions remained because the doses of E_2 needed to mimic T exceeded what could be formed from T in a developing male. This paradox was resolved with the discovery that the species under study had a protein, alpha-fetoprotein, in their blood during the period of sexual differentiation that binds E_2 (MacLusky and Naftolin, 1981; Plapinger and McEwen, 1978). Once bound to alpha-fetoprotein, E_2 apparently cannot enter brain cell nuclei. Thus, unless one injects enough EB to swamp the binding capacity of alpha-fetoprotein, the hormone does not reach the chromatin acceptor sites. By injecting EB with a drug, prednisolone, that disrupts the synthesis of alpha-fetoprotein, Whalen and Olsen (1978b) showed that female rats can be defeminized with very low doses of EB. Alpha-fetoprotein can also be bypassed by placing the hormone directly in the brain. Female rats given E_2 implants in the HPOA mount more often in adulthood, and/or have lower LQ scores, than controls (Christensen and Gorski, 1978; Nordeen and Yahr, 1982). Similarly, one can masculinize female hamsters with picogram doses of an estrogen analogue (RU-2858) that is not bound by alpha-fetoprotein (Whalen and Etgen, 1978).

Yet aromatization is not responsible for all of T's sexually differentiating effects on behavior. Even if we consider only sexual behaviors, the importance of E_2 varies across species and phenotypes. In particular, aromatization may be less important in masculinizing sexual behavior than in defeminizing it. The potency of RU-2858 in hamsters suggests that E_2 does mediate the masculinization of copulatory behavior in this species. In contrast, masculinization proceeds normally in ferrets when brain aromatase activity is blocked (Baum, Canick, Erskine, Gallagher, and Shim, 1983). In accord with this latter observation, exposing female ferrets to E_2 neonatally only slightly masculinizes mounting and neck gripping (Baum, Gallagher, Martin, and Damassa, 1982). In rats, a requirement for E_2 in masculinization is brought into question by the effects of ATD and another aromatase inhibitor, androst-4-ene-3,6,17-trione (ADT). Whether given to males before or after birth, neither decreases the frequencies of mounts or intromissions shown in adulthood in response to T. However, the rate at which males mount and intromit is lower after prenatal exposure to ATD, and either pre- or postnatal treatment can disrupt ejaculation or affect the latency to resume mating after ejaculation (Booth, 1978; Davis *et al.*, 1979a; Gladue and Clemens, 1980; Olsen, 1985; Olsen and Whalen, 1981; Thomas *et al.*, 1980; Vreeburg, van der Vaart, and van der Schoot, 1977). The possibility that E_2 is sufficient to masculinize mounting is suggested by the fact that mounting increases when female rats receive implants of E_2 in the HPOA neonatally (Christensen and Gorski, 1978; Nordeen and Yahr, 1982).

Now that it is clear that T is readily metabolized in the brain, it is difficult to determine if any of T's effects on sexual differentiation reflect a direct action (i.e., one that does not involve metabolism). This possibility is raised by the observation that the HPOA of neonatal rats binds an unaromatized androgen that does not appear to be DHT (Sheridan, 1981). Assessing the role of DHT is also difficult. Fetal brains do contain 5-alpha-reductase (Denef, Magnus, and McEwen, 1984; Massa, Justo, and Martini, 1975; Tobet, Shim, Osiecki, Baum, and Canick, 1985), DHT (Butte, Moore, and Kakihana, 1979) and androgen receptors (Lieberburg, MacLasky, and McEwen, 1980a; Vito, Baum, Bloom, and Fox, 1985), although the receptor concentration is relatively low for the first week after birth in rats. Yet, like adult brains, fetal brains may also contain enzymes that rapidly metabolize DHT (Gustafsson, Pousette, and Svensson, 1976; Whalen and Rezek, 1972). Some metabolites of DHT do not bind as well as DHT to androgen receptors in the HPOA; others bind to the receptors for estrogen (Doering and Gladue, 1982). Thus, if exogenous DHT does alter sexual differentiation, it could be because one of its metabolites mimics E_2 (Södersten and Gustafsson, 1980). If exogenous DHT does not affect sexual differentiation, it could be because it is not available long enough to interact with the androgen receptors (Gay, 1975). Such an availability problem need not imply, though, that the same fate befalls endogenous DHT. The reductase and androgen receptor systems could be coupled in such a way that the DHT formed by the metabolism of T passes efficiently between the two.

Research on the role of DHT and/or unmetabolized T has been aided by the development of the synthetic androgen R1881, which binds to androgen but not to estrogen receptors, and which is not metabolized in the brain (Bonne and Raynaud, 1976; Doering and Leyra, 1984; Olsen, 1985; Raynaud and Moguilewsky, 1977). The data available to date suggest that androgens alone cannot fully masculinize copulatory behavior, and that the effects they do have may be mediated by changes in the genitalia. Neonatally castrated male rats that receive R1881 for 5–10 days after birth are no more likely to mount females when given T in adulthood than are neonatal castrates that receive no steroids after birth (Olsen, 1985), although their copulatory efficiency (number of intromissions/number of mounts + intromissions) at least doubles. R1881-treated males intromit during 37%–52% of their attempts, whereas vehicle-treated controls do so during 8%–19% of their attempts. Thus, the copulatory efficiency of males exposed only to androgens neonatally approaches that of males exposed to endogenous T (53%–65%). The ability of R1181 to mimic T's effect on copulatory efficiency may reflect androgenic effects of R1881 on the penis. Yet, despite their efficient intromissive behavior, neonatally castrated males given R1881 do not show the ejaculatory response. This result is reminiscent of the data discussed earlier in which males that were presumably exposed only to androgens postnatally because of the presence of ATD or ADT sometimes showed impairments in ejaculation or related behaviors. The possibility that both E_2 and DHT are necessary to masculinize this aspect of copulatory behavior in rats is suggested by data showing that neonatally castrated males given both steroids shortly after birth do show the ejaculatory pattern when treated with T in adulthood (Booth, 1977; Hart, 1977, 1979). R1881 only slightly masculinizes the copulatory behavior of hamsters (Olsen, 1985), a finding that reinforces the earlier conclusion that masculinization is particularly sensitive to E_2 in this species. In ferrets, the masculinization of copulatory behavior proceeds normally when 5-alpha-reduction is curtailed, just as it does when aromatization is curtailed (Baum et al., 1983). Defeminization of the social preferences of female ferrets follows neonatal exposure to T, but not to DHT or E_2 (Martin and Baum, 1986). Thus, T may masculinize and defeminize ferrets by itself.

Similar analyses have been undertaken to determine the role of T metabolism in the sexual differentiation of other social and nonsocial behaviors. Singing by zebra finches, for example, differentiates primarily under the control of E_2 (Gurney, 1982; Gurney and Konishi, 1980; Pohl-Apel and Sossinka, 1984). So far, though, it appears that one must determine empirically which metabolite, if either, is involved in the sexual differentiation of any particular behavioral phenotype. Even knowing the form of the hormone that stimulates the behavior in adulthood does not necessarily provide a clue. In zebra finches, early exposure to E_2 masculinizes later sensitivity to DHT, which enables the bird to sing.

THE ROLE OF E_2 IN THE DEVELOPMENT OF FEMININE PHENOTYPES

The discovery that E_2 contributes to the sexual differentiation of the brain and behavior stimulated interest in the role of E_2 in other aspects of sexual development. In particular, E_2's role in the development of feminine functions is being explored. Unfortunately, the fact that E_2 defeminizes many phenotypes of mammals has made it difficult to test in vivo the hypothesis that low levels of E_2 must reach the brain during the period of sexual differentiation in order for the feminine versions of these phenotypes to develop (Dohler et al., 1984). Attempts to test this hypothesis have encountered the conceptual problem that the defeminized version of the phenotype is difficult to distinguish from the version supposedly caused by estrogen deficiency. Both would produce females that are anovulatory and that do not show lordosis. Attempts to test this hypothesis have also encountered a technical problem when using antiestrogens, such as tamoxifen, to decrease estrogen activity, namely, that estrogen antagonists can also be estrogen agonists. Thus, when one determines how much tamoxifen must be given perinatally to produce anovulatory females that do not display lordosis, it is difficult to know if that dose is sufficiently estrogenic to cause defeminization. Yet despite these problems, the data suggest that E_2 may contribute to the development of feminine phenotypes. Giving tamoxifen to newborn female rats suppresses their ability to ovulate and to show lordosis in adulthood, even when special care is taken to prevent the drug from dissociating into its more estrogenic cis-isomer. Tamoxifen impairs feminine development more effectively than its cis-isomer does, even though the cis-isomer is more estrogenic. Moreover, small doses of E_2 counteract the disruptive effects of tamoxifen on both lordosis and ovulation. Neonatal exposure to tamoxifen (Dohler et al., 1984b) also reduces the size of the sexually dimorphic nucleus

(SDN) of the rat POA, which is already smaller in females than in males. On the other hand, neonatal ovariectomy produces no effect on SDN volume other than that caused by surgery *per se* (Jacobson, Csernus, Shryne, and Gorski, 1981). Other evidence indicating that E_2 present during and/or after sexual differentiation promotes feminine development is that neonatally castrated male rats show more feminine sexual behavior in adulthood when given EB and P if they receive ovarian transplants shortly after castration than if they do not (Gerall, Dunlap, and Hendricks, 1972).

The effects of E_2 have also been studied *in vitro* by monitoring neurite outgrowth from explants of fetal mouse brains (Toran-Allerand, 1976, 1980, 1984). Supplementing the E_2 normally available in the tissue culture medium (serum) by providing E_2 directly, or by providing its precursor T, increases the density of neurite outgrowth from the HPOA. Reducing E_2 levels by adding antibodies to E_2 brings neurite outgrowth below baseline. This approach to studying E_2 action in the developing brain is promising; however, it does not tell us whether E_2 is specifically required for the development of feminine phenotypes or whether it is a general growth factor needed for HPOA development in either sex. Indeed, many aspects of mammalian development may require E_2. Mammalian embryos of both sexes temporarily synthesize E_2 before they implant in the uterine wall, and doing so may be essential for their survival (George and Wilson, 1978). The possiblity that E_2 is essential in mammals is supported by the fact that no mutations have been identified in the synthetic pathway for E_2 or for E_2 receptors (Wilson *et al.*, 1981), whereas such mutations are known for other steroid hormones. E_2 is also essential for the survival of hypothalamic neurons cultured in defined media (Puymirat, Loudes, Faivre-Bauman, Tixier-Vidal, and Bourre, 1982). Thus, in regard to sexual development, E_2 may be necessary for the differentiation of the sexually indifferent primordia or for the developmental events that follow sexual differentiation, in addition to mediating some of the sexually differentiating effects of T. These possibilities are supported by the observation that cells in most areas of the brain take up the alpha-fetoprotein–E_2 complex (Schachter and Toran-Allerand, 1982). However, certain cells within the HPOA specifically lack this uptake system (Toran-Allerand, 1982). It is not clear which cells contribute to the neurite outgrowth seen in tissue culture, but it is clear that the process requires E_2, other than what can be derived from aromatization. Neurite outgrowth does not occur in response to T when E_2 is missing. If the cells in which E_2 can reach the nucleus cannot take up E_2 that is bound to alpha-fetoprotein, then some of their responses to E_2 may be mediated indirectly, such as through estrogenic effects on the synthesis of a neuronotrophic factor in other cells.

WHICH NEURAL TISSUES CONTRIBUTE TO SEXUAL DIFFERENTIATION OF BEHAVIOR?

One of the most interesting challenges facing psychobiology is to identify specific cell groups and pathways in the brain that contribute to the sexual differentiation of specific behaviors. A system that is proving to be a model for such analyses is the motor pathway for singing in the songbird brain. In zebra finches and canaries, the syrinx, or vocal organ, is innervated by a branch of the hypoglossal nerve. For singing to occur, the motoneurons, which are located in the tracheo-syringeal portion of the hypoglossal nucleus (nXIIts), must receive an input from the robust nucleus of the archistriatum (RA), which, in turn, must receive an input from a portion of the telencephalic cortex, the caudal nucleus of the ventral hyper-striatum (HVc). Lesioning either HVc or RA, like cutting the tracheosyringeal branch of the hypoglossal nerve, severely disrupts singing in adult male canaries (Nottebohm *et al.*, 1976, 1979). In adults of both species, these nuclei accumulate T (Arnold, 1980b; Arnold, Nottebohm, and Pfaff, 1976) and are larger in males than in females (Nottebohm and Arnold, 1976). In addition, three other nuclei connected to this pathway (Gurney, 1981, 1982; Gurney and Konishi, 1980; Not-tebohm, Kelley, and Paton, 1982) are larger in males and/or accumulate T. The midbrain nucleus intercollicularis (ICo), which is often implicated in the control of avian vocalizations, but which is not essential for singing in canaries, receives a projection from RA and projects to nXIIts. It accumulates T in both species. In canaries, the dorsomedial portion of ICo (Dm/ICo), which receives the input from RA, is also twice as large in males as in females. Area X, which receives a projection from HVc, is nearly four times as large in male as in female canaries. In zebra finches, X is prominent in males but is not even recognizable in females. However, X does not take up T. The magnocellular nucleus of the anterior neostriatum (MAN), which projects to both HVc and RA, does accumulate T. In zebra finches, it is also larger in males. MAN is not necessary for adult male zebra finches to sing. It is important, though, for the development of song in adolescence (Bottjer, Mies-ner, and Arnold, 1984), when males compare the sounds that they are starting to produce with memories of their father's songs.

Some of these sex differences reflect sex differences in the adult steroid environment. Giving female zebra finches DHT causes nXIIts and Dm/ICo to become as large as they are in males (Gurney, 1981). In canaries, both RA and HVc shrink in males that are castrated or exposed to short days (Nottebohm, 1980, 1981; Not-tebohm, Nottebohm, and Crane, 1986). Conversely, when adult female canaries receive T, RA and HVc enlarge. However, the system includes examples of sexual differentiation that parallel the sexual differentiation of the behavior. Even when given T in adulthood, female canaries sing much less than males do. Similarly, RA and HVC do not become as large as they are in males. Normal female zebra finches never sing a malelike song when given T in adulthood, even though they occasion-ally produce other sounds in the context in which males would produce a courtship song (Pohl-Apel and Sossinka, 1984). Similarly, adult exposure to T or DHT does not affect the volumes of RA or HVc in this species (Arnold, 1980a; Gurney, 1982; Gurney and Konishi, 1980). In order to sing and to show an enlargement of RA, HVc, MAN, and X when exposed to T or DHT as adults, female zebra finches must be exposed to T or E_2 earlier in development, such as shortly after hatching. The song-control system provides the clearest and most extensive correlations available to date between the sexual differentiation of the brain and of behavior. However, it appears that some of the neural parameters can be dissociated from effects on singing. In particular, the critical period for masculinizing song seems to terminate earlier than the critical period for masculinizing the hormone binding patterns in MAN and HVc (Nordeen, Nordeen, and Arnold, 1987; Pohl-Apel and Sossinka, 1984), although parameters that can affect the critical period (e.g., hormone dose) were not identical in the two studies. If such dissociations are found, they may prove useful for determining which features of a masculinized song-control system are essential for masculinization of the behavior and which are not.

The vocalizations of the amphibian species *Xenopus laevis* provide another example of a sexually dimorphic, hormonally modulated communication behavior for which it has been possible to trace connections from the vocal organ (larynx) into the brain (Kelley, 1986). The laryngeal muscles and the nuclei of the motor pathway, which in this case includes the POA, are all larger in males than in females. Sexual differentiation involves the masculinizing effects of T after metamorphosis.

In mammals, efforts to identify neural targets for sexual differentiation have focused on the HPOA because it is involved in the adult expression of so many sexually differentiated behaviors, including male and female copulatory behavior (Hart and Leedy, 1985; Kelley and Pfaff, 1978), scent marking (Yahr, 1983), food intake (Wade and Zucker, 1970), and maternal behavior (Numan, 1985), as well as in the control of gonadotropin secretion in some species. These efforts have revealed a wide variety of biochemical and morphological differences between the sexes (DeVries, DeBruin, Uylings, and Corner, 1984b). Where their developmental bases have been sought, it has been shown that the neural systems sexually differentiate under the control of T, although in some cases the adult hormone environment contributes as well. Yet, because so many sexually differentiated functions are controlled by the HPOA, it has been difficult to associate specific cell groups or pathways with specific functions.

For example, several aspects of POA morphology are sexually dimorphic in adult rats as a result of differential exposure to T perinatally. One aspect is the volume of the SDN, which is a portion of the medial preoptic nucleus (MPN) that is several times larger in males than in females (Döhler *et al.*, 1982, 1984b; Gorski *et al.*, 1978, 1980; Jacobson *et al.*, 1981; Simerly, Swanson, and Gorski, 1984b). Another is the synaptic organization of a region dorsolateral to the MPN (i.e., near the bed nucleus of the stria terminalis). In this region, females have a higher proportion of nonstrial inputs (source unknown) synapsing onto dendritic spines than males do (Raisman and Field, 1971, 1973). Because the POA is the locus for positive feedback control of LH secretion in rats, each of these structural sex differences was a candidate for being the neural correlate of this sex difference in POA function. However, in each case, the sexual differentiation of morphology can be dissociated from the sexual differentiation of LH secretion. More TP is needed to defeminize the synaptic organization of the region studied by Raisman and Field than is needed to defeminize LH secretion. Similarly, the critical period for masculinizing the SDN does not coincide with the critical period for disrupting positive feedback. As the POA also mediates T's effects on masculine sexual behavior, the anatomical sex differences could be related, instead, to this behavior. This possibility has been tested only for the SDN. Unfortunately, SDN size is no greater among females that mount than among those that do not (Nordeen and Yahr, 1982). Moreover, bilateral lesions of the SDN have no effect on the sexual behavior of adult male rats, although similar-sized lesions dorsomedial to it do (Arendash and Gorski, 1983). More recently, though, it was reported that the SDN is larger in males that ejaculate than in males that do not (Anderson, Fleming, Rhees, and Kinghorn, 1986).

Neither structural dimorphism of the POA appears to be involved in the control of lordosis, as perinatal hormonal manipulations that usually eliminate this behavior do not necessarily affect these anatomical parameters. This lack of correlation is not surprising because the defeminizing effects of T on sexual behavior are mediated primarily by the MBH, particularly the ventromedial nucleus (VMN). Interestingly, VMN volume is also sexually dimorphic in rats, and again, the sex difference develops perinatally under the control of T (Matsumoto and Arai, 1983). However, if this anatomical sex difference produces the sex difference in lordosis, then the defeminization of lordosis must involve an active inhibition of the behavior in males, as the VMN is smaller in females than in males.

In the gerbil HPOA, a sexually dimorphic area (SDA) has been identified that does appear to be involved in the control of two sexually dimorphic behaviors: scent marking and masculine sexual behavior (Commins and Yahr, 1984a,b,c, 1985). Bilateral lesions of the adult male SDA produce greater deficits in these behaviors than do lesions either anterior or posterior to it. However, we do not yet know what role hormones play in the sexual differentiation of the SDA. One subdivision of the SDA, the SDA pars compacta (SDApc), which is extremely dimorphic (males have SDApcs, but females do not), does differentiate sexually under the control of T (see Figure 1; Ulibarri and Yahr, 1988), but its function is not known. SDApc volume correlates significantly, though, with copulatory efficiency in adult males (Yahr and Stephens, 1987).

The spinal cord has also been explored for pathways mediating the sexual differentiation of copulatory behavior. Clear sex differences are seen in two nuclei in the lumbar cord of rats—the spinal nucleus of the bulbocavernosus (SNB) and the dorsolateral nucleus (DLN)—that innervate four striated penile muscles that exist only in males in adulthood. Both nuclei, but particularly the SNB, contain more motoneurons in males than in females (Breedlove and Arnold, 1980, 1981; Breedlove, Jacobson, Gorski, and Arnold, 1982; Jordan, Breedlove, and Arnold, 1982; McKenna and Nadelhoft, 1986). The number of cells in SNB differentiates sexually under the control of T acting as DHT (Breedlove and Arnold, 1983a,b; Breedlove et al., 1982). In adult males, SNB cells accumulate T, largely and perhaps exclusively as DHT (Breedlove and Arnold, 1980), and respond to it by enlarging their somas (Breedlove and Arnold, 1981) and extending their dendrites (Kurz, Sengelaub, and Arnold, 1986). The few SNB cells in female rats also enlarge when exposed to T in adulthood, but they do not attain the size seen in males. SNB cells of adult females may be less responsive to T because they do not accumulate as much hormone per cell as SNB cells of males do (Breedlove and Arnold, 1983c). The SNB neuromuscular system is not involved, though, in the sexual differentiation of the major body movements involved in masculine copulatory behavior. The muscles innervated by SNB are important for the reproductive success of males because they enable males to deposit tight copulatory plugs and to dislodge plugs deposited by other males (Hart and Melese d'Hospital, 1983; Sachs, 1982, 1983; Wallach and Hart, 1983). Nonetheless, the sexual differentiation of the SNB has been dissociated from the sexual differentiation of mounting, intromission, and ejaculation (Breedlove and Arnold, 1983a,b). In contrast, it seems likely that sensory pathways in the spinal cord will prove to be important in the sexual differentiation of masculine copulatory behavior, as the most sexually dimorphic components of this behavior are the ones that depend most heavily on tactile feedback from the genitalia. Even female rats that mount are less likely than males to display the intromissive pattern (i.e., copulatory efficiency is low) and rarely display the ejaculatory pattern. Similarly, in males, mounting rates are high but intromissive and ejaculatory patterns are rare if the penis is anesthetized or the dorsal penile nerves are cut (Adler and Bermant, 1966; Carlsson and Larsson, 1964; Larsson and Södersten, 1973). Sex differences in the display of feminine sexual behavior probably also reflect differences in the possibility of sensory feedback from the cervix or the vagina (Dixson, 1986; Rodriquez-Sierra, Crowley, and Komisaruk, 1975).

WHAT PROPERTIES OF NEURAL TISSUES DIFFERENTIATE SEXUALLY?

Almost every property of neuronal structure and function has been shown to be sexually dimorphic somewhere in the central nervous system. Sex differences in the volumes of brain nuclei can reflect differences in cell number, somal size, or somal density. In RA of zebra finches, for example, exposure to DHT at hatching increases the number of neurons, whereas exposure to E_2 increases their average size and enables them to increase their spacing when they are later exposed to DHT (Gurney, 1981, 1982; Gurney and Konishi, 1980). Dendritic arbors can differ as well. The dendrites of at least some RA neurons extend further from the soma, branch more often, and have more synapses on their surfaces in males than in females (DeVoogd and Nottebohm, 1981a,b; DeVoogd, Nixdorf, and Nottebohm, 1985; Gurney, 1981); however, these sex differences do not seem to reflect sexual differentiation. When adult female canaries receive T, their RA dendrites become as long and as branched as those of males, and the number of synapses increases. Thus, the dendritic arbor may simply reflect the adult hormonal environment. Alternatively, it is possible that the critical period for this phenotype does not terminate until the cells are exposed to T. In other words, it is not known whether the dendritic trees of male canaries, or of females exposed to T, retract when T is removed from the circulation. This possibility seems highly likely, though, given that the total RA volume of males decreases in the fall of each year, when T levels decline (Nottebohm, 1981; Nottebohm et al., 1986). In rats, the electrical properties of the SDN and the surrounding POA sexually differentiate under the control of T (Dyer, 1984). POA cells that have no direct connection to the MBH are more spontaneously active in females and in neonatally castrated males than in normal males or in neonatally androgenized females. In contrast, POA cells that project to the MBH are less likely to respond to electrical stimulation of the corticomedial amygdala in the two former groups than in the two latter.

Because sexual differentiation is often detected as a sex difference in adult responsiveness to gonadal steroids, sex differences in steroid binding have received special attention. In particular, sex differences in E_2 binding in the HPOA have been sought as correlates for sex differences in the sensitivity of lordosis and positive feedback to E_2. In rats, sex differences have been detected in the number of receptors available to bind E_2 (Rainbow *et al.*, 1982) and in the amount of E_2 bound to cell nuclei (Whalen and Massicci, 1975) or chromatin at various times after E_2 injection (Olsen and Whalen, 1980; Whalen and Olsen, 1978a). However, other studies have found no differences in the E_2 uptake systems of males and females (Lieberburg and McEwen, 1977; Lieberburg *et al.*, 1980b; Maurer and Woolley, 1974). This variability probably reflects the actual heterogeneity of the HPOA, and even of its subdivisions. For example, we noted earlier that the POA of rats mediates both positive feedback, for which responsiveness to E_2 is greater in females, and mounting, for which responsiveness to E_2 is greater in males (Pfaff, 1970; Pfaff and Zigmond, 1971). Therefore even if E_2 binding correlated with responsiveness to E_2 for each of these two phenotypes, their sex differences might cancel each other out when E_2 binding is assayed in the POA as a whole, or one might obscure the other. Indeed, when E_2 binding to cell nuclei is measured in the POA 30 min after an E_2 injection, males bind more E_2 than females do (Nordeen and Yahr, 1983). At this time point, the binding properties of the cells that control mounting may dominate total E_2 binding. By 60 min after an E_2 injection, E_2 binding in the POA is greater in females. At this time point, total E_2 binding may be dominated by the cells responsible for positive feedback. The latter suggestion is supported by data on the sexual differentiation of E_2 binding. The E_2 binding seen after 60 min is malelike in female rats whose gonadotropin secretion has been defeminized, regardless of whether their mounting behavior has been masculinized or not. In contrast, the binding pattern is femalelike in ovulatory female rats whose mounting behavior has been masculinized.

In regard to feminine sexual behavior and positive feedback in rats, sexual differentiation affects adult responsiveness to P as well as to E_2. Therefore, sex differences in P binding have been explored (Etgen, 1984). These analyses have been particularly interesting because they suggest that apparent differences in responsiveness to P actually represent differences in responsiveness to E_2, because in some cells (e.g., those of the hypothalamus and/or POA), the receptor that binds P is one of the proteins whose synthesis is increased by E_2 (Baum, Gerlach, Krey, and McEwen, 1986; MacLusky and McEwen, 1978; MacLusky, Lieberburg, Krey, and McEwen, 1980; Moguilewsky and Raynaud, 1979a). In other cells with P receptors (e.g., those of the amygdala, the cortex, or the midbrain), synthesis is not modulated by E_2. From the standpoint of sexual differentiation, interest in the E_2 induction of P receptor synthesis has centered on the claim that male rats are less capable than females of showing this response in the HPOA (Moguilewsky and Raynaud, 1979b; Rainbow, Parsons, and McEwen, 1982). Others have obtained different results (Etgen, 1981; Graf, Kirchoff, Grunke, Reinhardt, Ball, and Knuppen, 1983; Kirchoff, Grunke, and Ghraf, 1983). Yet, even if P receptor synthesis in the HPOA does turn out to be sexually differentiated, the question of what behavioral or physiological difference has just been explained will remain unanswered until P receptor synthesis is studied in groups in which the various functional phenotypes have been dissociated. The analyses undertaken to date indicate that E_2-induced P receptor synthesis in the HPOA does not correlate with the display of feminine sexual behavior (Baum *et al.*, 1986; Etgen, 1981, 1982, 1984). On the other hand, male rats given EB and methysergide, a serotonin antagonist that facilitates lordosis when P receptors are unavailable, obtain higher LQ scores than they do when given EB and P (Crowley, Ward, and Margules, 1975). The same is true of some neonatally androgenized females (Ulibarri and Yahr, 1987); however, other neonatally androgenized females respond better to EB and P than to EB and methysergide. Together, these observations suggest that the defeminization of lordosis may involve the defeminization of several aspects of neural function. For example, within the HPOA, male and female rats differ in their ability to synthesize type 1 serotinin receptors in response to E_2 (Bigeon and McEwen, 1982; Fischette, Biegon, and McEwen, 1983). This phenotype may sexually differentiate independently of various others.

Because some gonadal steroids, notably T, must be metabolized by target tissues before binding, sex differences in metabolizing enzymes have also been explored. In adult quail, aromatase activity in the POA is higher in males than in females because of a sex difference in the ability of T to activate the enzyme (Schumacher and Balthazart, 1986). The sexes do not differ after castration, when activity is low, but they do differ after receiving T. The sensitivity of the aromatase system of the POA therefore corresponds to the sensitivity of masculine sexual behavior to T. It has not yet been demonstrated, though, that this sex difference can be reversed developmentally.

When sex differences are observed on a regional basis, as in biochemical analyses of hormone binding or metabolism, two possibilities arise about the properties of the tissue that may account for them. Each cell that displays the phenotype may do so to a different degree in each sex. Alternatively, the number of cells with that phenotype in the region sampled may differ in males and females. Clearly, both situations may obtain. A standard method for correcting for differing numbers of cells in different biochemical samples is to express the phenotype per milligram of DNA. However, this approach corrects for differences in the total number of cells, not for differences in the number of cells with the phenotype of interest. Because the cells of interest (those contributing to the numerator) may not be a constant fraction of the total (those contributing to the denominator), this "correction" could cause some interesting sex differences to be overlooked because they are overshadowed by an unknown sex difference in cell density. One also runs the risk of falsely attributing an unsuspected sex difference in the denominator to a sex difference in the numerator. Another approach is to take smaller samples by using more specific anatomical landmarks (Palkovitz, 1973). Yet, even this strategy may not overcome the heterogeneity of the HPOA (e.g., see Fahrbach, Morrell, and

Pfaff, 1986; Morrell and Pfaff, 1982). Moreover, as one decreases the size of the area sampled, one runs the risk of mistaking a sex difference in the anatomical distribution of cells displaying a particular phenotype for a sex difference in the total number of cells with that phenotype. Because of these problems, resolving the bases for sex differences in the brain will benefit from histological and immunocytochemical approaches that enable the investigator to distinguish phenotypes on a cell-by-cell basis. The approach is already being fruitfully used in attempts to identify HPOA and related pathways that may subserve sexually differentiated patterns of behavior or hormone secretion (DeVries et al., 1984; Fahrbach et al., 1986; Morrell and Pfaff, 1982; Simerly and Swanson, 1986; Simerly et al., 1984a,b, 1985a,b, 1986; Wray and Hoffman, 1986). None of these analyses has provided an example of a pathway or cell group that differentiates sexually (independent of, or in addition to, adult hormonal effects) and that is associated with a specific sexually differentiated behavior, but hopefully this will happen soon.

In regard to steroid uptake, autoradiographic analyses show that the sexes can differ in either the number of cells that accumulate hormones or in the hormone accumulation per cell. Male rats, for example, have a higher percentage of SDN cells that accumulate T than female rats do (Jacobson, Arnold, and Gorski, 1987). They also have more SDN cells in total (Gorski et al., 1980). The sexes do not differ in the percentage of SDN cells that accumulate E_2 or DHT, although in the HPOA surrounding the SDN, the percentages of T-accumulating and E_2-accumulating cells are both greater in males than in females. In the SNB of rats (Breedlove and Arnold, 1983c) and in MAN and HVc of zebra finches (Nordeen, Nordeen, and Arnold, 1986), the DHT accumulation per cell is greater in males than in females. In the finches, this cellular phenotype is masculinized by earlier exposure to E_2. The percentage of cells in MAN and HVc that accumulate T or its metabolites is also greater in males than in females (Arnold and Saltiel, 1979).

How Do Hormones Establish Sex Differences in Neural Structure and Function?

One mechanism by which T or its metabolites may lead to sex differences in the number of cells displaying a particular phenotype is by influencing neuronal death or survival. The development of the nervous system often involves an "exuberant" overproduction of cells and connections from which the mature system is "sculpted" as axons compete for synaptic space and trophic factors (Cowan, Fawcett, O'Leary, and Stanfield, 1984). It would not be surprising, then, to find that the hormonal mechanisms of sexual differentiation have tapped into or capitalized on the same morphogenetic mechanisms. Some cells in the central nervous system synthesize essential growth factors only if exposed to T. Other cells may do so unless exposed to T. T may also affect the rate at which a cell extends its processes. Changes in this parameter may determine whether the axon reaches its target before or after axons from other cells arrive and, hence, may determine whether the cell will compete successfully for a synaptic site. Failure to extend enough dendrites, or extending them too late, could mean that the cell will not receive enough stimulation from other neurons to survive.

Several of the systems we have discussed sexually differentiate, at least in part, via cell death. The SNB cells of rats are one example. On Day 20 of gestation, which is a week after SNB cells are born (Breedlove, Jordan, and Arnold, 1983), male and female rat fetuses have an equal number of SNB cells (Nordeen, Nordeen, Sengelaub, and Arnold, 1985). Starting around the time of birth, females have fewer healthy SNB cells and more dying ones than males do, unless the females receive T. However, the motor neurons themselves are not the target for T action. Although SNB cells have androgen receptors, at least in adulthood, SNB cells that lack these receptors survive if the penile muscles they innervate survive. The ability of SNB cells to survive without their own androgen receptors was shown elegantly by Breedlove (1986), who produced XX male mice that carried the *tfm* allele on one of their X chromosomes and an allele, *Sxr*, for sex reversal on one of their autosomes. Because of the clonal nature of X chromosome inactivation in mammalian cells, such males are chimeras for the presence or absence of androgen receptors in different tissues. As a result, Breedlove found some males with well-developed penile muscles (in these cells, the *tfm*-bearing X was apparently inactive) innervated by SNB cells that lacked androgen receptors (in these cells, the *tfm*-bearing X was apparently active). Thus, during sexual differentiation, the effects of T on the SNB are determined indirectly via its effects on the musculature. As noted above, T's effects on the genital muscles are mediated by DHT. Yet, without undergoing metabolism, T may also affect the migration of motoneurons into the SNB from lateral parts of the cord (Nordeen *et al.*, 1985). Such migration could explain why female rats given DHT prenatally have masculinized penile muscles that are innervated by laterally situated motor neurons (Breedlove, 1985).

Sexual differentiation of the zebra finch song-control nuclei also involves selective cell death. By 19–26 days after hatching, females are losing more HVc cells than males are (DeVoogd, 1986). At this age, cell loss in RA is the same in both sexes. However, about 30 days after hatching, the RA of males quite suddenly becomes innervated by axons from HVc and begins to grow (Konishi and Akutagawa, 1985). In contrast, the female RA remains uninnervated and starts to lose cells. It is not clear if the lack of innervation causes cell death in RA, if some property of the female RA prevents innervation by HVc, or if both situations pertain. In MAN of this species, E_2 masculinizes the later pattern of androgen accumulation by selectively preserving DHT-accumulating neurons in the face of massive overall cell loss (Nordeen *et al.*, 1987). In contrast, in HVc, E_2 promotes the addition of DHT-accumulating cells. It is not clear whether it does this by affecting the proliferation, migration, or survival of cells that migrate into this region during development, or by inducing more cells to express the gene that codes for the androgen receptor.

The sex difference in the presence or absence of the gerbil SDApc may also result from the selective loss of cells in females. The SDApc appears to be present in both sexes at birth. Over the next 2–3 weeks, the cell group becomes more prominent in males but disappears in females. This sexual differentiation is controlled by T because giving female gerbils TP before they are 4 days old increases the probability that they will have an SDApc at 2 weeks of age or in adulthood (Ulibarri and Yahr, 1988; Yahr, 1988). Thus T preserves the integrity of this nucleus. This has also been proposed as a mechanism for the sexual differentiation of the rat SDN (Gorski, 1984; Jacobson, Davis, and Gorski, 1985). However, one must be cautious about attributing such changes to cell death. Cells that have been lost from the nucleus may have differentiated a different biochemical phenotype, may have migrated to a different location, or may have become distributed more diffusely in the same area, so that they are not recognized as cells that would have been part of the nucleus if they had been exposed to T.

By affecting the rate (Hammer and Jacobson, 1984) or direction (Greenough, Carter, Steerman, and DeVoogd, 1977) of dendritic extension, or by altering the cell's ability to accept synapses from other cells, T could affect the neural systems to which the cell will respond in adulthood. The sexual differentiation of lordosis behavior in rats, for example, may reflect a differential sensitivity to efferents. A lordosis-inhibiting system appears to project into the HPOA from a more dorsal site, possibly the septum. When this projection was removed, males and some neonatally androgenized females showed as much lordosis as normal females (Kondo, Shinoda, Yamanouchi, and Arai, 1986; Yamanouchi and Arai, 1985), although the doses of E_2 used to induce lordosis were relatively large. Thus, defeminization may involve increased inputs from this system into the HPOA.

It is also possible that the biochemical phenotype that a neuron differentiates can be modified by effects of T on its morphology (e.g., via effects on the synaptic connections formed). Alternatively, T could sexually differentiate neurons by the mechanisms discussed at the beginning of this chapter (e.g., by altering the segments of the genome that will be available for transcription, or by altering their ability to respond to inducers or suppressors). The synthesis of P receptors provides a good example here. Nearly all cells contain the gene that codes for this protein, but few transcribe it. In the cells that do not transcribe the P-receptor gene, the polymerase presumably can not gain access to the gene because of the chromatin proteins in which it or its regulatory locus is wrapped. Cells that do make P receptors are subdivided, in turn, into those in which P receptor synthesis can be induced by E_2 and those in which it cannot. Even if these two subsets use the same gene (i.e., if it is represented only once per haploid genome), only the former subset may surround this gene or its regulatory locus with chromatin proteins that include an acceptor site for the E_2–receptor complex. If T does sexually differentiate these cells, it could do so by functionally deleting this acceptor site.

The genetic mechanisms that underlie the sexual differentiation of behavior are poorly understood, but in rats, the sexual differentiation of feminine sexual behavior and gonadotropin secretion do involve effects of T on the synthesis of mRNA, particularly poladenylated (poly-A^+) mRNA, within the HPOA. By infusing cordycepin, an adenosine analogue that preferentially disrupts the synthesis of poly-A^+ mRNA, into the HPOA of newborn female rats within an hour of when they receive TP, we can protect them from defeminization, as shown in Figure 3 (Ulibarri and Yahr, 1987). As adults, these females ovulate and obtain high LQ scores when given EB and P. The mRNA(s) that may be involved are not known, but they are not limited to the mRNA for aromatase, as cordycepin also curtails the defeminizing effects of R2858, the artificial estrogen that is not sequestered by alpha-fetoprotein. In adult rats, cordycepin does not affect the uptake of E_2 by cell nuclei in the HPOA (Yahr and Ulibarri, 1986), so there is no reason to believe that it protects developing animals simply by keeping E_2 out of cells. These observations help to clarify a confusing body of knowledge on the effects of metabolic inhibitors on the sexual differentiation of gonadotropin secretion by suggesting that only those compounds that inhibit eukaryotic mRNA synthesis can prevent the anovulatory sterility induced by TP. They also provide the first demonstration that similar genetic mechanisms underlie the sexual differentiation of behavior.

Finally, we should keep in mind that probably only some of T's sexually differentiating effects on the brain occur directly (i.e., in cells that have receptors for T or its metabolites). Like T's effects on the SNB, others may follow secondarily, through the interactions of cells with others that accumulate the steroid. Area X of the songbird brain, for example, sexually differentiates, although it does not accumulate T or its metabolites, at least not in adulthood. Perhaps it simply mirrors the sexual differentiation of HVc. Implanting E_2 near HVc shortly after hatching is sufficient to masculinize singing behavior and is more effective than implanting the hormone subcutaneously (Hutchison and Hutchison, 1985). Thus, hormone action at one site may initiate a cascade with consequences for other cell groups.

Yet more distant targets of early hormone action must also be considered. It appears, for example, that sex differences in the masculine copulatory behavior of rats develop, in part, through differences in the amount of anogenital licking that mother rats direct toward male versus female pups (Moore, 1984; Moore and Morelli, 1979). The greater licking is a response to a urinary cue controlled by T

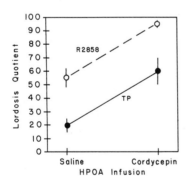
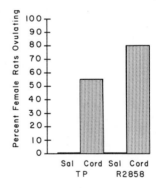

Figure 3. The ability of cordycepin, an adenosine analogue that preferentially inhibits the synthesis of poly-A$^+$ mRNA, to protect female rats from the defeminizing effects of TP or R2858, an E_2 analogue that is not sequestered by alpha-fetoprotein. The females received 50 μg TP or 5 μg R2858 subcutaneously on the day after birth. They also received an infusion of cordycepin (Cord) or the saline (Sal) vehicle into the HPOA an hour before the TP injection or immediately before the injection of R2858. As adults, they were ovariectomized and tested for female sexual behavior after receiving EB and P. Their ovaries were also examined for corpora lutea, an index of ovulation. (Adapted from Ulibarri and Yahr, 1987.)

(Moore, 1981, 1982). As the pups approach puberty, males groom their own genitalia more than females do. This behavior is stimulated by T and may promote T secretion (Moore, 1986a,b; Moore and Rogers, 1984). Thus, the possibility exists that some sex differences in behavioral and neural development result indirectly from hormonal effects on social signals that cause males and females to elicit different reactions from conspecifics. Still other sex differences may result from self-perpetuating cycles of hormonal effects on behavior and behavioral effects on hormone secretion. Determining how hormones act at the cellular and the molecular level, and determining which aspects of sexual differentiation occur directly and which occur as part of a cascade, illustrates the range of intriguing questions open for study when one explores the sexual differentiation of behavior in the context of developmental psychobiology.

Acknowledgments

This review was prepared while the author was supported by Research Scientist Development Award MH-00478. Research from the author's laboratory was supported by MH 26481. Dr. Brad Powers and Dr. Barry Keverne commented on an earlier version of this review. It is a pleasure to acknowledge their help.

REFERENCES

Adler, N., and Bermant, G. Sexual behavior of male rats: Effects of reduced sensory feedback. *Journal of Comparative and Physiological Psychology*, 1966, *61*, 240–243.

Anderson, J. N. The effect of steroid hormones on gene transcription. In R. F. Goldberger and K. R. Yamamoto (Eds.), *Biological regulation and development*. Vol. 3B. *Hormone action*. New York: Plenum Press, 1982.

Anderson, R. H., Fleming, D. E., Rhees, R. W., and Kinghorn, E. Relationships between sexual activity, plasma testosterone, and the volume of the sexually dimorphic nucleus of the preoptic area in prenatally stressed and non-stressed rats. *Brain Research*, 1986, *370*, 1–10.

Andrews, W. W., Mizcjewski, G. J., and Ojeda, S. R. Development of estradiol-positive feedback on luteinizing hormone release in the female rat: A quantitative study. *Endocrinology*, 1981, *109*, 1404–1413.

Arendash, G. W., and Gorski, R. A. Effects of discrete lesions of the sexually dimorphic nucleus of the preoptic area or other medial preoptic regions on the sexual behavior of male rats. *Brain Research Bulletin*, 1983, *10*, 147–154.

Arnold, A. P. The effects of castration and androgen replacement on song, courtship, and aggression in zebra finches *(Poephila guttata)*. *Journal of Experimental Zoology*, 1975, *191*, 309–326.

Arnold, A. P. Effects of androgens on volumes of sexually dimorphic brain regions in the zebra finch. *Brain Research*, 1980a, *185*, 441–444.

Arnold, A. P. Quantitative analysis of sex differences in hormone accumulation in the zebra finch brain: Methodological and theoretical issues. *Journal of Comparative Neurology*, 1980b, *189*, 421–436.

Arnold, A. P., and Saltiel, A. Sexual difference in pattern of hormone accumulation in the brain of a songbird. *Science*, 1979, *205*, 702–705.

Arnold, A. P., Nottebohm, F., and Pfaff, D. W. Hormone concentrating cells in vocal control and other areas of the brain of the zebra finch *(Poephila guttata)*. *Journal of Comparative Neurology*, 1976, *165*, 487–512.

Barbarino, A., DeMarinis, L., and Mancini, A. Estradiol modulation of basal and gonadotropin-releasing hormone-induced gonadotropin release in intact and castrated men. *Neuroendocrinology*, 1983, *36*, 105–111.

Barraclough, C. A. Production of anovulatory sterile rats by single injections of testosterone propionate. *Endocrinology*, 1961, *68*, 62–67.

Baum, M.J. Effects of testosterone propionate administered perinatally on sexual behavior of female ferrets. *Journal of Comparative and Physiological Psychology*, 1976, *90*, 399–410.

Baum, M. J. Differentiation of coital behavior in mammals: A comparative analysis. *Neuroscience and Biobehavioral Reviews*, 1979, *3*, 265–284.

Baum, M. J., and Erskine, M. S. Effects of neonatal gonadectomy and administration of testosterone on coital masculinization in the ferret. *Endocrinology*, 1984, *115*, 2440–2444.

Baum, M. J., and Gallagher, C. A. Increasing dosages of estradiol benzoate activate equivalent degrees of sexual receptivity in gonadectomized male and female ferrets. *Physiology and Behavior*, 1981, *26*, 751–753.

Baum, M. J., and Tobet, S. A. Effect of prenatal exposure to aromatase inhibitor, testosterone, or antiandrogen on the development of feminine sexual behavior in ferrets of both sexes. *Physiology and Behavior*, 1986, *37*, 111–118.

Baum, M. J., Gallagher, C. A., Martin, J. T., and Damassa, D. A. Effects of testosterone, dihydrotestosterone, or estradiol administered neonatally on sexual behavior of female ferrets. *Endocrinology*, 1982, *111*, 773–780.

Baum, M. J., Canick, J. A., Erskine, M. S., Gallagher, C. A., and Shim, J. H. Normal differentiation of masculine sexual behavior in male ferrets despite neonatal inhibition of brain aromatase or 5-alpha-reductase activity. *Neuroendocrinology*, 1983, *36*, 277–284.

Baum, M. J., Stockman, E. R., and Lundell, L. A. Evidence of proceptive without receptive defeminization in male ferrets. *Behavioral Neuroscience*, 1985, *99*, 742–750.

Baum, M. J., Gerlach, J. L., Krey, L. C., and McEwen, B. S. Biochemical and autoradiographic analysis of estrogen-inductible progestin receptors in female ferret brain: Correlations with effects of progesterone on sexual behavior and gonadotropin-releasing hormone-stimulated secretion of luteinizing hormone. *Brain Research*, 1986, *368*, 296–309.

Beach, F. A. Hormonal factors controlling the differentiation, development, and display of copulatory behavior in the ramstergig and related species. In E. Tobach, L. R. Aronson, and E. Shaw (Eds.), *The biopsychology of development*. New York: Academic Press, 1971.

Beach, F. A. Effects of gonadal hormones on urinary behavior in dogs. *Physiology and Behavior*, 1974, *12*, 1005–1013.

Beach, F. A. Sexual attractivity, proceptivity, and receptivity in female mammals. *Hormones and Behavior*, 1976, *7*, 105–138.

Beatty, W. W. Gonadal hormones and sex differences in nonreproductive behaviors in rodents: Organizational and activational influences. *Hormones and Behavior*, 1979, *12*, 112–163.

Berg, D. K. New neuronal growth factors. *Annual Review of Neuroscience*, 1984, *7*, 149–170.

Bigeon, A., and McEwen, B. S. Modulation by estradiol of serotonin₁ receptors in brain. *Journal of Neuroscience*, 1982, *2*, 199–205.

Black, I. B., Adler, J. E., Dreyfus, C. F., Jonakait, J. M., Datz, D. M., La Gamma, E. F., and Markey, K. M. Neurotransmitter plasticity at the molecular level. *Science*, 1984, *225*, 1266–1270.

Bonne, C., and Raynaud, J.-P. Assay of androgen binding sites by exchange with methyltrienolone (R1881). *Steroids*, 1976, *27*, 497–507.

Booth, J. E. Sexual behavior of neonatally castrated rats injected during infancy with oestrogen and dihydrotestosterone. *Journal of Endocrinology*, 1977, *72*, 135–141.

Booth, J. E. Effects of the aromatization inhibitor androst-4-ene-3,6,17-trione on sexual differentiation induced by testosterone in the neonatally castrated rat. *Journal of Endocrinology*, 1978, *79*, 69–76.

Bottjer, S. W., Miesner, E. A., and Arnold, A. P. Forebrain lesions disrupt development but not maintenance of song in passerine birds. *Science*, 1984, *224*, 901–903.

Breedlove, S. M. Hormonal control of the anatomical specificity of motoneuron-to-muscle innervation in rats. *Science*, 1985, *227*, 1357–1359.

Breedlove, S. M. Cellular analyses of hormone influence on motoneuronal development and function. *Journal of Neurobiology*, 1986, *17*, 157–176.

Breedlove, S. M., and Arnold, A. P. Hormone accumulation in a sexually dimorphic motor nucleus of the rat spinal cord. *Science*, 1980, *210*, 564–566.

Breedlove, S. M., and Arnold, A. P. Sexually dimorphic motor nucleus in the rat lumbar spinal cord: Response to adult hormone manipulation, absence in androgen-insensitive rats. *Brain Research*, 1981, *225*, 297–307.

Breedlove, S. M., and Arnold, A. P. Hormonal control of a developing neuromuscular system. I. Complete demasculinization of the spinal nucleus of the bulbocavernosus in male rats using the antiandrogen, flutamide. *Journal of Neuroscience*, 1983a, *3*, 417–423.

Breedlove, S. M., and Arnold, A. P. Hormonal control of a developing neuromuscular system. II. Sensitive periods for the androgen induced masculinization of the rat spinal nucleus of the bulbocavernosus. *Journal of Neuroscience*, 1983b, *3*, 424–432.

Breedlove, S. M., and Arnold, A. P. Sex differences in the pattern of steroid accumulation by motoneurons of the rat lumbar spinal cord. *Journal of Comparative Neurology*, 1983c, *215*, 211–216.

Breedlove, S. M., Jacobson, C. D., Gorski, R. A., and Arnold, A. P. Masculinization of the female rat spinal cord following a single neonatal injection of testosterone propionate but not estradiol benzoate. *Brain Research*, 1982, *237*, 173–181.

Breedlove, S. M., Jordan, C. L., and Arnold, A. P. Neurogenesis of motoneurons in the sexually dimorphic spinal nucleus of the bulbocavernosus in rats. *Developmental Brain Research*, 1983, *9*, 39–43.

Bronson, F. H., and Desjardins, C. H. Aggression in adult mice: Modification by neonatal injections of gonadal hormones. *Science*, 1968, *161*, 705–706.

Bronson, F. H., and Desjardins, C. H. Neonatal androgen administration and adult aggressiveness in female mice. *General and Comparative Endocrinology*, 1970, *15*, 320–322.

Buhl, A. E., Norman, R. L., and Resko, J. A. Sex differences in estrogen-induced gonadotropin release in hamsters. *Biology of Reproduction*, 1978, *18*, 592–597.

Bull, J. J. Sex determination in reptiles. *Quarterly Review of Biology*, 1980, *55*, 3–21.

Burns, R. K. Experimental reversal of sex in the gonads of the opossum *Didelphis virginiana. Proceedings of the National Academy of Sciences*, 1955, *41*, 669–676.

Butte, J. C., Moore, J. A., and Kakihana, R. Brain and plasma levels of testosterone, dihydrotestosterone and estradiol in the one-day-old rat. *Life Sciences*, 1979, *24*, 2343–2350.

Carlsson, S. G., and Larsson, K. Mating in male rats after local anesthetization of the glans penis. *Zeitschrift für Tierpsychologie*, 1964, *21*, 854–856.

Christensen, L. W., and Gorski, R. A. Independent masculinization of neuroendocrine systems by intracerebral implants of testosterone or estradiol in the neonatal female rat. *Brain Research*, 1978, *146*, 325–340.

Clemens, L. G. Neurohormonal control of male sexual behavior. In W. Montagna, and W. A. Sadler (Eds.), *Reproductive behavior*. New York: Plenum Press, 1974.

Clemens, L. G., and Gladue, B. H. Feminine sexual behavior in rats enhanced by prenatal inhibition of androgen aromatization. *Hormones and Behavior*, 1978, *11*, 190–201.

Clemens, L. G., Shryne, J., and Gorski, R. A. Androgen and development of progesterone responsiveness in male and female rats. *Physiology and Behavior*, 1970, *5*, 673–678.

Clemens, L. G., Gladue, B. A., and Coniglio, L. P. Prenatal endogenous androgenic influences on masculine sexual behavior and genital morphology in male and female rats. *Hormones and Behavior*, 1978, *10*, 40–53.

Commins, D., and Yahr, P. Acetylcholinesterase activity in the sexually dimorphic area of the gerbil brain: Sex differences and influences of adult gonadal steroids. *Journal of Comparative Neurology*, 1984a, *224*, 123–131.

Commins, D., and Yahr, P. Adult testosterone levels influence the morphology of a sexually dimorphic area in the Mongolian gerbil brain. *Journal of Comparative Neurology*, 1984b, *224*, 132–140.

Commins, D., and Yahr, P. Lesions of the sexually dimorphic area disrupt mating and marking in male gerbils. *Brain Research Bulletin*, 1984c, *13*, 185–193.

Commins, D., and Yahr, P. Autoradiographic localization of estrogen and androgen receptors in the sexually dimorphic area and other regions of the gerbil brain. *Journal of Comparative Neurology*, 1985, *231*, 473–489.

Cotman, C. W., and Nieto-Sampedro, M. Cell biology of synaptic plasticity. *Science*, 1984, *225*, 1287–1294.

Coulombe, J. N., and Bronner-Fraser, M. Cholinergic neurons acquire adrenergic neurotransmitters when transplanted into an embryo. *Nature*, 1986, *324*, 569–572.

Cowan, W. M., Fawcett, J. W., O'Leary, D. D. M., and Stanfield, B. B. Regressive events in neurogenesis. *Science*, 1984, *225*, 1258–1265.

Crowley, W. R., Ward, I. L., and Margules, D. L. Female lordotic behavior mediated by monoamines in male rats. *Journal of Comparative and Physiological Psychology*, 1975, *88*, 62–68.

Davidson, E. H., and Britten, R. J. Organization, transcription and regulation in the animal genome. *Quarterly Review of Biology,* 1973, *48,* 565–613.

Davidson, J. M., Rodgers, C. H., Smith, E. R., and Block, G. J. Stimulation of female sex behavior in adrenalectomized rats with estrogen alone. *Endocrinology,* 1968, *82,* 193–195.

Davis, P. G., and Barfield, R. J. Activation of feminine sexual behavior in castrated male rats by intra-hypothalamic implants of estradiol benzoate. *Neuroendocrinology,* 1979a, *28,* 228–233.

Davis, P. G., and Barfield, R. J. Activation of masculine sexual behavior by intracranial estradiol benzoate implants in male rats. *Neuroendocrinology,* 1979b, *28,* 217–227.

Davis, P. G., Chaptal, C. V., and McEwen, B. S. Independence of the differentiation of masculine and feminine sexual behavior in rats. *Hormones and Behavior,* 1979a, *12,* 12–19.

Davis, P. G., McEwen, B. S., and Pfaff, D. W. Localized behavioral effects of tritiated estradiol implants in the ventromedial hypothalamus of female rats. *Endocrinology,* 1979b, *104,* 898–903.

DeBold, J. F., and Whalen, R. E. Differential sensitivity of mounting and lordosis control systems to early androgen treatment in male and female hamsters. *Hormones and Behavior,* 1975, *6,* 197–209.

Denef, C., Magnus, C., and McEwen, B. S. Sex-dependent changes in pituitary 5α-dihydrotestosterone and 3α-androstanediol formation during postnatal development and puberty in the rat. *Endocrinology,* 1974, *94,* 1265–1274.

DeVoogd, T. J. Steroid interactions with structure and function of avian song control regions. *Journal of Neurobiology,* 1986, *17,* 177–201.

DeVoogd, T., and Nottebohm, F. Gonadal hormones induce dendritic growth in the adult avian brain. *Science,* 1981a, *214,* 202–204.

DeVoogd, T., and Nottebohm, F. Sex differences in dendritic morphology of a song control nucleus in the canary: A quantitative Golgi study. *Journal of Comparative Neurology,* 1981b, *196,* 309–316.

DeVoogd, T., Nixdorf, B., and Nottebohm, F. Synaptogenesis and changes in synaptic morphology related to acquisition of a new behavior. *Brain Research,* 1985, *329,* 304–308.

DeVries, G. J., Buijs, R. M., and Sluiter, A. A. Gonadal hormone actions in the morphology of the vasopressinergic innervation of the adult rat brain. *Brain Research,* 1984a, *298,* 141–145.

DeVries, G. J., DeBruin, J. P. C., Uylings, H. B. M., and Corner, M. A. (Eds.), *Progress in brain research.* Vol. 61. *Sex differences in the brain.* Amsterdam: Elsevier, 1984b.

Dixson, A. F. Genital sensory feedback and sexual behavior in male and female marmosets *(Callithrix jacchus). Physiology and Behavior,* 1986, *37,* 447–450.

Döcke, F., and Dörner, G. Anovulation in adult female rats after neonatal intracerebral implantation of oestrogen. *Endokrinologie,* 1975, *65,* 375–377.

Doering, C. H., and Gladue, B. A. 5α-Androstane-3β, 17β-diol binds to androgen and estrogen receptors without activating copulatory behavior in female rats. *Pharmacology, Biochemistry and Behavior,* 1982, *16,* 837–840.

Doering, C. H., and Leyra, P. T. Methyltrienolone (R1881) is not aromatized by placental microsomes or rat hypothalamic homogenates. *Journal of Steroid Biochemistry,* 1984, *20,* 1157–1162.

Dohanich, G. P., Witcher, J. A., Weaver, D. R., and Clemens, L. G. Alteration of muscarinic binding in specific brain areas following estrogen treatment. *Brain Research,* 1982, *241,* 347–350.

Döhler, K. D., Coquelin, A., Davis, F., Hines, M., Shryne, J. E., and Gorski, R. A. Differentiation of the sexually-dimorphic nucleus in the preoptic area of the rat brain is determined by the perinatal hormone environment. *Neuroscience Letters,* 1982, *33,* 295–298.

Döhler, K. D., Hancke, J. L., Srivastava, S. S., Hofmann, C., Shryne, J. E., and Gorski, R. A. Participation of estrogens in female sexual differentiation of the brain; Neuroanatomical, neuroendocrine and behavioral evidence. In G. J. DeVries, J. P. C. DeBruin, H. B. M. Uylings, and M. A. Corner (Eds.), *Progress in brain research.* Vol. 61. *Sex differences in the brain.* Amsterdam: Elsevier, 1984a.

Döhler, K. D., Srivastava, S. S., Shryne, J. E., Jarzab, B., Sipos, A., and Gorski, R. A. Differentiation of the sexually dimorphic nucleus in the preoptic area of the rat brain is inhibited by postnatal treatment with an estrogen antagonist. *Neuroendocrinology,* 1984b, *38,* 297–301.

Dyer, R. G. Sexual differentiation of the forebrain—Relationship to gonadotropin secretion. In G. J. DeVries, J. P. C. DeBruin, H. B. M. Uylings, and M. A. Corner (Eds.), *Progress in brain research.* Vol. 61. *Sex differences in the brain.* Amsterdam: Elsevier, 1984.

Edwards, D. A. Mice: Fighting by neonatally androgenized females. *Science,* 1968, *161,* 1027–1028.

Edwards, D. A. Early androgen stimulation and aggressive behavior in male and female mice. *Physiology and Behavior,* 1969, *4,* 333–338.

Edwards, D. A., and Thompson, M. L. Neonatal androgenization and estrogenization and the hormonal induction of sexual receptivity in rats. *Physiology and Behavior*, 1970, *5*, 115–119.

Edwards, D. A., Whalen, R. E., and Nadler, R. D. The induction of estrus: Estrogen-progesterone interactions. *Physiology and Behavior*, 1968, *3*, 29–33.

Elsaesser, F., and Parvizi, N. Estrogen feedback in the pig: Sexual differentiation and the effect of prenatal testosterone treatment. *Biology of Reproduction*, 1979, *20*, 1187–1193.

Etgen, A. M. Estrogen induction of progestin receptors of the hypothalamus of male and female rats which differ in their ability to exhibit cyclic gonadotropin secretion and female sexual behavior. *Biology of Reproduction*, 1981, *25*, 307–313.

Etgen, A. M. 1-(o-chlorophenyl)-1-(p-chorophenyl)-2,2,2-trichloroethane: A probe for studying estrogen and progestin receptor mediation of female sexual behavior and neuroendocrine responses. *Endocrinology*, 1982, *111*, 1498–1504.

Etgen, A. M. Progestin receptors and the activation of female reproductive behavior: A critical review. *Hormones and Behavior*, 1984, *18*, 411–430.

Fadem, B. H., and Barfield, R. J. Neonatal hormonal influences on the development of proceptive and receptive feminine sexual behavior in rats. *Hormones and Behavior*, 1981, *15*, 282–288.

Fadem, B. H., and Tesoriero, J. V. Inhibition of testicular development and feminization of the male genitalia by neonatal estrogen treatment in a marsupial. *Biology of Reproduction*, 1986, *34*, 771–776.

Fadem, B. H., Barfield, R. J., and Whalen, R. E. Dose-response and time-response relationships between progesterone and the display of patterns of receptive and proceptive behavior in the female rat. *Hormones and Behavior*, 1979, *13*, 40–48.

Fahrbach, S. E., Morrell, J. I., and Pfaff, D. W. Identification of medial preoptic neurons that concentrate estradiol and project to the midbrain in the rat. *Journal of Comparative Neurology*, 1986, *247*, 364–382.

Feder, H. H. Experimental analysis of hormone actions on the hypothalamus, anterior pituitary, and ovary. In N. T. Adler (Ed.), *Neuroendocrinology of reproduction*. New York: Plenum Press, 1981a.

Feder, H. H. Hormonal actions on the sexual differentiation of the genitalia and the gonadotropin-regulating systems. In N. Adler (Ed.), *Neuroendocrinology of Reproduction*. New York: Plenum Press, 1981b.

Feder, H. H. Perinatal hormones and their role in the development of sexually dimorphic behaviors. In N. Adler (Ed.), *Neuroendocrinology of reproduction*. New York: Plenum Press, 1981c.

Fischette, C. T., Biegon, A., and McEwen, B. S. Sex differences in serotonin 1 receptor binding in rat brain. *Science*, 1983, *222*, 333–335.

Ford, J. J. Testicular control of defeminization in male pigs. *Biology of Reproduction*, 1982, *27*, 425–430.

Ford, J. J. Postnatal differentiation of sexual preferences in male pigs. *Hormones and Behavior*, 1983, *17*, 152–162.

Gandleman, R. Uterine position and the activation of male sexual activity in testosterone propionate-treated female guinea pigs. *Hormones and Behavior*, 1986, *20*, 287–293.

Gandelman, R., and Graham, S. Singleton female mouse fetuses are subsequently unresponsive to the aggression-activating property of testosterone. *Physiology and Behavior*, 1986, *37*, 465–467.

Gandelman, R., vom Saal, F. S., and Reinisch, J. M. Contiguity to male foetuses affects morphology and behaviour of female mice. *Nature*, 1977, *266*, 722–724.

Gay, V. L. Ineffectiveness of DHT treatment in producing increased serum DHT in orchidectomized rats: Evidence for rapid *in vivo* metabolism of DHT to androstanediol. *Federation Proceedings*, 1975, *34*, 303.

Gentry, R. T., and Wade, G. N. Sex differences in sensitivity of food intake, body weight, and running-wheel activity to ovarian steroids in rats. *Journal of Comparative and Physiological Psychology*, 1976, *90*, 747–754.

George, F. W., and Wilson, J. D. Estrogen formation in the early rabbit embryo. *Science*, 1978, *199*, 200–201.

Gerall, A. A., and Kenney, A. M. Neonatally androgenized females' responsiveness to estrogen and progesterone. *Endocrinology*, 1970, *87*, 560–566.

Gerall, A. A., and Ward, I. L. Effects of prenatal exogenous androgen on the sexual behavior of the female albino rat. *Journal of Comparative and Physiological Psychology*, 1966, *62*, 370–375.

Gerall, A. A., Hendricks, S. E., Johnson, L. L., and Bounds, T. W. Effects of early castration in male rats on adult sexual behavior. *Journal of Comparative and Physiological Psychology*, 1967, *64*, 206–212.

Gerall, A. A., Dunlap, J. L., and Hendricks, S. E. Effect of ovarian secretions in female behavioral potentiality in the rat. *Journal of Comparative and Physiological Psychology*, 1972, *82*, 449–465.

Ghru, R., Kirchoff, J., Grunke, W., Reinhardt, W., Ball, P., and Knuppen, R. Estrogen responsiveness of progestin receptor induction in the pituitary, preoptic-hypothalamic brain and uterus of neonatally estrogenized female rats. *Brain Research*, 1983, *258*, 133–138.

Gibori, G., and Sridaran, R. Sites of androgen and estradiol production in the second half of pregnancy in the rat. *Biology of Reproduction*, 1981, *24*, 249–256.

Gladue, B. A., and Clemens, L. G. Masculinization diminished by disruption of prenatal estrogen biosynthesis in male rats. *Physiology and Behavior*, 1980, *25*, 589–593.

Goldman, B. D. Developmental influences of hormones on neuroendocrine mechanisms of sexual behaviour: Comparisons with other sexually dimorphic behaviors. In J. B. Hutchison (Ed.), *Biological determinants of sexual behavior*. Chichester: Wiley, 1978.

Goodman, R. L. The site of the positive feedback action of estradiol in the rat. *Endocrinology*, 1978, *102*, 151–159.

Gordon, J. W., and Ruddle, F. H. Mammalian gonadal determination and gametogenesis. *Science*, 1981, *211*, 1265–1271.

Gorski, J., and Gannon, F. Current models of steroid hormone action: A critique. *Annual Review of Physiology*, 1976, *38*, 425–450.

Gorski, R. A. Influence of age on the response to paranatal administration of a low dose of androgen. *Endocrinology*, 1968, *82*, 1001–1004.

Gorski, R. A. Critical role for the medial preoptic area in the sexual differentiation of the brain. In G. J. DeVries, J. P. C. DeBruin, H. B. M. Uylings, and M. A. Corner (Eds.), *Progress in brain research.* Vol. 61. *Sex differences in the brain.* Amsterdam: Elsevier, 1984.

Gorski, R. A., and Wagner, J. W. Gonadal activity and sexual differentiation of the hypothalamus. *Endocrinology*, 1965, *76*, 226–239.

Gorski, R. A., Gordon, J. H., Shryne, J. E., and Southam, A. M. Evidence for a morphological sex difference within the medial preoptic area of the rat. *Brain Research*, 1978, *148*, 333–346.

Gorski, R. A., Harlan, R. E. Jacobson, C. D., Shryne, J. E., and Southam, M. Evidence for the existence of a sexually dimorphic nucleus in the preoptic area of the rat. *Journal of Comparative Neurology*, 1980, *193*, 529–539.

Goy, R. W. Development of play and mounting behavior in male rhesus virilized prenatally with esters of testosterone or dihydrotestosterone. In D. J. Chivers and J. Herbert (Eds.), *Recent advances in primatology.* Vol. 1. *Behaviour.* London: Academic Press, 1978.

Goy, R. W., and Phoenix, C. H. The effects of testosterone propionate administered before birth and the development of behavior in genetic female rhesus monkeys. In C. Sawyer and R. Gorski (Eds.), *Steroid hormones and brain function.* Berkeley: University of California Press, 1971.

Goy, R. W., Bridson, W. E., and Young, W. C. Period of maximal susceptibility of the prenatal female guinea pig to masculinizing actions of testosterone propionate. *Journal of Comparative and Physiological Psychology*, 1964, *57*, 166–174.

Grady, K. L., Phoenix, C. H., and Young, W. C. Role of the developing rat testis in differentiation of the neural tissues mediating behavior. *Journal of Comparative and Physiological Psychology*, 1965, *59*, 176–182.

Greenough, W. T., Carter, C. S., Steerman, C., and DeVoogd, T. J. Sex differences in dentritic patterns in hamster preoptic area. *Brain Research*, 1977, *126*, 63–72.

Gurdon, J. B. Nuclear transplantation and the control of gene activity in animal development. *Proceedings of the Royal Society of London B*, 1970, *176*, 303–314.

Gurdon, J. B., and Woodland, H. R. The cytoplasmic control of nuclear activity in animal development. *Biological Reviews*, 1968, *43*, 233–267.

Gurney, M. E. Hormonal control of cell form and number in the zebra finch song system. *Journal of Neuroscience*, 1981, *1*, 658–673.

Gurney, M. E. Behavioral correlates of sexual differentiation in the zebra finch song system. *Brain Research*, 1982, *231*, 153–172.

Gurney, M., and Konishi, M. Hormone-induced sexual differentiation of brain and behavior in zebra finches. *Science*, 1980, *208*, 1380–1383.

Gustafsson, J.-Å, Pousette, A., and Svensson, E. Sex specific occurrence of androgen receptors in the rat. *Journal of Biological Chemistry*, 1976, *247*, 4047–4054.

Hamilton, T. H. Control by estrogen of genetic transcription and translation. *Science*, 1968, *161*, 649–661.

Hammer, R. P., Jr., and Jacobson, C. D. Sex difference in dendritic development of the sexually dimorphic nucleus of the preoptic area in the rat. *International Journal of Developmental Neuroscience,* 1984, *2,* 77–85.

Hardy, D. F., and DeBold, J. F. The relationship between levels of exogenous hormones and the display of lordosis by the female rat. *Hormones and Behavior,* 1971, *2,* 287–297.

Harris, G. W., and Levine, S. Sexual differentiation of the brain and its experimental control. *Journal of Physiology,* 1965, *181,* 379–400.

Hart, B. L. Neonatal castration: Influence on neural organization of sexual reflexes in male rats. *Science,* 1968, *160,* 1135–1136.

Hart, B. L. Neonatal dihydrotestosterone and estrogen stimulation: Effects on sexual behavior of male rats. *Hormones and Behavior,* 1977, *8,* 193–200.

Hart, B. L. Sexual behavior and penile reflexes of neonatally castrated male rats treated in infancy with estrogen and dihydrotestosterone. *Hormones and Behavior,* 1979, *13,* 256–268.

Hart, B. L. and Leedy, M. S. Neurological bases of male sexual behavior: A comparative analysis. In N. Adler, D. Pfaff, and R. W. Goy (Eds.), *Handbook of behavioral neurobiology,* Vol. 7. *Reproduction.* New York: Plenum Press, 1985.

Hart, B. L., and Melese-d'Hospital, P. Y. Penile mechanisms and the role of the striated penile muscles in penile reflexes. *Physiology and Behavior,* 1983, *31,* 807–813.

Haseltine, F. P., and Ohno, S. Mechanisms of gonadal differentiation. *Science,* 1981, *211,* 1272–1278.

Hauser, G. A. Testicular feminization. In C. Overzur (Ed.), *Intersexuality.* New York: Academic Press, 1963.

Hayashi, S. Sterilization of female rats by neonatal placement of estradiol micropellets in anterior hypothalamus. *Endocrinologia Japonica,* 1976, *23,* 55–60.

Hayashi, S., and Gorski, R. A. Critical exposure time for androgenization by intracranial crystals of testosterone propionate in neonatal female rats. *Endocrinology,* 1974, *94,* 1161–1167.

Hodges, J. K. Regulation of oestrogen-induced LH release in male and female marmoset monkeys *(Callithrix jacchus). Journal of Reproduction and Fertility,* 1980, *60,* 389–398.

Hutchison, J. B., and Hutchison, R. E. Phasic effects of hormones in the avian brain during behavioral development. In R. Gilles and J. Balthazart (Eds.), *Neurobiology: Current comparative approaches.* Berlin: Springer-Verlag, 1985.

Imperato-McGinley, J., Guerrero, L., Gautier, T., and Peterson, R. E. Steroid 5α-reductase deficiency in man: An inherited form of male pseudohermaphroditism. *Science,* 1974, *186,* 1213–1215.

Imperato-McGinley, J., Peterson, R. E. Leshin, M., Griffin, J. E., Cooper, G., Draghi, S., Berenyi, M., and Wilson, J. D. Steroid 5α-reductase deficiency in a 65-year-old male pseudohermaphrodite: The natural history, ultrastructure of the testes, and evidence for inherited enzyme heterogeneity. *Journal of Clinical Endocrinology and Metabolism,* 1980, *50,* 15–22.

Jacobson, C. D., Csernus, V. J., Shryne, J. E., and Gorski, R. A. The influence of gonadectomy, androgen exposure, or a gonadal graft in the neonatal rat on the volume of the sexually dimorphic nucleus of the preoptic area. *Journal of Neuroscience,* 1981, *10,* 1142–1147.

Jacobson, C. D., Davis, F. C., and Gorski, R. A. Formation of the sexually dimorphic nucleus of the preoptic area: Neuronal growth, migration and changes in cell number. *Developmental Brain Research,* 1985, *21,* 7–18.

Jacobson, C. D., Arnold, A. P., and Gorski, R. A. Steroid autoradiography of the sexually dimorphic nucleus of the preoptic area. *Brain Research,* 1987, *414,* 349–356.

Jacobson, M. *Developmental Neurobiology.* New York: Plenum Press, 1978.

Jordan, C. L., Breedlove, S. M., and Arnold, A. P. Sexual dimorphism in the dorsolateral motor nucleus of the rat lumbar spinal cord and its response to neonatal androgen. *Brain Research,* 1982, *249,* 309–314.

Joslyn, W. D. Androgen-induced social dominance in infant female rhesus monkeys. *Journal of Child Psychology and Psychiatry,* 1973, *14,* 137–145.

Jost, A. A new look at the mechanisms controlling sex differentiation in mammals. *Johns Hopkins Medical Journal,* 1972, *130,* 38–53.

Jost, A., and Magre, S. Testicular development phases and dual hormonal control of sexual organogenesis. In M. Serio, M. Motta, M. Aznisi, and L. Martini (Eds.), *Sexual differentiation: Basic and clinical aspects.* New York: Raven Press, 1984.

Karsch, F. J., and Foster, D. L. Sexual differentiation of the mechanism controlling the preovulatory discharge of luteinizing hormone in sheep. *Endocrinology,* 1975, *97,* 373–379.

Karsch, F. J., Dierschke, D. J., and Knobil, E. Sexual differentiation of pituitary function: Apparent difference between primates and rodents. *Science*, 1973, *179*, 484–486.

Kelley, D. B. Neuroeffectors for vocalization in *Xenopus laevis:* Hormonal regulation of sexual dimorphism. *Journal of Neurobiology*, 1986, *17*, 231–248.

Kelley, D. B., and Pfaff, D. W. Generalizations from comparative studies on neuroanatomical and endocrine mechanisms of sexual behaviour. In J. B. Hutchison (Ed.), *Biological determinants of sexual behaviour.* Chichester, England: Wiley, 1978.

King, W. J., and Green, G. L. Monoclonal antibodies localize oestrogen receptor in the nuclei of target cells. *Nature*, 1984, *307*, 745–747.

Kirchoff, J., Grunke, W., and Ghraf, R. Estrogen induction of progestin receptors in pituitary, hypothalamic and uterine cytosol of androgenized female rats. *Brain Research*, 1983, *275*, 173–177.

Knobil, E., and Plant, T. M. The hypothalamic regulation of LH and FSH secretion in the rhesus monkey. In S. Riechlin, R. J. Baldessarini, and J. B. Martin (Eds.), *The hypothalamus.* New York: Raven Press, 1978.

Kondo, Y., Shinoda, A., Yamanouchi, K., and Arai, Y. Recovery of lordotic activity by dorsal deafferentation of the preoptic area in male and androgenized female rats. *Physiology and Behavior*, 1986, *37*, 495–498.

Konishi, M., and Akutagawa, E. Neuronal growth, atrophy and death in a sexually dimorphic song nucleus in the zebra finch brain. *Nature*, 1985, *315*, 145–147.

Kurz, E. M., Sengelaub, D. R., and Arnold, A. P. Androgens regulate the dendritic length of mammalian motoneurons in adulthood. *Science*, 1986, *232*, 395–398.

Larsson, K. Effects of neonatal castration upon the development of mating behavior of the male rat. *Zeitschrift für Tierpsychologie*, 1966, *13*, 867–873.

Larsson, K., and Södersten, P. Mating in male rats after section of the dorsal penile nerve. *Physiology and Behavior*, 1973, *10*, 567–571.

LeDouarin, N. M. A model for cell-line divergence in the ontogeny of the peripheral nervous system. In I. B. Black (Ed.), *Cellular and molecular biology of neuronal development.* New York: Plenum Press, 1984.

Levi-Montalchini, R. Developmental neurobiology and the natural history of nerve growth factor. *Annual Review of Neuroscience*, 1982, *5*, 341–362.

Liao, S., Tymoczko, J. L., Casteneda, E., and Liang, T. Androgen receptors and androgen-dependent initiation of protein synthesis in the prostate. *Vitamins and Hormones*, 1975, *33*, 297–317.

Lieberburg, I., and McEwen, B. S. Brain cell nuclear retention of testosterone metabolites, 5α-dihydrotestosterone and estradiol-17β, in adult male rats. *Endocrinology*, 1977, *100*, 588–597.

Lieberburg, I., MacLusky, N. J., and McEwen, B. S. Androgen receptors in the perinatal rat brain. *Brain Research*, 1980a, *196*, 125–138.

Lieberburg, I., MacLusky, N., and McEwen, B. S. Cytoplasmic and nuclear estradiol-17β binding in male and female rat brain: Regional distribution, temporal aspects and metabolism. *Brain Research*, 1980b, *193*, 487–503.

Luck, D. N., and Hamilton, T. H. Early estrogen action: Stimulation of the synthesis of methylated ribosomal and transfer RNAs. *Biochimica et Biophysica Acta*, 1975, *383*, 23–29.

Luine, V. N., and McEwen, B. S. Effects of an estrogen antagonist on enzyme activities and ^{3}H-estradiol nuclear binding in uterus, pituitary and brain. *Endocrinology*, 1977, *100*, 903–910.

Luine, V. N., and Rhodes, J. C. Gonadal hormone regulation of MAO and other enzymes in hypothalamic areas. *Neuroendocrinology*, 1983, *36*, 235–241.

Luine, V. N., McEwen, B. S., and Black, I. B. Effect of 17β-estradiol on hypothalamic tyrosine hydroxylase activity. *Brain Research*, 1977, *120*, 188–192.

MacLusky, N. J., and McEwen, B. S. Oestrogen modulates progestin receptor concentrations in some brain regions and not others. *Nature*, 1978, *274*, 276–277.

MacLusky, N. J., and Naftolin, F. Sexual differentiation of the central nervous system. *Science*, 1981, *211*, 1294–1303.

MacLusky, N. J., Lieberburg, I., Krey, L. C., and McEwen, B. S. Progestin receptors in the brain and pituitary of the bonnet monkey *(Macaca radiata):* Differences between the monkey and the rat in the distribution of progestin-binding sites. *Endocrinology*, 1980, *106*, 185–191.

Maenpaa, P. H. Seryl transfer RNA alterations during estrogen-induced phosvitin synthesis: Quantitative assay of the hormone-responding species by ribosomal binding. *Biochemical and Biophysical Research Communications*, 1972, *47*, 971–974.

Martin, J. T., and Baum, M. J. Neonatal exposure of female ferrets to testosterone alters sociosexual preferences in adulthood. *Psychoneuroendocrinology*, 1986, *11*, 167–176.

Massa, R., Justo, L., and Martini, L. Conversion of testosterone into 5α-reduced metabolites in the anterior pituitary and in the brain of maturing rats. *Journal of Steroid Biochemistry*, 1975, *6*, 567–571.

Matsumoto, A., and Arai, Y. Sex difference in volume of the ventromedial nucleus of the hypothalamus in the rat. *Endocrinologia Japonica*, 1983, *30*, 277–280.

Maurer, R. A., and Woolley, D. E. Demonstration of nuclear ^{3}H-estradiol binding in hypothalamus and amygdala of female, androgenized-female and male rats. *Neuroendocrinology*, 1974, *16*, 137–147.

McEwen, B. S., Krey, L. C., and Luine, V. N. Steroid hormone action in the neuroendocrine system: When is the genome involved? In S. Reichlin, R. J. Baldessarini, and J. B. Martin (Eds.), *The hypothalamus.* New York: Raven Press, 1978.

McKenna, K. E., and Nadelhaft, I. The organization of the pudental nerve in the male and female rat. *Journal of Comparative Neurology*, 1986, *248*, 532–549.

McLaren, A., Simpson, E., Tomonari, K., Chandler, P., and Hogg, H. Male sexual differentiation in mice lacking H-Y antigen. *Nature*, 1984, *312*, 552–555.

Meany, M. J., and Stewart, J. A descriptive study of social development in the rat *(Rattus norvegicus)*. *Animal Behaviour*, 1981a, *29*, 34–45.

Meany, M. J., and Stewart, J. Neonatal androgens influence the social play of prepubescent rats. *Hormones and Behavior*, 1981b, *15*, 197–213.

Meisel, R. L., and Ward, I. L. Fetal female rats are masculinized by male littermates located caudally in the uterus. *Science*, 1981, *213*, 239–242.

Moguilewsky, M., and Raynaud, J. P. Estrogen-sensitive progestin-binding sites in the female rat brain and pituitary. *Brain Research*, 1979a, *164*, 165–175.

Moguilewsky, M., and Raynaud, J. P. The relevance of hypothalamic and hypophyseal progestin receptor regulation in the induction and inhibition of sexual behavior in the female rat. *Endocrinology*, 1979b, *105*, 516–522.

Money, J., and Ehrhardt, A. A. *Man and woman, boy and girl.* Baltimore: Johns Hopkins University Press, 1972.

Moore, C. L. An olfactory basis for maternal discrimination of sex of offspring in rats *(Rattus norvegicus)*. *Animal Behaviour*, 1981, *29*, 383–386.

Moore, C. L. Maternal behavior of rats is affected by hormonal condition of pups. *Journal of Comparative and Physiological Psychology*, 1982, *96*, 123–129.

Moore, C. L. Maternal contributions to the development of masculine sexual behavior in laboratory rats. *Developmental Psychobiology*, 1984, *17*, 347–356.

Moore, C. L. A hormonal basis for sex differences in the self-grooming of rats. *Hormones and Behavior*, 1986a, *20*, 155–165.

Moore, C. L. Sex differences in self-grooming of rats: Effects of gonadal hormones and context. *Physiology and Behavior*, 1986b, *36*, 451–455.

Moore, C. L., and Morelli, G. A. Mother rats interact differently with male and female offspring. *Journal of Comparative and Physiological Psychology*, 1979, *93*, 677–684.

Moore, C. L., and Rogers, S. A. Contribution of self-grooming to onset of puberty in male rats. *Developmental Psychobiology*, 1984, *17*, 243–253.

Moreines, J., McEwen, B., and Pfaff, D. Sex differences in response to discrete estradiol injections. *Hormones and Behavior*, 1986, *20*, 445–451.

Morrell, J. I., and Pfaff, D. W. Characterization of estrogen-concentrating hypothalamic neurons by their axonal projections. *Science,* 1982, *217*, 1273–1276.

Moss, R. L., and Dudley, C. A. Molecular aspects of the interaction between estrogen and the membrane excitability of hypothalamic nerve cells. In G. J. DeVries, J. P. C. DeBruin, H. B. M. Uylings, and M. A. Corner (Eds.), *Progress in brain research.* Vol. 61. *Sex differences in the brain.* Amsterdam: Elsevier, 1984.

Nadler, R. D. Further evidence on the intrahypothalamic locus for androgenization of female rats. *Neuroendocrinology*, 1973, *12*, 110–119.

Naftolin, F., and MacLusky, N. Aromatization hypothesis revisited. In M. Serio, M. Motta, M. Zanisi, and L. Martini (Eds.), *Sexual differentiation: Basic and clinical aspects.* New York: Raven Press, 1984.

Neill, J. D. Sexual differences in the hypothalamic regulation of prolactin secretion. *Endocrinology*, 1972, *90*, 1154–1159.

Nordeen, E. J., and Yahr, P. Hemispheric asymmetries in the behavioral and hormonal effects of sexually differentiating mammalian brain. *Science*, 1982, *218*, 391–394.

Nordeen, E. J., and Yahr, P. A regional analysis of estrogen binding to hypothalamic cell nuclei in relation to masculinization and defeminization. *Journal of Neuroscience*, 1983, *3*, 933–941.

Nordeen, E. J., Nordeen, K. W., Sengelaub, D. R., and Arnold, A. P. Androgens prevent normally occurring cell death in a sexually dimorphic spinal nucleus. *Science*, 1985, *229*, 671–673.

Nordeen, K. W., Nordeen, E. J., and Arnold, A. P. Estrogen establishes sex differences in androgen accumulation in zebra finch brain. *Journal of Neuroscience*, 1986, *6*, 734–738.

Nordeen, E. J., Nordeen, K. W., and Arnold, A. P. Sexual differentiation of androgen accumulation within the zebra finch brain through selective cell loss and addition. *Journal of Comparative Neurology*, 1987, *259*, 393–399.

Nottebohm, F. Testosterone triggers growth of brain vocal control nuclei in adult female canaries. *Brain Research*, 1980, *189*, 429–436.

Nottebohm, F. A brain for all seasons: Cyclical anatomical changes in song control nuclei of the canary brain. *Science*, 1981, *214*, 1368–1370.

Nottebohm, F., and Arnold, A. P. Sexual dimorphism in vocal control areas of the songbird brain. *Science*, 1976, *194*, 211–213.

Nottebohm, F., Stokes, T. M., and Leonard, C. M. Central control of song in the canary, *Serinus canarius. Journal of Comparative Neurology*, 1976, *165*, 457–486.

Nottebohm, F., Manning, E., and Nottebohm, M. E. Reversal of hypoglossal dominance in canaries following unilateral syringeal denervation. *Journal of Comparative Physiology, A*, 1979, *134*, 227–240.

Nottebohm, F., Kasparian, S., and Pandazis, C. Brain space for a learned task. *Brain Research*, 1981, *213*, 99–109.

Nottebohm, F., Kelley, D. B., and Paton, J. A. Connections of vocal control nuclei in the canary telencephalon. *Journal of Comparative Neurology*, 1982, *207*, 344–357.

Nottebohm, F., Nottebohm, M. E., and Crane, L. Developmental and seasonal changes in canary song and their relation to changes in the anatomy of song-control nuclei. *Behavioral and Neural Biology*, 1986, *46*, 445–471.

Numan, M. Brain mechanisms and parental behavior. In N. Adler, D. Pfaff, and R. W. Goy (Eds.), *Handbook of behavioral neurobiology*. Vol. 7. *Reproduction*. New York: Plenum Press, 1985.

Olsen, K. L. Androgen-sensitive rats are defeminized by their testes. *Nature*, 1979a, *279*, 238–239.

Olsen, K. L. Induction of male mating behavior in androgen-insensitive *(tfm)* and normal (King-Holtzman) male rats: Effect of testosterone propionate, estradiol benzoate, and dihydrotestosterone. *Hormones and Behavior*, 1979b, *13*, 66–84.

Olsen, K. L. Aromatization: Is it critical for the differentiation of sexually dimorphic behaviours? In R. Gilles and J. Balthazart (Eds.), *Neurobiology: Current comparative approaches*. Berlin: Springer-Verlag, 1985.

Olsen, K. L., and Whalen, R. E. Sexual differentiation of the brain: Effects on mating behavior and [^{3}H]estradiol binding by hypothalamic chromatin in rats. *Biology of Reproduction*, 1980, *22*, 1068–1072.

Olsen, K. L., and Whalen, R. E. Hormonal control of the development of sexual behavior in androgen-insensitive *(tfm)* rats. *Physiology and Behavior*, 1981, *27*, 883–886.

Olsen, K. L., and Whalen, R. E. Estrogen binds to hypothalamic nuclei of androgen-insensitive *(tfm)* rats. *Experientia*, 1982, *38*, 139–140.

O'Malley, B. W., and Means, A. R. Female steroid hormones and target cell nuclei. *Science*, 1974, *183*, 610–620.

Palkovitz, M. Isolated removal of hypothalamic or other brain nuclei of the rat. *Brain Research*, 1973, *59*, 449–450.

Perez-Palacios, G., Ulloa-Aguirre, A., and Kofman-Alfaro, S. Inherited male pseudohermaphroditism: Analogies between the human and rodent models. In M. Serio, M. Motta, M. Zanisi, and L. Martini (Eds.), *Sexual differentiation: Basic and clinical aspects. New York: Raven Press, 1984.*

Peters, P. J., Bronson, F. H., and Whitsett, J. M. Neonatal castration and intermale aggression in mice. *Physiology and Behavior*, 1972, *8*, 265–268.

Pfaff, D. W. Nature of sex hormone effects on rat sex behavior: Specificity of effects and individual patterns of response. *Journal of Comparative and Physiological Psychology*, 1970, *73*, 349–358.

Pfaff, D. W., and Zigmond, R. E. Neonatal androgen effects on sexual and non-sexual behavior of adult rats tested under various hormone regimes. *Neuroendocrinology,* 1971, *7,* 129–145.

Phoenix, C. H., Goy, R. W., Gerall, A. A., and Young, W. C. Organizing action of prenatally administered testosterone propionate on the tissues mediating mating behavior in the female guinea pig. *Endocrinology,* 1959, *65,* 369–382.

Plapinger, L., and McEwen, B. S. Gonadal steroid-brain interactions in sexual differentiation. In J. B. Hutchison (Ed.), *Biological determinants of sexual behaviour.* Chicester, England: Wiley, 1978.

Pohl-Apel, G., and Sossinka, R. Hormonal determination of song capacity in females of the zebra finch: Critical phase of treatment. *Zeitschrift für Tierpsychologie,* 1984, *64,* 330–336.

Puymirat, J., Loudes, C., Faivre-Bauman, A., Tixier-Vidal, A., and Bourre, J. M. Expression of neuronal function by mouse hypothalamic cells cultured in hormonally defined medium. In G. H. Sato, A. B. Pardee, and D. A. Sirbosky (Eds.), *Cold Spring Harbor conferences on cell proliferation.* Vol. 9. *Growth of cells in hormonally defined media.* Cold Spring Harbor, NY: Cold Spring Harbor Laboratory, 1982.

Rainbow, T. C., DeGroff, V., Luine, V. N., and McEwen, B. S. Estradiol-17β increases the number of muscarinic receptors in hypothalamic nuclei. *Brain Research,* 1980, *198,* 239–243.

Rainbow, T. C., Parsons, B., and McEwen, B. S. Sex differences in rat brain oestrogen and progestin receptors. *Nature,* 1982, *300,* 648–649.

Raisman, G., and Field, P. M. Sexual dimorphism in the preoptic area of the rat. *Science,* 1971, *173,* 731–733.

Raisman, G., and Field, P. M. Sexual dimorphism in the neurophil of the preoptic area and its dependence on neonatal androgen. *Brain Research,* 1973, *54,* 1–29.

Ranson, E., and Beach, F. A. Effects of testosterone on ontogeny of urinary behavior in male and female dogs. *Hormones and Behavior,* 1985, *19,* 36–51.

Raynaud, J.-P., and Moguilewsky, M. Steroid competition for estrogen receptors in the central nervous system. *Progress in Reproductive Biology,* 1977, *2,* 78–87.

Resko, J. A. Gonadal hormones during sexual differentiation in vertebrates. In N. Adler, D. Pfaff, and R. W. Goy (Eds.), *Handbook of behavioral neurobiology.* Vol. 7. *Reproduction.* New York: Plenum Press, 1985.

Resko, J. A., and Ellinwood, W. E. Sexual differentiation of the brain of primates. In M. Serio, M. Motta, M. Zanisi, and L. Martini (Eds.), *Sexual differentiation: Basic and clinical aspects.* New York: Raven Press, 1984.

Richmond, G., and Sachs, B. D. Further evidence for masculinization of female rats by males located caudally *in utero. Hormones and Behavior,* 1984a, *18,* 484–490.

Richmond, G., and Sachs, B. D. Maternal discrimination of pup sex in rats. *Developmental Psychobiology,* 1984b, *17,* 87–89.

Robertson, D. R. Social control of sex reversal in a coral-reef fish. *Science,* 1972, *177,* 1007–1009.

Rodriquez-Sierra, J. F., Crowley, W. R., and Komisaruk, B. R. Vaginal stimulation in rats induces prolonged lordosis responsiveness and sexual receptivity. *Journal of Comparative and Physiological Psychology,* 1975, *89,* 79–85.

Ronnekleiv, O. K., Ojeda, S. R., and McCann, S. M. Undernutrition, puberty and the development of estrogen positive feedback in the female rat. *Biology of Reproduction,* 1978, *19,* 414–434.

Rosenfeld, M. G., Amara, S. G., and Evans, R. M. Alternative RNA processing: Determining neuronal phenotype. *Science,* 1984, *225,* 1315–1320.

Sachs, B. D. Role of striated penile muscle in penile reflexes, copulation, and induction of pregnancy in the rat. *Journal of Reproduction and Fertility,* 1982, *66,* 433–443.

Sachs, B. D. Potency and fertility: Hormonal and mechanical causes and effects of penile actions in rats. In J. Balthazart, E. Pröve, and R. Gilles (Eds.), *Hormones and behaviour in higher vertebrates.* Berlin: Springer-Verlag, 1983.

Savikurki, H., and de la Chapelle, A. Etiology of XX males. H-Y antigen studies in seven probands and their families. In M. Serio, M. Motta, M. Zanisi, and L. Martini (Eds.), *Sexual differentiation: Basic and clinical aspects.* New York: Raven Press, 1984.

Schachter, B. S., and Toran-Allerand, C. D. Intraneuronal α-fetoprotein and albumin are not synthesized locally in developing brain. *Developmental Brain Research,* 1982, *5,* 93–98.

Schumacher, M., and Balthazart, J. Testosterone-induced brain aromatase is sexually dimorphic. *Brain Research,* 1986, *370,* 285–293.

Shander, D., and Barraclough, C. A. Role of the preoptic area in the regulation of preovulatory gonadotropin surges in the hamster. *Experimental Brain Research,* 1980, *40,* 123–130.

Shapiro, B. H., Levine, D. C., and Adler, N. T. The testicular feminized rat: A naturally occurring model of androgen independent brain masculinization. *Science*, 1980, *209*, 418–420.

Shapiro, D. Y. Serial female sex changes after simultaneous removal of males from social groups of a coral reef fish. *Science*, 1980, *209*, 1136–1137.

Sheridan, P. J. Unaromatized androgen is taken up by the neonatal rat brain: Two receptor systems for androgen. *Developmental Neuroscience*, 1981, *4*, 46–54.

Shivers, R. D., Harlan, R. E., Morrell, J. I., and Pfaff, D. W. Immunocytochemical localization of luteinizing hormone-releasing hormone in male and female rat brains: Quantitative studies on the effect of gonadal steroids. *Neuroendocrinology*, 1983, *361*, 1–12.

Simerly, R. B., and Swanson, L. W. The organization of neural inputs to the medial preoptic nucleus of the rat. *Journal of Comparative Neurology*, 1986, *246*, 312–342.

Simerly, R. B., Swanson, L. W., and Gorski, R. A. The cells of origin of a sexually dimorphic serotonergic input to the medial preoptic-nucleus of the rat. *Brain Research*, 1984a, *324*, 185–189.

Simerly, R. B., Swanson, L. W., and Gorski, R. A. Demonstration of a sexual dimorphism in the distribution of serotonin-immunoreactive fibers in the medial preoptic nucleus of the rat. *Journal of Comparative Neurology*, 1984b, *225*, 151–166.

Simerly, R. B., Swanson, L. W., and Gorski, R. A. The distribution of monoaminergic cells and fibers in a periventricular nucleus involved in the control of gonadotropin release: Immunohistochemical evidence for a dopaminergic sexual dimorphism. *Brain Research*, 1985a, *330*, 55–64.

Simerly, R. B., Swanson, L. W., Handa, R. J., and Gorski, R. A. Influence of perinatal androgen on the sexually dimorphic distribution of tyrosine hydroxylase-immunoreactive cells and fibers in the anteroventral periventricular nucleus of the rat. *Neuroendocrinology*, 1985b, *40*, 501–510.

Simerly, R. B., Gorski, R. A., and Swanson, L. W. The neurotransmitter specificity of cells and fibers in the medial preoptic nucleus: An immunohistochemical study in the rat. *Journal of Comparative Neurology*, 1986, *246*, 364–381.

Simpson, E., Chandler, P., Goulmy, E., Disteche, C., Ferguson-Smith, M. A., and Page, D. C. Separation of the genetic loci for the H-Y antigen and for testis determination on human Y chromosome. *Nature*, 1987, *326*, 876–878.

Slob, A. K., and Van der Shoot, P. Testosterone induced mounting behavior in adult female rats born in litters of different female to male ratios. *Physiology and Behavior*, 1982, *28*, 1007–1010.

Slob, A. K., and Vreeburg, J. T. M. Prenatal androgens in female rats and adult mounting behavior. In R. Gilles and J. Balthazart (Eds.), *Neurobiology: Current comparative approaches*. Berlin: Springer-Verlag, 1985.

Södersten, P. Sexual differentiation: Do males differ from females in behavioral sensitivity to gonadal hormones? In G. J. DeVries, J. P. C. DeBruin, H. B. M. Uylings, and M. A. Corner (Eds.), *Progress in brain research*. Vol. 61. *Sex differences in the brain*. Amsterdam: Elsevier, 1984.

Södersten, P., and Gustafsson, J.-Å. A way in which estradiol might play a role in the sexual behavior of male rats. *Hormones and Behavior*, 1980, *14*, 271–274.

Södersten, P., Pettersson, A., and Eneroth, P. Pulse administration of estradiol-17β cancels sex differences in behavioral estrogen sensitivity. *Endocrinology*, 1983, *112*, 1883–1885.

Spelsberg, T. C., Littlefield, B. A., Seelke, R., Dani, G. M., Torjoda, H., Boyd-Leinen, P., Thrall, C., and Kon, O. L. Role of specific chromosomal proteins and DNA sequences in the nuclear binding sites for steroid receptors. *Recent Progress in Hormone Research*, 1983, *39*, 463–517.

Sridaran, R., Basuray, R., and Gibori, G. Source and regulation of testosterone secretion in pregnant and pseudo-pregnant rats. *Endocrinology*, 1981, *108*, 855–861.

Steiner, R. A., Schiller, H. S., Barber, J., and Gale, C. C. Luteinizing hormone regulation in the monkey (*Macaca nemestrina*): Failure of testosterone and dihydrotestosterone to block the estrogen-induced gonadotropin surge. *Biology of Reproduction*, 1978, *19*, 51–56.

Sutcliffe, J. G., Milner, R. J., Gottesfeld, J. M., and Reynolds, W. Control of neuronal gene expression. *Science*, 1984, *225*, 1308–1315.

Tennent, B. J., Smith, E. R., and Davidson, J. M. The effects of estrogen and progesterone on female rat proceptive behavior. *Hormones and Behavior*, 1980, *14*, 65–75.

Terasawa, E., and Wiegand, S. J. Effects of hypothalamic deafferentiation on ovulation and estrous cyclicity in the female guinea pig. *Neuroendocrinology*, 1978, *26*, 229–248.

Thiessen, D. D., Friend, H. C., and Lindzey, G. Androgen control of territorial marking in the Mongolian gerbil. *Science*, 1969, *160*, 26–30.

Thomas, D. A., McIntosh, T. K., and Barfield, R. J. Influence of androgen in the neonatal period on ejaculatory and postejaculatory behavior in the rat. *Hormones and Behavior*, 1980, *14*, 153–162.

Thomas, D. A., Barfield, R. J., and Etgen, A. M. Influence of androgen on the development of sexual behavior in rats. I. Time of administration and masculine copulatory responses, penile reflexes, and androgen receptors in females. *Hormones and Behavior*, 1982, *16*, 443–454.

Thomas, D. A., Howard, S. B., and Barfield, R. J. Influence of androgen on the development of sexual behavior in the rat. II. Time and dosage of androgen administration during the neonatal period and masculine and feminine copulatory behavior in females. *Hormones and Behaviors*, 1983, *17*, 308–315.

Tiefer, L. Gonadal hormones and mating behavior in the adult golden hamster. *Hormones and Behavior*, 1970, *1*, 189–202.

Tobet, S. A., Dunlap, J. L., and Gerall, A. A. Influence of fetal position on neonatal androgen-induced sterility and sexual behavior in female rats. *Hormones and Behavior*, 1982, *16*, 251–258.

Tobet, S. A., Shim, J. T., Osiecki, S. T., Baum, M. J., and Canick, J. A. Androgen accumulation and 5α-reduction in ferret brain: Effects of sex and testosterone manipulation. *Endocrinology*, 1985, *116*, 1869–1877.

Toran-Allerand, C. D. Sex steroids and the development of the newborn mouse hypothalamus and preoptic area *in vitro:* Implications for sexual differentiation. *Brain Research*, 1976, *106*, 407–412.

Toran-Allerand, C. D. Sex steroids and the development of the newborn mouse hypothalamus and preoptic area *in vitro.* II. Morphological correlates and hormonal specificity. *Brain Research*, 1980, *189*, 413–427.

Toran-Allerand, C. D. Regional differences in intraneuronal localization of alpha-fetoprotein in developing mouse brain. *Developmental Brain Research*, 1982, *5*, 213–217.

Toran-Allerand, C. D. On the genesis of sexual differentiation of the central nervous system: Morphogenetic consequences of steroidal exposure and possible role of α-fetoprotein. In G. J. DeVries, J. P. C. DeBruin, H. B. M. Uylings, and M. A. Corner (Eds.), *Progress in brain research.* Vol. 61. *Sex differences in the brain.* Amsterdam: Elsevier, 1984.

Turner, J. W. Influence of neonatal androgen on the display of territorial marking behavior in the gerbil. *Physiology and Behavior,* 1975, *15*, 265–270.

Ulibarri, C., and Yahr, P. Poly-A$^+$ mRNA and defeminization of sexual behavior and gonadotropin secretion in rats, *Physiology and Behavior,* 1987, *39*, 767–774.

Ulibarri, C., and Yahr, P. Role of neonatal androgens in sexual differentiation of brain structure, scent marking, and gonadotropin secretion in gerbils. *Behavioral and Neural Biology,* 1988, in press.

Vacas, M. J., and Cardinali, D. P. Effect of estradiol on α- and β-adrenoceptor density in medial basal hypothalamus and pineal gland of ovariectomized rats. *Neuroscience Letters,* 1980, *17*, 73–77.

Vergnaud, G., Page, D. C., Simmler, M.-C., Brown, L., Rouyer, F., Noel, B., Botstein, D., de la Chapelle, A., and Weissenbach, J. A deletion map of the human Y chromosome based on DNA hybridization. *American Journal of Human Genetics*, 1986, *38*, 109–124.

Vito, C. C., Baum, M. J., Bloom, C., and Fox, T. O. Androgen and estrogen receptors in perinatal ferret brain. *Journal of Neuroscience,* 1985, *5*, 268–274.

vom Saal, F. S., and Bronson, F. H. In utero proximity of female mouse fetuses to males: Effect on reproductive performance during later life. *Biology of Reproduction,* 1978, *19*, 842–853.

vom Saal, F. S., and Bronson, F. H. Sexual characteristics of adult female mice are correlated with their blood testosterone levels during prenatal development. *Science,* 1980a, *208*, 597–599.

vom Saal, F. S., and Bronson, F. H. Variation in length of the estrous cycle in mice due to former intrauterine proximity to male fetuses. *Biology of Reproduction,* 1980b, *22*, 777–780.

vom Saal, F. S., Grant, W. M., McMullen, C. W., and Laves, K. S. High fetal estrogen concentrations: Correlation with increased adult sexual activity and decreased aggression in male mice. *Science,* 1983, *220,* 1306–1309.

Vreeburg, J. T. M., van der Vaart, P. D. M., and van der Schoot, P. Prevention of central defeminization but not masculinization in male rats by inhibition neonatally of estrogen biosynthesis. *Journal of Endocrinology,* 1977, *74*, 375–382.

Wachtel, S. S. *H-Y antigen and the biology of sex determination.* New York: Grune & Stratton, 1983.

Wade, G. N., and Zucker, I. Modulation of food intake and locomotor activity in female rats by diencephalic hormone implants. *Journal of Comparative and Physiological Psychology,* 1970, *72,* 328–336.

Wallach, S. J. R., and Hart, B. L. The role of the striated penile muscles of the male rat in seminal plug dislodgement and deposition. *Physiology and Behavior,* 1983, *31*, 815–821.

Wallis, C. J., and Luttge, W. G. Influence of estrogen and progesterone on glutamic acid decarboxylase activity in discrete regions of rat brain. *Journal of Neurochemistry,* 1980, *34*, 609–613.

Ward, I. L., and Ward, O. B. Sexual behavior differentiation: Effects of prenatal manipulations in rats.

In N. Adler, D. Pfaff, and R. W. Goy (Eds.), *Handbook of behavioral neurobiology*. Vol. 7. *Reproduction*. New York: Plenum Press, 1985.

Welshons, W. V., Lieberman, M. E., and Gorski, J. Nuclear localization of unoccupied oestrogen receptors. *Nature*, 1984, *307*, 747–749.

Weston, J. A., Girdlestone, J., and Ciment, G. Heterogeneity in neural crest cell populations. In I. B. Black (Ed.), *Cellular and molecular biology of neuronal development*. New York: Plenum Press, 1984.

Whalen, R. E., and Edwards, D. A. Hormonal determinants of the development of masculine and feminine behavior in male and female rats. *Anatomical Record*, 1967, *157*, 173–180.

Whalen, R. E., and Etgen, A. M. Masculinization and defeminization induced in female hamsters by neonatal treatment with estradiol benzoate and RU-2858. *Hormones and Behavior*, 1978, *10*, 170–177.

Whalen, R. E., and Massicci, J. Subcellular analysis of the accumulation of estrogen by the brain of male and female rats. *Brain Research*, 1975, *89*, 255–264.

Whalen, R. E., and Olsen, K. L. Chromatin binding of estradiol in the hypothalamus and cortex of male and female rats. *Brain Research*, 1978a, *152*, 121–131.

Whalen, R. E., and Olsen, K. L. Prednisolone modifies estrogen-induced sexual differentiation. *Behavioral Biology*, 1978b, *24*, 549–553.

Whalen, R. E., and Olsen, K. L. Role of aromatization in sexual differentiation: Effects of prenatal ATD treatment and neonatal castration. *Hormones and Behavior*, 1981, *15*, 107–122.

Whalen, R. E., and Rezek, D. L. Localization of androgenic metabolites in the brain of rats administered testosterone and dihydrotestosterone. *Steroids*, 1972, *20*, 717–722.

Whalen, R. E., Luttge, W. G., and Gorzalka, B. B. Neonatal androgenization and the development of estrogen responsivity in male and female rats. *Hormones and Behavior*, 1971, *2*, 83–90.

Whalen, R. E., Yahr, P., and Luttge, G. G. The role of metabolism in hormonal control of sexual behavior. In N. Adler, D. Pfaff, and R. W. Goy (Eds.), *Handbook of behavioral neurobiology*. Vol. 7. *Reproduction*. New York: Plenum Press, 1985.

Whalen, R. E., Gladue, B. A., and Olsen, K. L. Lordotic behavior in male rats: Genetic and hormonal regulation of sexual differentation. *Hormones and Behavior*, 1986, *20*, 73–82.

Wicks, W. D., Greenman, D. L., and Kenney, F. T. Stimulation of ribonucleic acid synthesis by steroid hormones. I. Transfer ribonucleic acid. *Journal of Biological Chemistry*, 1965, *240*, 4414–4419.

Wiegand, S. J., and Terasawa, E. Discrete lesions reveal functional heterogeneity of suprachiasmatic structures in regulation of gonadotropin secretion in the female rat. *Neuroendocrinology*, 1982, *34*, 395–404.

Williams, C. L. Estradiol benzoate facilitates lordosis and ear wiggling of 4- to 6-day old rats. *Behavioral Neuroscience*, 1987, *101*, 718–723.

Wilson, J. D., George, F. W., and Griffin, J. E. The hormonal control of sexual development. *Science*, 1981, *211*, 1278–1284.

Witcher, J. A., and Clemens, L. G. A prenatal source for defeminization of female rats is the maternal ovary. *Hormones and Behavior*, 1987, *21*, 36–43.

Wray, S., and Hoffman, G. A developmental study of the quantitative distribution of LHRH neurons within the central nervous system of postnatal male and female rats. *Journal of Comparative Neurology*, 1986, *252*, 522–531.

Yahr, P. Hormonal influences on territorial marking behavior. In B. B. Svare (Ed.), *Hormones and aggressive behavior*. New York: Plenum Press, 1983.

Yahr, P. Pars compacta of the sexually dimorphic area of the gerbil hypothalamus: Postnatal ages at which development responds to testosterone. *Behavioral and Neural Biology*, 1988, in press.

Yahr, P., and Stephens, D. R. Hormonal control of sexual and scent marking behaviors of male gerbils in relation to the sexually dimorphic area of the gerbil brain. *Hormones and Behavior*, 1987, *21*, 331–346.

Yahr, P., and Ulibarri, C. Estrogen induction of sexual behavior in female rats and synthesis of polyadenylated messenger RNA in the ventromedial nucleus of the hypothalamus. *Molecular Brain Research*, 1986, *1*, 153–165.

Yamanouchi, K., and Arai, Y. Presence of a neural mechanism for the expression of female sexual behaviors in the male rat brain. *Neuroendocrinology*, 1985, *40*, 393–397.

7

Learning in Infancy
A Mechanism for Behavioral Change during Development

INGRID B. JOHANSON AND LESLIE M. TERRY

INTRODUCTION

Several decades ago, the prevailing view of how learning and memory mechanisms might develop was based on the idea that altricial neonates are simply incompletely formed adults. Infant learning tasks were designed with the adult in mind, and performance differences between infants and adults were considered proof of the immature learning and performance capacities of infants. These immature capacities were attributed, in turn, to an immature nervous system (e.g., Cornwell and Fuller, 1961; Fuller, Easler, and Banks, 1950).

More recently, the study of infant learning and memory has benefited from a contrasting approach—one drawn from both developmental biology and psychology—that infants are not simply less complex versions of adults but have sensory and motoric capabilities that are uniquely adapted to the changing demands of their own special environments (Oppenheim, 1981; Turkewitz and Kenny, 1982). Rather than emphasizing the infant's deficiencies relative to the adult norm, this approach views "limitations" in perceptual and motor function as requisites for the normal integration that must develop among the emerging sensory and motor systems (Turkewitz and Kenny, 1982). An increasing awareness of the *Umwelt* of young animals has led scientists to use species-typical behaviors (e.g., simple approach–withdrawal, suckling, and components of maternal search behavior) and

INGRID B. JOHANSON Department of Psychology, Florida Atlantic University, Boca Raton, Florida 33431.   LESLIE M. TERRY Department of Psychology, Duke University, Durham, North Carolina 27706.

their eliciting thermotactile and olfactory stimuli to identify and better understand learning mechanisms during infancy (cf. Rosenblatt, 1983).

Ingenious methodologies for testing motorically and sensorially immature organisms have yielded evidence of learning in the infants (e.g., Amsel, Burdette, and Letz, 1976; Bacon and Stanley, 1970; Blass, Ganchrow, and Steiner, 1984; Brake, 1981; Bulut and Altman, 1974; DeCasper and Fifer, 1980; Johanson and Hall, 1979; Kenny and Blass, 1977; Martin and Alberts, 1982; Rovee-Collier, Sullivan, Enright, Lucas, and Fagen, 1980; Rudy and Cheatle, 1977) and even the fetuses (Leader, Baillie, Martin, and Vermeulen, 1982; Smotherman, 1982; Stickrod, Kimble, and Smotherman, 1982) of a number of mammalian species. These successes have undoubtedly stemmed from two sources: first, the *use of stimuli from the mother and the nest* (such as contact, warmth, home odors, and suckling odors) that infants are prepared to learn about and, as we will discuss later, most probably do learn about in the course of normal behavioral development; and second, the judicious *selection of age-appropriate responses* (such as simple approach and sucking) with which to assess infant learning. The focus of research is shifting from asking simple questions about capability (e.g., "Can infants learn?") to posing the more difficult questions about the mechanisms of learning and memory during development, and about how such mechanisms may help infants meet the needs that naturally arise during normal behavioral ontogeny.

Accordingly, we first describe some advances in our understanding of infant learning and memory, emphasizing those studies that have used natural contextual cues and reinforcers. Because most developmental psychobiological studies of mammalian learning have used rat neonates, our review will be limited, for the most part, to this species. Next, we assess whether infant rats actually learn in the normal context provided by mother, littermates, and nest, and whether such learning influences the development of certain species-typical behaviors in rats. Recent work from our laboratory, for example, demonstrates the sensory and experiential basis for rat pups' responsiveness to milk and implicates mechanisms of associative learning, specifically classical conditioning, in the development of this responsiveness. The implications of these findings for the development of incentive and motivational systems will be discussed.

RECENT PROGRESS IN LEARNING AND MEMORY RESEARCH

Altricial mammalian infants are exposed during early development to numerous nurturing stimuli and events, such as warmth, maternal and sibling odors, maternal care, and the opportunity to suckle and to obtain milk. Many of these stimuli provide significant cues that (a) modulate infantile response patterns and (b) are rewarding in both classical and instrumental conditioning paradigms.

AMBIENT SENSORY INFLUENCES ON LEARNING

WARMTH. Because of the physiological vulnerability of altricial mammalian infants (which is due to their large surface-to-mass ratio and poor brown fat deposits; Brody, 1943; Leon, 1986), their body temperature is regulated behaviorally (e.g., by huddling with mother and siblings, Alberts, 1978; Cosnier, 1965; and by avoiding cool temperatures and approaching sources of warmth, Freeman and Rosenblatt, 1978; Johanson, 1979; Kleitman and Satinoff, 1982; Leonard, 1974). This responsiveness of infants to thermal cues and the thermal modulation of maternal–infant contact (Leon, Croskerry, and Smith, 1978) acts to ensure protracted contact between infants and their siblings and dam and perhaps accounts for the importance of thermotactile stimulation in early affective development and the development of incentive and motivational systems (Jeddi, 1979; Rosenblatt, 1983). Although warmth is not essential for a wide variety of infantile behaviors (e.g., suckling occurs readily at cooler temperatures; Blass, Teicher, Cramer, Bruno, and Hall, 1977), providing a warm environment (i.e., nest) during behavioral assessment has revealed a number of more "adultlike" capabilities in altricial neonates that had remained hidden at cooler temperatures. Deprived rats 1 to 10 days of age, which normally ingest only by suckling from their dam, can feed independently of their mother if they are given milk in a warm environment (Hall, 1979). This independent ingestion is not displayed if pups are given milk in a cool (22°C) environment. Further, pups fed at cool ambient temperatures fail to display the intense externalized excitement seen in pups fed in a warm environment (Hall, 1979; Johanson and Hall, 1980), a finding suggesting that warmth may enhance the rewarding properties of milk. The lack of ingestion and activation is most likely due to the pups' perception (via peripheral thermal receptors) of a cool ambient temperature, and not to a general debilitation produced by a low core temperature. Although the effect of warm temperatures on ingestion decreases with age, it is still apparent in 15- and 20-day-old rat pups, which are much more able than younger pups to defend their core body temperatures (Adolph, 1957; Brody, 1943; Gulick, 1937). Furthermore, young (3- and 6-day-old) pups that had their body temperatures lowered to 29°C (34–36°C is normal nest temperature) before being infused with milk immediately ingested diet and became activated when placed in a warm incubator, before any apparent increase in body temperature occurred. In contrast, pups with warm body temperatures immediately refused to ingest when they were offered food in a cool environment (Johanson and Hall, 1980). Thus, behavioral responsiveness to milk is modulated by the perceived thermal context in which the milk is presented. Other types of behavioral patterns also depend on a warm ambience for their occurrence. For example, 6-day-old rats display lordosis in response to flank stimulation, but only in a warm (34–35°C) ambience (Williams, 1979). Thus, infant rats are capable of emitting a variety of adultlike response patterns (such as feeding and sexual reflexes) if stimulated in an appropriate thermal environment.

A warm ambient temperature is likewise essential for the infants' learning of tasks in which the reward or reinforcer is milk provided away from the dam. Thus, a normally aversive odor signaling infusions of milk became strongly preferred, but only if the odor–milk pairing occurred in a warm environment (Johanson and Hall, 1982; Johanson and Teicher, 1980). Similarly, performance in instrumental conditioning tasks that use milk as the reward is influenced by the temperature at which training occurs. One-day-old pups tested at 32–34°C probed into a paddle for milk reward and even learned a two-choice odor discrimination (Johanson and Hall, 1979). In contrast, 10- to 15-day-old pups trained at room temperature in a T maze did not acquire the spatial discrimination task for milk reward, even though they learned this discrimination when they were rewarded with suckling (Smith and Bogomolny, 1983).

PRESENCE OF FAMILIAR ODORS. Familiar olfactory cues (usually in the form of home or maternal odors) also influence how infants respond to other stimuli. Home odor cues enhanced milk intake and the behavioral activation elicited by milk in 6-day-old rat pups fed through oral cannulas (Johanson and Hall, 1981). Likewise, an artificial odor previously paired with an activating stimulus (stroking with a soft brush) resulted in an increased intake of milk by pups (Sullivan, Brake, Hofer, and Williams, 1986). Familiar odors can also facilitate learning in infants. Infant rats trained in the presence of home environment cues acquired shock-escape (Smith and Spear, 1981) and passive-avoidance (Smith and Spear, 1978) responses more quickly than pups trained without home environment cues. Similarly, the presence of siblings (which provide thermotactile, as well as olfactory, stimulation) facilitated odor aversion learning in 2-day-old infant rats (Smith and Spear, 1980). Associations between two tastes are more readily learned in the home environment. Preweanling rats provided with previous exposure to a two-taste compound in their home environment, and then made ill (with LiCl) in association with only one of the tastes, later displayed greater aversion to the second taste in the compound than pups initially exposed to the compound in a novel environment (Spear, 1984).

It appears that the pups' prior experiences with maternal or sibling odors may be responsible, in part, for facilitating learning in infants. The presence of a botanical odor (banana) to which pups had been previously exposed (for even brief periods) facilitated the pups' learning a shock-escape task (Wigal, Kucharski, and Spear, 1984). Because the prior odor exposure had occurred in a warm environment, subsequent effects on learning may have been due to the presence of conditioned associations of the odor with warmth (see below) instead of or in addition to simple familiarity with the odor.

There are some learning situations, however, in which pups' learning is actually hampered by the presence of familiar olfactory cues. For example, the presence of home environment odors interfered with the acquisition of a taste aversion in 18-day-old rat pups, though it did not have this effect in slightly older (21-day-old) pups or in adults (Infurna, Steinert, and Spear, 1979; Spear, 1984).

In attempting to explain these differences in the effects of home environmental cues, Wigal et al. (1984) suggested that the association of home odors with reinforcing events lends a "positive valence" to these odors. Their presence may thus facilitate the learning of tasks with similar positive consequences and should interfere with learning about aversive events involving solely negative consequences (such as taste aversion learning). For certain conditioning tasks, Wigal et al. suggested that escape from aversive consequences such as shock may have "positive" consequences, thus explaining why the presence of home odor enhances escape and avoidance learning.

There is no question that infant rats can learn about positive events while suckling from the mother (e.g., 11-day-old pups learned a preference for a novel odor that had been paired with milk infusions received while suckling; Brake, 1981). However, the ability of preweanlings to learn about aversive events while suckling their dam was called into question by Martin and Alberts (1979). They found that preweanling (10-day-old) pups did not learn an illness-induced aversion to flavored milk obtained while suckling from a lactating foster mother, although weanling (21-old-day) pups did. The lack of aversion in the preweanlings was apparently not due to an inability to learn taste aversions. Ten-day-old pups exposed to flavored milk infused via oral cannulas located far back in the mouth, where the tip of the nipple normally extends during suckling, developed strong aversions to the milk if the training occurred off the nipple. However, they showed no aversion to the milk if it was infused through a cannula while they were suckling. Martin and Alberts proposed that the preweanlings' inability to acquire taste aversions in the suckling context results from an inability to associate taste cues with illness, perhaps because of the "blocking" effect of the suckling context.

It has recently been demonstrated, however, that the blocking effect of suckling can be overcome by simply changing the site of the intraoral infusion (Kehoe and Blass, 1986). This finding would suggest that the failure of preweanlings to acquire learned taste aversions in the suckling situation may be due in large part to the failure to adequately detect the taste cues while suckling (perhaps because of something fairly simple, such as the presence of the nipple in the mouth), rather than to a blocking effect of the suckling context *per se* on the pups' ability to associate illness with tastes perceived while suckling.

SUMMARY. In summary, the presence of cues associated with "mother" or "nest" appears to facilitate the learning of certain types of events in young infants and actually to interfere with their learning about other types of events. The suggestion made by Wigal *et al.* (1984) that the "positive valence" attached to home odors enhances learning about positive events and interferes with learning about aversive events could explain, as well, the effects on learning of other types of ambient cues that may be positive in nature (e.g., warmth and the suckling context). If this is the case, then it may be possible that the effects of these other ambient cues on learning would be similar. For example, the presence of home odors may facilitate the learning of preferences for odors associated with milk infusions, whereas taste aversion learning may occur less readily in a warm environment than in a cool environment. Alternatively, these ambient cues may elicit behaviors that are incompatible with the learned responses.

STUDIES OF ASSOCIATIVE LEARNING IN INFANTS

Warmth, exposure to home and maternal odors, and suckling have served, as well, as reinforcers in both classical and instrumental conditioning paradigms. Some of these cues may be what learning theorists have called *primary reinforcers* (i.e., they are reinforcing to the infant on first encounter), and others may have acquired their reinforcing properties only after the infant has had certain experiences with them (i.e., they are secondary or conditioned reinforcers).

WARMTH AS REWARD. Warmth appears to be a significant reinforcing stimulus to altricial mammalian infants. Odors can acquire "positive" or "negative" incentive value, depending on the temperatures associated with them. Alberts (1981; Brunjes and Alberts, 1979) provided infant rats with several hours of contact daily with a warm and a cool cylinder, each with a different scent. In a test of huddling preferences, pups overwhelmingly chose the object scented with the odor previously associated with the warm cylinder. Absence of warmth may, in fact, be punishing to young infants. Odors associated with exposure to severe cold have been found to evoke acceleratory heart-rate changes similar to those elicited by odors associated with another "aversive" consequence, LiCl-induced illness (Martin and Alberts, 1982).

Additional evidence that warmth has reinforcing value to infants comes from the studies of Guenaire and colleagues in which "warmth" is used as a reward in instrumental learning tasks. Rat pups 4 days old learned a spatial discrimination reinforced by a puff of warm air (Guenaire, Costa, and Delacour, 1982a). Further, pups reinforced with warm air for raising their heads above a certain level showed an increased frequency of head rasing relative to noncontingent controls (Guenaire, Costa, and Delacour, 1982b).

EXPOSURE TO FAMILIAR ODORS. Infants are strongly attracted to home odors, an attraction that is manifested in their orienting to dam and nest (e.g., kittens, Freeman and Rosenblatt, 1978; Rosenblatt, Turkewitz and Schneirla, 1969; rat pups, Altman, Sudarshan, Das, McCormick, and Barnes, 1971; Sczerenie and Hsiao, 1977). The tendency of infant rats to approach and maintain contact with sources of home odor was exploited by Altman and his colleagues to assess neonatal learning (Altman, Brunner, Bulut, and Sudarshan, 1972; Bulut and Altman, 1974). They found that 6-day-old pups learned a two-choice spatial or tactile discrimination to gain access to their home cage.

Rosenblatt (1983) convincingly argued that olfactory cues, particularly those from the nest and the mother, may have acquired incentive value (i.e., may have become secondary reinforcers) by their early association with certain primary reinforcers, such as thermal and tactile stimulation. The findings that infant rats come to strongly prefer odors associated with warmth (Alberts, 1981; Brunjes and Alberts, 1979) and selectively attach to nipples labeled with an odor associated with the activating effects of tactile stimulation (Pedersen, Williams, and Blass, 1982) certainly support this possibility. However, the situation is complicated by the fact that simple exposure to novel odors, at room temperatures and without tactile stimulation, can alter infant rats' later preferences for those odors. For example, Leon, Galef and Behse (1977) found that isolated rat pups exposed to a mildly aversive odor (peppermint) for 3 h daily were as likely to approach this odor in a preference test as normally reared pups were to approach the normal odors of their dam. In fact, even a brief (3-min) exposure to a novel odor was sufficient to increase rat pups' preference for that odor 24 h later (Caza and Spear, 1984).

Although simple exposure to an odor may be sufficient to induce changes in responding to that odor, it is clear that certain experiences may produce more permanent and qualitatively different types of behavioral changes. Along this line, Galef and Kaner (1980) found that pups that received simple exposure to peppermint odor each day following birth displayed a preference for peppermint at age 21 days, but not at age 33 days. However, considerably longer lasting preferences could be established in pups by painting the odorous solution on the ventrum of their dam (Fillion and Blass, 1986b; Galef and Kaner, 1980), a finding suggesting (as we will elaborate later) the involvement of associative learning mechanisms, in addition to simple exposure effects, in the establishment of learned olfactory preferences.

SUCKLING AS REINFORCEMENT. One of the more ubiquitous responses in the behavioral repertoires of mammalian infants is suckling, and this behavior has been exploited in studies of infant learning and memory. Sucking has proved to be a particularly malleable operant. For example, human newborns can alter various parameters of their sucking behavior to maximize their obtaining either milk reinforcement from a nipple (Sameroff, 1973) or the opportunity to hear a recording of their mothers' voices (DeCasper and Fifer, 1980).

Moreover, the opportunity to suckle (from either an artificial nipple or an anesthetized dam) is a potent reinforcer in both classical and instrumental conditioning paradigms. Human infants displayed conditioned sucking responses to a tone paired with a nonnutritive artificial nipple (Lipsitt and Kaye, 1964) or to a light touch paired with the presentation of a pipette filled with sucrose (Blass *et al.*, 1984). Beagle puppies could learn (Stanley, Bacon, and Fehr, 1970) and reverse (Bacon and Stanley, 1970) a tactile discrimination when the opportunity to suckle from a nutritive artificial nipple was the reinforcer. Amsel and his colleagues (Amsel *et al.*, 1976; Amsel, Letz, and Burdette, 1977a) have shown that infant rats about 10–11 days old increased their runway running speed to suckle the nonlactating nipples of their anesthetized dam. Similarly, Kenny and Blass (1977) found that 7-day-old rat pups were able to learn a spatial Y-maze discrimination for the opportunity to suckle. In these studies, either reversal or extinction of the response was also demonstrated. In fact, rat pups indicated their presumed "frustration" at the lack of reinforcement during extinction by emitting ultrasound vocalizations (Amsel, Radek, Graham, and Letz, 1977b).

Of particular significance in establishing the reinforcing value of suckling stimulation was the finding reported by Blass and his colleagues (Kenny, Stoloff, Bruno, and Blass, 1979) that pups younger than age 12 days were motivated by the opportunity to suckle and were seemingly oblivious to the nutritive consequences of their choice. When the infants were reinforced with nonnutritive suckling in one arm of the maze, and with suckling accompanied by milk infusion in the other arm, they failed to discriminate between the two arms until the were 12–15 days old, at which time they began to prefer the arm that led to nutritive suckling. The milk was clearly irrelevant to the younger pups in this situation, whereas suckling— apparently for its own sake and independent of its nutritive consequences—was reinforcing to the young infant.

SUMMARY. Warmth, exposure to home odors, and suckling can all serve as reinforcers to the young infant in various laboratory learning paradigms. In many cases, the learning that these reinforcers promote endures for days or weeks (Fillion and Blass, 1986b; Galef and Kaner, 1980). These sources of reinforcement are present in the natural environment of the infant, and we believe that they contribute to normal behavioral change in part through the mechanisms of associative learning. Evidence for this proposition comes from studies we have conducted on learning in both experimental and "natural" situations.

MILK AS INCENTIVE FOR ASSOCIATIVE LEARNING IN INFANT RATS

Our studies in the last few years demonstrate that, under certain conditions, milk is a potent reinforcer for infant rats. Furthermore, recent work from our laboratory (discussed below) suggests that *milk is rewarding to the deprived infant in part because its odor has been associated with stimulation provided by the dam;* the nutritive properties of the milk may, in fact, contribute little to its rewarding properties in the very young infant. That is, an infant's early experiences with the odor of milk—perceived in concert with other rewarding stimulation provided by the dam—can influence the infant's subsequent behaviors, and, more generally, can gain control over a variety of behaviors (social and sexual, as well as ingestive), both during infancy and in adulthood (e.g., Alberts and Brunjes, 1978; Fillion and Blass, 1985, 1986; Pedersen and Blass, 1981, 1982).

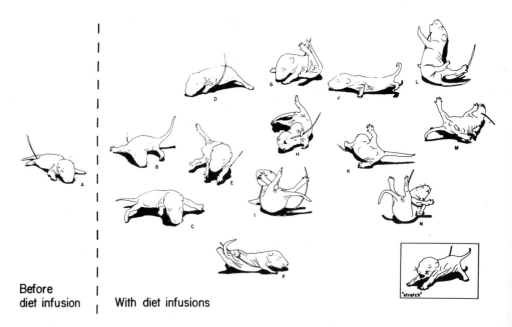

Before diet infusion | With diet infusions

Figure 1. Diagram of some of the behaviors shown by 3-day-old rat pups in response to milk infusions and milk odor. The individual drawings do not portray an actual sequence; rather, they provide examples of pups' initial response to milk with mouthing and probing of the floor (B, C) that becomes more vigorous and is extended to twisting and locomotion (D, E, F, G). Pups often roll and curl (H, I) and exhibit forms of locomotion, probing, reaching and posturing (J–N). Some of these responses (G, L) may be components of maternal "search" behaviors. ,

Our studies in infant learning and memory have, as their basis, the independent ingestive behavior system described in infant rats by Hall (1979). The basic features of this system are as follows: From birth, infant rats can be induced to ingest milk infused into their mouths through oral cannulas (Hall, 1979) or spread on the floor beneath them (Hall and Bryan, 1980). Milk intake is directly related to the pups' deprivational state. In deprived infants younger than 9 days of age, milk intake is accompanied by a dramatic behavioral activation, depicted in Figure 1. This activation is characterized by mouthing, probing, rolling, and excited locomotion. As pups grows older, these global activational responses disappear, and food elicits the more discrete and focused behaviors that typify adult ingestion. Ingestion of milk and the accompanying behavioral activation occur only in the context of a warm ambient temperature (Hall, 1979; Johanson and Hall, 1980).

OPERANT CONDITIONING IN NEONATES. We began our studies of infant learning with the speculation that the behavioral activation shown by young deprived pups in response to milk infusions was an external manifestation of positive affect and "reward." We (Johanson and Hall, 1979) evaluated this possibility by determining whether pups would learn to perform some task in order to obtain infusions of

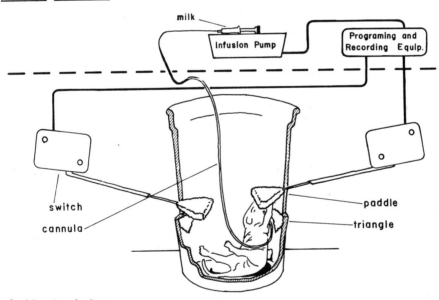

Figure 2. Diagram of the apparatus used for the operant learning experiments. The test container was a styrofoam cup. Terrycloth-covered paddles extended into the container and were mounted 3–4 cm from the floor. An upward force of 3–3.5 g was required to activate an infusion. In the simple learning paradigm, pups were provided with one paddle. In the discrimination situation (shown here), two different odors were placed on terrycloth triangles below the paddles. An upward probe into one paddle produced a small milk infusion, and a probe into the other paddle only triggered a counter. The test container was placed inside an incubator maintained at 34°C. An infusion pump and recording equipment were located outside the incubator.

milk. One- and three-day-old pups were placed in a 32–34°C incubator and were required to probe up into a terrycloth-covered paddle to obtain a small amount of milk delivered into the pup's mouth via an intraoral cannula. A diagram of the apparatus used for these studies is shown in Figure 2.

Pups as young as 1 day were very capable of appetitive operant learning for milk reward (Johanson and Hall, 1979; reviewed in Johanson and Hall, 1984). Initially, the experimental pups responded at rates similar to those observed in yoked controls (which received milk whenever the experimental pup responded, but whose own paddles were ineffective) and deprived controls (which did not receive milk). After a few hours of training, however, the experimental pups probed at much higher rates, as can be seen in the reconstructed cumulative record of a representative 1-day-old pup (see Figure 3a). One- and three-day-old pups also readily learned to discriminate between a paddle that yielded milk from one that did not, and they restricted their probing to the paddle that produced milk (Figure 3b). In both the simple and the discriminative operant paradigms, the experimental pups generally responded to the rewarding paddle several hundred times over the course of 12–16 h of testing—not a mean feat, considering a force of approximately 50% of their body weight was required to receive 1–2 μl of milk.

Our success in obtaining learning in these very young pups was undoubtedly due to our selection of ambient, discriminative, and reinforcing stimuli and instrumental responses that are highly related. Specifically, the upward probing response that was rewarded is also on occasion elicited by milk and milk odor, a situation reminiscent of the phenomenon of autoshaping. We now believe that this probing may, in fact, be a component of the infants' "maternal search" behavior; that is, it can be elicited in maternally deprived pups by a variety of cues (especially olfactory

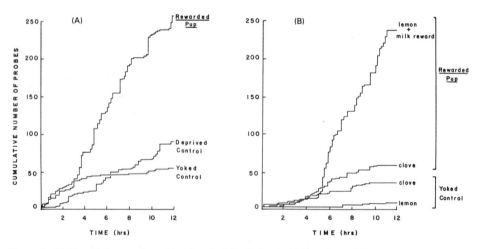

Figure 3. (a) Cumulative number of probes (in 10-min intervals) into the paddle made by a representative 1-day old pup that was rewarded with a milk infusion for each probe. The littermate yoked-control and deprived-control pups made fewer probes over the 12 h of testing. (b) Cumulative number of upward probe (in 10-min intervals) made by a representative pup in the discrimination situation. This pup's littermate yoked control responded very little overall and did not discriminate between the paddles.

and tactile cues) that have been associated with the mother (discussed further below).

CONDITIONED ORIENTATION PREFERENCE TO ODORS ASSOCIATED WITH MILK. Rat pups undoubtedly form many associations in the operant paradigm that we developed, for example, classically conditioned associations between the odor that labels the rewarding paddle and the milk. In an attempt to isolate one of the associations that the pups might be learning, we next developed a classical conditioning paradigm in which a novel odor was explicitly paired with milk infusions (Johanson and Hall, 1982; Johanson and Teicher, 1980).

For the experimental group (C/M pups), a cedar-scented airstream was presented for 15 sec before a brief milk infusion, for a total of 10 trials. One control group received cedar exposure only (C); another group received milk infusions only (M); a third group received milk infusions followed 20 min later by cedar exposure (M C); and fourth group was untreated (UNT). For all of these groups, training occurred inside a warm (34°C) incubator. An additional group recieved C/M pairings at room temperature (26°C). Pups were then given a two-choice olfactory preference test similar to the one used by Cornwell (1975) and Rudy and Cheatle (1977). They were placed in the middle of a plastic screen suspended over a container that had fresh bedding on one side and cedar-scented bedding on the other. For each pup, the time spent over the unscented bedding and the cedar-scented bedding was measured in five 1-min trials.

Three-day-old pups that were exposed to cedar before receiving milk infusions (C/M pups in Figure 4) clearly preferred the cedar-scented bedding to the unscented bedding, and they spent much more time over the cedar-scented side than any of the controls. Conditioning at 6 days of age was less robust than at 3 days, but it still occurred: after training, 6-day-old pups no longer showed the marked aversion to cedar seen in their controls, though they did not come to prefer cedar to pine as the 3-day-olds did. At 9 days of age, pups given cedar–milk pairings did not differ from pups receiving control treatments on any of the measures of preference. The treatment had no apparent effect on the pups' tendency to orient toward cedar, though, as we shall see below, pups at this age display components of ingestive responding to an olfactory CS associated with milk infusions.

The altered response to cedar odor was retained by both 3- and 6-day-old pups for at least 24 h (the maximum retention interval tested in this study), a finding indicating good retention after just a few training trials. Subsequent experiments on the emergence of conditioned ingestive responses (activity, mouthing, and probing) to an odor CS (conditioned stimulus) using this paradigm indicated substantially longer retention intervals (from 6 to 9 days; discussed below). Enduring memory has been demonstrated in other types of olfactory conditioning tasks, as well (see, for example, Rudy and Cheatle, 1977; Stickrod et al., 1982), the findings suggesting that infants' memories may be much better than we previously suspected.

The conditioned preference was specific to the odor used during training. Three-day-old pups for whom the cedar odor was paired with milk oriented to

INGRID B.
JOHANSON AND
LESLIE M. TERRY

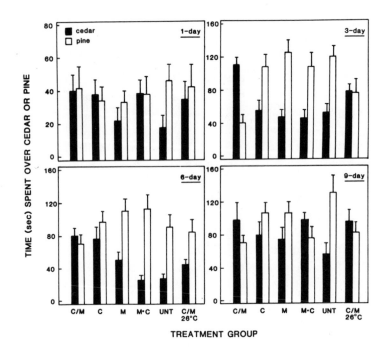

Figure 4. Mean total time spent over cedar (black bars) or pine (unfilled bars) for 1- to 9-day-old pups. Experimental pups (C/M) were given 10 cedar–milk pairings. Controls received cedar exposure alone (C); milk infusions alone (M); milk infusions followed by cedar exposure (M/C); or no treatment (UNT); or they were trained with cedar–milk pairings at 26°C.

cedar but behaved similarly to controls in avoiding another strong odor (clove). Conversely, pups trained with clove used as the conditioned odor cue oriented to clove but avoided cedar. The conditioned orientation preference clearly did not generalize to any strong, novel odor; it was specific to the odor associated with milk.

Both deprivation and warmth were necessary in order for the ingestion of milk and its accompanying behavioral activation to occur (Hall, 1979; Johanson and Hall, 1980), and both were critical determinants of the altered responsiveness to an odor paired with milk. Nondeprived pups and pups trained in a cool (26°C) ambient temperature both showed no preference for cedar-scented bedding over unscented bedding.

RESPONSE CONDITIONING TO ODORS ASSOCIATED WITH MILK. Not only did pups learn to orient to an odor that was paired with milk delivery, but they also showed conditioning of some of the components of their ingestive behavior (i.e., activation, mouthing, and probing) to the odor cue (Johanson, Hall, and Polefrone, 1984). In another series of experiments, a cedar-scented airstream (CS) was presented for 5 s before a brief milk infusion (US), for a total of 20 trials, 4 min apart. One control group received cedar exposure only; another group received milk infusions only; and a third group (which served as a control for pseudoconditioning) received milk infusions for the first 15 trials and cedar–milk pairings for the last 5 trials. Training occurred inside a warm (34°C) incubator. We rated the pups' level of activity on a scale of 0 (no activity) to 6 (frenzied locomotion around the test container, including vigorous probing, rolling, and wall climbing), and we also noted the occurrence of mouthing and probing, both during the 5-s CS interval during training and in five CS-only trials after training.

From 3 to 12 days of age, pups that had been exposed to a cedar odor CS before receiving milk showed components of their ingestive behavior in response to the onset of the CS. Figure 5 shows the magnitude of activity, mouthing, and probing that occurred during the CS interval over the course of training a group of 6-day-old pups. At each age, the pattern of conditioned responses (CRs) elicited by an odor paired with milk clearly reflected the pattern of unconditioned responses (URs) shown to milk. That is, 3- and 6-day-old trained pups responded to the CS onset with a marked behavioral activation, including mouthing and probing, the type of response shown by pups of these ages to milk infusions. Similarly, in CS-only trials conducted after training, 3- and 6-day-old pups responded to the odor CS with activity, mouthing, and probing. In contrast to younger pups, trained 9- and 12-day-old pups did not become active to the odor in CS-only trials, though they did mouth and probe. This lack of activation to the CS may have reflected the more subdued unconditioned responses shown by older animals to milk.

Surprisingly, there were no obvious differences in how readily pups of the various ages acquired some form of conditioned response. The younger pups

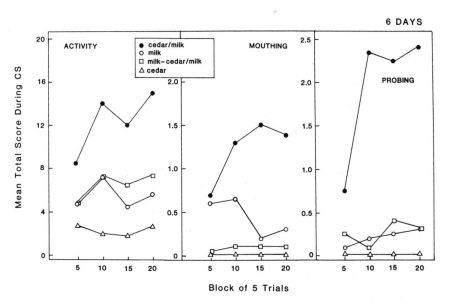

Figure 5. Mean activity, mouthing, and probing scores in the CS interval during training of 6-day-old rat pups. Trials are presented in blocks of 5 trials. The maximum activity score is 30; the maximum mouthing and probing score is 5.

seemed to acquire the association as readily as the older pups. The development of conditioned responding during training was sometimes obscured in very young pups by the activation produced by the milk. Both 1- and 3-day-old pups appeared to become fatigued, satiated, or simply less reactive by the end of training, so that previously high levels of response to the CS declined toward the end of training. This pattern of responding paralleled the young pups' unconditioned response to milk, with both conditioned and unconditioned activity reaching a peak between 5 and 15 trials, and declining somewhat thereafter.

The pups retained their conditioned responsiveness to the odor CS for several days following training. Although 1-day-olds did not show clear evidence of conditioned responding on the day they were trained, the trained pups became active and mouthed and probed when they were presented with the odor CS 24 h after training. Pups trained at age 3 days showed some retention for up to 6 days later, and those trained at 6 days showed retention of conditioned mouthing at age 15 days (i.e., a retention interval of 9 days).

Significantly, as these trained pups grew older, the types of responses that were shown to a previously conditioned stimulus seemed to change to reflect the infants' now more mature ingestive behavior. For example, when tested for retention at 9 days of age, pups trained at 6 days responded to the CS just as 9-day-olds would respond to milk infusions: they mouthed and probed, but they did not become very active. This finding suggests a certain plasticity in the organization of learning and memory in infants, in that it appears that a conditioned stimulus that elicits certain conditioned motor responses at younger ages can, at a later point in development, gain access to the now more mature motor patterns of which the infant is capable.

As with altered odor preference, the conditioned responses did not generalize to other odor stimuli. Infants trained with cedar odor as the CS, and then tested in CS-only trials with cedar, clove, or unscented air, responded only to the cedar odor, and not the other stimuli. The olfactory component of the CS was clearly important in eliciting the conditioned responding, in that the somatosensory stimulation of the unscented airstream elicited no response.

A variety of factors can affect the form or strength of a conditioned response, including the nature of the conditioned stimulus (e.g., Holland, 1977). We initially chose an odor for the conditioned stimulus because infant rats can readily detect odors (Alberts and May, 1980), and odors may be particularly associable with feeding. However, CSs in other modalities may also be capable of being associated with ingestion. For example, Rudy and Hyson (1982) found that an auditory stimulus paired with sucrose infusions came to elicit conditioned mouthing in 12- to 15-day-old pups. We found that vibrotactile stimulation can also serve as an effective CS in this conditioning paradigm; 3-, 6-, and 9-day-old rat pups trained with a vibration CS preceding milk infusion responded to the CS with some probing (and in 3- and 6-day-olds, mouthing), but the CS elicited little increased activity. Here, the forms of conditioned and unconditioned responses differed; the former involved only certain components of the unconditioned response to milk. The different pattern of responding from what was found with an olfactory CS may have reflected differences in the relative intensity of the stimulation provided by the CS. Alternatively, olfactory stimuli might be particularly associable with food, so that a pattern of conditioned responding results that is very similar to the pattern of unconditioned responding. The finding (discussed below) that the odor of milk without any accompanying oral infusions can elicit ingestive responses such as activation, mouthing, and proving gives added support to the idea that olfactory cues may be particularly important in the sensory control of these behaviors.

Internal state determined to a large extent the development of conditioned responding. We attempted to condition ingestive responding in pups in two different deprivational states: nondeprived pups and pups dehydrated with 1% NaCl. Dehydrated 3-day-olds showed some probing to the odor CS, but they did not become active, nor did they mouth. Nondeprived pups failed to show any evidence of conditioning, even if they were subsequently deprived during a retention test. Significantly, the only reliable conditioned responding was seen in pups that had been deprived of both food and maternal care for 24 h before training.

ACTIVATION AND LEARNING. The failure to obtain reliable orientation and response conditioning in nondeprived and dehydrated pups may be due, at least in part, to their lack of activation in response to milk infusions. This interpretation is supported by the growing evidence that activation may be necessary—though perhaps it is not sufficient—for early olfactory learning to occur. Pedersen *et al.* (1982) reported that stimulating pups (by amphetamine injection or by anogenital stroking with a soft brush) in the presence of an odor resulted in the pups' preferentially attaching to nipples scented with that odor, though the stimulant caffeine did not result in preferential attachment. Also, Sullivan *et al.* (1986) reported that any of several methods for producing activation (e.g., tail pinch, exposure to salivary gland odor, or stroking) could be paired with a novel odor to produce a relative preference for that odor, but a contingency must exist between the odor and the activation to produce altered preference. Together, these studies suggest that certain types of stimulation provided by the mother (e.g., anogenital licking) may serve as significant sources of reinforcement in the normal nest context, in part because they "activate" or "arouse" the infant.

SUMMARY. From the research discussed so far, it is clear that even very young infants are capable of quite complex learning, especially when the learning situation is constructed to incorporate some of the unique aspects of the infants' environment. In particular, evidence of infant learning has been obtained most readily when the infant has been provided with some or all aspects of the mother or the nest environment, either as an ambient cue or as an incentive for learning. Given the availability in the natural environment of the infant of such reinforcers as warmth, home odors, and the opportunity to suckle, we are left with the question of whether infants actually use their demonstrated learning capabilities as a mechanism for behavioral change during normal development.

INGRID B.
JOHANSON AND
LESLIE M. TERRY

ASSOCIATIVE LEARNING AND THE DEVELOPMENT OF SOCIAL, SEXUAL, AND INGESTIVE BEHAVIOR

There is abundant—though somewhat indirect—evidence that associative learning mechanisms may contribute to the normal development of certain vital behaviors, particularly in the development of the social, sexual and ingestive behaviors of rats.

DEVELOPMENT OF HUDDLING PREFERENCES. During the first few weeks after birth, infant rats huddle with objects solely on the basis of thermotactile stimulation (Alberts, 1978; Alberts and Brunjes, 1978; Cosnier, 1965). By the end of the second week, rat pups prefer to huddle with warm objects that also bear appropriate (i.e. conspecific) olfactory cues (Alberts and Brunjes, 1978). Alberts and his colleagues have provided evidence that the pups' preferences for conspecific odors are acquired as a result of specific experiences with their dam. Pups that had been reared by mothers scented with an artificial (nonrat) odor displayed, at age 15 days, a preference to huddle with objects scented with the odor to which they had been exposed.

Although simple exposure to an odor was sufficient to induce an olfactory preference, it did not induce the same degree of preference as that produced from olfactory experiences associated with some aspects of maternal care. Infants given equivalent amounts of exposure to two artificial odors, one of which had been experienced in a "simple exposure" situation and the other of which had been painted on their dam, overwhelmingly preferred the odor associated with the dam (Alberts, 1981).

What aspect of "mother" was necessary to induce olfactory huddling preferences? It turned out that experience with odors associated with the opportunity to suckle and obtain milk added little to the development of olfactory preference: pups alternated between a dam whose nipples were involuted, so that suckling could not occur, and a lactating dam, each labeled with a different odor, and showed no differences in preference for the two odors. On the other hand, odors associated with a warm tube were as effective in inducing an olfactory preference as a lactating dam.

These studies provide strong evidence that associative learning mechanisms may play an important role in the development of early filial behaviors. Specifically, it seems that, during the first two weeks after birth, infants learn an association between conspecific odors and the warmth provided by the dam that is critical to their later preference for huddling with conspecifics (Alberts, 1981).

SUCKLING AND OLFACTORY LEARNING. Infant rats rely primarily on olfactory cues in their search for nipples to suckle, and the cues that they use appear to be modulated, as well, by early olfactory experiences.

Evidence of the critical importance of olfactory cues in mediating suckling behavior in infant rats comes from two sources. First, olfactory bulbectomy or zinc sulfate lavage eliminates suckling and can prove fatal to pups (e.g., Hill and Almli, 1981; Singh and Tobach, 1975; Singh, Tucker, and Hofer, 1976; Teicher, Flaum, Williams, Eckhert, and Lumia, 1978; Tobach, Rouger, and Schneirla, 1967). The survival rate of pups following bulbectomy can be considerably enhanced by performing the procedure shortly after birth (Hill and Almli, 1981) or by favorable postoperative rearing conditions (Teicher *et al.*, 1978), both of which apparently promote a compensatory reliance on tactile cues for attaching to the nipple.

Second, removal or alteration of the olfactory cues that normally elicit attachment completely disrupts the suckling behavior of young pups. Blass and his colleagues (Blass *et al.*, 1977; Bruno, Teicher, and Blass, 1980) found that rat pups from 2 to 28 days of age would not attach to a nipple thoroughly washed of olfactory cues. Returning a distillate of the wash of pup saliva to the nipples reliably reinstated suckling (see also Hofer, Shair, and Singh, 1976). The active ingredient in pup saliva that appears to be responsible for saliva-eliciting attachment has been identified as dimethyl disulfide (DMDS; Pedersen and Blass, 1981), a sulfur compound also found in the vaginal secretions of estrous female hamsters (Singer, Agosta, O'Connell, Pfaffman, Bowen, and Field, 1976).

Like what occurs with older pups, the first nipple attachment is also eliminated by washing the dam's nipples, and in this case the application of amniotic fluid, newly parturient mother's saliva, or wash distillate to the nipples returns attachment by newborns to normal levels (Teicher and Blass, 1977). A combination of amniotic fluid and maternal saliva is undoubtedly applied to the nipples by the female, as she licks the vaginal and nipple areas during the delivery of her pups (Roth and Rosenblatt, 1965), and these substances then guide the newborn to the nipples.

What is the evidence for the involvement of learning mechanisms in the development of the olfactory control of suckling behavior? Pedersen and Blass (1981, 1982) reasoned that the infants' prenatal and early postnatal experiences with amniotic fluid may be responsible for establishing it as an elicitor of the infants' first nipple attachment, based on observations that fetuses ingest and probably detect chemical substances in amniotic fluid (by taste, Farbman, 1965; or by vomeronasal stimulation, Pedersen, Stewart, Greer, and Shepherd, 1983). To test this idea, Pedersen and Blass (1982) altered the odorous quality of the amniotic fluid by injecting a citral solution into the uterus of pregnant rats. Then, to mimic the dam's vigorous licking of the pup that occurs shortly after birth, the pups were stroked with an artist's brush in a citral-scented environment for an hour following birth. Pups that received this pre- and postnatal exposure to citral odor subsequently attached to nipples that were washed, but they did so only in the presence of citral odor. Moreover, only the combination of pre- and postnatal exposure to citral elicited suckling of washed nipples scented with citral; neither prenatal nor postnatal experience alone was effective. Although these results could be accounted for by simple exposure learning, it is certainly likely that a learned association between odorous substances in amniotic fluid and maternal saliva, as well as the activating effects of maternal licking and handling, contributed to the establishment of these initial preferences. Associations formed between the odorous components of amniotic fluid and pup saliva may, then, serve to subsequently establish pup saliva (and its component DMDS) as an elicitor of nipple attachment behavior.

OLFACTORY EXPERIENCE AND SEXUAL BEHAVIOR. Such early olfactory learning experiences—especially those associated with suckling—seem to bias adult sexual preferences, as Fillion and Blass (1985, 1986 a,b) have demonstrated. They found that pups are as responsive to odors from estrous (but not diestrous) virgin females as they are to the nipple and vaginal odors of the lactating dam; in both cases, pups probe and attempt to suckle (Fillion & Blass, 1986a). Further, pups' responsiveness to estrous odors appears to be dependent, by 10 days of age, on specific olfactory experience. Infants reared by dams whose nipple and vaginal odors were altered with citral did not probe at 10 days of age in response to estrous odors, except when they occurred in combination with citral, whereas infants reared by dams whose backs, only, were citral-scented probed normally in response to estrous odors (Fillion and Blass, 1986a).

Of particular interest are the long-term consequences of such early rearing experiences for later sexual preferences. As adults, males reared by dams whose nipple and vaginal odors were altered with citral were slow to mate with normal estrous females, but they mated readily when such females were scented vaginally with citral (Fillion and Blass, 1986b). Normally reared males, on the other hand, or those reared by dams whose backs, only, were citral-scented, mated as readily or more readily with normal estrous females. Fillion and Blass speculated that the response of the virgin adult male to estrous odors is determined by its infantile experience with the similar odors of the dam's nipples and vagina—odors that become activating for the infant in the context of suckling. In this connection, these authors suggested the possibility that estrous odors may include that of dimethyl disulfide (DMDS), which has been found in vaginal secretions of estrous female hamsters (Singer *et al.*, 1976) and which has been implicated as well in the elicitation of nipple attachment in infant rats (Pedersen and Blass, 1981).

Another possible explanation is that young pups may be exposed to activating stimuli (maternal licking and handling) in the presence of vaginal odors from their dam's postpartum estrus. Anogenital licking of male pups by their dam has been shown to stimulate the development of their secondary sexual organs and to affect their competency in mating (Moore, 1984), so this explanation is certainly plausible.

Together, these findings suggest that associations that infants form between odors and other stimuli provided by the dam may persist well past the preweaning period and gain control over adult sexual behavior patterns.

DEVELOPMENT OF FOOD PREFERENCES. The enduring effects of the associations that infants acquire between odors and other stimuli provided by the dam are revealed as well in the development of food preferences. Considerable evidence suggests that food choice at weaning is modified by the olfactory and gustatory stimuli experienced during the preweaning period. Cues concerning the mother's diet are transmitted through her milk and her fecal and cecal material and determine, in part, the pup's choice of food at weaning (Capretta and Rawls, 1974; Galef and Clark, 1972; Galef and Henderson, 1972).

Altered food preferences are reflected in the electrical activity of the olfactory bulbs, as well. Rat pups reared by mothers fed a eucalyptol-adulterated diet display, as adults, electrophysiological responses in the mitral cell layer to the odor of eucalyptol that normally reared animals display to food odors (Pager, 1974). Exposure to the odor must occur during the preweaning period in order to induce the change in electrophysiological responsiveness; adult rats placed on a eucalyptol-scented diet for the same length of time as the weanlings do not display altered responsiveness to eucalyptol.

Associative learning helps to account for the establishment of olfactory-based food preferences (Galef and Kaner, 1980). Although simple exposure to an odor induced a preference for the odor at 21 days of age, considerably longer lasting preferences could be induced by placing the odor on the ventrum of the dam. It seems likely that, when the odor was painted directly on the dam, the infants were provided with specific associations between the odor and the thermotactile, olfactory, suckling, or other stimulation provided by the dam. At this point, however, it is not clear what specific learned associations mediate this long-term change in olfactory-guided food preferences.

SUMMARY. Together, these studies indicate that associations that the infants acquire between odors and other stimulation provided by the dam (e.g., warmth, the opportunity to suckle, the activation produced by licking and cleaning, and even other odors) not only may influence infantile behaviors, such as huddling or suckling but may also persist well past the preweaning period to gain control over adult behavioral patterns (such as sexual and feeding behavior). The findings from these studies clearly suggest that infant rats actually use the impressive learning capabilities that we have described above—especially their ability to acquire classically conditioned olfactory associations—in the natural context of mother and nest.

OLFACTORY CONTROLS OF INGESTIVE BEHAVIOR: CLASSICAL CONDITIONING IN THE NEST?

We believe that we now have some more direct evidence that infant rats use their learning abilities in the nest. This evidence stems from a paradigm of "olfactory learning" in the home environment that has direct parallels to the milk-reinforced classical conditioning paradigms that we have described above. Specifically, artificial odors that have been associated with the dam come to elicit behavioral activation and probing similar to that shown to milk and milk odor, in much the same way that artificial odors explicitly associated with milk infusions in a classical conditioning paradigm come to elicit these same responses.

PUPS' RESPONSES TO MILK ODOR. The finding that certain components of pups' response to milk—namely, activity, mouthing, and probing—can come under olfactory control raised the possibility that milk odor might also come to elicit behavioral activation. Accordingly, we evaluated the extent to which the olfactory qualities of milk contributed to behavioral excitement in young pups.

To test the possibility that pups may respond to the odor of milk in much the same way that they respond to oral infusions of milk, 24-h-deprived pups from 1 to 12 days of age were presented with either an airstream scented with the odor of commercially available heavy cream or an unscented airstream. These airstreams were presented alone or were accompanied by intraoral infusions of water, sucrose, quinine, or milk. Pups received a total of five exposures to the odor–infusion combination in a standard 12-min test. The first odor–infusion presentation began at the end of a 2-min adaptation period, with subsequent presentations occurring every 2 min. During each 15-s interval of the 12-min test, the pups' level of activity was scored on a scale of 0 (no activity) to 6 (frenzied locomotion), and the occurrence of mouthing and probing was noted. The activity data are presented as a total activity score for the 10 min in which the odor–infusion presentations occurred. For both mouthing and probing, the data are presented as the total number of 15-sec intervals in which mouthing or probing was observed.

The results from this experiment are shown in Figure 6, which indicates the levels of activity, mouthing, and probing to milk odor (black bars) or no odor (cross-hatched bars) in 1- to 12-day-old pups *without* accompanying intraoral infusions), and in Figure 7, which depicts the level of probing to milk odor or no odor in pups receiving infusions of water, sucrose, quinine, or milk. One-day-old rats

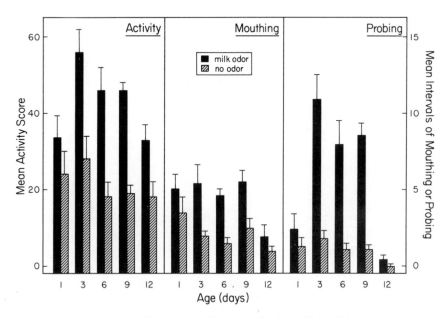

Figure 6. Mean activity, mouthing, and probing scores for 1- to 12-day-old pups exposed to milk odor (black bar) or no odor (cross-hatch bar).

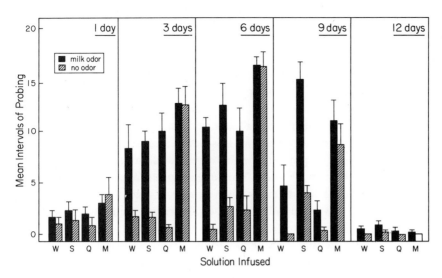

Figure 7. Mean total intervals of probing of 1- to 12-day-old pups exposed to milk odor (black bar) or no odor (cross-hatch bar) while receiving infusions of water, sucrose, quinine, or milk.

showed little response to milk odor and were, for that matter, relatively unresponsive, behaviorally, to oral infusions of milk. However, by age 3 days, milk odor elicited high levels of activity and vigorous mouthing and probing, even when no oral infusions were made (see Figure 6). In fact, accompanying infusions of water, sucrose, or quinine did not further enhance the pups' response to milk odor (Figure 7; Terry and Johanson, 1987).

Probing, in particular, was specifically elicited by the odor of milk: infusions of sucrose or water that were paired with the odor of milk elicited two to three times as much probing as infusions without accompanying milk odor (Figure 7). In some cases (e.g., in the 3- and 9-day-olds), milk odor without any concomitant gustatory stimulation elicited as much probing as an infusion of milk, a finding suggesting that it is the odor of the milk that is primarily responsible for eliciting probing and other aspects of behavioral activation. Although the effects on mouthing behavior were not quite as pronounced as the effects on activity and probing and tended to be obscured when oral infusions were made, we nevertheless found that 3- to 9-day-old pups mouthed in response to milk odor. The effects of exposing pups to milk odor extended beyond eliciting these specific components of pups' ingestive behavior: 6- and 9-day-old pups increased their intake of various sapid solutions by 20%–25% in the presence of milk odor, thereby providing additional evidence that milk odor may serve as a CS linked to ingestive behavior.

Age-related changes in behavior elicited by milk odor parallel those observed in pups during independent feeding (Hall, 1979; Hall and Bryan, 1980). Pups less than 1 week old are the most active and probe most vigorously to oral infusions of milk, and it was these younger pups that responded most to milk odor. By age 9 days, the diffuse activation elicited by milk tends to be replaced by more directed

ingestive behavior, and again, this change from generalized activation to less frenzied and more discrete behavior was also seen in response to milk odor.

The pups' responsiveness to milk odor was also modulated by two factors—
deprivational state and ambient temperature—that influence pups' intake and
behavioral activation during oral infusions of milk (Hall, 1979; Johanson and Hall,
1980). Nondeprived pups and pups that had been removed from their dams 24 h
before testing were exposed to the odor of milk, at either 32°C or 24°C, whereas
littermate controls were exposed to an unscented airstream. Only 24-h-deprived
pups tested in a warm environment became active and mouthed and probed when
they were presented with milk odor. Nondeprived pups and deprived pups tested
in a cool environment failed to show this vigorous activity when exposed to milk
odor (Figure 8). This is essentially the same pattern of results found with young
pups receiving oral infusions of milk (Hall, 1979; Johanson and Hall, 1980), finding supporting the view that the effects of milk odor on behavioral activation are
very much like the effects of oral infusions of milk in rat pups.

Finally, these effects—the behavioral activation, the increased probing, and
the enhanced ingestion of sapid fluids—were elicited only by the odor of milk and
were not observed in response to other strong odors (cedar, clove, or rat chow).
Pups were not simply reacting to the presence of any strong odor, therefore, but
were showing rather specific responsiveness to the odor of milk.

We believe that milk odor may acquire its activating effects by being associ-

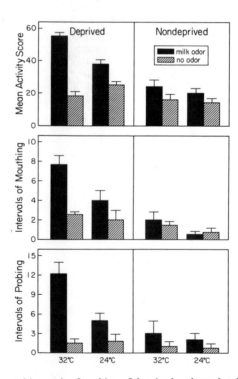

Figure 8.   Mean total intervals of probing of deprived and nondeprived 6-day-old pups,
exposed to milk odor or no odor at either 24°C or 34°C.

ated, via the mechanism of classical conditioning, with other types of reinforcing stimulation provided by the dam, for example, her warmth, the tactile stimulation she provides, or the opportunity to engage in suckling and its various components behaviors (nipple search, attachment, sucking, and stretching). That is, milk odor may be established during the first few days after birth as a CS for "mother" or some component of "mother." We base this hypothesis on two lines of research from our lab. First, destruction of the main olfactory and vomeronasal systems (which appears to disrupt pups' "maternal recognition" behavior; Teicher, Shaywitz, and Lumia, 1984) disrupts pups' responsiveness to milk odor. Second, a novel odor that has been associated with the dam during the first few days after birth comes to elicit activation and probing in deprived infants. The remainder of this chapter describes these studies and their implications in detail.

THE ROLE OF MAIN AND ACCESSORY OLFACTORY SYSTEMS IN MEDIATING PUPS' RESPONSES TO MILK ODOR. We found that intact functioning of both the main and the accessory olfactory systems is necessary in order for the odor of milk to elicit high levels of behavioral activation, and specifically probing (Terry, 1985). In these experiments, 5-day-old pups were rendered anosmic with a $ZnSO_4$ lavage of the nasal mucosa (Singh, *et al.*, 1976) or were deprived of vomeronasal input by a sectioning of the vomeronasal nerve as it passes through the medial portion of the olfactory bulbs (using the technique described by Powers, Fields, and Winans, 1979). Controls either received a NaCl lavage of the nares (as a control for $ZnSO_4$ lavage) or were sham-operated (as a control for the vomeronasal nerve cut; sham-operated pups were treated identically to vomeronasal nerve-sectioned pups, except that the scissors were inserted into the bulb and then removed without cutting the nerve). The day after either main or accessory deafferentation, following 24 h of deprivation, the pups were tested for their responsiveness to oral infusions of milk, or to oral infusions of water accompanied by milk odor, a novel odor (eucalyptol), or unscented air (as a "no-odor" condition). Odor–infusion exposures (15s in duration) occurred every 2 min for a total of 10 min, or five exposures. Pups' activity, mouthing, and probing were scored in each 15-s interval.

Pups made anosmic by $ZnSO_4$ lavage displayed reduced activity to milk infusions and to milk odor accompanied by water infusions, although their levels of activity in response to "no odor" or eucalyptol odor were similar to the activity levels of controls. Intake of both milk and water was somewhat suppressed in $ZnSO_4$-treated pups, though the level of intake was still substantial (they ingested an average of 59.7% of the infusion volume versus 78.3% for controls). This difference in intake was not due to any gastric distress produced by ingestion of the $ZnSO_4$ during the lavage, in that pups given $ZnSO_4$ orally ingested as much as controls. Most striking, $ZnSO_4$-induced anosmia virtually eliminated the high levels of probing normally shown to milk infusions or to the odor of milk (Figure 9).

Vomeronasal deafferentation also markedly reduced activity and probing in response to milk or its odor (Figure 10). Infants that had had their vomeronasal nerve sectioned ingested as much as sham-operated controls, but they were less active. Although vomeronasal deafferentation may depress general activity, the

INGRID B.
JOHANSON AND
LESLIE M. TERRY

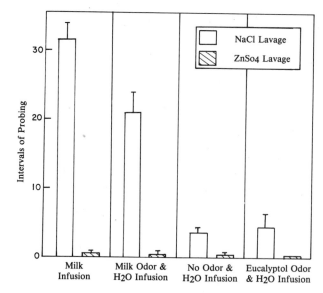

Figure 9. Mean total intervals of probing in ZnSO$_4$-treated or sham-treated 6-day-old pups, in response to milk odor, no odor, or eucalyptol odor.

effect that we observed was specific to activity elicited by milk or milk odor; sectioning of the vomeronasal nerve had no depressive effect on the levels of activity elicited by eucalyptol odor or unscented air. Although the technique for sectioning the vomeronasal nerve inevitably produced a small amount of damage to the main olfactory bulbs, vomeronasally deafferented pups were able to detect at least some odors (as indicated by their increased sniffing and turning away from a cotton swab dipped in cedar oil). That is, they did not seem to be anosmic.

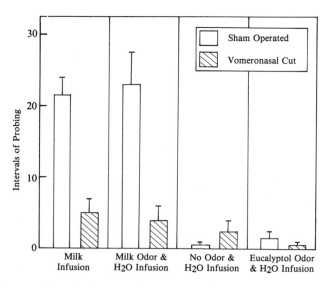

Figure 10. Mean total intervals of probing in vomeronasal-deafferented or sham-operated 6-day-old pups, in response to milk odor, no odor, or eucalyptol odor.

The pups' brains were removed five days following testing, and the effectiveness of the ZnSO₄ lavage and the vomeronasal nerve cues was assessed by examining the main and accessory olfactory bulbs for glomerular degeneration and absence of the mitral cell layer. Histological analysis using cresyl violet staining (Fleming, Vaccarino, Tambosso, and Chee, 1979) revealed no sign of glomerular shrinkage or degeneration in the main olfactory bulbs of any of the lavage controls (see Figure 11a); in contrast, the main olfactory bulbs of ZnSO₄-treated pups showed pronounced glomerular as well as mitral cell degeneration (Figure 11b). There was no evidence of any degeneration in the accessory olfactory bulb of these animals, a finding indicating that the deafferentation was limited to the main olfactory system in ZnSO₄-treated pups.

Analysis of the olfactory bulbs of vomeronasal-sectioned pups indicated poor lamination of the accessory olfactory bulb, as well as absence of the mitral cell layer (Figure 11d), but very little degeneration of the main olfactory glomeruli (less than 10% shrinkage in 5 of 29 vomeronasal-sectioned animals, with the remaining animals showing no evidence of shrinkage of glomeruli in the main bulbs). In other words, the histological evidence supports the behavioral evidence in indicating that the main olfactory system of these pups was essentially intact, whereas the vomeronasal system was not. Sham-operated controls displayed no signs of degeneration in either the main or the accessory olfactory bulbs. Incidentally, most of the ZnSO₄-treated and vomeronasal-sectioned pups survived for the five days between deafferentation and sacrifice for histology, though the ZnSO₄-treated pups all lost significant amounts of weight (pups with vomeronasal nerve section, on the other hand, weighed only slightly less than their sham-operated controls).

Given the lack of evidence of the involvement of the vomeronasal system in adult feeding behavior, why should deafferentation of the accessory olfactory system have this pronounced effect on pups' activational and probing responses to milk? One possible explanation for the importance of vomeronasal input in mediating behavioral activation is that the activity and probing are actually components of a system of behavioral responsiveness to the dam. The vomeronasal system has been implicated in the social and sexual behavior of adults (e.g., see Wysocki, 1979), and there is evidence that it is involved, as well, in infantile behaviors elicited by the dam, specifically suckling and maternal "recognition."

As discussed earlier, infant rats' perinatal experiences with amniotic fluid may facilitate nipple-attachment behavior, and the vomeronasal system may mediate this effect (Pedersen et al., 1983; 1986). Vomeronasal nerve sectioning, as well as bilateral olfactory bulbectomy, also appears to disrupt other facets of responsiveness to the mother in rat pups (Teicher et al., 1984). Pups normally show a high level of arousal to the ventral surface of their mother, but elimination of vomeronasal or both vomeronasal and main olfactory input caused pups to be most responsive to the dorsal surface of their mother. Teicher et al., (1984) suggested that, following vomeronasal deafferentation, the infants relied more on tactile cues (the long hair on the dorsal surface) than olfactory cues to assist them in directing their responses to the mother.

Consistent with the interpretation that the activity and probing are components of behavior elicited by maternal cues, it now appears that the activation that

INGRID B.
JOHANSON AND
LESLIE M. TERRY

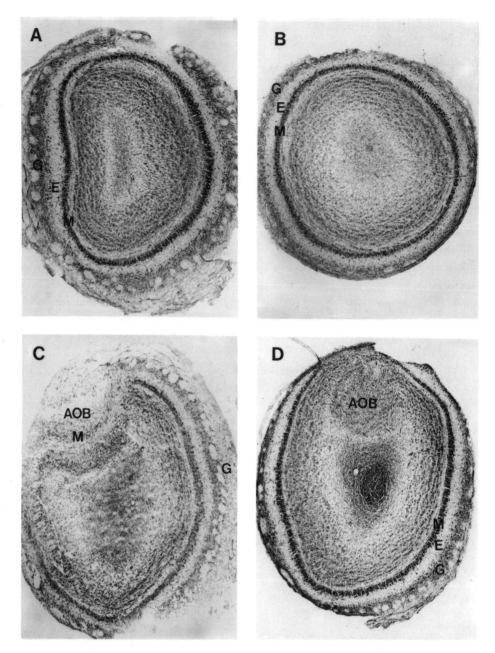

Figure 11. Coronal section through the olfactory bulb of 10- to 11-day-old rat pups. Pups were sacrificed for histology approximately five days after olfactory deafferentation (ZnSO₄ lavage or vomeronasal nerve cut). (a) Section through the main olfactory bulb (MOB) of a pup that had received a sham lavage (NaCl) of the nares. (b) Section through the MOB of a pup that had received a ZnSO₄ lavage of the nares five days earlier. Note the pronounced glomerular degeneration, indicating the effectiveness of the deafferentation procedure. (c) Section through the accessory olfactory bulb (AOB) of a sham-operated pup. (d) Section through the AOB of a pup in which the vomeronasal nerve had been sectioned five days earlier. Note the poor lamination of the AOB, and the absence of the mitral cell layer. Abbreviations: AOB, accessory olfactory bulb; MOB, main olfactory bulb; G, glomerular layer; E, external plexiform layer; M, mitral cell layer.

deprived pups display when they are fed is more a result of the deprivation of maternal care than a result of nutritive deprivation. Hall and his co-workers (Bornstein, Terry, Browde, Assimon, and Hall, 1987) found that the behavioral activation shown by deprived pups in response to milk infusions was critically dependent on their deprivation of maternal stimulation and was relatively unaffected by the dam's nutritional contribution to her pups. Six-day-old pups that were left with an anesthetized dam overnight, so that they had the opportunity to suckle and to remain in the presence of the dam's fur and odors, were, for the most part, behaviorally unresponsive to oral milk infusion, although their intake was equivalent to that of pups deprived of both maternal and nutritional care. One obvious possibility is that maternal deprivation consists of "suckling" deprivation, and that it is the lack of the opportunity to suckle during the 24-h deprivation period that results in pups' activational response to milk. However, deprivation of suckling *per se* appears to have little effect on pups' responses to milk. Pups that remained with a maternal virgin female (whose undeveloped nipples prevented suckling) over the typical 24-h deprivation period showed no behavioral excitement in response to milk infusions, though they still ingested large quantities of milk. These studies support the idea that the activation seen in response to milk is not a purely ingestive phenomenon but may be intimately tied to the stimulation that the infant receives from its dam.

Together, these studies indicate that the odor of milk is the powerful stimulus for eliciting components of pups' activational response to milk. This olfactory cue appears to be mediated through the main and accessory olfactory systems, with intact function in both being necessary for obtaining full responsiveness to the odor. Further, these studies support the growing evidence that the behavioral activation and probing elicited by milk and milk odor are actually a component of pups' responsiveness to the dam.

LEARNING ABOUT ODORS. Next, we speculated that these components of behavioral responsiveness to the mother had become conditioned to milk odor. Milk odor may have acquired its behavioral activating effects on pups through association with other types of reinforcing stimulation provided by the dam, for example, warmth, activating tactile stimulation, the opportunity to suckle, or even other odors from the dam, the siblings, and the nest environment.

The following evidence suggests the acquisition of olfactory significance by milk odor: First, behavioral responsiveness to milk and milk odor developed gradually. The 1-day-old pups in our studies had only limited contact with their dam being tested for their responsiveness to milk odor, and they failed to show significant activation. Perhaps the period of exposure to the necessary stimuli was not sufficient to establish olfactory learning in these very young pups. These results are, incidentally, in complete agreement with Hall's findings (1979) that 1-day-old pups showed much less activity and probing to milk infusions than slightly older pups, though their intakes of milk were substantially the same. Second, we knew that the behavioral activation shown by young pups to milk can readily come under the control of an olfactory conditioned stimulus. Pups come to display behavioral activation to a neutral odor cue that has been explicitly paired with oral milk infusions (Johanson *et al.*, 1984), and they also develop a marked orientation preference for that odor (Johanson and Hall, 1982; Johanson and Teicher, 1980). If the odor of milk has acquired its ability to elicit behavioral activation through the normal mother–infant relationship, then a novel odor that has been associated with the dam during the first few days after birth, like the odor of milk, should come to elicit activity, mouthing, and probing in deprived infant rats.

We attempted to alter the pups' early olfactory experiences with their dam by adding a distinctive odor (eucalyptol) to the dam's diet (assuming that this odor would adulterate her milk). We chose this paradigm based in part on Pager's finding (1974) that rats reared by dams fed a diet containing eucalyptol showed, as adults, the same electrophysiological responses in the mitral cell layer of their olfactory bulbs to eucalyptol odor that normally reared rats showed to food odors. Would young infants react to novel odor experienced in this way in the same way that they reacted to milk odor?

We examined the responses elicited by the odor of eucalyptol in 3-, 6-, 9-, and 12-day-old rat pups whose dams had been assigned, before mating, to one of three conditions: eucalyptol-reared, eucalyptol-exposed, or normally reared. Pups assigned to the "eucalyptol-reared" condition were reared by dams that had been maintained on eucalyptol-adulterated food and water throughout pregnancy and lactation. Pups in the "eucalyptol-exposed" condition were reared by dams maintained on a normal, unadulterated diet, but the air in their colony room was scented with eucalyptol to control for effects of simple exposure to the odor during rearing. Normally reared pups were born to dams maintained on a normal, unadulterated diet, and these litters were housed in a separate colony room, to ensure that they would have no experience with eucalyptol odor. At the time of testing, the pups from these three treatment groups were exposed to milk odor, unscented air, or eucalyptol odor while receiving oral infusions of distilled water. The pups' activity, mouthing, and probing were scored, and their intake of water was measured (to determine whether the presence of eucalyptol odor increased intake of water in eucalyptol-reared and/or eucalyptol-exposed pups, in the same way that the presence of milk odor increases water intake in normally reared pups). Immediately following the odor–infusion test, those pups that were exposed to unscented air during the odor–infusion test were given the two-choice olfactory orientation preference test (described above and in Johanson and Hall, 1982, and Johanson and Teicher, 1980).

Pups reared by dams fed a eucalyptol-adulterated diet responded to the odor of eucalyptol in much the same way that normally reared pups responded to milk (Terry, Craft, and Johanson, 1983). Eucalyptol-reared pups became very active when the odor of eucalyptol was introduced into their test container. This increased activity was seen even at 3 days of age and continued to occur, though to a lesser extent, in the 12-day-olds. Eucalyptol-reared pups also responded to the odor of eucalyptol with intense probing (Figure 12), similar to the level of probing elicited by the odor of milk in normal pups. In contrast, normally reared pups and

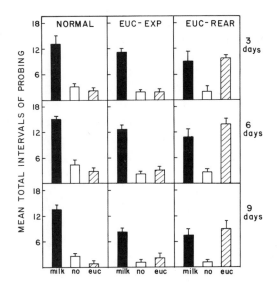

Figure 12. Mean total intervals of probing in normally reared, eucalyptol-exposed, and eucalyptol-reared 3- to 9-day-old pups, as a function of odor (milk odor, no odor, or eucalyptol odor) presented during a water infusion test.

eucalyptol-exposed pups showed very little activity or probing in response to eucalyptol odor (the levels of probing were similar for unscented air and eucalyptol.

The finding that an odor associated with the dam elicited specific behaviors in her offspring is consistent with the findings of Fillion and Blass (1986a,b; discussed above) in rat pups and Ivanitskii (1958; cited in Rosenblatt, 1983) and Hudson (1985) in rabbit pups. Ivanitskii placed an artificial odor on the ventrum of a lactating rabbit and observed that her offspring, after one or two nursing episodes, lifted their heads to the odor alone. When older, the pups approached the entrance to the nest box—presumably to meet the doe—in response to a presentation of the odor. This finding was replicated by Hudson (1985). Together, these studies provide additional support for the idea that odors associated with the dam can come to elicit specific behaviors in her offspring.

Besides influencing activity and probing, the early experiences with eucalyptol odor also influenced behaviors that were more purely ingestive in character. Whereas normally reared pups ingested less water if infusions were accompanied by eucalyptol odor, 6- and 9-day-old eucalyptol-reared pups ingested more water and showed higher levels of mouthing when infusions were accompanied by the odor of eucalyptol, and a similar effect occurred in 9-day-old eucalyptol-exposed pups. Recall that the presence of milk odor during oral infusions of various sapid solutions also tends to increase levels of intake by 6- and 9-day-old pups.

Not surprisingly, 3- to 9-day-old eucalyptol-reared pups overwhelmingly preferred the eucalyptol-scented bedding over the unscented bedding, spending over 80% of their time on the eucalyptol-scented side (Figure 13). Normally reared pups, on the other hand, spent very little time (from 14% to 22% of the total) over eucalyptol-scented bedding. The eucalyptol-exposed pups were indifferent: they spent approximately equal amounts of time over the eucalyptol-scented and unscented beddings. Thus, although simple exposure to the odor of eucalyptol in the rearing environment was sufficient to eliminate the pups' normal aversion to the odor, simple exposure was not sufficient to establish eucalyptol as an elicitor of activation and probing in deprived pups. By age 12 days of age, the pups were indifferent to the odor of eucalyptol, regardless of their rearing condition.

The eucalyptol-reared pups in this experiment had received both pre- and postnatal exposure to eucalyptol (remember that the dams were maintained on eucalyptol during pregnancy and lactation), so it was not clear when the exposure to eucalyptol odor had to occur to be effective. In a follow-up cross-fostering study, half of the pups that had been born to dams on a eucalyptol-adulterated diet were fostered to dams maintained on a normal diet, and half of the pups born to dams fed a normal diet were fostered to eucalyptol-fed mothers. The cross-fostering occurred within 6 h of birth, so that the "prenatal"-exposed pups actually may have had some limited postnatal experience, but this turned out to be unimportant. At 6 days of age, when pups' activational response to milk or milk odor is robust, these cross-fostered pups were tested for their response to eucalyptol odor, milk odor, or unscented air.

Postnatal exposure to eucalyptol clearly determined whether the pups responded to the odor with activity and probing. Pups reared by dams maintained on a eucalyptol-adulterated diet, regardless of their prenatal treatment, became active and probed to eucalyptol. Prenatal exposure alone had no effect on the pups' behavior, and the combined pre- and postnatal exposure was no more effective in eliciting probing than postnatal exposure alone (Figure 14). This finding provides additional support for the idea that the eucalyptol odor acquired its ability to elicit probing because the pups had associated the odor with stimuli provided

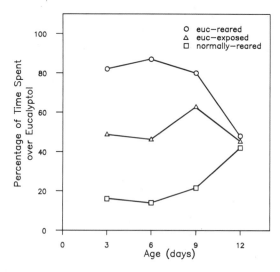

Figure 13. Percentage of total time spent over eucalyptol-scented bedding (versus unscented bedding) by normally reared, eucalyptol-exposed, and eucalyptol-reared 3- to 12-day-old pups.

by their dam in the first few days after birth, perhaps by the same type of mechanism—appetitive classical conditioning—by which novel odors come to elicit activation and probing when they are paired with milk infusions.

SUMMARY. Behavioral activation and probing that deprived infant rats' display to milk and milk odor may reflect classically conditioned associations between milk odor and certain classes of rewarding stimulation (warmth, suckling, nonspecific tactile stimulation, or other odor cues) provided by the dam in the first few days after birth. Through these acquired associations, milk odor comes to elicit components of the complex infant–mother interaction. This conclusion is based, in part, on the results of an olfactory learning paradigm in which behavioral activation and probing come to be elicited by a novel odor associated with the dam during the early postpartum period.

This "natural" learning paradigm has some direct parallels with our classical conditioning paradigm, in which activation and probing responses come to be elicited by novel odor stimuli explicitly associated with milk infusions (Johanson *et al.*, 1984). In both of these paradigms, a novel odor comes, as a result of association either with milk or with the dam, to elicit specific behavioral responses (activation and probing).

SUMMARY AND CONCLUSIONS

What is particularly evident—both from our own work and from other recent studies in infant learning—is the remarkable capability of infants to learn. Since the mid-1970s, we have progressed from questioning whether infants can form *any* type of learned association to asking about the extent to which neonatal and even

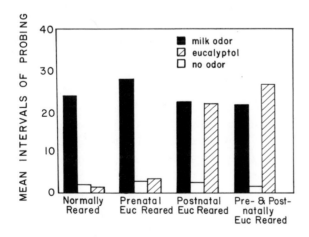

Figure 14. Mean intervals of probing in 6-day-old pups as a function of odor exposure (milk odor, no odor, or eucalyptol odor) and rearing condition. Pups were reared with prenatal eucalyptol exposure only, postnatal eucalyptol exposure only, or both pre- and postnatal eucalyptol exposure, or they were normally reared, with no exposure to eucalyptol.

fetal learning contributes to the progression of normal behavioral development. Much of this progress has stemmed from realizing that infants are not miniature adults and that paradigms that assess infants' abilities must especially consider their unique sensory and motor capabilities. The recent successes enjoyed by developmental psychobiologists stems from using stimuli, responses, and contexts that infants normally encounter in some form. As an example, we cited research from our laboratory that suggests that the same type of classically conditioned association that develops when novel odors are explicitly paired with milk infusions in a highly structured experimental setting may also develop to a novel odor associated with the dam during normal rearing. More generally, we believe that classically conditioned associations between odors and the stimulation provided by the dam play an important role in the development of a broad range of olfactory-mediated social, sexual, and ingestive behaviors, as we described earlier.

The special role of olfaction and olfactory learning in mammalian behavioral development was discussed by Rosenblatt (1983). He proposed that olfactory cues become established as "incentives" during early development because they have been associated with stimulation provided by the mother. Odors, he argued, elicit fewer "inherent" responses than do thermotactile stimuli, and so they are particularly well-suited, during early development, to being associated with thermotactile stimulation and to mediating the behavioral transition from responses based purely on the quantitative aspects of stimuli (e.g., their intensity) to responses that depend on the qualitative aspects of stimuli, including their specific ability to predict or signal significant events.

What stimulation might the dam be providing to effect changes in responsiveness to odors associated with her? We believe that the studies cited here support the possibility that infant rats associate the various odors of their dam (for example, the odors of maternal saliva, amniotic fluid, pup saliva on nipples, milk, vaginal secretions, and the food that the dam ingests) with the warmth or tactile stimulation that the dam provides, or—through second-order conditioning—with other odors that have previously been established as incentives. As a result of the infants' early reinforcing experiences with these various odors, they acquire a positive hedonic valence, eventually coming to serve as "incentive" stimuli for other goal objects that they label (e.g., early in development, huddling partners and their dam's nipples, and later in development, food and sexual partners).

Learned associations between odors and the warmth provided by the dam may underlie the development of all of the various motivated behaviors that we have discussed here, and that subsequent learned associations derive from higher order conditioning processes that occur later in development. Supporting this possibility is research that demonstrates that associations between a novel odor and warmth induce strong huddling preferences for objects scented with the odor, that warmth is a significant contextual cue for learning in young infants, and that warmth is rewarding or reinforcing in its own right. Indeed, both Jeddi (1979) and Rosenblatt (1983) have argued that infants' responsiveness to thermal stimulation provides a basis for early affective and motivational development.

Alternatively, there may be specific classes of maternal stimulation that are particularly effective in establishing olfactory cues as incentives for specific behavior patterns. For example, the effects of early odor experiences on the olfactory mediation of adult sexual behavior may derive from infants' associating vaginal odors from their dam with the stimulation that she provides as she licks their anogenital areas to stimulate urination and defecation, and these effects may be relatively unaffected by odor–warmth associations. On the other hand, olfactory preferences in the choice of huddling partner may depend primarily on odor–warmth associations and may be unaffected by odor–anogenital-stimulation associations, whereas olfactory preferences in food choice may depend on odor–suckling associations rather than on associations between odors and warmth or anogenital stimulation.

With respect to this last point, we believe that future research aimed at identifying the extent to which different behavioral systems share, in ontogeny, the same underlying conditioned associations has the potential to reveal which behavioral systems are "tied together" developmentally and can indicate how early learning experiences may exert their later effects on behavior.

Acknowledgment

Preparation of this chapter was supported by a grant from the National Institute of Child Health and Human Development (HD 16712).

REFERENCES

Adolph, E. F. Ontogeny of physiological regulations in the rat. *Quarterly Review of Biology*, 1957, *32*, 89–137.

Alberts, J. R. Huddling by rat pups: Multisensory control of contact behavior. *Journal of Comparative and Physiological Psychology*, 1978, *92*, 220–230.

Alberts, J. R. Ontogeny of olfaction: Reciprocal roles of sensation and behavior in the development of perception. In R. N. Aslin, J. R. Alberts, and M. R. Peterson (Eds.,) *Development of Perception: Psychobiological Perspectives*, Vol. 1. New York: Academic Press, 1981.

Alberts, J. R., and Brunjes, P. C. Ontogeny of thermal and olfactory determinants of huddling in the rat. *Journal of Comparative and Physiological Psychology*, 1978, *92*, 897–906.

Alberts, J. R., and May, B. Ontogeny of olfaction: Development of the rats' sensitivity to urine and amyl acetate. *Physiology and Behavior*, 1980, *24*, 965–970.

Altman, J., Brunner, R. L., Bulut, F. G., and Sudarshan, K. The development of behavior in normal and brain damaged infant rats studied with homing (nest-seeking) as motivation. In A. Vernadakis and N. Weiner (eds.), *Drugs and the developing nervous system*. New York: Plenum Press, 1972.

Altman, J., Sudarshan, K., Das, G. D., McCormick, N., and Barnes, D. The influence of nutrition on neural and behavioral development, III. The development of some motor, particularly locomotor, patterns during infancy. *Developmental Psychobiology*, 1971, *4*, 97–114.

Amsel, A., Burdette, D. R., and Letz, R. Appetitive learning, patterned alternation, and extinction in 10-d-old rats with non-lactating suckling as reward. *Nature*, 1976, *262*, 816–818.

Amsel, A., Letz, R., and Burdette, D. R. Appetitive learning and extinction in 11-day-old rat pups: Effects of various reinforcement conditions. *Journal of Comparative and Physiological Psychology*, 1977a, *91*, 1156–1167.

Amsel, A., Radek, C. C., Graham, M., and Letz, R. Ultrasound emission in infant rats as an indicant of arousal during appetitive learning and extinction. *Science*, 1977b, *197*, 786–788.

Bacon, W. E., and Stanley, W. C. Reversal learning in neonatal dogs. *Journal of Comparative and Physiological Psychology*, 1970, *70*, 344–350.

Blass, E. M., Ganchrow, J., and Steiner, J. Classical conditioning in newborn humans 2–48 hours of age. *Infant Behavior and Development*, 1984, *7*, 223–235.

Blass, E. M., Teicher, M. H., Cramer, C. P., Bruno, J. P., and Hall, W. G. Olfactory, thermal, and tactile controls of suckling in preaudial and previsual rats. *Journal of Comparative and Physiological Psychology*, 1977, *91*, 1248–1260.

Bornstein, B. H., Terry, L. M., Browde, J. A., Assimon, S. A., and Hall, W. G. Maternal and nutritional contributions to infant rats' activational responses to ingestion. *Developmental Psychobiology*, 1987, *20*, 147–163.

Brake, S. C. Suckling infant rats learn a preference for a novel olfactory stimulus paried with milk delivery. *Science*, 1981, *211*, 506–508.

Brody, E. B. Development of homeothermy in suckling rats. *American Journal of Physiology*, 1943, *139*, 230–232.

Brunjes, P. C. and Alberts, J. R. Olfactory stimulation induces filial huddling preferences in rat pups. *Journal of Comparative and Physiological Psychology*, 1979, *93*, 548–555.

Bruno, J. P., Teicher, M. H., and Blass, E. M. Sensory determinants of suckling behavior in weanling rats. *Journal of Comparative and Physiological Psychology*, 1980, *94*, 115–127.

Bulut, F. G., and Altman, J. Spatial and tactile discrimination learning in infant rats motivated by homing. *Developmental Psychobiology*, 1974, *7*, 465–473.

Capretta, P. J., and Rawls, L. H. Establishment of a flavor preference in rats: Importance of nursing and weaning experience. *Journal of Comparative and Physiological Psychology*, 1974, *86*, 670–673.

Caza, P. A., and Spear, N. E. Short-term exposure to an odor increases its subsequent preference in preweanling rats: A descriptive profile of the phenomenon. *Developmental Psychobiology*, 1984, *17*, 407–422.

Cornwell, A. C., and Fuller, J. L. Conditioned responses in young puppies. *Journal of Comparative and Physiological Psychology*, 1961, *54*, 13–15.

Cornwell, c. A. Golden hamster pups adapt to complex rearing odors. *Behavioral Biology*, 1975, *14*, 175–188.

Cosnier, J. *Le comportement gregaire du rat d'élévage (Étude éthologique)*. Unpublished doctoral dissertation, University of Lyon, France, 1965.

DeCasper, A. J., and Fifer, W. P. Of human bonding: Newborns prefer their mothers' voices. *Science*, 1980, *208*, 1174–1176.

Farbman, A. I. Electron microscope study of the developing taste bud in rat fungiform papillae. *Developmental Biology*, 1965, *11*, 110–135.

Fillion, T. J., and Blass, E. M. Responsiveness to estrous chemostimuli in male rats *(Rattus norvegicus)* of different ages. *Journal of Comparative Psychology*, 1985, *99*, 328–335.

Fillion, T. J., and Blass, E. M. Infantile behavioural reactivity to oestrous chemostimuli in Norway rats. *Animal Behaviour*, 1986a, *34*, 123–133.

Fillion, T. J., and Blass, E. M. Infantile experience with suckling odors determines adult sexual behavior in male rats. *Science*, 1986b, *231*, 729–731.

Fleming, A., Vaccarino, F., Tambosso, L., and Chee, P. Vomeronasal and olfactory modulation of maternal behavior in the rat. *Science*, 1979, *203*, 372–374.

Freeman, N. C. G., and Rosenblatt, J. S. The interrelationship between thermal and olfactory stimulation in the development of home orientation in newborn kittens. *Developmental Psychobiology*, 1978, *11*, 437–457.

Fuller, J. L., Easler, C. A., and Banks, E. M. Formation of conditioned avoidance responses in young puppies. *American Journal of Physiology*, 1950, *160*, 462–466.

Galef, B. G., and Clark, M. M. Mother's milk and adult preference. Two factors determining initial dietary selection by weanling rats. *Journal of Comparative and Physiological Psychology*, 1972, *78*, 220–225.

Galef, B. G., and Henderson, P. W. Mother's milk: A determinant of the feeding preferences of weaning rat pups. *Journal of Comparative and Physiological Psychology*, 1972, *78*, 213–219.

Galef, B. G., and Kaner, H. C. Establishment and maintenance of preference for natural and artificial olfactory stimuli in juvenile rats. *Journal of Comparative and Physiological Psychology*, 1980, *94*, 588–596.

Guenaire, C., Costa, J. C., and Delacour, J. Discrimination spatiale avec renforcement thermique chez le jeune rat. *Physiology and Behavior*, 1982a *29*, 725–731.

Guenaire, C., Costa, J. C., and Delacour, J. Conditionnement operant avec renforcement thermique chez le rat nouveau-né. *Physiology and Behavior*, 1982b, *29*, 419–424.

Gulick, A. The development of temperature control in infant rats. *American Journal of Physiology*, 1937, *119*, 322.

Hall, W. G. The ontogeny of feeding in rats: I. Ingestion and behavioral responses to oral infusions. *Journal of Comparative and Physiological Psychology*, 1979, *93*, 977–1000.

Hall, W. G., and Bryan, T. E. The ontogeny of feeding in rats. II. Independent ingestive behavior. *Journal of Comparative and Physiological Psychology*, 1980, *94*, 746–756.

Hill, D. L., and Almli, C. R. Olfactory bulbectomy in infant rats. *Physiology and Behavior*, 1981, *27*, 811–817.

Hofer, M. A., Shair, H., and Singh, P. Evidence that maternal skin substance promotes suckling in infant rats. *Physiology and Behavior*, 1976, *17*, 131–136.

Holland, P. C. Conditioned stimulus as a determinant of the form of the Pavlovian conditioned response. *Journal of Experimental Psychology: Animal Behavior Processes*, 1977, *3*, 77–104.

Hudson, R. Do newborn rabbits learn the odor stimuli releasing nipple-search behavior? *Developmental Psychobiology*, 1985, *18*, 575–585.

Infurna, R. N., Steinert, P. A., and Spear, N. E. Ontogenetic changes in the modulation of taste aversion learning by home environmental cues in rats. *Journal of Comparative and Physiological Psychology*, 1979, *93*, 1097–1108.

Ivanitskii, A. M. The morphophysiological investigation of development of higher conditioned alimentary reaction in rabbits during ontogenesis. *Works of the Institute of Higher Nervous Activity*, 1958, *4*, 126–141.

Jeddi, E. Ontogenesis of thermal comfort. Its role in affective development. In J. Durand and J. Raynaud (Eds.), *Thermal comfort: physiological and psychological bases*. Paris: Institut National de la Santé et de la Récherche Medicale, 1979.

Johanson, I. B. Thermotaxis in neonatal rat pups. *Physiology and Behavior*, 1979, *23*, 871–874.

Johanson, I. B., and Hall, W. G. Appetitive learning in 1-day-old rat pups. *Science*, 1979, *205*, 419–421.

Johanson, I. B., and Hall, W. G. The ontogeny of feeding in rats. III. Thermal determinants of early ingestive responding. *Journal of Comparative and Physiological Psychology*, 1980, *94*, 977–992.

Johanson, I. B., and Hall, W. G. The ontogeny of feeding in rats. V. Influence of texture, home odor, and sibling presence on ingestive behavior. *Journal of Comparative and Physiological Psychology*, 1981, *95*, 837–847.

Johanson, I. B., and Hall, W. G. Appetitive conditioning in neonatal rats: Conditioned orientation to a novel odor. *Developmental Psychobiology*, 1982, *15*, 379–397.

Johanson, I. B., and Hall, W. G. Ontogeny of appetitive learning: Independent ingestion as a model motivational system. In R. Kail and N. E. Spear (Eds.), *Comparative Perspectives on the Development of Memory*. Hillsdale, NJ: Erlbaum, 1984.

Johanson, I. B., Hall, W. G., and Polefrone, J. M. Appetitive conditioning in neonatal rats: Conditioned ingestive responding to stimuli paired with oral infusions of milk. *Developmental Psychobiology*, 1984, *17*, 357–382.

Johanson, I. B., and Teicher, M. H. Classical conditioning of an odor preference in 3-day-old rats. *Behavioral and Neural Biology*, 1980, *29*, 132–136.

Kehoe, P., and Blass, E. M. Conditioned aversions and their memories in 5-day-old rats during suckling. *Journal of Experimental Psychology: Animal Behavior Processes*, 1986, *12*, 40–47.

Kenny, J. T., and Blass, E. M. Suckling as incentive to instrumental learning in preweanling rats. *Science*, 1977, *196*, 898–899.

Kenny, J. T., Stoloff, M. L., Bruno, J. P., and Blass, E. M. The ontogeny of preferences for nutritive over nonnutritive suckling in albino rats. *Journal of Comparative and Physiological Psychology*, 1979, *93*, 752–759.

Kleitman, N., and Satinoff, E. Thermoregulatory behavior in rat pups from birth to weaning. *Physiology and Behavior*, 1982, *29*, 537–541.

Leader, L. R., Baillie, P., Martin, B., and Vermeulen, E. The assessment and significance of habituation to a repeated stimulus by the human fetus. *Early Human Development*, 1982, *7*, 211–219.

Leon, M. Development of thermoregulation. In E. M. Blass (Ed.), *Handbook of behavioral neurobiology: Developmental psychobiology and developmental neurobiology*, Vol. 8. New York: Plenum Press, 1986.

Leon, M., Galef, B. G., and Behse, J. H. Establishment of phermonal bonds and diet choice in young rats by odor pre-exposure. *Physiology and Behavior*, 1977, *18*, 387–391.

Leonard, C. M. Thermotaxis in golden hamster pups. *Journal of Comparative and Physiological Psychology*, 1974, *86*, 458–469.

Lipsitt, L. P., and Kaye, H. Conditioned sucking in the human newborn. *Psychonomic Science,* 1964, *1,* 29–30.

Martin, L. T., and Alberts, J. R. Taste aversions to mother's milk: The age-related role of nursing in acquisition and expression of a learned association. *Journal of Comparative and Physiological Psychology,* 1979, *93,* 430–445.

Martin, L. T., and Alberts, J. R. Associative learning of neonatal rats revealed by heartrate response patterns. *Journal of Comparative and Physiological Psychology,* 1982, *96,* 668–675.

Moore, C. L. Maternal contributions to the development of masculine sexual behavior in laboratory rats. *Developmental Psychobiology,* 1984, *17,* 347–356.

Oppenheim, R. W. Ontogenetic adaptations and retrogressive processes in the development of the nervous system and behavior: A neuroembryological perspective. In K. J. Connolly and H. F. R. Prechtl (Eds.), *Maturation and development: Biological and psychological perspectives.* Philadelphia: Lippincott, 1981.

Pager, J. A selective modulation of the olfactory bulb electrical activity in relation to the learning of palatability in hungry and satiated rats. *Physiology and Behavior,* 1974, *12,* 189–195.

Pedersen, P. E., and Blass, E. M. Olfactory control over suckling in albino rat. In R. N. Aslin, J. R. Alberts, and M. R. Peterson (Eds.), *Development of perception: Psychobiological perspectives,* Vol. 1. New York: Academic Press, 1981.

Pedersen, P. E., and Blass, E. M. Prenatal and postnatal determinants of the 1st suckling episode in albino rats. *Developmental Psychobiology,* 1982, *15,* 349–355.

Pedersen, P. E., Greer, C. A., and Shepherd, G. M. Early development of olfactory function. In E. M. Blass (Ed.), *Handbook of behavioral neurobiology: Developmental psychobiology and developmental neurobiology* (Vol. 8). New York: Plenum Press, 1986.

Pedersen, P. E., Stewart, W. B., Greer, C. A., and Shepherd, G. M. Evidence for olfactory function in utero. *Science,* 1983, *221,* 478–480.

Pedersen, P. E., Williams, C. L., and Blass, E. M. Activation and odor conditioning of suckling behavior in 3-day-old albino rats. *Journal of Experimental Psychology: Animal Behavior Processes,* 1982, *8,* 329–341.

Powers, J. B., Fields, R. B., and Winans, S. S. Olfactory and vomeronasal system participation in male hamsters' attraction to female vaginal secretions. *Physiology and Behavior,* 1979, *22,* 77–84.

Rosenblatt, J. S. Olfaction mediates developmental transition in the altricial newborn of selected species of mammals. *Developmental Psychobiology,* 1983, *16,* 347–375.

Rosenblatt, J. S., Turkewitz, G., and Schneirla, T. C. Development of home orientation in newly born kittens. *Transactions of the New York Academy of Science,* 1969, *31,* 231–250.

Roth, L. L., and Rosenblatt, J. S. Mammary glands of pregnant rats: Development stimulated by licking. *Science,* 1965, *151,* 1403–1404.

Rovee-Collier, C. K., Sullivan, M. W., Enright, M., Lucas, D., and Fagen, J. W. Reactivation of infant memory. *Science,* 1980, *208,* 1159–1161.

Rudy, J. W., and Cheatle, M. D. Odor-aversion learning in neonatal rats. *Science,* 1977, *198,* 845–846.

Rudy, J. W., and Hyson, R. L. Consummatory response conditioning to an auditory stimulus in neonatal rats. *Behavioral and Neural Biology,* 1982, *34,* 209–214.

Sameroff, A. J. Reflexive and operant aspects of sucking behavior in early infancy. In J. F. Bosma (Ed.), *Oral sensation and perception: Development in the fetus and infant.* Bethesda: U.S. Department of Health, Education, and Welfare, 1973.

Sczerenie, V., and Hsiao, S. Development of locomotion toward nesting material in neonatal rats. *Developmental Psychobiology,* 1977, *10,* 315–321.

Singer, A. C., Agosta, W. C., O'Connell, R. J., Pfaffman, C., Bowen, D. V., and Field, F. H. Dimethyl disulfide: An attractant pheromone in hamster vaginal secretion. *Science,* 1976, *191,* 948–950.

Singh, P. J., and Tobach, E. Olfactory bulbectomy and nursing behavior in rat pups (Wistar DAB). *Developmental Psychobiology,* 1975, *8,* 151–164.

Singh, P. J., Tucker, A. M., and Hofer, M. A. Effects of nasal $ZnSO_4$ irrigation and olfactory bulbectomy on rat pups. *Physiology and Behavior,* 1976, *17,* 373–382.

Smith, G. J., and Bogomolny, A. Appetitive instrumental training in preweanling rats. I. Motivational determinants. *Developmental Psychobiology,* 1983, *16,* 119–128.

Smith, G. J., and Spear, N. E. Effects of the home environment on withholding behaviors and conditioning in infant and neonatal rats. *Science,* 1978, *202,* 327–329.

Smith, G. J., and Spear, N. E. Facilitation of conditioning in two-day-old rats by training in the presence of conspecifics. *Behavioral and Neural Biology,* 1980, *28,* 491–495.

Smith, G. J., and Spear, N. E. Home environmental stimuli facilitate learning of shock escape discrimination in rats 7–11 days of age. *Behavioral and Neural Biology*, 1981, *31*, 360–365.

Smotherman, W. P. Odor aversion learning in the rat fetus. *Physiology and Behavior*, 1982, *29*, 769–771.

Spear, N. E. Ecologically determined dispositions control the ontogeny of learning and memory. In R. Kail and N. E. Spear (Eds.), *Comparative perspectives on the development of memory*. Hillsdale, NJ: Erlbaum. 1984.

Stanley, W. C., Bacon, W. E., and Fehr, C. Discriminated instrumental learning in neonatal dogs. *Journal of Comparative and Physiological Psychology*, 1970, *70*, 335–343.

Stickrod, G., Kimble, D. P., and Smotherman, W. P. In utero taste/odor aversion and conditioning in the rat. *Physiology and Behavior*, 1982, *28*, 5–8.

Sullivan, R. M., Brake, S. C., Hofer, M. A., and Williams, C. L. Huddling and independent feeding of neonatal rats can be facilitated by a conditioned change in behavioral state. *Developmental Psychobiology*, 1986, *19*, 625–635.

Teicher, M. H., and Blass, E. M. First suckling response of the newborn albino rats: Roles of olfaction and amniotic fluid. *Science*, 1977, *198*, 635–636.

Teicher, M. H., Flaum, L. E., Williams, M., Eckhert, S. J., and Lumia, A. R. Survival, growth, and suckling behavior of neonatally bulbectomized rats. *Physiology and Behavior*, 1978, *21*, 553–561.

Teicher, M. H., Shaywitz, B. A., and Lumia, A. R. Olfactory and vomeronasal system mediation of maternal recognition in the developing rat. *Developmental Brain Research*, 1984, *12*, 97–110.

Terry, L. M. *Olfactory contributions to the ingestive behavior of infant rats: Effects of olfactory and vomeronasal deafferentation*. Unpublished master's thesis, Florida Atlantic University, Boca Raton, 1985.

Terry, L. M., and Johanson, I. B. Olfactory influences on the ingestive behavior of infant rats. *Developmental Psychobiology*, 1987, *20*, 313–332.

Terry, L. M., Craft, G., and Johanson, I. B. *Early olfactory experiences modulate infant rats' ingestive behaviors*. Paper presented at the annual meeting of the International Society for Developmental Psychobiology, Hyannis, MA, 1983.

Tobach, E., Rouger, Y., and Schneirla, T. C. Development of olfactory functions in the rat pup. *American Zoologist*, 1967, *7*, 792–793.

Turkewitz, G., and Kenny, P. Limitations on input as a basis for neural organization and perceptual development: A preliminary theoretical statement. *Developmental Psychobiology*, 1982, *15*, 357–368.

Wigal, T., Kucharski, D., and Spear, N. E. Familiar contextual odors promote discrimination learning in preweanling but not in older rats. *Developmental Psychobiology*, 1984, *17*, 555–570.

Williams, C. L. *The ontogeny of steroid-facilitated lordosis and ear wiggling in infant rats*. Paper presented at the meeting of the International Society for Developmental Psychobiology, Atlanta, 1979.

Wysocki, C. J. Neurobehavioral evidence for the involvement of the vomeronasal system in mammalian reproduction. *Neuroscience and Biobehavioral Reviews*, 1979, *3*, 301–341.

8

The Neurobiology of Early Olfactory Learning

ROBERT COOPERSMITH AND MICHAEL LEON

INTRODUCTION

Young organisms emerge into a world of extraordinary complexity and yet must begin to function immediately in that world. Rather than dealing with the barrage of new stimuli in their new surround, some neonates filter much of it by restricting the number and sophisticaton of senses that are functional at birth. Altricial rodents, for example, are born with their eyes and ears sealed to external stimulation; their olfactory sense is their primary window to their world. As we shall see, even this system, although functional, is still a far less complex system than will eventually develop to process the complexities of the olfactory world. Rather, the system may be just competent enough to deal with the dominant odors in the surround, thus filtering the complexity in the olfactory environment by limitations in the sensory system. Because the important aspects of the olfactory world and the organization of the olfactory nervous system are unique to the neonatal period, there must be mechanisms to ensure a reliable response to the olfactory cues that are critical to the survival of the young.

In the one mammalian species that we have studied, such a unique mechanism appears to involve a reorganization of the olfactory circuitry which responds to the significant odors experienced early in life. This neural reorganization appears to underlie the sensory processing that may be involved in the special behavioral responses to such odors. Thus, rather than having subtle neural mechanisms available

---

ROBERT COOPERSMITH AND MICHAEL LEON   Department of Psychobiology, University of California, Irvine, California 92717.

for responses to an evanescent and complex sensory world, the sensory cues impinging on the neonate are obvious and limited. The young brain forms so as to have those cues evoke large, reliable responses when the cues are subsequently encountered. There is also some reason to believe that the neurobehavioral responses to these olfactory cues that are imprinted in these young animals persist throughout their lifetime and may mediate important social responses in adulthood.

We will first discuss the plasticity of the behavioral responses to odors experienced early in life. We will then discuss the organization and development of rodent olfactory systems. Finally, we will describe the changes that can occur in the young olfactory nervous system in response to early olfactory learning.

EARLY OLFACTORY LEARNING

The olfactory system of rats can be modified by experience at least as early as 2 days before birth (Pedersen and Blass, 1982). Citral, a lemon scent, was injected into the amniotic fluid on prenatal Day 20, and the pups were exposed to citral odor immediately after birth. These pups would not suckle either washed or unwashed nipples in a clean air ambience. In a citral ambience, however, these pups suckled both washed and unwashed nipples. It should be noted that both the prenatal and postnatal odor experiences were necessary to specify the odor that would elicit the first suckling episode, a condition that mimics the normal course of odor exposure. Also of interest is the fact that it was not necessary to paint the citral odor directly on the nipples to elicit suckling in the pups preexposed to citral; a citral ambience was sufficient. Because rats ingest birth fluids and lick their nipples during the birth process, it would seem that the pups normally attach in the presence of familiar uterine odors.

Washing the nipples of a newly parturient rat eliminated suckling by her pups (Teicher and Blass, 1976). If the nipples were then painted with either an extract of the wash fluid, the mother's saliva, or amniotic fluid, suckling was reinstated (Teicher, and Blass, 1977). By the second postnatal day, suckling could be reinstated after nipple washing by painting the nipples with pup saliva (Teicher and Blass, 1976). By 3 days of age, conditions slightly different from those needed on Day 1 were necessary in order for a novel odor to gain control over suckling (Pedersen, Williams, and Blass, 1982). Specifically, postnatal preexposure to citral odor accompanied by either stroking the pups with a small brush (which mimics maternal contact), or what may have been a state of heightened arousal induced by amphetamine administration, was sufficient to cause citral odor to elicit nipple attachment without prenatal exposure. Perhaps this change in responsiveness reflected the transition from amniotic fluid to pup saliva as the salient cue for nipple attachment.

Pedersen *et al.* (1982) also found that pups would acquire this olfactory preference only when they were stimulated in ways that mimicked the maternal presence. Stimulation could be provided by stroking, amphetamine administration, a warm ambience (33°C) during exposure, or an increased citral odor concentration, but not by caffeine. Overstimulation (perineal stroking and amphetamine administration and high temperature or odor concentration) did not facilitate suckling of citral-scented nipples, although there was an optimal combination of conditions that induced virtually all of the pups to attach. The authors suggested that this pattern of learning may have arisen because suckling becomes paired with the state of arousal caused by maternal stimulation.

Odors experienced by male rats within a specific context of maternal stimulation also appear to affect their sexual orientation in adulthood. Fillion and Blass (1986a) demonstrated that rat pups responded to odors from estrous females as they did to suckling-significant maternal odors, by probing. However, this response to estrous odors disappeared by Day 10 in pups reared by dams whose nipple and vaginal odors—odors that normally elicit probing—had been altered with citral. Such pups probed in response to estrous odors only when they were presented in combination with citral (Fillion and Blass, 1986a). In a subsequent study, adult males that had been reared in this manner until weaning were slow to complete sexual encounters with normal estrous females but were quick to do so with citral-scented estrous females. Males reared by dams whose backs, only, were citral-scented, or whose nipples and vaginas were treated with saline, mated as readily or more readily with normal females (Fillion and Blass, 1986b). The authors suggested that initial adult male reactivity to estrous odors is normally determined in the course of infantile experience with similar odors, presumably including pup saliva, that gain significance through their association with suckling.

Rat pups can also learn an odor aversion prenatally (Strickrod, Kimble, and Smotherman, 1982). Apple juice or saline was injected into the amniotic fluid of a pregnant rat on prenatal Day 20, followed 5 min later by an intraperitoneal (IP) injection of lithium chloride (LiCl) or saline to the fetus. The pups were tested for an aversion to the apple juice by determining their response to nipples that were painted either with apple juice or saline. Pups receiving the apple-juice-LiCl pairing *in utero* showed significantly less suckling on apple-juice painted nipples than did pups from the three control groups (apple-juice–saline, saline–LiCl, or saline–saline). It should be noted that the experiment did not separate olfactory from gustatory learning.

In contrast to vision and audition, some olfactory functions are present at birth. Nipple attachment is prevented if olfactory cues are removed from the nipples of a parturient rat (Hofer, Shair, and Singh, 1976; Teicher and Blass, 1976, 1977). Similarly, neonatal olfactory bulbectomy in rats (Hill and Almli, 1981; Teicher, Flaum, Williams, Eckhert, and Lumia, 1978), and rabbits (Hudson and Distel, 1984), or destruction of the neurosensory epithelium (Singh, Tucker, and Hofer, 1976), disrupts suckling in pups.

Schapiro and Salas (1970) also found that, at as early as 2 days of age, rat pups inhibited their spontaneous locomotor activity in response to maternal odors. The effect grew more robust over the next week. Using odor-induced sniffing as an indicator of detection, Alberts and May (1980) found that approximately 50% of 1-day-old, 90% of 3-day-old, and 100% of 6-day-old rat pups were capable of detecting a relatively strong concentration of amyl acetate.

Indeed, 1-day-old rat pups can even learn an odor discrimination task requiring an operant response (Johanson and Hall, 1979). Neonates were implanted with intraoral cannulas that could deliver microliter quantities of milk directly into their mouths. The pups were placed in a styrofoam cup that was fitted with a terrycloth-covered paddle, which, when pushed, closed a microswitch that delivered milk to the pup. The pups were milk-deprived overnight and testing was performed at the approximate temperature of the nest (33°C). The pups rapidly learned to probe into a single paddle without an odor cue. In the discrimination test, each of two paddles was paired with an odor (lemon versus clove or perfume versus cedar) with a reward for probing against only one of the paddles. The pups learned this discrimination within 5 or 6 h. Thus, when a relevant stimulus and a response appropriate to the pup's state of motor development are chosen, it can be shown that 1-day-old rats are capable of using olfactory cues in a relatively complex learning task.

Johanson and Teicher (1980) then examined the effects of pairing milk delivery (using the intraoral catheter) with odor exposure on the development of odor preferences in 3-day-old rats. Pups were given 20-second exposures to cedar odor (normally an aversive odor), the last 5 s of which coincided with a milk infusion. Each pup received 10 such pairings in a warm ambience (33°C). Control groups received (a) odor only; (b) milk only; (c) odor and milk separated by 20 minutes; or (d) no treatment. One hour later, pups were tested for their preference between cedar and pine odors. The preference was measured as the amount of time spent over pine- or cedar-scented shavings in a screen-covered container. Pups that had received cedar–milk pairings spent almost 75% of their time over cedar; the control groups all showed aversions to the cedar odor. The warm ambience proved to be necessary for learning to develop, as pups that received cedar–milk pairings at 26°C showed no cedar odor preference.

Although familiar olfactory cues can control suckling behavior, odors experienced during suckling are also preferred by rat pups. Brake (1981) exposed 11- to 14-day-old rat pups to orange or pine odor under several conditions. Pups, deprived for 24 h, suckled a passive dam and either did or did not receive milk through an intraoral cannula. Other pups were isolated in a tub either with or without milk delivered through the cannula. Pups exposed to the orange odor developed a preference for it when exposure occurred during suckling, whether or not milk was delivered. Pups exposed in isolation developed a preference for orange only if they had received milk delivery during exposure. The strongest preference occurred in pups that had had their suckling accompanied by milk delivery, followed by the pups that had received milk delivery in isolation. Pups suckling without milk delivery showed slightly less preference for the orange odor. Thus, suckling alone or milk ingestion alone was sufficient to cause a conditioned odor preference, and the combination of both was even more effective. It would have been interesting to measure the relative effectiveness of the odor experience in nondeprived pups; perhaps, in this case, suckling would have been a relatively more effective reinforcer.

Neonates can also learn a conditioned odor-aversion (Rudy and Cheatle, 1977). Two-day-old rat pups were exposed to the odor of lemon for 30 min, that was paired with an ip injection of lithium chloride, a substance that induces a mild toxicosis in rats. Pups were tested on Day 8 on an odor preference apparatus similar to those described above. The pups receiving the odor–illness pairing spent significantly less time over lemon-scented shavings than did control pups, which had either been poisoned while exposed to clean shavings, injected with saline while exposed to lemon-scented shavings, or injected with saline while exposed to clean shavings. In this odor–toxicosis study, there was no ambiguity in the olfactory nature of the training or the testing stimuli.

Rat pups become mobile by the beginning of the third week postpartum, and they soon begin to investigate areas further and further from their nest. Despite their forays into new areas, the pups must still return to their mother until they are weaned, weeks later. Although olfactory cues are still necessary to elicit nipple attachment (Bruno, Teicher, and Blass, 1980), the pups must now also have a mechanism for locating and/or remaining in the nest until they can be fully independent of their mother. Olfactory learning and memory may continue to play an important role in the maintenance of a bond between the pups and their mother (cf. Leon, 1983), as well as between the littermates themselves (cf. Alberts, 1981).

When given a chance to approach either their own mother or a virgin female, 16-day-old rat pups overwhelmingly (93%) approached their dam (Leon and Moltz, 1971). The olfactory nature of the maternal attraction was demonstrated in two ways. A goal box that the mother had recently occupied was also approached by the pups, whereas pups would not approach a mother that was not visible to them when they were upwind of her. The mothers begin to be attractive to the pups by days 12–14 of lactation and remain attractive until Day 27. By independently varying pup age and lactational age of the dam, it was found that this time course represented both a developmental change in the attraction of the pups to maternal odor and a change in the attractiveness of the mothers to pups of a given age (Leon and Moltz, 1971).

Leon (1974) went on to show that the maternal odor is emitted in the cecotroph portion of maternal anal excreta. The attraction-producing element of the cecotroph odor is diet-specific, and pup attraction is dependent on prior experience with that odor (Leon, 1975). This fact was shown by feeding mothers rearing pups one of two arbitrarily selected diets (A or B). In a two-choice test, pups raised by dams eating Diet A approached only the anal excreta of A-fed mothers. Pups of B-fed dams approached anal excreta from B-fed dams.

The odor does not have to be associated with the mother. One can rear pups with a mother that has had a suppression of her own cecal odor (Leon, 1974) and expose isolated pups either to the odor of another dam or to an arbitrarily selected odor such as peppermint. Pups develop strong attractions to odors experienced in this manner (Leon, Galef, and Behse, 1977).

Weanlings of other rodent speices show similar odor preferences based on early experience. Spiny mice *(Acomys cahirinus)* are a precocial murid species that are born furred, sighted, and mobile. Spiny mice pups exposed to the odor of cinnamon or cumin in their home cage for the first 24–36 h of life developed a preference for the familiar odor when tested shortly after exposure (Porter and Etscorn, 1974). Twelve-hour-old pups were also separated from their parents and exposed to cinnamon or cumin odor for 1 h. When tested 24 h later, the pups showed a preference for the odor to which they had previously been exposed (Porter and Etscorn, 1974).

Spiny mice pups are also attracted to a diet-dependent olfactory cue emitted by lactating dams (Porter and Doane, 1976, 1977). One-day-old pups were attracted to bedding soiled by 3- to 5-day postpartum lactating females. Furthermore, using an experimental design similar to that of Leon (1975), Porter and Doane (1976) fed spiny mouse dams one of two different diets. Pups tested on Day 3 showed a preference for bedding soiled by dams eating the same diet as their own mothers. The pups even preferred the bedding of a lactating female of another species, *Mus musculus,* that had been eating the same diet as their own dam, to the bedding of a conspecific dam eating a different diet.

There appears to be an early sensitive period for spiny mice during which exposure to an odor induces a subsequent preference (Porter and Etscorn, 1976). Thus, pups exposed to cinnamon odor on Days 1 or 2 and tested on Day 3, as well as pups exposed on Day 3 and tested on Day 6, all showed a preference for cinnamon. Pups exposed on Days 4 or 5 and tested on Day 6, however, no longer showed a cinnamon preference.

Sensitive periods during which odor exposure leads to a subsequent preference have also been demonstrated in guinea pigs (Carter, 1972; Carter and Marr, 1970) and golden hamster pups (Cornwell-Jones, 1979). Guinea-pigs, a precocial species, were most sensitive to the effects of odor exposure during the first 3 days of life, and showed a pattern of experience-dependent olfactory preference development very similar to that of precocial spiny mice. Hamsters, an altricial species, developed strongest attraction for odors that were experienced at the beginning of the second postnatal week.

Mongolian gerbil pups preferentially approach maternal nest odors by 3 weeks of age (Gerling and Yahr, 1982; Yahr and Anderson-Mitchell, 1983). The major olfactory cue is a product of the mother's ventral scent gland; pups showed a decreased attraction to nest odors from glandectomized dams. Pups 2 to 3 weeks old show some attraction to maternal nest odors, although the effect is much less robust than during the third week. This earlier attraction is eliminated if pups are raised by glandectomized dams, a finding suggesting that prior experience is necessary for the preference to develop. Older pups still show some attraction to glandectomized dams, a finding suggesting that other sources of odor can act as attractants. Moreover, by 40 days of age, gerbil pups begin to discriminate between their own mother and other dams.

Rats, gerbils, and spiny mice are similarly attracted to maternal odors, and the time course of the period of attraction varies in accordance with the general precocity of the species. Moreover, it was found that the onset of the attraction was correlated with a particular stage of olfactory bulb development (Leon, Coopers-mith, Ulibarri, Porter, and Powers, 1984). Specifically, pups of each species began to be attracted to maternal odor at the same time that the organization of their olfactory bulbs appeared to reach its adult level.

Alberts and May (1984) compared the effectiveness of mere exposure to an odor with exposure paired with maternal contact in inducing olfactory prefer-ences. Preference was measured as time spent in contact with each of two scented, fur-covered huddling surrogates during a 5-h test. Alberts and May found that 4 h of daily exposure to an odor (on Days 1–19) was sufficient to induce a significant preference for the familiar odor on Day 20. Similarly, 4 h of daily exposure to an odor in the presence of the mother induced a strong preference. However, when the two modes of preexposure were directly compared by exposing pups on alter-nate days to one odor in isolation and a second odor in the presence of the dam, the pups preferred the latter odor. Thus, although the mere exposure of pups to an odor is sufficient to induce a subsequent preference, this preference is strength-ened if the odor is paired with maternal contact.

Alberts and May (1984) then determined that a very specific component of maternal care, thermotactile contact, was just as effective in inducing an olfactory preference as the odor experienced with the mother herself. When pups were exposed on alternate days to one odor painted on a warm furry tube and a second odor painted on their dam, they spent equal amounts of time huddling with stim-ulus objects of either scent. When mere exposure was alternated daily with odor painted on a warm surrogate, the pups preferred the odor paired with the warm object.

Early olfactory learning of the kind that normally deals with the acquisition of attraction to maternal odors may be reinforced by a nonspecific arousal of neo-nates by any of a variety of stimuli. This kind of stimulation would normally be provided by the mother during the course of her contact with the young. Other kinds of olfactory learning, such as aversive conditioning, may have different underlying neural substrates, even in neonates.

OLFACTORY SYSTEM ORGANIZATION

The laminar organization of the bulb has allowed a detailed study of different classes of its input, output, and intrinsic neurons. The olfactory receptor neurons, which sense and transduce the olfactory stimuli in the olfactory turbinates, enter the bulb and synapse with three types of second-order neurons; the mitral, tufted, and periglomerular cells. The connections between the olfactory receptor neurons and the second-order neurons occur in large synaptic conglomerations called *glo-meruli*. The neural signal from the bulb is then projected to the olfactory cortex and other basal forebrain areas (Figure 1). This information can then be passed on to the frontal and entorhinal cortex, where complex processing and integration may be mediated. The many levels of processing that the olfactory information is subjected to may allow rats to extract different levels of complexity from environmental olfactory cues. Just how these different levels of neural processing affect olfactory perception is still not known, and it is the subject of an intensified research effort in several laboratories.

The olfactory receptor cells reside in the sensory neuroepithelium, which lines the turbinates and the lateral walls of the posterior nasal cavity (Bojsen-Moller, 1975; Leonard and Tuite, 1981). The sensory neurons lie interspersed among supporting cells, above a layer of basal cells. They are bipolar neurons that have a single unbranched, ciliated dendrite extending to the epithelial surface, as well as an unmyelinated axon (Graziadei and Monti Graziadei, 1978; Monti Graziadei and Graziadei, 1979). The axons travel in bundles, the fila olfactoria, through the cribriform plate of the ethmoid bone, to the olfactory bulb; the projections remain unbranched until reaching the olfactory glomeruli.

The olfactory receptor neurons form the outermost layer around the bulb and are the thickest on the anterior and ventral surfaces. There is a great deal of convergence in the projections from the receptors to the glomeruli; in the rabbit, approximately 50 million primary neurons project to 2,000 glomeruli in each bulb (Allison, 1953). It should also be noted that the projection from the sensory epi-

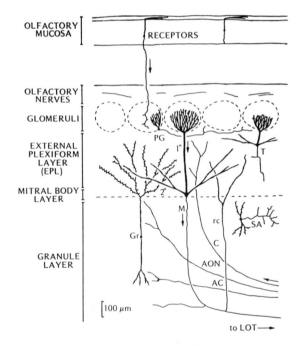

Figure 1. Neuronal elements of the olfactory bulb. Inputs: Afferent fibers from the olfactory receptors; central fibers from three sources: centrifugal fibers (C) from the nucleus of the horizontal limb of the diagonal band; ipsilateral fibers from the anterior olfactory nucleus (AON); contralateral fibers from the anterior commissure (AC). Principal Neurons: Mitral cell (M), with primary (1°) and secondary dendrites (2°) and recurrent axon collaterals (rc); tufted cell (T). Intrinsic neurons: Periglomerular (PG); deep short axon (SA); granule cell (Gr). LOT, lateral olfactory tract. (Used with permission. From *Synaptic Organization of the Brain,* by G. Shepherd, Oxford University Press, 1984).

thelium to the glomerular sheet is at least moderately topographic (cf. Jastreboff, Pedersen, Greer, Stewart, Kauer, Benson, and Shepherd, 1984; Land, 1973; Le Gros Clark, 1951) in that specific areas of the receptor sheet project to specific areas of the glomerular layer. In the glomerulus, the olfactory axon ramifies and terminates on the primary dendrite of a mitral or tufted cell or on a periglomerular cell dendrite (Shepherd, 1972). Mitral cells, the major projection neurons in the bulb, are relatively large ($20–30\mu m$ diameter) and their cell bodies form a layer internal to the glomerular lamina. Mitral cells send primary apical dendrites radially through the external plexiform layer, to the glomerular layer. In addition, sets of secondary dendrites are given off, which spread tangentially within the external plexiform layer, which lies between the glomerular and mitral cell layers (Price and Powell, 1979c). The axon from each mitral cell joins the centripetally projecting lateral olfactory tract, the only output from the bulb.

There seems to be no clear topographic map in the projection of the mitral cells to the olfactory cortex. Small patches of mitral cells project to large areas of the olfactory cortex, and conversely, small areas of the olfactory cortex receive projections from widely spaced mitral cells (cf. Scott, McBride, and Schneider, 1980).

Internal to the mitral-cell-body lamina is the granule cell layer. Granule cells are small, axonless, inhibitory interneurons that send dendrites into the external plexiform layer, where they make dendrodendritic synapses with the secondary dendrites of mitral cells. The synapses are believed to occur in reciprocal pairs, the mitral-to-granule synapses being excitatory and the granule-to-mitral synapses inhibitory (Price and Powell, 1970d; Shepherd, 1972). This arrangement provides for both self-inhibition of the mitral cells and, when other mitral cells contact the same granule cell, lateral inhibition (Shepherd, 1963, 1972).

The other main class of inhibitory interneurons in the bulb are the periglomerular (PG) cells. These are small cells whose perikarya lie just outside the glomeruli. PG cells send dendrites into one, or occasionally two, glomeruli, and their laterally spreading axons can span up to four glomeruli. PG cell dendrites receive input from olfactory axons and have been observed to make dendrodendritic reciprocal synapses with the primary dendrites of mitral cells (Pinching and Powell, 1971a,c).

The tufted cells have both intra- and extrabulbar connections. These cells are dispersed within the external plexiform and glomerular layers, and like the mitral cells, each sends a primary dendrite into a glomerulus. Tufted cells are morphologically similar to mitral cells (Pinching and Powell, 1971b), although there is some heterogeneity in form both within the tufted cell population and between the mitral and the tufted cells (Macrides and Schneider, 1982). The projections from the tufted cells to the olfactory cortex course via the lateral olfactory tract and overlap with, but are more limited than, those of mitral cells (Haberly and Price 1977).

Mitral cell axons project to a number of limbic system areas (Figure 2). The most rostral of these is the anterior olfactory nucleus (AON), which, in turn, projects to the contralateral bulb and to most of the primary projection areas of the mitral cells themselves. These areas are the olfactory tubercle, the prepyriform cortex, the periamygdaloid cortex, the lateral entorhinal cortex, and both the anterior and posterolateral cortical nuclei of the amygdala (Haberly and Price, 1977; MacLeod, 1971; Powell, Cowan, and Raisman, 1965). There are also projections to the lateral, anterior, and preoptic areas of the hypothalamus, the lateral habenula, and the dorsomedial thalamus, although some of these connections may be polysynaptic (Powell *et al.*, 1965). There appears to be no topographic organization for the mitral cell projections (cf. Scott *et al.*, 1980), although the projection to the ipsilateral AON, as well as the projection from the AON to the contralateral olfactory bulb, appears to be topographically arranged (Schoenfeld and Macrides, 1984).

The tufted cells show a systematic projection pattern, based on their depth from the surface of the bulb, rather than with respect to the rostrocaudal or dorsoventral axes. These output cells can be divided into three categories: internal, middle, and external. The term *external* is used by some authors to refer to the middle tufted cells and by some to refer to the peripheral cells, depending on their position in the external plexiform or glomerular layer. The axons of some external tufted cells project through the internal plexiform layer to the opposite side of the same bulb (Schoenfeld, Marchand, and Macrides, 1985). Some external tufted cells project axon collaterals to the internal plexiform layer on the same side of the bulb (Orona, Rainer, and Scott, 1984). Projections leaving the bulb from deep tufted cells are limited to the more rostral of the mitral cell projection areas, namely, the olfactory tubercle and the prepyriform cortex (Haberly and Price, 1977). The deeper the cell body lies, the more caudal is its projection to the olfactory cortex (Haberly and Price, 1977). The function of this projection pattern is uncertain and

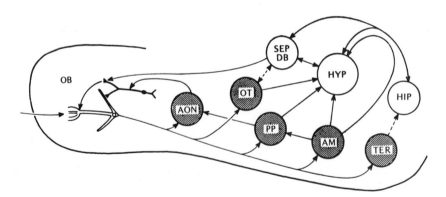

Figure 2. Relations between olfactory and limbic parts of the brain. The primary olfactory areas, which receive input from the mitral cells of the olfactory bulb (OB), are shown as shaded circles: anterior olfactory nucleus (AON); olfactory tubercle (OT); prepyriform cortex (PP); amygdaloid complex (AM); and transitional entorhinal cortex (TER). Limbic structures are shown as open circles: septum and diagonal band (SEP-DB); hypothalamus (HYP); and hippocampus (HIP). Note the multiplicity of connections, including centrifugal pathways to the granule cells of the olfactory bulb. (Used with permission. From *Synaptic Organization of the Brain,* by G. Shepherd, Oxford University Press, 1984).

will probably remain so until the specific role of the tufted cells in olfactory processing is better understood.

The bulb receives a considerable afferent projection from caudal sites (Davis and Macrides, 1981; Pinching and Powell, 1972; Price and Powell, 1979a). Although early degeneration studies indicated centrifugal afferent fibers only from the horizontal limb of the diagonal band (HLDB; Price and Powell, 1970b), more recent studies using the neural transport of horseradish peroxidase (HRP) and autoradiographic techniques indicate a more widespread source of the projections. Specifically, the bulb receives afferents from the anterior olfactory nucleus (ipsilateral and contralateral), the nucleus of the lateral olfactory tract, the ventral hippocampal rudiment (tenia tecta), the pyriform cortex, the hypothalamus, the locus coeruleus, and the dorsal and median raphe nuclei. Projections from the HLDB are cholinergic (Macrides, Davis, Youngs, Nadi, and Margolis, 1981), and evidence indicates that the locus coeruleus afferents are probably noradrenergic and the raphe projections serotonergic (Macrides *et al.*, 1981; Margolis, 1981; Shipley, Halloran, and De La Torre, 1985). Input from the rest of the brain to the bulb may allow the animal to modulate the olfactory bulb's responsiveness to particular cues based on previous experience of the organism, its physical state, its emotional state, and its stage of development. The massive centrifugal influences on olfactory bulb function suggest that olfactory function depends on the function of other parts of the brain.

There is a segregation of the terminal fields of the different projections within the bulb. In general, projections from the anterior olfactory nucleus and the most rostral areas of the pyriform cortex appear to terminate on both granule cells and periglomerular cells, whereas the more caudal forebrain areas seem to terminate mostly on granule cells alone (Macrides *et al.*, 1981). The serotonergic input terminates in the glomerular layer (Moore, Halaris, and Jones, 1978). Indeed, serotonergic terminals from the raphe have been localized within individual glomeruli (Schumacher, McLean and Shipley, 1984). The noradrenergic projection is confined mostly to the external plexiform layer (Jaffe and Cuello, 1980).

In many vertebrates, there is an accessory olfactory structure known as the vomeronasal, or Jacobsohn's, organ, which is a pouch in the nasal chamber, usually connected to the nasal cavity, sometimes opening into the oral cavity. Output from the vomeronasal organ forms the vomeronasal nerve, which terminates in the accessory olfactory bulb, a laminated structure in the dorsocaudal part of the main olfactory bulb (MacLeod, 1971). Projections from output cells of the accessory olfactory bulb are limited to the medial cortical nucleus of the amygdala; the main olfactory bulb also sends projections to the amygdala (Scalia and Winans, 1975).

In summary, the olfactory receptor cells project to the glomerular layer of the olfactory bulb, where they synapse with mitral and tufted cells. Mitral-cell and some tufted-cell excitability is mediated, in part, through inhibitory interneurons, the granule and periglomerular cells, which are themselves influenced by centrifugal afferents from some of the same limbic areas to which the output cells project. The accessory olfactory system appears to be independent of the main bulb.

ROBERT
COOPERSMITH AND
MICHAEL LEON

The complexity of the adult olfactory network is in line with the sensory complexities of the adult world. The relatively simple olfactory world of neonates, however, may require a simplified, but highly reliable, system for responding to the few, but critical, odors in its life. Below, we describe such a system.

The neurosensory epithelium, which is formed by the olfactory receptor neurons, develops prenatally in rodents, starting as early as embryonic Day 10 (E10) and attaining an adultlike appearance by E18 (Cuschieri and Bannister, 1975a,b; Farbman and Margolis, 1980). In the mouse, receptor cell dendrites are first visible on E11, and cilia formation occurs from E12 to E16. Basal and supporting cells appear on E17. Hinds (1968a) reported that olfactory axons reach the bulb by E13 and possibly by E12. Monti Graziadei, Stanley, and Graziadei (1980) observed sensory axons leaving the neuroepithelium by E10 and reaching the future olfactory bulb site, the telencephalic wall, by E11. The development of the vomeronasal organ parallels that of the epithelium, except that it begins 2 days later (Cushieri and Bannister, 1975a).

In both rats and mice, olfactory bulb neurogenesis begins on Day E10 (Altman, 1969; Bayer, 1983; Hinds, 1968a,b). By the use of tritiated thymidine autoradiography, to date cell birth by its incorporation into the DNA of dividing cells, the mitral cells have been found to be the first to be born in the bulb. In mice, mitral cells are born from E11 to E15; the majority being born on E12 and E13. In rats, mitral cells are generated on Days E12 to E18, with a peak occurring on E15 and E16. The next group of cells to be born are the tufted cells. Of interest is that these cells, which show a projection pattern based on their depth from the surface of the bulb, originate along a temporal gradient based on the same axis. Thus, internal tufted cells, located near the mitral cell layer, are born first (mouse: E11–E16, peak on E15; rat: E12–E20, peak on E17), followed by middle tufted cells (mouse: E10–E18, peak on E16; rat: E12–E22, peak on E19), and peripheral tufted cells are born last (mouse: E10–E18, peak on E17; rat: E17–P1, peak on E20). The system therefore appears to start out with a crude form of the organization that it has in adulthood.

Cells of the accessory olfactory bulb (AOB) are born earlier than cells of the main olfactory bulb. In mice, AOB output cells are generated on Days 10–12, with a peak on Day 10 (Hinds, 1968a). Rats show the same pattern with a peak on Day 13. AOB granule cells are also born prenatally; in mice, they peak on Day E17 (Hinds, 1968a), and in rats on Day E20 (Bayer, 1983).

Consistent with the early neurogenesis of AOB cells, neural activity has been demonstrated *in utero* in the AOB of rat fetuses (Pedersen, Stewart, Greer, and Shepherd, 1983). Rats were injected with ^{14}C-2-deoxyglucose (2DG) an Day 22 of pregnancy, and their pups were deliver by cesarean section 1 h later. High 2DG uptake, probably reflecting neural activity, was observed in the accessory bulb, but not in the main bulb.

In mice, the first synapses in the bulb are seen in the presumptive glomerular layer on Day E15 (Hinds and Hinds, 1976a,b). Most of these synapses were axodendritic, presumably from olfactory nerve terminals onto mitral cells. A few dendrodendritic synapses were observed; it was not certain whether these were mitral-to-periglomerular or periglomerular-to-mitral cell synapses. No dendrodendritic synapses were seen in the external plexiform layer until E18, the same day that the first synapse was seen in the granule cell layer.

In rats, presynaptic sites were not observable in the glomerular layer until E21 (Friedman and Price, 1984). This finding corresponds well with the time course in mice, if the 3-day difference in the time course of neurogenesis between the species is considered.

At E15–E16 in mice, some of the olfactory axons, which normally terminate within the glomerular layer, penetrate this lamina and reach the area of the mitral cell bodies (Hinds and Hinds, 1976b). This phenomenon was further described by Monti Graziadei *et al.* (1980), who noted that some olfactory axons still reached the mitral cell layer by postnatal Day 1 (P1). None were observable by P5. During this same period (E15–P1), mitral cells were seen to undergo a major change in orientation (Hinds and Ruffett, 1973). At E14, almost all mitral cells were oriented tangentially within the olfactory bulb. Over the next 5 days, the neurons seemed to rotate 90° to a radial orientation. This reorganization included the atrophy and regrowth of dendritic processes resulting in the radially directed apical dendrite observed in the adult. This observation is particularly intriguing because regenerating olfactory axons in the adult appear to be able to induce a reorientation of mitral cell dendrites (Graziadei and Samanen, 1980). The relationship between the two phenomena remains to be demonstrated.

Anterograde transport of ^{3}H-leucine has revealed that the lateral olfactory tract projects to the pyriform cortex as early as E16 in rats (Schwob and Price, 1984a). A similar projection was observed in mice at E13 (Derer, Caviness, and Sidman, 1977). It should be noted that this time corresponds well with the peak of mitral cell neurogenesis in mice (Hinds, 1968a) and is a few days before the first observable synapses onto mitral cell dendrites (Hinds and Hinds, 1976a). Similarly, E16 represents the peak of mitral cell generation in rats (Bayer, 1983), several days before presynaptic elements are observable in the olfactory bulb glomerular layer (Friedman and Price, 1984).

At E16 and E17, the rat olfactory bulb efferents are limited to the lateral olfactory tract itself. Over the next 2 weeks, the projection fields widens, gradually reaching its adult form. Periamygdaloid and entorhinal cortices are not fully innervated until P5–P6, and the adult projection field is not realized until P9, when the medial edge of the olfactory tubercle receives its fibers. The projections of the accessory olfactory bulb arise several days earlier and are adultlike by day P1 (Schwob and Price, 1978, 1984a). The areas that are innervated first are those that show the densest terminal fields as adults.

In rats, synapses have been observed in prepyriform cortex as early as P0 (Westrum, 1975b), although presynaptic terminals, as demonstrated by Timm staining, do not develop through the extent of the olfactory cortex until the first postnatal week (Friedman and Price, 1984). In mice, synapses were observed in pyriform cortex at E13, although these were very rare (Derer *et al.*, 1977). At E15, still not more than a handful of synapses were seen, a finding indicating that synaptogenesis begins in earnest not earlier than the last few prenatal days of development. Again, this would be consistent with the time course observed in rats. The olfactory system of mice and rats, particularly the accessory olfactory system, is therefore at least partially functional even before birth. The main olfactory system appears to be functional at birth and continues to develop during the mother–young episode.

In contrast to the olfactory bulb output cells, the majority of the bulb interneurons are born postnatally. In rats, approximately half of the granule and periglomerular cells originate during the first postnatal week; after this peak, the remainder of the cells are born over the next 2 weeks (Altman, 1969; Bayer, 1983). In mice, the same time course of granule and periglomerular cell birth is evident, except that the peak begins 2–3 days before birth (Hinds, 1968a,b).

The granule cells of rat pups continue to divide and migrate out from the periventricular core of the bulb after the second postnatal week. Although the rate of granule cell formation plateaus, granule cell neurogenesis continues into adulthood, possibly as part of a slow cell turnover (Bayer, 1983). In mice, the synapse number in the granule and the external plexiform layers continues to increase, apparently past Day 44 (Hinds and Hinds, 1976a). However, when the ontogeny of individual granule cells was examined in rats, they appeared to grow, as measured by several parameters (including width of dendritic field, dendritic length, and number of dendritic spines) until 14–21 days postnatally, when dendritic field size began to decline (Brunjes, Schwark, and Greenough, 1982). Thus, the increase in total granule synapse number, even after 3 weeks postnatally, may be a result of granule cell proliferation outstripping the decline in individual dendritic fields. After the end of the second week, both the efferent and the afferent bulbar projections have reached their adult pattern (Schwob and Price 1984a).

During the first 2 weeks, the number of synapses in the bulb increases rapidly. The number of synapses in the glomerular layer peaks 2–3 weeks postnatally, whereas the number of external plexiform and granule layer synapses is still rising at this point (Hinds and Hinds, 1976a,b).

In adult rats, olfactory bulb efferent fibers terminate in the outermost lamina of the olfactory cortex, Layer Ia. The inner half of Layer I (Layer Ib) receives intracortical associational fibers (Price 1973). These two lamina correspond to the distal and proximal segments, respectively, of the cortical pyramidal-cell apical dendrites (Westrum, 1975a). In neonates, however, this pattern is not apparent (Schwob and Price, 1984b). On Day P1, these sets of projections overlap extensively, and not until P7 were they segregated as in the adult cortex. A competition for postsynaptic sites was suggested by an experiment by Westrum (1975a). In adult rats, lesions were placed in the olfactory cortex, which resulted in terminal degeneration restricted to Layer Ib of the olfactory cortex rostral to the lesion (the site of termination of the intracortical association fibers). If, however, the same lesions were placed in rats that had been unilaterally olfactory-bulbectomized at birth (on the same side as the lesion), then degeneration was seen throughout

Layer I, a finding suggesting that the intracortical fibers had innervated the post-synaptic sites left vacant by the missing olfactory fibers. Perhaps there is also a competition among the olfactory fibers themselves, although this possibility remains to be demonstrated.

It appears that the order in which the mitral cells send axons into the lateral olfactory tract is spatially determined (Grafe and Leonard, 1982). Horseradish per-oxidase (HRP) was injected into the olfactory cortex or the lateral olfactory tract of neonatal hamsters, and the pattern of labeled olfactory bulb mitral and tufted cells was examined. At 3 and 7 days of age, almost half of the labeled cells occurred in the medial quadrant of the bulb; this segregation of labels disappeared by Day 8.

Most of the centrifugal projections to the bulb appear to develop during the first postnatal week (Schwob and Price, 1984a). HRP injected into the bulb on Day P1 labels only part of the anterior olfactory nucleus, the HLDB and the rostral pyriform cortex. The remainder of the afferents develop over the next 6 days. In addition, there appears to be a shift in the terminal fields of fibers arising from the contralateral anterior olfactory nucleus. On P3, these fibers terminate in the deep part of the granule cell layer; by the end of the second postnatal week, the terminals are observed in their adult position, in the superficial aspect of the granule layer.

The development of rat olfactory bulb electrical activity, recorded as surface EEG, appears to lag several days behind the first behavioral observation of olfactory function. Activity was not observed until the fifth or sixth day postpartum, at which time bursts of 8-Hz waves were seen after each inspiration. The frequency of waves within these bursts increased daily, reaching adult EEG patterns after about 4 weeks (Almli, Henault, Velozo, and Morgane, 1985; Oishi, Sano, Yang, and Takahashi, 1973; Salas, Schapiro, and Guzman-Flores, 1970). The apparent paradox that behavioral activity precedes observable electrical activity may be resolved if one considers Shepherd's analysis (1972) of current flow through the olfactory bulb; the major contributors to surface-recorded EEG are probably the granule cells, a population of postnatally developing inhibitory interneurons. The time course of development of these cells corresponds well with the development of olfactory bulb EEG activity. In contrast, spontaneous spike activity was recorded extracellularly from single mitral cells hours after birth (Math and Davrainville, 1980). The spontaneous activity of individual mitral cells increases during the first 3 weeks postpartum (Shafa, Shineh, and Bidanjiri, 1981; Wilson and Leon, 1986). Individual mitral cells respond differentially to odors on the day of birth, and their responses preserve the temporal patterns of activity exhibited by the receptor neu-rons (Mair and Gesteland, 1982).

The picture that emerges of the olfactory system early in life in Norway rats is one in which all the components are in place to form a system competent to deal with olfactory stimuli. The changes that occur in the system over the course of development may add to the ability of these animals to perform an increasingly sophisticated processing of incoming olfactory information. In addition, the large changes that develop postnatally in this system raise the possibility that differential olfactory experience during this period may permanently modify the system during its formation.

CHANGES IN NEURAL ACTIVITY WITH OLFACTORY EXPERIENCE

We tested the hypothesis that familiarization with an odor might change the olfactory bulb response to that odor (Coopersmith and Leon, 1984). The technique of 2-deoxyglucose (2DG) autoradiography was used to measure relative neural activity in the olfactory bulbs of 19-day-old odor-familiar and odor-unfamiliar rat pups during a peppermint odor exposure. One group of pups had been previously exposed to peppermint for 10 min per day, accompanied by perineal stimulation on Days 1–18, and a second group was exposed to clean air under the same conditions. In response to the peppermint test-stimulus on Day 19, the pups that had previously received daily exposure to peppermint showed 64% higher uptake of 2DG in three complexes of glomeruli, 1.5–2.2 mm from the rostral pole of the bulb, on its lateral aspect (Figure 3).

The enhanced neural response is not due to the increased stimulus availability caused by increased respiration of the familiar odor during the 2DG test. Neither the total number of respirations nor the frequency pattern of respirations differed between odor-familiar and odor-unfamiliar pups (Coopersmith and Leon, 1984; Figure 4).

The response is long-lived. Pups exposed to peppermint odor on Days 1–18

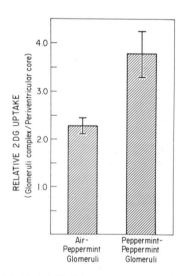

Figure 3.   Mean uptake of 14-C labeled 2DG in response to peppermint odor in focal areas of the glomerular layer 1.5–2.2 mm from the rostral pole of the bulb of odor-familiar (peppermint–peppermint) and odor-unfamiliar (air–peppermint) animals. Uptake is expressed as a ratio of glomerular to periventricular core activity. (Used with permission. Coopersmith and Leon, 1984).

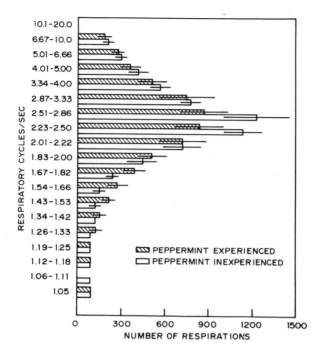

Figure 4. Mean number of respirations for different respiratory frequencies (respiratory CPS) in 20 arbitrarily selected bins for peppermint-experienced and peppermint-inexperienced 19-day-old pups.

and then tested for relative 2DG uptake to peppermint odor on Day 90 have an enhanced neural response to that odor (Coopersmith and Leon, 1986).

The response is odor-specific. Daily experience with cyclohexanone odor does not induce an enhanced response to peppermint odor. Experience with cyclohexanone odor, however, does induce an enhanced response to cyclohexanone, although in a different part of the bulb (Coopersmith, Henderson, and Leon, 1986). Thus, it appears that early experience with an odor induces a specific enhanced olfactory-bulb response to that odor. The fact that the concentration of cyclohexanone used would not have evoked a significant trigeminal response (Silver and Moulton, 1982) suggests that that system is not involved in the development of the enhanced neural response.

We have also determined that the enhanced glomerular response does not develop after simple olfactory experience. In the above experiments, all of the animals were stroked with an artist's brush during odor presentation because this procedure (which mimics maternal contact) had been shown to facilitate the acquisition of olfactory preferences in young rats (Pedersen, et al., 1982; Sullivan, et al., 1986). We found that brief odor exposure by itself was ineffective in inducing either a behavioral preference or an enhanced neural response. Only those pups that had experienced concurrent odor exposure and stroking had the special behavioral and neural responses (Sullivan and Leon, 1986; Figure 5). Sullivan and Hall (1985) found that the stroking stimulation acts as a reinforcer that is as effec-

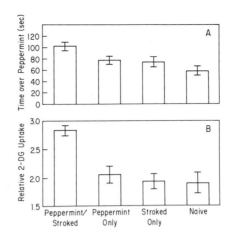

Figure 5. (A) Mean time spent over peppermint odor in a two-odor choice test for pups that were previously exposed to peppermint and stroking, peppermint only, stroking only, and neither stimulus. (B) Mean relative 2DG uptake in the focal areas of the glomerular layer during test exposure to peppermint odor for each of the groups. (Used with permission. Sullivan and Leon, 1986).

tive as milk in facilitating olfactory learning. The enhanced response therefore seems to be a correlate of early olfactory learning.

The enhanced response does not accompany all forms of olfactory learning. Specifically, we found that pups that experienced the peppermint odor associated with toxicosis subsequently avoided that odor but, despite its behavioral significance, did not develop an enhanced glomerular response (Coopersmith, Lee, and Leon, 1986). The enhanced olfactory bulb response therefore appears to depend on the type of olfactory learning encountered during development. The mother may therefore restrict the development of olfactory attractions to her own odors, as she is normally the only source of reinforcing stimulation for the pups.

Mechanism of the Enhanced Neural Response

In order to begin to understand the mechanism underlying the enhanced neural response, we decided to first verify our assumption that the increase in glomerular activity associated with early olfactory learning would be reflected in an increase in mitral cell activity. We reasoned that, if there were increased dendritic stimulation of the mitral cells, we should see increased firing in the output signal from the bulb generated by mitral cells. We therefore recorded single-unit activity from the portion of the mitral body cell layer associated with the active glomerular sites in odor-familiar and odor-unfamiliar pups with either peppermint or orange odor on Day 19 (Wilson, Sullivan, and Leon, 1985; 1987).

Rather than an increase in activity, we found that mitral cells of peppermint-familiar pups had significantly more inhibitory responses and significantly fewer excitatory responses to peppermint than did the peppermint-unfamiliar pups. No differences were found in response to the orange odor, which does not appear to be processed in that glomerular area. Odor familiarity also decreased the number of cells that responded to peppermint with either an excitatory or an inhibitory response and increased the number of cells that did not respond to peppermint odor. Again, simple exposure to peppermint without the reinforcing stroking stimulation did not produce the neurophysiological changes found in those pups that had experienced concurrent odor-stroking stimulation (Wilson, *et al.,* 1987; Figure 6). The signal from the bulb in response to familiar odors is therefore not reflected in an increase, but rather in a decrease in neural activity. The pyriform cortex therefore must be able to recognize a decrease in the ongoing activity from the olfactory bulb to identify the familiar odor.

These data also suggest that the change in the bulb that is induced by olfactory experience could not be primarily or solely due to changes in the mitral cells because it seems highly unlikely that either the mitral cell dendrites or the olfactory receptor neurons synapsing with those dendrites in the glomeruli would increase their activity while the mitral cells themselves decreased their activity. It seemed more likely that another cell type was increasing its glomerular activity and then somehow inhibiting neighboring mitral cell activity. We therefore looked more closely at the glomerular areas associated with the enhanced 2DG uptake in odor-familiar pups and compared its morphology to that of the odor-unfamiliar pups to gain a clue about how an increase in glomerular activity could be reflected in a decrease in mitral cell activity.

Alternate olfactory bulb sections of odor-familiar and odor-unfamiliar pups were therefore processed for autoradiography and histochemically treated for either cytochrome oxidase or succinic dehydrogenase. These are two activity-dependent mitochondrial enzyme stains with finer resolution than 2DG, but without its ability to reveal quantifiable differences between brain areas. We then aligned the sections to determine whether there were identifiable structural modifications associated with early olfactory learning. Although the glomerular areas associated with the 2DG uptake in odor-unfamiliar pups seemed to be unchanged, those of the odor-familiar pups often had a glomerulus protruding into the exter-

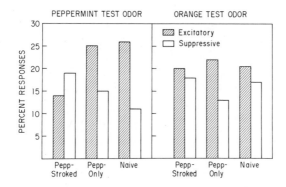

Figure 6. Percentage of excitatory and suppressive responses of presumed mitral cells to peppermint and orange odors in each group.

nal plexiform layer. Sometimes, we could observe two or three of these glomeruli in a cluster. These glomeruli typically do not have the uniform staining of other glomeruli but are lighter staining in the interior, with staining heavier on the periphery of the glomerulus. We then found that, although there are no differences in the number of glomeruli associated with the focal 2DG areas between odor-familiar and odor-unfamiliar pups, the size of the glomeruli and the width of the glomerular layer increased dramatically within these areas in odor-familiar pups (Woo, Coopersmith, and Leon, 1987; Figure 7). The increased neuropil focused in a glomerular area may partially mediate the increased neural response.

We then stained the bulbs of odor-familiar and odor-unfamiliar pups with both a fiber stain and a Nissl stain to examine the glomeruli more closely. We very often found large numbers of glomerular layer neurons in association with modified glomerular complexes. This finding suggested a model of how olfactory learning could produce the observed changes in the olfactory bulb of young rats. Increases in the activity of tufted cells surrounding the glomeruli may account for the 2DG uptake commonly observed in the olfactory bulb (Macrides, Schoenfeld, Marchand, and Clancy, 1985). These cells have a low threshold for activation and become particularly active during olfactory system stimulation (Schneider and Scott, 1983; Onoda and Mori, 1980). Early odor experience appears to be impor-

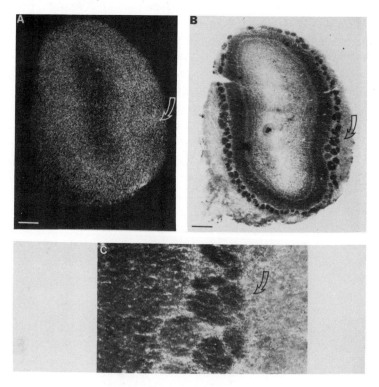

Figure 7. (A) 2DG autoradiograph of peppermint-familiar pups exposed to peppermint, with an arrow showing a glomerular area of heightened activity. (B) Adjacent section stained for succinic dehydrogenase with the arrow in the corresponding area. (C) Magnified view of this area, showing the modified glomerular cluster shown in B. Scale bars: A and B = 400 μm; C = 100 μm. (Used with permission, Woo, Coopersmith, & Leon, 1987.)

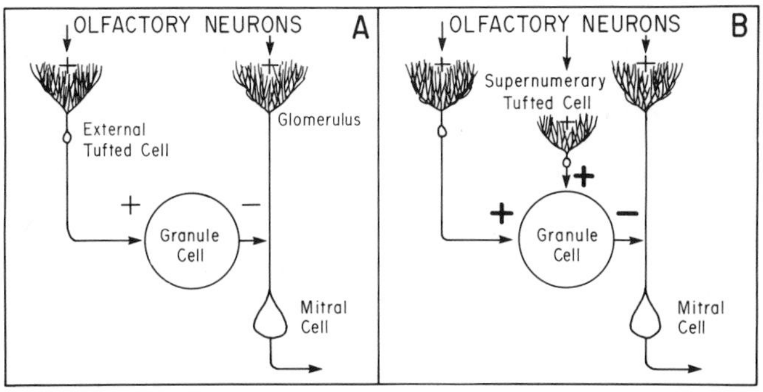

Figure 8. A model for the development of the enhanced neural response and its consequences for the neural coding of learned attractive odors. (A) Odor-unfamiliar pups may have many of their external tufted cells die in the glomerular area coding for a particular odor. The remaining tufted cells may be unable to effectively inhibit the firing of neighboring mitral cells via the granule cells. (B) Early olfactory learning with a particular odor may save and increase the effectiveness of tufted cells in that area. The increased activation of granule cells by tufted cells in response to the learned odor would inhibit local mitral cells.

tant for tufted-cell survival (Meisami and Safari, 1981), and it seems possible that olfactory learning may stabilize tufted-cell interactions with other neurons in the focal glomerular areas. Increased dendritic arborization or an increased number of arbors of tufted cells would then increase the size of the glomeruli in that region. Recall that a subpopulation of tufted cells may project deep to the glomerular layer and synapse with granule cells (Orona *et al.*, 1984). In odor-unfamiliar pups, the relatively lower activity of tufted cells would not provoke the granule cells to inhibit neighboring mitral cells. Odor-familiar pups, however, would have a relatively large number of tufted cells to stimulate local granule cells and to effectively inhibit local mitral cells (Figure 8).

If this model is correct, one would expect to see increased activity in glomerular layer neurons during odor exposure. As both periglomerular cells and tufted cells may have an increase in activity to odors, one would also want to see an increase in neural activity in the internal plexiform layer, where some tufted cells, but no periglomerular cells, project. Using a stain for glycogen phosphorylase, an activity-dependent stain with cellular resolution, we found that there was an increase in glomerular activity and an activity increase in a restricted area deep to the focal 2DG area only in odor-familiar pups and only during odor presentation (Coopersmith and Leon, 1987). These data are consistent with the proposed model.

SUMMARY

We have described behavioral and neural plasticity that can occur in the olfactory system of young mammals. Early olfactory learning, of the type normaly associated with the acquisition of preferences for maternal odors, produces large anatomical changes that appear to reorganize the neural circuitry so that an altered signal is emitted by the olfactory bulb in response to an odor that has acquired attractive value following learning. Because our data indicate that the brain may be permanently modified in a way that would make individuals respond differently to the same stimulus over the course of their lives, it is tempting to speculate that early experience can permanently modify the brain areas that may underlie individual differences in behavior. It would be of interest to extend this type of analysis to other learning paradigms in other species at different ages.

References

Alberts, J. R. Ontogeny of olfaction: Reciprocal roles of sensation and behavior in the development of perception. In R. N. Aslin, J. R. Alberts, and M. R. Petersen (Eds.), *The development of perception: Psychobiological perspectives,* Vol. 1. New York: Academic Press, 1981.

Alberts J. R., and May, B. Ontogeny of olfaction: Development of the rats' sensitivity to urine and amyl acetate. *Physiology and Behavior.* 1980, *24,* 965–970.

Alberts, J. R., and May, B. Nonnutritive, thermotactile induction of filial huddling in rat pups. *Developmental Psychobiology,* 1984, *17,* 161–181.

Allison, A. C. The structure of the olfactory bulb and its relationship to the olfactory pathways in the rabbit and the rat. *Journal of Comparative Neurology,* 1953, *98,* 309–353.

Almli, C. R., Henault, M. A., Velozo, C. A., and Morgane, P. J. Ontogeny of electrical activity of main olfactory bulb in freely moving normal and malnourished rats. *Developmental Brain Research,* 1985, *18,* 1–12.

Altman, J. Autoradiographic and histological studies of postnatal neurogenesis. IV. Cell proliferation and migration in the anterior forebrain, with special reference to persisting neurogenesis in the olfactory bulb. *Journal of Comparative Neurology,* 1969, *137,* 433–458.

Bayer, S. A. 3H-Thymidine-radiographic studies of neurogenesis in the rat olfactory bulb. *Experimental Brain Research,* 1983, *50,* 329–340.

Bojsen-Moller, F. Demonstration of terminalis, olfactory, trigeminal and perivascular nerves in the rat nasal septum. *Journal of Comparative Neurology,* 1975, *159,* 245–256.

Brake, S. C. Suckling infant rats learn a preference for a novel olfactory stimulus paired with milk delivery. *Science,* 1981, *211,* 506–508.

Brunjes, P. C., Schwark, H. D., and Greenough, W. T. Olfactory granule cell development in normal and hyperthyroid rats. *Developmental Brain Research,* 1982, *5,* 149–159.

Bruno, J. P., Teicher, M. H., and Blass, E. M. Sensory determinants of suckling behavior in weanling rats. *Journal of Comparative and Physiological Psychology,* 1986, *94,* 115–127.

Carter, C. S. Effects of olfactory experience on the behavior of the guinea pig *(Cavia porcellus). Animal Behavior,* 1972, *20,* 54–60.

Carter, C. S., and Marr, J. N. Olfactory imprinting and age variables in the guinea-pig, *Cavia porcellus, Animal Behavior,* 1970, *18,* 236–244.

Coopersmith R., and Leon, M. Enahnced neural response to familiar olfactory cues. *Science,* 1984, *225,* 849–851.

Coopersmith, R., and Leon, M. Enhanced neural response by adult rats to odors experienced early in life. *Brain Research,* 1986, *371,* 400–403.

Coopersmith, R., Henderson, S. R., and Leon, M. Odor specificity of the enhanced neural response following early odor experience in rats. *Developmental Brain Research,* 1986, *27,* 191–197.

Coopersmith, R., Lee, S., and Leon, M. Olfactory bulb responses after odor aversion learning by young rats. *Developmental Brain Research,* 1986, *24,* 271–277.

Coopersmith, M. R., and Leon, M. Glycogen phosphorylase and activity in the olfactory bulb of the young rat. *Journal of Comparative Neurology,* 1987, *261,* 148–154.

Cornwell-Jones, C. A. Olfactory sensitive periods in albino rats and golden hamsters. *Journal of Comparative Physiological Psychology,* 1979, *93,* 668–676.

Cuschieri, A., and Bannister, L. H. The development of the olfactory mucosa in the mouse: electron microscopy. *Journal of Anatomy,* 1975a, *119,* 471–498.

Cuschieri, A., and Bannister, L. H. The development of the olfactory mucosa in the mouse: light microscopy, *Journal of Anatomy,* 1975b, *119,* 277–286.

Davis, B. J., and Macrides, F. The organization of centrifugal projections from the anterior olfactory nucleus, ventral hippocampal rudiment, and piriform cortex to the main olfactory bulb in the hamster: an autoradiographic study. *Journal of Comparative Neurology*, 1981, *203*, 475–493.

Derer, P., Caviness, V. S., Jr., and Sidman, R. L. Early cortical histogenesis in the primary olfactory cortex of the mouse. *Brain Research*, 1977, *123*, 27–40.

Farbman, A. I., and Margolis, F. L. Olfactory marker protein during ontogeny: immunohistochemical localization. *Developmental Biology*, 1980, *74*, 205–215.

Fillion, T. J. and Blass, E. M. Infantile behavioral reactivity to oestrous chemostimuli in Norway rats. *Animal Behavior* 1986a, *34*, 123–133.

Fillion, T. J., and Blass, E. M. Infantile experience with suckling odors determines adult sexual behavior in male rats. *Science*, 1986b, *231*, 729–731.

Friedman, B., and Price, J. L. Fiber systems in the olfactory bulb and cortex: A study in adult and developing rats, using the Timm method with the light and electron microscope. *Journal of Comparative Neurology*, 1984, *223*, 88–109.

Gerling, S., and Yahr, P. Maternal and paternal pheromone in gerbils. *Physiol. Behavior*, 1982, *28*, 667–673.

Grafe, M. R., and Leonard, C. M. Developmental changes in the topographical distribution of cells contributing to the lateral olfactory tract. *Developmental Brain Research*, 1982, *3*, 387–400.

Graziadei, P. P. C., and Monti Graziadei, G. A. The olfactory system: A model for the study of neurogenesis and axon regeneration in mammals. In C. W. Cotman (Ed.), *Neuronal plasticity* New York: Raven Press, 1978.

Graziadei, P. P. C., and Samanen, D. W. Ectopic glomerular structures in the olfactory bulb of neonatal and adult mice. *Brain Research*, 1980, *187*, 467–472.

Haberly, L. B., and Price, J. L. The axonal projection patterns of the mitral and tufted cells of the olfactory bulb in the rat. *Brain Research*, 1977, *129*, 152–157.

Hill, D. L., and Almli, C. R. Olfactory bulbectomy in infant rats: Survival, growth and ingestive behaviors. *Physiology and Behavior*, 1981, *27*, 811–817.

Hinds, J. W. Autoradiographic study of histogenesis in the mouse olfactory bulb. I. Time of origin or neurons and neuroglia. *Journal of Comparative Neurology*, 1968a, *134*, 287–304.

Hinds, J. W. Autoradiographic study of histogenesis in the mouse olfactory bulb. II. Cell proliferation and migration. *Journal of Comparative Neurology*, 1968b, *134*, 305–322.

Hinds, J. W., and Hinds, P. L. Synapse formation in the mouse olfactory bulb. I. Quantitative studies. *Journal of Comparative Neurology*, 1976a, *169*, 15–40.

Hinds, J. W., and Hinds, P. L. Synapse formation in the mouse olfactory bulb. II. Morphogenesis. *Journal of Comparative Neurology*, 1976b, *169*, 41–62.

Hinds, J. W., and Ruffett, T. L. Mitral cell development in the mouse olfactory bulb: Reorientation of the perikaryon and maturation of the axon initial segment. *Journal of Comparative Neurology*, 1973, *151*, 281–306.

Hofer, M. A., Shair, H., and Singh, P. Evidence that maternal ventral skin substances promote suckling in infant rats. *Physiology and Behavior*, 1976, *17*, 131–136.

Hudson, R., and Distel, H. Factors involved in eliciting nipple-search behavior in newborn rabbits. *Int. Society for Developmental Psychobiology Abstracts*, 1984, *56*.

Iwahari, S., Oishi, H., Sano, K., Yang, K-M., and Takahashi, T. Electrical activity of the olfactory bulb in the postnatal rat. *Japanese Journal of Physiology*, 1973, *23*, 361–370.

Jaffe, E. H., and Cuello, A. C. The distribution of catecholamines, glutamate decarboxylase and choline acetyltransferase in layers of the rat olfactory bulb. *Brain Research*, 1980, 232–237.

Jastreboff, P. J., Pedersen, P. E., Greer, C. A., Stewart, W. B., Kauer, J. S., Benson, T. E., and Shepherd, G. M. Specific olfactory receptor populations projecting to identified glomeruli in the rat olfactory bulb. *Proceedings of the National Academy of Science*, 1984, *81*, 5250–5254.

Johanson, I. B., and Hall, W. G. Appetitive learning in 1-day-old rat pups. *Science*, 1979, *205*, 419–421.

Johanson, I. B., and Teicher, M. H. Classical conditioning of an odor preference in 3-day-old rats. *Behavior and Neural Biology*, 1986, *29*, 132–136.

Land, L. J. Localized projection of olfactory nerves to rabbit olfactory bulb. *Brain Research*, 1973, *63*, 153–166.

Le Gros Clark, W. E. The projection of the olfactory epithelium on the olfactory bulb in the rabbit. *Journal of Neurology Neurosurgery and Psychiatry*, 1951, *14*, 1–10.

Leon, M. Maternal pheromone. *Physiology and Behavior*, 1974, *13*, 441–453.

Leon, M. Dietary control of maternal pheromone in the lactating rat. *Physiology and Behavior,* 1975, *14,* 311–319.

Leon, M. Chemical communication in mother-young interactions. In J. Vandenbergh (Ed.), *Pheromones and reproduction in mammals.* New York: Academic Press, 1983.

Leon, M., and Moltz, H. Maternal pheromone: Discrimination by pre-weanling albino rats. *Physiology and Behavior,* 1971, *14, 311–319.*

Leon, M., and Moltz, H. The development of the pheromonal bond in the albino rat. *Physiology and Behavior,* 1972, *8,* 683–686.

Leon, M., Galef, B. G., Jr., and Behse, J. Establishment of pheromonal bonds and diet chioce in young rats by odor pre-exposure. *Phusiology and Behavior,* 1977, *18* 387-391.

Leon, M., Coopersmith, R., Ulibarri, C., Porter, R. H., and Powers, J. B. Development of olfactory bulb organization in precocial and altricial rodents. *Developmental Brain Research,* 1984, *12,* 45–53.

Leonard, B. E., and Tuite, M. Anatomical, physiological, and behavioral aspects of olfactory bulbectomy in the rat. *International Review of Neurobiology,* 1981, *22,* 251–286.

MacLeod, P. Structure and function of higher olfactory centers. In L. M. Biedler (Ed.), *Handbook of sensory physiology: Olfaction,* Vol. 4. New York: Springer, 1971.

Macrides, F., and Schneider, S. P. Laminar organization of mitral and tufted cells in the main olfactory bulb of the adult hamster. *Journal of Comparative Neurology,* 1982, *208,* 419–430.

Macrides, F., Davis. B. J., Youngs, W. M., Nadi, N. S., and Margolis, F. L. Cholinergic and catecholaminergic afferents to the olfactory bulb in the hamster: a neuroanatomical, biochemical, and histochemical investigation. *Journal of Comparative Neurology,* 1981, *203,* 495–514.

Macrides, F., Schoenfeld, T. A., Marchand, J. E., and Clancy, A. N. Evidence for morphologically, neurochemically and functionally heterogeneous classes of mitral and tufted cells in the olfactory bulb. *Chemical Senses,* 1985, *10,* 175–202.

Mair, R. G., and Gesteland, R. C. Response properties of mitral cells in the olfactory bulb of the neonatal rat. *Neuroscience,* 1982, *7,* 3117–3125.

Margolis, F. L. Neurotransmitter biochemistry of the mammalian olfactory bulb. In R. Cagan (Eds)., *Biochemistry of taste and olfaction.* New York: Academic Press, 1981.

Meisami, E., and Safari, L. A quantitative study of the effects of early unilateral olfactory deprivation on the number and distribution of mitral and tufted cells and of glomeruli in the rat olfactory bulb. *Brain Research,* 1981, *221,* 81–107.

Monti Graziadei, G. A., and Graziadei, P. P. C. Studies in neuronal plasticity and regeneration in the olfactory system: morphologic and functional characteristics of the olfactory sensory neuron. In E. Meisami and M. A. B. Brazier (Eds.), *Neural growth and regeneration.* New York: Raven Press, 1979.

Monti Graziadei, G. A., Stanley, R. S., and Graziadei, P. P. C. The olfactory marker protein in the olfactory system of the mouse during development. *Neuroscience,* 1980, *5,* 1239–1252.

Moore, R. Y., Halaris, A. E., and Jones, B. E. Serotonin neurons of the midbrain raphe: Ascending projections. *Journal of Comparative Neurology,* 1978, *180,* 417–438.

Onoda, N., and Mori, K. Depth distribution of temporal firing patterns in olfactory bulb related to air-intake cycles. *Journal of Neurophysiology,* 1980, *44,* 29–39.

Orona, E., Rainer, E. C., and Scott, J. W. Dendritic and axonal organization of mitral and tufted cells in the rat olfactory bulb. *Journal of Comparative Neurology,* 1984, *226,* 346–356.

Pedersen, P. E., and Blass, E. M. Prenatal and postnatal determinants of the first suckling episode in albino rats. *Developmental Psychobiology,* 1982, *15,* 349–356.

Pedersen, P. E., Williams, C. L., and Blass, E. M. Activation and odor conditioning of suckling behavior in 3-day-old albino rats. *Journal of Experimental Psychology: Animal Behavior Proceedings,* 1982, *8,* 329–341.

Pedersen, P. E., Stewart, W. B., Greer, C. A., and Shepherd, G. M. Evidence for olfactory function in utero. *Science,* 1983, *221,* 478–480.

Pinching, A. J., and Powell, T. P. S. The neuron types of the glomerular layer of the olfactory bulb. *Journal of Cell Science,* 1971a, *9,* 305–345.

Pinching, A. J., and Powell, T. P. S. The neuropil of the glomeruli of the olfactory bulb. *Journal of Cell Science,* 1971b, *9,* 347–377.

Pinching, A. J., and Powell, T. P. S. The neuropil of the periglomerular region of the olfactory bulb. *Journal of Cell Science,* 1971c, *9,* 379–409.

Pinching, A. J., and Powell, T. P. S. The termination of centrifugal fibers in the glomerular layer of the olfactory bulb. *Journal of Cell Science,* 1972, *10,* 621–635.

Porter, R. H., and Doane, H. M. Maternal pheromone in the spiny mouse *(Acomys cahirinus). Physiology and Behavior,* 1976, *16,* 75–78.

Porter R. H., and Doane, H. M. Dietary-dependent cross-species similarities in maternal chemical cues. *Physiology and Behavior,* 1977, *19,* 129–131.

Porter, R. H., and Etscorn, F. Olfactory imprinting resulting from brief exposure in *Acomys cahirinus. Nature,* 1974, *250,* 132–133.

Porter, R. H., and Etscorn, F. A sensitive period for the development of olfactory preference in *Acomys cahirinus. Physiology and Behavior,* 1976, *17,* 127–130.

Powell, T. P. S., Cowan, W. M., and Raisman, G. The central olfactory connections. *Journal of Anatomy,* 1965, *99,* 791–813.

Price, J. L. An autoradiographic study of complementary laminar patterns of termination of afferent fibers to the olfactory cortex. *Journal of Comparative Neurology,* 1973, *150,* 87–108.

Price, J. L., and Powell, T. P. S. An electron-microscopic study of the termination of the afferent fibres to the olfactory bulb from the cerebral hemisphere. *Journal of Cell Science,* 1970a, *7,* 157–187.

Price, J. L., and Powell, T. P. S. An experimental study of the site of origin and the course of the centrifugal fibers to the olfactory bulb in the rat. *Journal of Anatomy,* 1970b, *107,* 215–237.

Price, J. L., and Powell, T. P. S. The mitral and short axon cells of the olfactory bulb. *Journal of Cell Science,* 1970c, *7,* 631–651.

Price, J. L., and Powell, T. P. S. The morphology of the granule cells of the olfactory bulb. *Journal of Cell Science,* 1970d, *7,* 91–123.

Rudy, J. W., and Cheatle, M. D. Odor-aversion learning in neonatal rats. *Science,* 1977, *198,* 845–846.

Salas, M., Schapiro, S., and Guzman-Flores, C. Development of olfactory bulb discrimination between maternal and food odors. *Physiology and Behavior,* 1970, *5,* 1261–1264.

Scalia, F., and Winans, S. S. The differential projection of the olfactory bulb and accessory olfactory bulb in mammals. *Journal of Comparative Neurology,* 1975, *161,* 31–56.

Schapiro, S., and Salas, M. Behavioral response of infant rats to maternal odor. *Physiology and Behavior,* 1970, *5,* 815–817.

Schneider, S. P., and Scott, J. W. Orthodromic response properties of ray olfactory bulb mitral and tufted cells correlate with their projection patterns. *Journal of Neurophysiology,* 1983, *50,* 358–378.

Schoenfled, T. A., and Macrides, F. Topographic organizaton of connections between the main olfactory bulb and pars externa of the anterior olfactory nucleus in the hamster. *Journal of Comparative Neurology,* 1984, *227,* 121–135.

Schoenfeld, T. A., Marchand, J. E., and Macrides, F. Topographic organization of tufted cell axonal projections in the hamster main olfactory bulb: An intrabulbar associational system. *Journal of Comparative Neurology,* 1985, *235,* 503–518.

Schumacher, S., McLean, J., and Shipley, M. T. Serotonergic-raphe terminations in the main olfactory bulb of the rat. *Society for Neuroscience Abstracts,* 1984, *10,* 657.

Schwob, J. E., and Price, J. L. The cortical projection of the olfactory bulb: development in fetal and neonatal rats correlated with quantitative variations in adult rats. *Brain Research,* 1978, *151,* 369–374.

Schwob, J. E., and Price, J. L. The development of axonal connections in the central olfactory systems of rats. *Journal of Comparative Neurology,* 1984a, *223,* 177–202.

Schwob, J. E., and Price, J. L. The development of lamination of afferent fibers to olfactory cortex in rats, with additional observations in the adult. *Journal of Comparative Neurology,* 1984b, *223,* 203–222.

Scott, J. W., McBride, R. L., and Schneider, S. P. The organization of projections from the olfactory bulb to the piriform cortex and olfactory tubercle in the rat. *Journal of Comparative Neurology,* 1980, *194,* 519–534.

Shafa, F., Shineh, S. N, and Bidanjiri, A. Development of spontaneous activity in the olfactory bulb neurons of the postnatal rat. *Brain Research,* 1981, *223,* 409–412.

Shepherd, G. M. Neuronal systems controlling mitral cell excitability. *Journal of Physiology,* 1963, *168,* 101–117.

Shepherd, G. M. Synaptic organization of the mammalian olfactory bulb. *Physiological Reveiw,* 1972, *52,* 864–916.

Shepherd, G. M. *Synaptic organization of the brain.* Oxford: Oxford University Press, 1984.

Shipley, M. T., Halloran, F. J., and De La Torre, J. Suprisingly rich projections from locus coeruleus to the olfactory bulb in the rat. *Brain Research,* 1985, *329,* 294–299.

Silver, W. L., and Moulton, D. G. Chemosensitivity of rat nasal trigeminal receptors. *Physiology and Behavior,* 1982, *28,* 927–930.

Singh, P. J., Tucker, A. M., and Hofer, M. A. Effects of nasal ZnSO4 irrigation and olfactory bulbectomy on rat pups. *Physiology and Behavior*, 1976, *17*, 373–382.

Stickrod, G., Kimble, D. P., and Smotherman, W. P. In utero taste/odor aversion conditioning in the rat. *Physiology and Behavior*, 1982, *28*, 5–7.

Sullivan, R. M., and Hall, W. G. Classical conditioning of behavioral activation using intra-oral infusions of milk or stroking as reward in infant rats. *International Society for Developmental Psychobiology Abstracts*, 1985, 78.

Sullivan, R. M., and Leon, M. Early olfactory learning induces an enhanced olfactory bulb response in young rats. *Developmental Brain Research*, 1986, *27*, 278–282.

Sullivan, R. M., Hofer, M. A., and Brake, S. C. Olfactory-guided orientation in neonatal rats is enhanced by a change in behavioral state. *Developmental Psychobiology*, 1986, *19*, 615–623.

Teicher, M. H., and Blass, E. M. Suckling in newborn rats: eliminated by nipple lavage, reinstated by pup saliva. *Science*, 1976, *193*, 442–425.

Teicher, M. H., and Blass, E. M. First suckling response of the newborn albino rat: the roles of olfaction and amniotic fluid. *Science*, 1977, *198*, 635–636.

Teicher, M. H., Flaum, L. E., Williams, M., Eckhert, S. J., and Lumia, A. R. Survival, growth and suckling behavior of neonatally bulbectomized rats. *Physiology and Behavior*, 1978, *21*, 553–561.

Westrum, L. E. Axonal patterns in olfactory cortex after olfactory bulb removal in newborn rats. *Experimental Neurology*, 1975a, *47*, 442–447.

Westrum, L. E. Electron microscopy of synaptic structures in olfactory cortex of early postnatal rats. *Journal of Neurocytology*, 1975b, *4*, 713–732.

Wilson, D. A., and Leon, M. Early appearance of inhibition in the neonatal rat olfactory bulb. *Developmental Brain Research*, 1986, *26*, 289–292.

Wilson, D. A,, Sullivan, R. M., and Leon, M. Odor familiarity alters mitral cell response in the olfactory bulb of neonatal rats. *Developmental Brain Research*, 1985, *22*, 314–317.

Wilson, D. A., Sullivan, R. M., and Leon, M. Single unit analysis of postnatal olfactory learning: Altered mitral cell responsiveness to learned attractive odors. *Journal of Neuroscience*, 1987, *7*, 3154–3162.

Woo, C. C., Coopersmith, R., and Leon, M. Functional changes in olfactory bulb morphology following early learning. *Journal of Comparative Neurology*, 1987, *263*, 113–125.

Yahr, P., and Anderson-Mitchell, K. Attraction of gerbil pups to maternal nest odors: Duration, specificity and ovarian control. *Physiology and Behavior*, 1983, *31*, 241–247.

9

Opioids, Behavior, and Learning in Mammalian Development

PRISCILLA KEHOE

INTRODUCTION

Endogenous opioid peptides and their binding sites reside within systems found in the brain and spinal cord, the pituitary, the adrenal medulla, and the autonomic nervous system (Akil, Watson, Young, Lewis, Khachaturian, and Walker, 1984; Basbaum and Fields, 1984; Khachaturian, Lewis, Schafer, and Watson, 1985). These systems seem to be involved in the modulation of physiological and behavioral responsivity to endogenous and environmental demands. Morley (1981) suggested that the discovery of the opioid systems and their diverse functions concerning stress extends Cannon's flight-or-fight (1929) concept and Selye's theory of general adaptation (1976). Specifically, opioid physiology embraces thermal, cardiac, respiratory, miotic, and immune functions, among others (see Watson, Akil, Khachaturian, Young, and Lewis, 1984, for a review). Changes in opioid physiology and in derivative behaviors actually occur during stressful or emergency situations. For example, rats confronted with a novel experience and stressful handling demonstrate increased body temperature, which is naloxone-reversible and is correlated with increased beta-endorphin activity (Blasig, Holit, Bauerle, and Herz, 1978; Clark, 1979). Thermal fluctuations may thus reflect opioid preparation to meet environmental demands. Furthermore, evidence for opioid involvement in stress-induced enhancement of tumor growth has been found (Lewis, Shovit, Ternor, Nelson, Gale and Liebeskind, 1983).

Opioids exert cardiovascular control via the medulla, the pituitary, and the

---

PRISCILLA KEHOE   Department of Psychology, Trinity College, Hartford, Connecticut 06106.

sympathetic nervous system (Watson *et al.*, 1984), suggesting strategic visceral controls that can be situationally recruited. Some of these opioid-associated physiological responses, in fact, have been correlated with pain sensitivity. Changes in blood pressure, respiration, and blood glucose occur with changes in pain responsiveness during stressful situations (Amir and Bernstein, 1982; Isom and Elshowihy, 1982; Zamir, Simantov, and Segal, 1980). The large number of such diverse effects implicate a stress-related opioidergic physiology in need of more comprehensive analysis.

Behaviorally, opioids seem to mediate affective states and may participate in the mediation of appetitive behavior and reward phenomena, including responses to both positive and negative events. Specifically, rats lever-pressed for intracerebral enkephalin injections and self-stimulated at high rates at brainsites that demonstrate significant levels of enkephalinlike immunoreactivity (Beluzzi and Stein, 1977). Monkeys found the opiate hydormorphone reinforcing and self-administered without apparent tolerance or physical dependence (Ternes, Ehrman, and O'Brien, 1985). Furthermore, adult rats demonstrated a preference for an environment in which they had previously received morphine (Mucha and Van der Kooy, 1979; Rossi and Reid, 1976). Opioids may play a role in mediating the appetite for food and water consumption (Carr and Simon 1983; Cooper, 1980; Holtzman, 1979), possibly influencing food-seeking and eating behavior (Morley, Levine, Yim, and Lowy, 1983).

Opioids also recruit other neurochemical systems that mediate attentional and perceptual mechanisms. Thus, they may inhibit or modulate the sensory and motivational effects of aversive stimuli as well as determine the positive consequences of appetitive stimuli. Naloxone, an opioid antagonist, delivered subcutaneously in a dose from 1 to 10 mg/kg, reduced feeding induced by norepinephrine (20 μg ICV) in rats (Morley, Levine, Murray, and Kneip, 1982). Opioid-induced feeding can be blocked by dopamine antagonists, and suppression of tail-pinch-induced feeding by serotonin antagonism was reversed by enkephalin (Morley *et al.*, 1982).

Opioid systems seem to deal with behavioral adjustments to positive and negative events in an organism's environment that have both immediate and long-term consequences. Opiate antagonists have been shown to reduce social and exploratory activity in rats and mice in a novel environment (File, 1980; Katz, 1979; Katz, Carroll, and Baldrighi, 1978). Defensive behavior may be modulated in part by the endogenous opioid system (Bolles and Fanselow, 1980). The opioids dull perceptions of inflicted pain that might otherwise interfere with fight and flight behaviors. It is of considerable interest that stress, as opposed to pain *per se*, induces opioid release (Fanselow, 1984; Fanselow and Bolles, 1979; Whiteside and Devenport, 1985). Regardless of the origin of the opioid release, the same end point is achieved, as the injured animal is better able to locomote to safety.

This richness and diversity of function invites analyses of the possible contributions of opioid systems to behavior and physiology during development and of how these contributions may change over ontogenetic time. If, in fact, the opioid systems function in neonates as they do in adults, certain rewards and reinforcers of infant behavior may be identified. Thus, we can begin to explore the early functioning of opioid systems and how they may mediate particular aspects of mother–

infant bonding, early learning, and motivational and affective mechanisms. Infants can learn about relationships among maternal and environmental events that provide information affecting the performance of many classes of behavior. Therefore, it is most valuable to discover the underlying mechanisms and processes of such early capabilities, how they influence behavior during the neonatal period, and how they facilitate or constrain the expression of later capabilities.

This chapter focuses on how opioid peptides mediate and modulate infant affective states and reward mechanisms. As in adults, the opioid systems seem to mediate pain and stress. The interaction of pleasure and pain systems may be of great significance to neonatal learning and motivation. Because early learning influences mother–infant cohesion, the role of the opioids in this social context is explored. Evidence for early anatomical and biochemical developments of the opioid systems is reviewed first because it then becomes feasible to propose their possible behavioral functions.

Development of the Opioid System

Development of Opioid Peptides

Endogenous opioid systems seem to function as neurotransmitters and hormones and, as such, have a substantial role in brain and behavioral mechanisms. There are three biosynthetically and anatomically separate opioid peptide systems in the brain (Khachaturian *et al.*, 1985). On this basis, we can now begin to study the development as well as the anatomy and physiology of each of these systems functionally. In fact, ontological studies of the opioid peptide systems, among others, suggest that neurons containing beta-endorphin in rat brain exist separately from those containing enkephalin (Bloom, Battenberg, Rossier, Ling, and Guillemin, 1978).

The currently known opioid peptides are derived from three different biochemcial precursors: proopiomelanocortin (POMC), the beta-endorphin–ACTH precursor; proenkephalin, the enkephalin precursor; and prodynorphin, the dynorphin–neoendorphin precursor (see Watson *et al.*, 1984, for a review). POMC, or the beta-endorphin precursor, is localized in both the pituitary and the arcuate nucleus of the hypothalamus and the nucleus tractus solitarus in the caudal medulla. Proenkephalin is found in many widespread brain systems, both local circuits and long projections. In general, the enkephalins are located in neurons that are distinct from those containing beta-endorphin. The dynorphin peptide, although not as widespread as the enkephalins, is present in systems that may also contain enkephalinergic neurons.

Neurons containing the opioid peptides are scattered throughout various brain regions, thereby making specific mapping studies that much more difficult. Enkephalinergic neurons are widespread, with projections to the spinal cord from the medulla; high concentrations are found in the globus pallidus, the nucleus accumbens, the amygdala, and the hippocampus, with smaller amounts in the hypothalamus and the midbrain (Miller, 1983). These enkephalin-containing neurons are distinct from those with dynorphin, which are also widely distributed throughout the nervous system. They are especially found in the intermediate lobe of the pituitary, the hypothalamus, the caudateputamen, the dentate gyrus, and the pyramidal neurons of the hippocampus, as well as in the dorsal horn of the spinal cord (Chavkin, Bakhit, and Bloom, 1983; Haber and Watson, 1983). Beta-endorphin-containing neurons are localized in the pituitary and the basomedial and basolateral hypothalamus, particularly the arcuate nucleus and the periarcuate regions (Akil and Watson, 1983).

Several varieties of opiate receptors have been delineated within the central nervous system, a finding suggesting that specific opioid peptides may activate their own receptors (Chang and Cuatrecasas, 1979, 1981; Chavkin and Goldstein, 1981; Goodman, Snyder, Kuhar, and Young, 1980). Results of *in vivo* experimentation suggest that five separate types of opioid binding sites are present in the adult rat brain: mu, delta, kappa, and lambda receptors (Sadee, Richards, Grevel, and Rosenbaum, 1983), as well as sigma-opiate–PCP receptors (Sircar and Zukin, 1983).

Much research has been done on the neuroanatomical mapping of these opiate receptor systems and their specific agonists (Bloom *et al.*, 1978; Lubek and Wilber, 1980; Pert and Yaksh, 1974; Quirion, Weiss, and Pert, 1983; Simon and Hiller, 1984; Watson and Barchas, 1979), although final mapping has not yet been accomplished. In general, mu receptors are located in the cerebral cortex, the hippocampus, the periaqueductal gray, the thalamus, and the hypothalamus. Delta receptors are mainly found in the cerebral cortex, the limbic system, the pons, and the substantia gelatinosa. Kappa receptors are distributed throughout the caudate putamen, the nucleus accumbens, the amygdala, and the thalamus.

It is possible that the various receptor subtypes are functionally different when interacting with their selective ligands. (Synder, 1984). In fact, it has been suggested that mu receptors are morphine-selective and are localized in pain-modulating areas of the brain; that delta receptors are enkephalin-selective and are localized in the limbic regions possibly dealing with affective behaviors; and that kappa receptors mediating less addicting analgesia appear to be localized in the deep layers of the cerebral cortex.

All three types of opioid peptides appear during embryonic development and increase numerically postnatally. The levels of enkephalins, beta-endorphins, and dynorphins have been monitored during development by immunocytochemical and receptor autoradiographic techniques (Bayon, Shoemaker, Bloom, Mauss, and Guillemin, 1979; Khatchaturian, Alessi, Munfakh, and Watson, 1983; Loughlin, Massamiri, Kornblum, and Leslie, 1985; Patey, de la Baume, Gros, and Schwartz, 1980; Tsang, Ng, Ho, and Ho, 1982). Discrepancies occur between studies about whether the levels of peptides increase or decrease or remain the same during the first 3 weeks postnatally. Differences probably reflect the techniques and the region of the brain being examined (Bayon *et al.*, 1979).

On embryonic Day 16, endorphin levels are 10% of the level found in the weanling (Day 25); yet they display a basic adult pattern of distribution in the diencephalon, the telencephalon, and the midbrain (Bayon *et al.,* 1979; Khatchaturian *et al.,* 1983). Equivalent immunocytochemical studies have demonstrated endorphin immunoreactive cells in the brain of an 11-week human fetus (Bugnon, 1978). A more recent study found that beta-endorphin immunoreactivity in the neonatal rat telencephalon was markedly different from that of adults (Loughlin *et al.,* 1985). Specifically, cells and fibers were seen in germinal zones present only in neonates. Such observations are consistent with studies showing an opioid effect in cell division and changes in brain size (Vertes, Melegh, Vertes, and Kovacs, 1982; Zagon and McLaughlin, 1983). Agonists inhibit neuronal development, whereas antagonists increase brain size, neurons, glial cells, and the number of receptor binding sites. Opioids and their antagonists can alter opioid receptor levels in discrete brain areas (Bardo, Bhatnagar, and Gebhart, 1982; Handelman, 1983; Handelman and Quirion, 1983).

Enkephalin levels are very low on fetal Day 16, with a regional distribution unlike that of the adult (Bayon *et al.,* 1979). It has been suggested that the rat embryo's enkephalinergic system is not as differentiated as the endorphin system at that time (Bayon *et al.,* 1979; Khachaturian *et al.,* 1983). Small, local interneurons often migrate and differentiate later than the projectile type, and in fact, many of the enkephalin neurons fall into the former category. Enkephalin levels increase steadily with a gradual and continuous decrease of the endorphin–enkephalin ratio between embryonic Day 16 and postnatal Day 25, a finding suggesting that they are independent systems (Bayon *et al.,* 1979; Khachaturian *et al.,* 1983). Interestingly, both endorphin and enkephalin levels in the medulla and the midbrain are relatively high in the embryo, a finding suggesting a caudal-rostral development in the opioid systems. As the previous studies did not totally differentiate between leu- and met-enkephalin, a more recent study using antibodies directed at met-enkephalin specifically found a distribution of met-enkephalin in postnatal Day 2 rat brain similar to that found in the adult (Loughlin *et al.,* 1985). The olfactory tubercle and the globus pallidus exhibited especially dense areas, although hippocampal and cortical fibers seem to develop later.

Like leu-enkephalin, dynorphin immunoreactivity appears later in embryonic development when compared to beta-endorphin development in the brain (Khachaturian *et al.,* 1983). On embryonic Day 16, dynorphin is seen in the ventral brainstem and spinal cord. In the magnocellular hypothalamus and the posterior pituitary, dynorphin was detected prenatally, but the adult pattern wasn't seen until postnatal Day 1 or 2 (Khachaturian *et al.,* 1983). Striatal dynorphin is found perinatally, and pallidal, amygdalar, and hippocampal dynorphin develop later (Loughlin *et al.,* 1985).

DEVELOPMENT OF OPIOID BINDING SITES

The ontogenesis of opioid binding sites in the rat brain correlates well with the presence of opioid peptides. Opioid binding sites, using 3H-naltrexone, were present in embryonic Day 14 rat brain (Clendeninn, Petraitis, and Simon, 1976) and by birth had attained 40% of adult specific binding sites (Coyle and Pert,

1976). There is a six- to eight-fold increase in binding levels from midterm fetus to postnatal Day 20, with a more gradual increase from Day 21 to adulthood (Clendeninn *et al.*, 1976; Patey *et al.*, 1980). Saturation studies showed that this increase in binding is due to an increase in sites rather than to a change in the receptor affinity (Clendeninn *et al.*, 1976).

Using radioactive met-enkephalin as a ligand, Tsang and Ng (1980) found that binding differed significantly in different regions of the brain during development. Cerebellar binding was highest during the first week postpartum, brain stem binding was highest in the second week, and whole forebrain in the third week. As in the ontogeny of other neural systems, these opiate binding sites developed in a caudal-rostral sequence.

Opiate receptor density in the striatum increase only twofold (Clendeninn *et al.*, 1976; Coyle and Pert, 1976), whereas other types of striatal receptors show a more pronounced increase during development. Approximately one-third of the opiate binding sites in the adult striatum are localized on dopaminergic neurons, so that its density is increased sixfold during development (Coyle and Compochaiaro, 1976). Thus, dopamine neurons may contribute to the postnatal increase in striatal opiate binding sites. Apparently, this is only one example of multiple opiate–monoamine anatomical and physiological interactions in the central nervous system. Corresponding behavioral and functional interrelationships have been found in the opiate, dopamine, and norepinephrine influence on feeding, exploratory, and self-stimulating behaviors (Arbilla and Langer, 1978; Hoebel, 1977; Morely *et al.*, 1983).

The ligands used in the above-mentioned studies were not entirely site-specific, so that the developmental pattern of the subspecies of receptors was not identified. With the use of highly specific binding assays, the developmental profile of the three main opioid receptor types—mu, delta, and kappa—have been obtained (Spain, Roth and Coscia, 1985). In fact, the subspecies of opioid receptors exhibit differential postnatal developmental profiles. Mu and kappa binding sites are present at birth, whereas delta does not appear until 2 weeks postnatally (Spain *et al.*, 1985). In general, at parturition, mu binding sites in the rat brain are at 40% of adult levels (Coyle and Pert, 1976), and kappa receptors are at 65% of adult levels (Zhang and Pasternak, 1981). Subspecies of opiate binding sites have the characteristic of high- and low-affinity binding (Pasternak and Synder, 1975). Recent studies reveal a linear increase in the concentration of high-affinity kappa-binding sites similar to the ontogeny of mu receptors (Spain, Bennett, Roth, and Coscia, 1983). The low-affinity sites exhibit a large increase during the postnatal Days 7–14, developing like the delta receptors.

Autoradiography of postnatal Day 2 rat brains showed that mu labeling was dense in the striatum, the olfactory tubercle, and the nucleus accumbens, with a decrease throughout development until the adult distribution (Loughlin *et al.*, 1985). Kappa receptors were visible in the olfactory tubercle, the medial accumbens, and the ventral pallidum, with the density in these areas decreasing with development (Loughlin *et al.*, 1985). Delta receptors were very sparse at Day 2, visible only slightly in the anterior striatum, the nucleus accumbens, and the olfactory tubercle.

It is suggested that each receptor subtype functions differently in the developing rat. For example, saturation studies using 3H-morphine demonstrated high- and low-affinity binding sites. High-affinity sites may be associated with analgesia, and low-affinity sites with respiratory depression (Pasternak, Zhang, and Tecott, 1980). Low-affinity morphine binding was unchanged between 2 days of age and 14 days of age in rats, whereas the density of high-affinity binding increased 2.8 times. These results correlated with the two ages' demonstrating similar sensitivity to respiratory depression but a significant decreased analgesic sensitivity of the 2-day-old compared to the 14-day-old pup (Pasternak *et al.*, 1980). Thus, it appears that a differential ontogenetic appearance exists for high- and low-affinity opiate binding sites and their physiological functions.

Another reported developmental pattern of opiate binding sites using 3H-naloxone binding in the rat brain demonstrates a constancy during the first 10 days postnatally, then a rapid increase between 10 and 15 days of age and a slow rise between 2 weeks and adulthood (Auguy-Valette, Cros, Gouarderes, Gout, and Pontonnier, 1978). In this study, morphine was an effective analgesic agent on postnatal Day 5, demonstrating the dynamnic influence of the blood–brain barrier and its increasingly selective permeability.

Sigma-opiate–PCP binding sites are at adult level at birth (Sircar and Zukin, 1983). Sigma opiates have been shown to have psychomimetic effects in humans and may have a bearing on the ontogeny of neural systems related to emotions.

Opiate receptor binding in the rat spinal cord reveals the presence of synapses in the substantia gelatinosa on embryonic Days 16–17, with a linear increase of synaptic density until the third day postnatally (Kirby, 1981c). Binding in spinal cord homogenates first appears on embryonic Day 16 and increases linearly to prenatal Day 22, with a slight drop in Day 1 postnatally because of parturition (Kirby, 1981a). From postnatal Day 1, there is a linear increase in binding, with a slight reduction on Day 6 until Day 15, when adult levels of binding are attained (Kirby, 1981a). A biphasic binding curve is due to changes in receptor numbers rather than to binding affinity (Kirby 1981a).

PHARMACOLOGY OF OPIOIDS IN THE DEVELOPING ANIMAL

EFFECTS OF OPIATES ON THE FETUS

Antenatal exposure to morphine induced a transient increase in met-enkephalin binding in forebrain, brainstem, and cerebellum during the first postnatal week (Tsang and Ng, 1980). Subsequently, a lowering of binding was seen in the forebrain and the brainstem relative to controls, although no such effect was seen in the cerebellum. These results were obtained with morphine administration given from conception through pregnancy. However, binding to 3H-naloxone was unchanged if morphine was given only during the last week of gestation (Coyle and Pert, 1976). Apparently, opiates' pharmacological effects are most potent early in the development of the central nervous system.

Morphine crosses the placental barrier in pregnant ewes and has a primary drug effect in the fetus (Cohen, Rudolph, and Melmon, 1978, 1980). Fetal physiological changes occurred in response to a single intravenous injection of naloxone after continuous morphine. Fetuses exhibited increased arterial blood pressure, bradycardia, and a fall in partial oxygen in the blood. Morphological changes also occurred in the offspring of chronically morphine-exposed rats during gestation. At 1 day postnatally, these pups had lower body weights and lower brain weights, as well as lower total amounts of DNA, RNA, and protein in the brain (Steele and Johanssen, 1975; Zagon and McLaughlin, 1977). The growth retardation seems to have been a result of suppressed cell division. In addition to these changes, decreases in the cytoplasmic volume of selected brain nuclei and a decrease in cortical thickness resulted from antenatal exposure to morphine (McGinty and Ford, 1976).

In contrast to the suppressive effects of opioid agonists, antagonists increased total body weight and increased brain size and the numbers of naloxone binding sites and neuronal and glial cells (Slotkin, Seidler, and Whitmore, 1980; Zagon and McLaughlin, 1983). It is possible that these trophic effects may be receptor-mediated, as both agonists and antagonists can alter levels of opioid receptors in particular regions of neonatal brain (Bardo et al., 1982; Handelmann, 1983; Handelmann and Quirion, 1983). Moreover, female rats administered morphine for 5 days, allowed to withdraw for 5 days, and then mated gave birth to pups that demonstrated a delayed retardation in growth (Friedler and Cochin, 1972). The effect was not present at birth but was seen 3 to 4 weeks postnatally and was not eliminated by cross-fostering, a finding suggesting a prenatal origin. Whether the maternal influence that mediated the growth deficit was endocrinological, neurochemical, or behavioral remains to be uncovered as does the offspring's response to this maternal state.

These effects found with agonists and antagonists are not simply due to maternal nutritional status during gestation. The 18-day fetus after morphine exposure had a 20% reduction in spinal cord volume compared to controls, as well as a 10% reduction compared to yoked animals, those fed the identical amounts eaten by the morphine-injected animals (Kirby, 1980). Opiate receptors appear on the sixteenth day in fetal rat spinal cord (Kirby, 1981a), and these receptors mediate a dose-dependent decrease in fetal rat spontaneous activity that is naloxone-reversible (Kirby, 1979, 1981b). Normally, spontaneous activity begins late on the fifteenth embryonic day and peaks on Day 18, with a decrease thereafter until birth (Narayanan, Fox, and Hamburger, 1971). It is not known at present if endogenous opioids play a significant role in normal fetal activity (i.e., decreased movement immediately before parturition). However, this reduction in the spontaneous activity of the fetus, also seen in chicks, has been demonstrated to be naloxone-reversible (Newby-Schmidt and Norton, 1981).

The development of various behaviors and learning capabilities of the rat fetus is now being explored by the remarkable methodology of Smotherman and colleagues (Smotherman and Robinson, Chapter 5). Such information provides evidence for the ability of these immature neurotransmitter systems to be behaviorally functional, although how this might occur is not yet known.

Several aberrations have been seen in offspring that were antenatally exposed to opioids. These animals weighed significantly less at birth, with increased perinatal mortality (Davis and Lin, 1972; McGinty and Ford, 1976; Zagon and McLaughlin, 1977). The postnatal behavior of these animals was characterized by increased head shakes, tremors, and activity levels (Hutchings, 1980; Zagon and McLaughlin, 1977). Ambulation and rearing was increased at 1–3 months of age, as well as an incidence twice that of controls for minimal susceptibility to audiogenic seizures. Sobrian (1977) demonstrated that, although prenatally morphine-treated rats had decreased body weight and higher mortality, the appearance of behavioral disruption did not occur until the third and fourth postnatal week, at which time their weights were not different from those of controls. Fetal morphine-exposed rats demonstrated an increase in the analgesic effects of morphine at 3, 5, and 10 weeks of age (Johannesson and Becker, 1972; O'Callaghan and Holtzman, 1976; Zimmerberg, Charap, and Glick, 1974).

RESPONSE TO DIRECT OPIOID ADMINISTRATION

The only direct measurement of opioid response in the fetus looked at arterial blood pressure and partial oxygen pressure in fetal limbs (Cohen *et al.*, 1980). However, Stickrod, Kimbel, and Smotherman (1982) administered met-enkephalin directly into the fetus intraperitoneally in conjunction with a novel odor–taste substance (apple juice). Testing 2 weeks postnatally revealed a remarkable preference for the apple juice in these pups compared to saline controls. The opioid receptors present in the fetus, then, seem to be functional and perhaps able to mediate a reward state promoting associative learning.

Responses to opioids indicate that neonates exhibit greater sensitivity than adults, so that toxicity to opiate administration is higher the first 2 weeks postpartum than 4 weeks postpartum (Kupferberg and Way, 1963). Similarly, the analgesic effects of morphine increase from Day 5 to Day 15 and thereafter decrease (Auguy-Valette *et al.*, 1978): Day 20 rats are more than three time more sensitive than Day 26 rats (Johannesson and Becker, 1973). This change in morphine sensitivity correlates well with the age-dependent brain concentraions found in morphine-administered rats. Day 42 rats and adult rats had 20% lower brain concentrations of morphine than 26-day-old rats (Johannesson and Becker, 1973). The blood–brain ratio of opiate concentrations also correlated with analgesic sensitivity in that there was an apparent increase of specificity exhibited by the blood–brain barrier between 15 and 30 days (Auguy-Valette *et al.*, 1978).

Studies measuring the development of opioid analgesia have been largely confined to the tail flick response to heat (D'Amour and Smith, 1941). Morphine (1 mg/kg) was an effective analgesic agent in two studies at 5 days of age (Auguy-Valette *et al.*, 1978; Spear, Enters, Aswad and Louzan, 1985) but was relatively ineffective until Days 12–14 in two other studies (Barr, Paredes, Erickson, and Zukin, 1983; Pasternak *et al.*, 1980). Ketocyclozacine, a kappa agonist, produced analgesia in the tail flick method as early as 3 days of age (Barr *et al.*, 1983).

Reerach concerning measures other than analgesia in response to exogenous opioids has been scant. Caza and Spear (1980) examined the activity levels of pups 10, 17, and 24 days old after various doses of intraperitoneal morphine. Low doses (0.5 and 1 mg/kg) caused a depression of locomotion in Day 10 pups and hyperactivity in Day 17 pups. A dose of 5 mg/kg resulted in cataleptic responses in both ages.

Most of the behavioral research on opioid systems during ontogeny has been limited to the efforts of Panksepp and his colleagues and their studies of the mechanisms of social interactions. Morphine reduced distress vocalizations in newborn chicks and young guinea pigs (Herman and Panksepp, 1978; Panksepp, Vilberg, Bean, Coy, and Kastin, 1978b). An antagonist given intracranially increased the distress cries in chicks only 6–12 h old and reduced morphine's effect of inhibiting the vocalizations (Panksepp, Siviy, Normansell, White, and Bishop, 1982). Clonidine, a noradrenergic agonist, was also as effective as morphine in reducing separation distress (Panksepp, Meeker, and Bean, 1980), a finding suggesting an opioid interaction with other neurochemical systems in controlling these neonatal behaviors.

Low doses of opiates (0.1–0.5 mg/kg) also reduced crying and motor agitation in socially stressed puppies (Panksepp, Herman, Conner, Bishop, and Scott, 1978a). In dogs, however, naloxone did not increase vocalizations following simple isolation. However, naloxone administration did increase the frequency of socially induced tail wagging (Panksepp, 1981), perhaps a more sensitive index of canine social interaction. Management of timid, fearful kennel dogs (7–15 months old) improved following opioid treatment and was made worse after opioid antagonist treatment (Panksepp, Conner, Forster, Bishop, and Scott, 1983). Thus, opioid activity, when manipulated exogenously, modifies some aspects of the social responsivity of chicks, young guinea pigs, and puppies.

In addition to the role of brain opioids in the modulation of separation distress, other social behaviors have been affected by low doses of opiates administered to juvenile and adult rodents (see Panksepp, 1981, and Panksepp, Siviy, and Normansell, 1985b, for review). For example, low doses of morphine increase play fighting or rough-and-tumble play in juvenile rats 18–21 days of age, (Panksepp, 1981; Panksepp, Jalowiec, DeEskinazi, and Bishop, 1985a). Moreover, opioid blockade with naloxone reduced play activity, including dominance as measured by pinning. Beta-endorphin injected subcutaneously into adult rats also increased social activities (VanRee and Niesink, 1983). Specifically, the opioid peptide predominantly affected contact behavior, which meant crawling over, mounting, and social grooming. In these examples, the presence of opiates increased behaviors leading to contact, and antagonists caused a corresponding decrease in such responding. This finding contrasts with the suggestion that high central opioid activity creates a state of "social strength" (Panksepp, 1981). Because morphine-treated juvenile rats preferred a food reward over the home entrance in a T maze, it has been suggested that the juvenile need for social interaction is decreased by the presence of central opioids (Panksepp, 1981). However, in this case, an opioid influence on ingestive behavior, as well as the reward phenomenon, may have been an important factor in the animal's choice.

Morphine is capable of sustaining the expression of a learned behavior with a social reward in 15- and 27-day-old rats (Panksepp and DeEskinazi, 1980). Pups were trained on Day 15 to run to their home cage with the dam present through a T maze. Opiate-treated animals ran as quickly and accurately toward a clean cage for 12 days after they had reached criterion on this task. It is important to note that, in this experiment, the effects were most likely due to morphine's interaction with endogenous opioid binding sites, as naloxone alone facilitated extinction and also reversed the effects of morphine when given concurrently.

It is not known to what extent these opiate effects are due to social modulation in these young animals. Although these results were interpreted as an opioid capacity to sustain a social habit in the absence of reinforcement, it is quite possible that the pup had developed a conditioned place preference that was blocked by the opioid antagonist. Pairing a particular environment with an exogenous opioid leads to a preference for that place in the adult rat (Hunter and Reid, 1983; Mucha and Iversen, 1984; Mucha, Van der Kooy, O'Shaughnessy, and Bucenieks, 1982). An important issue, then, is whether the positively reinforcing properties of the opioid, evidenced by the adult rat's behavior, is experienced by the neonate.

The results of these pharmacological studies suggest true endogenous functions of the opioid systems in the young animal. First, the physiological and behavioral effects of the opiate morphine (0.5–1.0 mg/kg) are reversible with opioid antagonists, and more important, the antagonist naloxone (1 mg/kg) used alone often elicits an antithetical response from those effects hypothesized to be opioid-modulated. Second, brain-mapping studies, as localized by electrical stimulation, demonstrated that high-density opiate binding sites overlapped with the neural circuitry involved in the generation of distress vocalizations in adult guinea pigs (Herman and Panksepp, 1981). Vocalizations were produced by dorsal-thalamic electrical stimulation or the septum-preoptic area. Naloxone increased these vocalizations, and analgesic periventricular gray stimulation inhibited the calls. These results provide evidence for excitatory forebrain sites that mediate vocalizations and that can be inhibited by ascending opioid systems.

BEHAVIORIAL FUNCTIONING OF NEONATAL OPIOID SYSTEMS

Altricial mammals can form a remarkable variety of associations in circumstances that approximate the biological conditions of the nest (Brake, 1981; Johanson and Hall, 1979; Pedersen, Williams, and Blass, 1982; Rudy and Cheatle, 1979; Smith and Spear, 1978; Stoloff, Kenny, Blass, and Hall, 1980). For example, 5-day-old pups can form negative associations while suckling (Kehoe and Blass, 1986d). High doses of lithium chloride, when paired with a taste stimulus received while suckling, produced a taste aversion expressed 5 days later (Figure 1). Presumably, the negative effects were caused by the gastric toxicity and malaise that result from lithium chloride administration. Conversely, a low dose of lithium given on Day 5 very reliably produced positive consequences that led to an increased intake of a sweet solution while suckling on Day 10 (Kehoe, 1985).

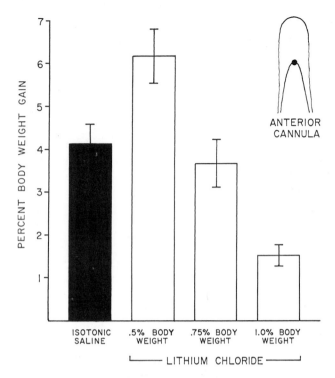

Figure 1. Mean percentage of body weight gain at the Day 10 suckling intake test of pups given saline or 0.5%, 0.75%, or 1.0% body weight of lithium (ip) subsequent to saccharin infusion on Day 5.

The basis of this finding was not immediately apparent. It seemed to us, however, that this very low dose of lithium chloride might have been subthreshold peceptually (i.e., the infants did not "experience" malaise), but suprathreshold physiologically (i.e., the mechanism of coping with malaise might have been activated). To the extent that the endogenous opioid systems seem to be involved in repsonses to pain and stress in adults (Akil, Madden, Patrick, and Barchas, 1976a; Amir, Brown and Amit, 1980; Chance, 1980; Fanselow and Baackes, 1982; Lewis, Cannon, and Liebeskind, 1980; Sherman and Liebeskind, 1980), it seems possible that this system might have been called into play in the immature infant in this possibly stressful situation. This scenario led to a testable hypothesis, namely, that low doses of naloxone should eliminate the exaggerated intake if administered before conditioning with the low-dose lithium on Day 5.

The positive affective state seen with lithium in low doses was blocked by pretreatment with an opioid antagonist, naloxone (Figure 2). The naloxone itself, at this particular dose (0.5 mg/kg), did not result in a decrease in the intake of the taste stimulus 5 days after conditioning relative to that of saline-treated rats. The combination of lithium and naloxone caused the intake to return to baseline levels and was not diminished compared to that of control rats. Presumably, naloxone's effect on the intake occurred via antagonism of the putative functional opioid system. These findings encouraged us to explore more fully the behavioral characteristics of the opioid systems in neonates as young as 5 days of age.

Kehoe and Blass performed a series of experiments to investigate the positively reinforcing properties of exogenous opioids in developing rats. In the first study we sought to determine whether neonatal rats could form an association between morphine injections and a novel taste while suckling (Kehoe and Blass, 1986a). Negative associations could be established during suckling if the taste stimulus could be detected (Kehoe and Blass, 1985, 1986d). Accordingly, 5-day-old rats received saccharin (0.5%), while suckling from an anesthetized dam, before an intraperitoneal injection of morphine. The sweet solution was infused via an anterior tongue cannula that apparently reaches lingual receptors during suckling (Kehoe and Blass, 1985). Five days later, when the pups were ten days of age, they were allowed to obtain saccharin again while suckling an anesthetized dam. The percentage of weight gain during this Day 10 test was the dependent measure. The amount of saccharin solution ingested in the Day 10 test differed significantly among groups, depending on the treatment given at 5 days of age (Kehoe and Blass, 1986a).

Specifically, 0.5 ml of a 0.5% saccharin solution was infused for 30 min during a nipple attachment to an anesthetized dam. Following the infusion, the 5-day-old pups were removed from the nipple and were immediately injected intraperitoneally with morphine sulfate in doses of 0.5mg/kg, 0.7mg/kg, 1.0mg/kg, or 2.0mg/kg, or with isotonic saline vehicle. The assessment of conditioning was done 5 days

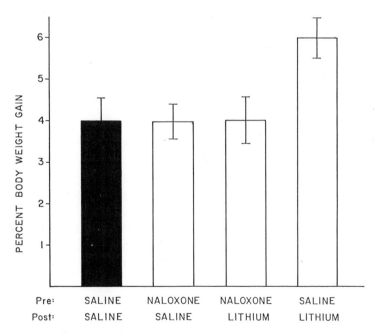

Figure 2. Mean percentage of body weight gain in the Day 10 test of pups that had received saline or 0.5 mg/kg of naloxone (sc) before and saline or 0.5 mg/kg of lithium (ip) after an oral saccharin infusion on Day 5.

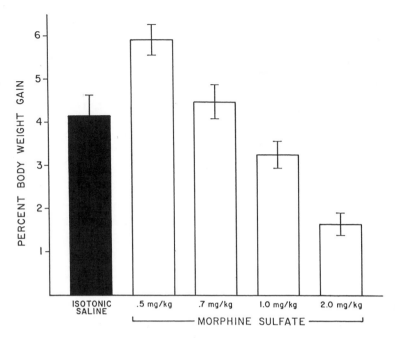

Figure 3. Mean percentage of body weight gain on the Day 10 suckling intake test of pups given saline or 0.5 mg/kg, 0.7 mg/kg, 1.0 mg/kg, or 2.0 mg/kg morphine after saccharin infusion on Day 5.

later, when the pups were allowed to ingest the saccharin under the same conditions as during acquisition.

The percentage of body weight gain, which directly reflected the amount of saccharin solution, was significantly different between the various groups (Figure 3). Pups that had received the highest dose of morphine (2.0 mg/kg) drank significantly less than all other groups on the Day 10 test. Pups given the intermediate doses of morphine (0.7mg/kg and 1.0 mg/kg) did not differ in percentage of weight gain from saline control littermates. In contrast, pups receiving 0.5mg/kg morphine after saccharin infusion on Day 5 drank significantly more than almost all other groups on Day 10.

The high dose of morphine used (2.0 mg/kg) may, in fact, have caused a malaise or a gastric toxicity that led to reduced intake and that paralleled findings with high dose administration (10–20 mg) in humans (Jaffee and Martin, 1975). In contrast to these negative associations, the lowest dose (0.5 mg/kg) may have produced positive consequences, as these pups gained 50% more weight during the test than control pups. Day 5 rats given various control treatments did not differ effectively and showed no evidence of associative learning. An experience with morphine after suckling, but without the infusion, resulted in a test weight-gain similar to that in saline-injected and no-injection controls. Thus, the positive affective consequences caused by the opiate were associated with the sweet taste specifically and not with the other aspects of the conditioning environment thus providing evidence for an associative learning process.

The positive consequences of the low morphine dose seems to be a result of the drug's action on the pup's opioid receptor system. This was demonstrated by the use of naloxone, an opioid antagonist, given to the pups before the morphine conditioning (Figure 4). In this study, pups that had received saline before and morphine after ingesting saccharin solution on Day 5 gained significantly more weight than the saline–saline control. The rat pups acquired the positive association if they experienced the state caused by the morphine after the novel taste stimulus. Pretreatment with saline had no effect on the formation and expression of the phenomenon. Naloxone, which binds to the opioid receptor sites and blocks opioid neural activity (Coyle and Pert, 1976), precluded the association formation. Thus, the administration of naloxone before the morphine treatment resulted in a subsequent test intake similar to that of the saline–saline control pups. Furthermore, naloxone treatment alone on Day 5 did not result in a reduced test intake on Day 10, a finding demonstrating that the antagonist did not inhibit positive associations by way of producing a conditioned taste aversion to the saccharin taste.

These results indicate that Day 5 infant rats have a component of the endogenous opioid system available (namely, the receptor) that appears to give rise to the affective state provided by an endogenous opioid. These experimental conditions, then, provide evidence in 5-day-old rats for functional behavioral properties

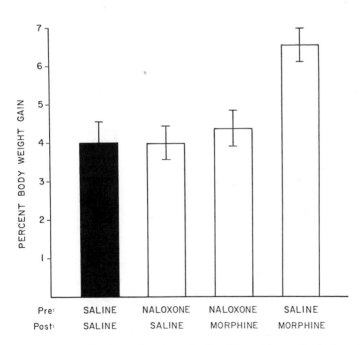

Figure 4. Mean percentage of body weight gain on the Day 10 test of pups that had received saline or naloxone (sc) before and saline or 0.5 mg/kg of morphine (ip) after a saccharin oral infusion on Day 5.

of opioid systems in providing positive reinforcement, at least at the receptor levels integrated with sensory-perceptual mechanisms.

The experimental circumstances that provided these results included the social context of suckling and the ingestion of a sweet substance, which in and of themselves may contain factors involved in endogenous opioid release (Lieblich, Cohen, Ganchrow, Blass, & Pergmann, 1983; Blass, Fitzgerald, Synder, and Kehoe, 1985). In a second series of studies, the elements of suckling and its social context, as well as the sweet taste of saccharin, were eliminated. Instead, an olfactory conditioning paradigm was undertaken in which the neonatal rat was treated with morphine after isolation in the presence of a novel odor (Kehoe and Blass, 1986a).

Each 5-day-old pup was placed individually for 30 min in a cup containing clean cage bedding mixed with orange extract, after which intraperitoneal morphine was administered. Five days later, the pups were given a preference test in which they were placed in a chamber with orange-scented pine bedding on one side and plain pine bedding on the other. The percentage of time (10 min) the pup spent over each area was the dependent measure. Pups that had experienced the state resulting from morphine administration after the orange odor spent 73.6% of the Day 10 test over the orange-scented bedding (Figure 5). In contrast, sibling control pups spent only 34% of the time over the orange odor. Thus, the novel odor of orange extract had taken on a positive value. It predicted morphine administration and became the preferred odor 5 days later. Just experiencing the morphine state at 5 days of age, however, without the presence of the novel odor, did not influence the pup's choice between that odor and the familiar bedding (pine) on the Day 10 test. The opioid antagonist naltrexone, given before the odor exposure, apparently blocked the positive association made between the morphine state and the orange odor. The unantagonized opioid system must be available for the morphine affective state to occur or at least to elicit a positive association.

The association between the novel odor and the morphine-induced state did

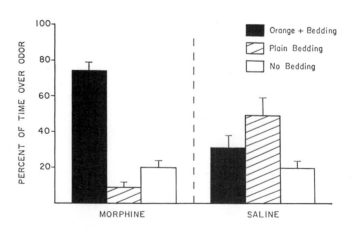

Figure 5. Mean percentage of time that Day 10 pups spent over each area in a chamber that contained three areas: orange, plain, or no bedding. Pups on Day 5 had received morphine or saline (ip) after exposure to orange-scented bedding.

not cause a generalized preference for any novel odor. Pups given morphine in association with the orange odor on Day 5 but tested with clove-scented bedding versus pine bedding were not significantly different from saline controls, choosing the more familiar pine scent. It appears likely then that the positive conditioning caused by morphine administration is specific to the environmental stimulus that predicts the opioid state.

Antagonizing opioid receptors with naltrexone does not alter olfactory perception. This effect was demonstrated by administering naltrexone or saline to 5-day-old pups before a choice test between soiled home-bedding and clean bedding. Both groups showd an overwhelming preference for the odor of soiled bedding, which presumably maintains important characteristics of the dam. Pups detected the odor differences within the chamber and demonstrated their preference for the maternal odor. Thus, pretreatment with this opioid antagonist did not interfere with either gross olfactory perception or the exhibition of a preference.

Central opioid receptors probably support the positive associative learning produced by morphine administration. Experimentation was undertaken to determine whether neonates could form an association between a novel odor and morphine administered directly into the brain (Kehoe and Blass, 1986c). Pups were conditioned in a manner similar to those that had received intraperitoneal morphine, except that the opiate, beginning with a dose 60 times less (.15 μg, .25 μg, and .35 μg), was administered directly into the cerebral ventricles (icv) of the 5-day-old pup. India ink comprised part of the solution injected icv. After the Day 10 test, postmortem examination of the brain revealed the presence of the ink in the lateral and third ventricles. All doses of morphine given intracerebrally in conjunction with the odor of orange extract caused a significant preference for the orange scent 5 days later as compared to the preference pups not injected or given saline icv (Figure 6). These results strongly implicate central opiate receptors as mediating such behavior.

Further evidence of central nervous system mediation in the neonate was obtained when the treatment of pups 5 days of age with icv naltrexone blocked the formation of positive associations acquired with peripherally administered morphine, as can be seen in Figure 7 (Kehoe and Blass, 1986c). Pups receiving naltrexone icv and morphine intraperitoneally after orange odor exposure on Day 5 preferred the orange scent significantly less than siblings that had received saline (icv) and morphine (ip). Thus, an opioid antagonist given intracerebrally apparently blocked the positive association made between the peripheral administration of morphine and orange odor. Therefore, positive consequences of peripheral morphine injections are a result of the drug's actions on the pup's central opioid receptor system. The unantagonized central opioid system must be available for the morphine affective state to occur or at least to elicit positive associations.

The results of these studies imply that central opioid systems are functional behaviorally in neonatal rats. Morphine (icv) in a dose markedly lower than that needed to support conditioning with peripheral administration was positively reinforcing. The formation of these associations was blocked with opioid antagonism given intracerebrally at the time of conditioning, a finding suggesting a central

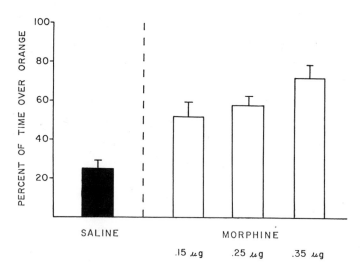

Figure 6. Mean percentage of time pups from each group spent over the orange-scented bedding on the Day 10 test. Pups on Day 5 had received 0.15 μg, 0.25 μg, or 0.35 μg of morphine intracerebrally in conjunction with the orange odor.

endogenous opioid receptor contribution to this learning. With the receptor occupation by the antagonist, morphine given peripherally was unable to elicit the neural activity needed for the affective state.

These studies provide the first evidence that neonatal rats, like adult rats, may, in fact, experience the postively reinforcing properties of exogenous opioids (Hunter and Reid, 1983; Katz and Gormezano, 1979; Mucha and Iversen, 1984; Mucha *et al.*, 1982). This state seems to be due to a brain component mediated by central opioid receptor systems. Furthermore, it is possible that neonatal central endogenous systems mediate affective responses in natural learning and conditioning. How do the endogenous opioid systems contribute to preference behavior, as

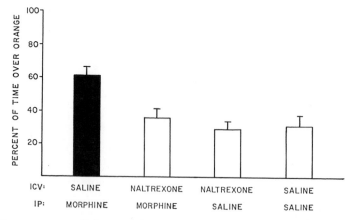

Figure 7. Mean percentage of time pups from each group spent over the orange-scented bedding on the Day 10 test. Pups on Day 5 had received a combination of intracerebral and intraperitoneal injection of drugs in conjunction with the orange odor.

exhibited by the pups in the above studies? Is a functional endogenous opioid system necessary for the neonate to express its acquired preference for an odor that is associated with morphine injection?

Presentation of the conditioned stimulus may reestablish two separate but interdependent processes in the organism; cognitive and affective. It is possible, by the use of the previously described paradigms, to separate the affective component from the informational component of this particular case of associative learning. The affective component of such learning may, in fact, be mediated by the endogenous opioid systems, in which case opioid antagonism should eliminate the conditioned affective state and presumably the demonstration of the acquired preference. Therefore, conditioned rats pretreated with an opioid antagonist should behave as do control rats, preferring the familiar odor of pine bedding to that of the conditioned orange scent, which now can no longer elicit an opioid state. If naltrexone does block the preference behavior, the implications are that the conditioned stimulus (orange) elicits, on subsequent presentations, an endogenous opioid release producing the preference exhibited by conditioned rats.

Five-day-old rats were trained as before with morphine injected after orange odor exposure. When the pups were 10 days old, they received an intraperitoneal injection of naltrexone before preference testing. Morphine-conditioned pups treated with naltrexone on Day 10 before the test no longer demonstrated the preference for orange and, in fact, were not different from controls (Figure 8). Naltrexone did not impair ambulation, as the pups were able to traverse the chamber. The conditioned pups avoided the orange side of the chamber, as did the control pups, thereby demonstrating unimpaired sensory-perceptual abilities. This effect was further verified by injecting Day 10 naive pups with naltrexone or saline before a choice test between soiled and clean home-beding. Both groups demonstrated a preference for the soiled home-bedding identical to the preference of the 5-day-old pups described earlier.

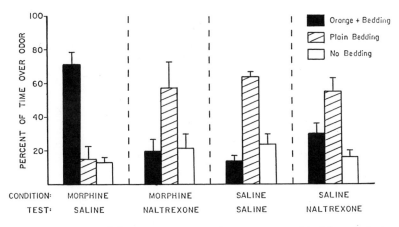

Figure 8. Mean percentage of time pups spent over the orange-scented bedding on the Day 10 test after administration of saline or 0.5 mg/kg naltrexone. Pups on Day 5 received saline or 0.5 mg/kg of morphine ip in conjunction with the orange odor.

Further validation was needed to support the conclusion that the exposure to the conditioned stimulus had caused a release of endogenous opioids. Such evidence was sought in the area of stress-induced analgesia. It is well established that morphine and other opiates produce decreased sensitivity to pain, which is often tested in rodents by means of a hotplate paw-lick method. The adult rat is placed on a heated plate, and the latency to licking a paw is the dependent measure. This method of measuring the efficacy of a substance in providing analgesia also seems sensitive to endogenous substances producing similar responses. In particular, endogenous opioids are released in response to various stressors and produce a reduced sensitivity to pain in animals tested after the stress stimulus.

This particular methodology was modified to accommodate the responses of 10-day-old rat pups, and in a series of experiments, its use was validated as a sensitive measure of pharmacological and physiological opioid levels (Kehoe and Blass, 1986b). With this behavioral bioassay of opioid levels in the neonate, we tested the hypothesis that exposure to the conditioned stimulus would cause an endogenous opioid release in the conditioned pups. On Day 10, pups that had been treated with morphine or saline after orange exposure on Day 5 were placed as a group in a bin containing the orange-scented clean bedding. After a 5-min exposure, each pup was tested for latency to remove its paw from a heated surface (48°C). Morphine-conditioned pups demonstrated elevated paw-lift latencies relative to the saline control pups (Figure 9). Thus, an olfactory stimulus previously associated

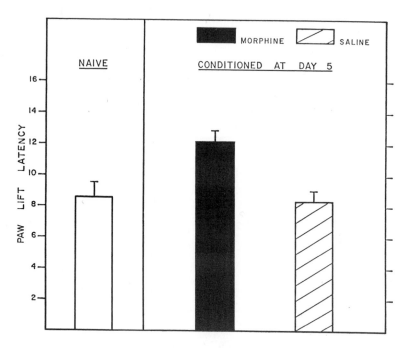

Figure 9. Mean paw-lift latency of pups exposed to orange-scented bedding on Day 10 that had experienced no orange-scented bedding on Day 5 (naive), morphine and orange scent, or saline and orange scent.

with an opioid state may cause a biochemical event in which the pup exhibits a decreased sensitivity to heat nociception. Thus far, the results have demonstrated (a) that there is a need for an unantagonized opioid system to be available in order for the animal to exhibit the acquired perference and (b) that the conditioned stimulus induced analgesia. Such converging evidence suggests that the associated olfactory stimulus produces a conditioned opioid release, or at least increased opioid sensitivity, which may instill an affective state in the organism and may influence its behavior toward that stimulus.

Negative Reinforcement of Opioids in Neonates

In adults, pain and stress mediation frequently involves the opioid system. Exogenous opioids decrease pain sensitivity and reactivity in a dose–response fashion. In addition, a wide variety of stressors, ranging from electric shock to odors of stressed conspecifics can activate the biochemical and physiological mechanisms that modulate pain sensitivity. This effect has been empircally demonstrated by measuring withdrawal responses from noxious stimuli, particularly heat (Akil, Mayer, and Liebeskind, 1976b; Amir *et al.*, 1980; Chance, White, Krynock, and Rosencrans, 1977; Chesher and Chan, 1977; Dewey and Harris, 1975; Fanselow, 1985; Fanselow and Baackes, 1982; Lewis *et al.*, 1980; Satoh, Kawajiri, Yamamoto, Makino, and Takagi, 1979; Sherman and Liebeskind, 1980). In particular, in adults rodents, the paw-lick response has proved to be sensitive to opioid treatment and induced stress (Bardo and Hughes, 1979; Frederickson, Burgis, and Edwards, 1977; Jacob, Tremblay, and Colombel, 1974; O'Callaghan and Holtzman, 1975; Sherman, Proctor, and Strub, 1982; Sherman, Strub, and Lewis, 1984). Modification of these heat-withdrawal responses was made in order to investigate the behavioral properties of a neonatal negative affective system and its association with endogenous opioids. An important issue here is whether the positive and negative systems develop apace with one another and, in fact, may be importantly interrelated.

As stated earlier, studies investigating the opioid modulation of pain sensitivity in neonatal rats have been scant and have most often been assessed by tail-flick response to heat nociception (Auguy-Valette *et al.*, 1978; Barr *et al.*, 1983; Pasternak *et al.*, 1980; Spear *et al.*, 1985; Zhang and Pasternak, 1981). In some cases, morphine-induced analgesia was obtained as early as Day 5 (Auguy-Valette *et al.*, 1978; Spear *et al.*, 1985); in others, it was not detected until Day 12 (Barr *et al.*, 1983; Pasternak *et al.*, 1980). Such contradictory results can possibly be explained by the variety of methodologies. Stressors produce opioid changes in adults, and if this is also true for neonates, then treatment before nociceptive testing may prove quite important, leading to a change in pain sensitivity. Using a modified version of the hotplate paw-lick test, we set out to determine the characteristics of the neonatal opioid system during stressful situations (Kehoe and Blass 1986b).

The method was changed so that the pup was required simply to remove its paw from the heat source (hotplate at 46 or 48°C), and the latency to remove the paw was the dependent measure. For this method to be valid, paw-lift latencies must reflect the pup's opioid state caused pharmacologically or physiologically through a stressful experience. If this test reflects opioid system participation, then opioid administration should cause elevated paw-withdrawal latencies in a dose-related fashion, and opioid blockade should reverse the responses in neonatal rats.

In this study, 10-day-old pups were removed from the nest, were injected subcutaneously with either saline or naloxone (0.5 mg/kg), and were returned to the nest (Kehoe and Blass, 1986b). Fifteen minutes later, the pups were removed for a second injection, either morphine (0.5 mg/kg) or saline, and half of each group was allowed to remain in the nest with the dam, while the other half was group-isolated at 32°C. Thirty minutes later, the pup was gently lifted out of the nest or the isolated group and lowered so that its left paw made contact with a heated steel plate (46°C). The experimenter's hand rested on an insulated part of the plate so that the pup had no downward pressure placed on it. The contact of the paw with the hotplate triggered an electronic counter/timer, and paw withdrawal terminated it. Each pup had axillary temperatures taken to assess drug-induced or housing-induced differences. None were demonstrated. The pup was returned to the nest or the group and tested again 1 and 2 h later. During this period, the pups were active and able to right themselves, displaying no signs of catalepsy. Caza and Spear (1980) also found that, after morphine treatment (0.5 mg/kg), 10-day-old rats did not exhibit catatonia.

Pups that were pretreated with saline and later received an injection of morphine exhibited significantly longer latencies than the control groups (Figure 10, left side). Thus, morphine affected the pain system in Day 10 rats. If this analgesia

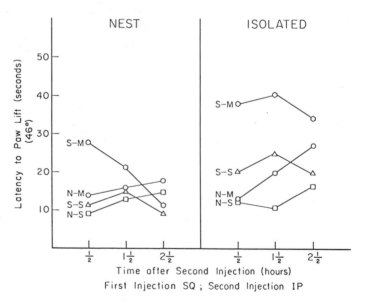

Figure 10. Mean paw-lift latency of pups that remained in the nest (left side) or were group-isolated (right side) and received saline–morphine, naloxone–morphine, saline–saline, or naloxone–saline combinations. Pups were tested 0.5, 1.5, and 2.5 h after the second injection.

reflects morphine's actions on an endogenous opioid system, then pretreatment with naloxone should attenuate or eliminate the effect. In fact, pups that received naloxone before morphine administration did not demonstrate the increased latencies and did not differ from the saline–saline and naloxone–saline control rats.

The only significant change over time was found in pups receiving the saline–morphine combination. Their paw withdrawal was much faster in the third-hour test than in the first. After 3 hours, they did not differ from any of the control groups. The results of this part of the study seemed quite straightforward. The exogenous opioid morphine, without any antagonistic pretreatment, caused 10-day-old rats to exhibit prolonged latencies to heat escape as compared to saline controls. This exaggeration was dissipated 3 h after morphine administration. As expected, pretreatment with naloxone blocked the morphine effect, producing latencies that did not differ from those of controls. Clearly, morphine provides analgesia against heat nociception in neonates. Furthermore, because the antagonist blocked the analgesic effects, it seems likely that the opiate worked at the receptor level of this system.

In adult rodents, opioid-induced analgesia in the heat withdrawal method has been well established. Apparently, a descending neural system from the brain stem to the spinal cord inhibits transmission in ascending pain systems. It has also been found that opiates can act directly on the spinal cord neurons (Yaksh and Rudy, 1978). Opiate receptor binding in the substantia gelatinosa of the rat spinal cord was found on the 18th day of fetal development (Kirby, 1981c). Thus, the neonatal opioid system may function in a manner similar to the mature system when dealing with pain stimuli.

Stress-induced analgesia may also be characteristic of the infantile pain system, as it is in the audlt. Exposure to a variety of stressors produces subsequent decreases in pain sensitivity and responsiveness. It appears that a probable neonatal stressor, maternal deprivation, results in a functional increase in opioid activity, as implied by the analgesic response of pups group-housed away from their dam (Kehoe and Blass, 1986b). By use of the paw-lift latency as the dependent measure, the characteristics of the neonatal opioid system during a distressful situation were determined.

Pups separated as a group from the dam after the second injection demonstrated response latencies similar to, but, in important ways, different from those of rats that had remained with the dam (Figure 10, right side). As in the nest group, saline pretreatment and morphine injection caused an initial elevated paw-withdrawal latency. No significant thermal changes occurred to confound the results because of drug and/or maternal separation. Naloxone pretreatment apparently blocked the morphine effects. Unlike the nest-housed pups, however, pups that received saline–saline treatment but were maternally deprived exhibited significantly longer latencies. Moreover, the elevated latency was blocked by naloxone pretreatment. Thus, maternal separation caused distress in group-isolated pups that was apparently sufficiently severe to release endogenous opioids within 30 min after separation. Similar results were obtained in the 6-day-old rat by the use of 30 min of individual isolation and assessment by tail-flick nociceptive response (Spear *et al.,* 1985).

An additional difference found between nest-housed and maternally isolated pups was demonstrated in those that received saline–morphine treatments. The mother-deprived pups showed no attenuation of the morphine effect. In fact, even 2.5 h after drug administration, their response latencies were remarkably longer than those of the isolated control pups. Thus, separation stress facilies drug-induced analgesia. It seems unlikely that this particualr response was due to an induced hypothermia, as the temperatures in these pups did not differ from that in any other group of pups. Furthermore, each pup was able to right itself, a finding reducing the likelihood of a cataleptic response in pups isolated from the dam after opioid treatment.

An endogenous response probably occurred in these stressed pups that may have enhanced and prolonged the decreased sensitivity to pain seen with exogenous opioids. Interestingly, adult rats repeatedly exposed to stress subsequently display enhanced analgesia to opiates (Belenky and Holaday, 1981; Grau, Hyson, Maier, Madden, and Barchas, 1981; Sherman *et al.*, 1982, 1984). Perhaps in a 10-day-old rat, maternal separation of several hours is sufficient to produce such an enhanced response to morphine. In fact, naloxone, which blocked the morphine analgesia for a short while, did not prevent the decreased pain sensitivity after 2.5 h of maternal isolation (Kehoe and Blass, 1986d). According to pharmacokinetics, an intravenous dose of naloxone in adult rats showed a rapid onset and decline in brain tissue, in contrast to the brain concentration of morphine that was sustained for 1 h (Ngai, Berkowitz, Yang, Hempstead, and Spector, 1976). The stressed organism administered these drugs may exhibit even more complex pharmacokinetics involving several hormonal and neurochemical systems (Akil *et al.*, 1976a; Bodnar, 1985; Lewis *et al.*, 1980; Mayer, 1985; Roth and Katz, 1979). Moreover, after maternal separation, infants demonstrate profound physiological changes indicative of stress (Hennessey and Kaplan, 1982; Smotherman, Hunt, McGinnis, and Levine, 1979).

Thus far, the nociceptive paradigm developed for infant rat testing reflected the pharmacological and physiological state of the nest-housed and maternally deprived pups. The results of this test provided evidence that 10-day-old rats' endogenous opioid system participates in pain and stress mediation (Kehoe and Blass, 1986b). The behavioral characteristics of the neonatal system bear a great resemblance to those of the adult system, such as (1) morphine-induced analgesia, which is naloxone-reversible, and (2) stress-induced analgesia, which is also naloxone-reversible. This methodology seemed appropriate to a further testing for the more severe stress of individual isolation and the physiological response it may engender.

Pups at 10 days of age were individually isolated for 5 min in a styrofoam cup that contained clean pine bedding and were then tested on the hotplate for paw withdrawal latency. As seen in Figure 11 (Kehoe and Blass, 1986e), these pups had significantly longer latencies than control pups tested immediately on removal from the nest. Pups that had naltrexone treatment before isolation demonstrated significantly shorter latencies than the other isolates but did not differ from the nonisolated rats. Adding the novel and pungent odor of orange extract to the pine bedding of the isolate did not significantly increase the latencies, although a trend toward longer latencies was seen. Again, naltrexone reversed the increased latencies.

Pups grouped together but maternally deprived for only 5 min did not differ in their paw withdrawal responses from those that remained in the nest before testing. Thus, individual isolation for even 5 min caused a naltrexone-reversible stress-induced analgesia, a finding suggesting an opioid-mediated response to this biosocial stress. Group housing away from the dam for 30 min, a seemingly mild social stress, decreased pain sensitivity to heat, a response not seen after 5 min. In contrast, individual isolation, an apparently more severe social stressor, produced a marked analgesia after only 5 min.

The stress of individual isolation is known to produce vocalizations in the young of many species. Neonatal rats emit ultrasonic cries under various social and thermal conditions (Allin and Banks, 1982; Noirot 1982). Furthermore, distress vocalizations can be pharmacologically manipulated by opiates and opiate antagonists; morphine decreases and naloxone increases vocalizations in neonatal chicks and young guinea pigs (Herman and Panksepp, 1978; Panksepp *et al.*, 1978b). In short, the endogenous opioid systems may influence the general stress response to naturally occurring maternal separation during development. Therefore, it was necessary to establish a relationship between distress vocalizations, response to nociception, and opioids in isolated 10-day-old rats.

Ten day old rat pups were individually isolated for 5 min in a cup with clean pine bedding ast 32°C. During the isolation, the pups' ultrasonic vocalizations were

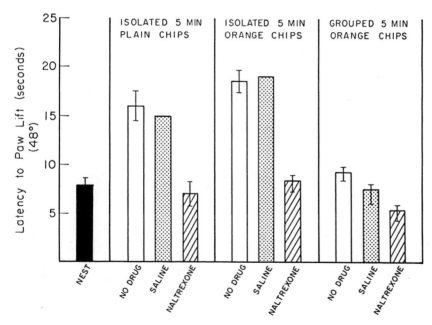

Figure 11. Mean paw-lift latency of pups taken right out of the nest and individually isolated for 5 min in clean bedding or orange-scented bedding or grouped in orange-scented bedding and given no injection, saline or naltrexone (sc) 15 min before the isolation.

made audible through a bat dectector and were counted and recorded. At the end of the 5 min, the pups were tested on the hotplate (48°C) for their paw withdrawal response. During the 5 min of isolation, the pups not pretreated emitted 300 ultrasonic vocalizations a response virtually identical to that of rats pretreated with saline (Figure 12). Naltrexone-treated rats emitted a remarkable number of calls (630), and the morphine-treated pups were relatively quiet (105).

The paw lift latencies reliably reflected the treatment of each group of pups. Isolated rat pups, either noninjected or pretreated with saline, demonstrated a decreased heat sensitivity (15 s) in comparison to the nonisolated pups (9 s). Naltrexone-treated pups had an extremely short mean latency of 6 s as opposed to morphine-treated pups, with a long mean latency of 22 s. Thus, an exogenous opioid significantly increased paw withdrawal latency and markedly decreased the number of distress vocalizations in isolated neonatal rats. In contrast, an opioid antagonist reduced paw lift latency and increased vocalizations. These data lend strong support to the hypothesis that endogenous opioid systems are recruited in the coping process of isolation distress in neonatal rats. Neonatal opioid systems appear to be functional: they detect the presence of opiates and their antagonists and are linked to the expression of pain sensitivity and ultrasonic vocalizations.

Perhaps the biological relevance of the infant vocalizations can be better emphasized when analyzed on a minute-by-minute basis (Kehoe and Blass, 1986b). Pups that had received the opiate or its antagonist did not change in their levels of vocalizations over the isolation period but maintained them over the 5 min, at low levels for the morphine-treated pups and at high levels for the naltrexone-treated ones (Figure 13). The most telling groups, however, were the untreated or saline-

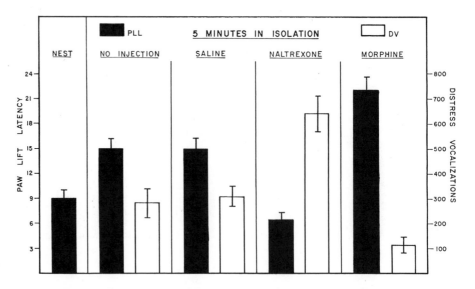

Figure 12. Mean paw-lift latency (black bars) to a hotplate for pups either removed directly from the nest or isolated for 5 min after pretreatment with no injection, saline, naltrexone, or morphine injections (ip). White bars represent the mean number of distress vocalizations during the 5-min isolation period for each group of pups.

treated pups. These rats demonstrated a significant linear decrease in their vocalizations over time. By the third minute of isolation, the vocalizations had significantly decreased compared to the first minute. It is possible that such a change in behavior reflects alterations in endogenous opioid activity, producing a quiet state in the pup. In fact, when heat withdrawal responses and vocalizations were examined in the 1st, 3rd, and 5th minute of isolation, a significant negative correlation was seen beginning at the 3rd minute (-0.69) and was even greater at the 5th minute (-0.83), in that the fewer calls, the greater the latency to withdrawing from the heat (Kehoe and Blass, 1986e). Thus, a commonality exists over time between these two behaviors, perhaps because of the release and processing of opioids affecting crying and pain sensitivity.

The profile of vocalizations of the isolated rat pup may, in fact, be an adaptive response for rodent ecology. The drugged pups may define the limits of the crying response (e.g., naltrexone causes continuous high levels of vocalizations and morphine continuous low levels). The undrugged pup cries profusely during the first few minutes and then becomes almost quiet. The dam achieves effective pup retrieval when she perceives the ultrasonic vocalizations (Hennessey, Kaplan, Mendoza, Lowe, and Levine, 1979). If she has not responded to these distress calls during the first few minutes, it becomes potentially dangerous for the pup to advertise its position to nearby predators.

As isolation from the dam seems to be a neonatal stressor that recruits the endogenous opioid systems, what are the events that apparently comfort the isolate, and what are their influence on vocalizations, pain sensitivity, and the opioid system? At issue, therefore, is the alleviation of isolation-induced stress by various

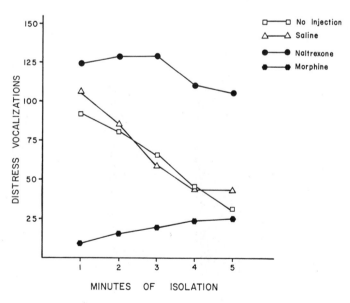

Figure 13. Mean number of distress vocalizations emitted by the pups in each treatment group for each minute of the 5-min isolation period.

stimuli that are meaningful to infant rats. In a counterexperiment, we evaluated paw withdrawal latencies and ultrasonic vocalizations after returning the dam or her component features to the isolated pup (Kehoe and Blass, 1986e).

After the initial 5 min of isolation in a cup with clean pine bedding, each pup was transferred to a second condition for 1, 3, or 5 min, during which its vocalizations were counted and after which it was paw-tested on the hotplate (48°C). The pups were placed on the ventrum of an anesthetized dam, or an anesthetized virgin, in a cup of soiled home bedding, or in one with clean bedding. Proximity and nipple attachment to the anesthetized dam caused responses that most closely resembled those of the nonisolated sibling (Figure 14), that is, virtually no vocalizations and short paw-lift latencies. However, the presence of the virgin female, which the pups did not suckle, was equally effective in relieving isolation stress.

Isolated pups placed in the familiar odor of soiled bedding demonstrated a profile over the 5 min that, although less dramatic than that of rats returned to a female, differed noticeably from that of pups placed in clean bedding. The salient odors of the dander and excreta, through their familiarity, served to reduce the separation-induced stress, but certainly not with the speed that a warm furry female could. In fact, the distress vocalizations of the pups put in the various conditions paralleled to a great extent, the profiles of pain sensitivity (Figure 15). Although, in general, all levels of crying were reduced, female contact was successful in producing almost virtual quiet, and familiar nest odor caused a relative reduction of calls compared to those of pups remaining in clean bedding.

These studies suggest that maternal separation causes neonatal behavioral re-

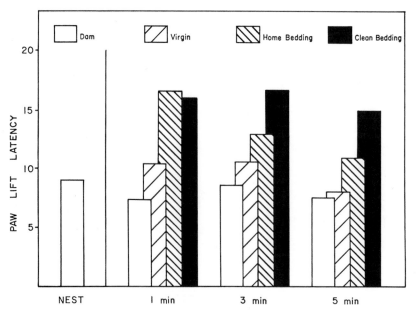

Figure 14. Mean paw-lift latency of pups taken directly from the nest or isolated for 5 min and then placed for 1, 3, or 5 min on clean bedding, home bedding, anesthetized virgin, or anesthetized dam.

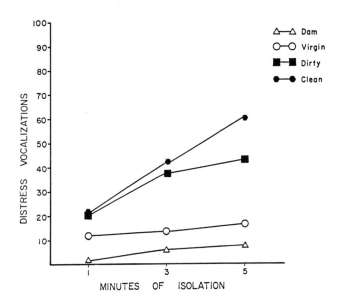

Figure 15. Mean number of distress vocalizations for pups during the 1-, 3-, or 5-min period on clean bedding, home bedding, anesthetized virgin, or anesthetized dam.

ponses that are, in part, mediated by endogenous opioids. If maternal separation caused an opioid response, then reversing the stress with maternal stimuli should reverse the biochemical profile. Stress reduction, in this case, was shown by normalization of pain sensitivity levels. Ultrasonic cries were virtually absent when contact was made with an anesthetized dam. This was also the case for pups with their dam in the nest.

This profile differs from that of isolated siblings treated with opiates. Although morphine-treated animals were also silent, their pain thresholds were enormously elevated. Furthermore, opioid antagonism did not initiate ultrasonic vocalizations in pups living in the nest (unpublished observations) nor reverse their measured response to pain (Kehoe and Blass, 1986c; Spear *et al.*, 1985). In short, it appears that, although isolation can activate the opioid system in neonates, comforting events probably do not act through the same system, or at least, the opioid system may be inhibited through the action of another affective mechanism. Moreover, because many of the responses measured were emitted in a graded manner, it is likely that the biochemical systems were likewise functioning in an incremental fashion, perhaps through the summation of several systems in harmony.

GENERAL DISCUSSION

Altricial neonates are capable of complex learning and conditioning, especially under ecologically valid circumstances (i.e., nest temperature). There seem to be classes of experiences through which the developing organism discovers relationships and consequences allowing for the recognition of home, parent, and siblings.

The information acquired can serve as an ontogenetic adaptation as well as significantly affect adult motivated behaviors. An extremely important class of experiences is those that lead to the development of a learned affectional relationship. It seems evident from our recent studies that one central mechanism that may in part mediate and/or modulate such behavior is the opioid system.

To date, we have demonstrated that the neonatal opioid system is functional behaviorally. Empirical evidence that central nervous system opioid mechanisms are an effective agent in neonatal behavior comes from two forms of evaluation: responsiveness to exogenous opiates and effective endogenous opioid release.

RESPONSES TO EXOGENOUS OPIATES

Rats preferred a novel taste that predicted the delivery of morphine and demonstrated the acquired preference some 5 days after the initial experience. Pretreatment with an opioid antagonist blocked the acquisition of such learning. Moreover, the neonate was sensitive to the toxic qualities of higher doses of morphine, which probably caused an unpleasant sensation leading to a conditioned aversion. It was only at a relatively low dose that morphine produced a state in the infant that was positively associated with its predicting taste or odor. Such a dose may well have produced the phenomenologically pleasant state reported by human subjects.

Exogenous morphine administration was positively associated with a novel, otherwise aversive, odor (orange), present during such administration. Again, conditioning was not successful with opioid receptor antagonism. Unlike the previous experiment, in which the pup ingested either more or less, the present study required the neonate to move in space and to locate what had become salient and apparently preferred through its previous predictive association. Control pups actually avoided the odor, whereas the morphine-injected pups approached it, even though both groups had been previously exposed to it and were therefore equally familiar with it. The affective state produced by the morphine is likely to be mediated by central systems, as intracerebral injections successfully supported the positive association.

Not only did morphine promote a positive state, but it seemed to effectively reduce pain sensitivity to heat nociception. Latencies to escape from heat were measurably longer after relatively low doses of morphine treatment that did not reduce mobility in the pups. Such prolonged responses to nociception were never seen when the morphine was preceded by an opioid antagonist. Thus, the same dose of morphine that promoted a preference for a particular novel stimulus present in the pups' environment was able to reduce discomfort to pain and to promote analgesia. It appears, then, that, at least in the former case, the pup had to be attentive to certain cues in its surroundings. It therefore seems unlikely that the analgesia was due to reduced perceptual mechanisms, at least not to reduced perception of environmental stimuli.

Although morphine reduced sensitivity to pain from heat, it also seems to attenuate the stress of maternal separation. Pups pretreated with morphine were relatively quiet during isolation, whereas their untreated siblings emitted frequent ultrasonic vocalizations, and the naltrexone-treated pups cried at extremely high rates. Morphine at a dose of 0.5 mg/kg promoted a positive state, attenuated crying during isolation, and promoted analgesia in the neonatal rat pup.

EFFECTIVE ENDOGENOUS OPIOID RELEASE

In exploring the capabilities of the neonatal opioid system, overt behavioral responses provided evidence of instances of its spontaneous activation. The most significant and dramatic exhibition was the effects of reexposure to a conditioned stimulus. Specifically, rats given the morphine–orange pairing on Day 5 did not exhibit the preference on Day 10 if they were pretreated with naltrexone before the test. Furthermore, a substantially decreased pain sensitivity accompanied reexposure to the conditioned stimulus. Taken together, these results imply that a positively associated stimulus causes a release of endogenous opioids influencing pain systems and directing choice. Whether such a response is peculiar to morphine conditioning or is due to positive associative learning in general remains to be explored.

Although the aforementioned endogenous release seems to occur under positive circumstances, the negative situation of maternal separaton also involves opioid activity. Exogenous opiates and opioid antagonists force distress vocalizations to their extremes; naloxone increased and sustained emitted cries; and morphine exerted the opposite effect. Nontreated isolates vocalized within this range and, more importantly, decreased their crying linearly over time, a finding suggesting a quieting effect of endogenous opioids as they are released. Because this finding correlated well with the time-dependent change in pain sensitivity, it seems that maternal separation is a natural circumstance sufficient to produce behaviorally functional endogenous opioid release.

Opioid release in reponse to maternal separation was evident in mild form when pups were group-housed. The more severe individual isolation produced a greater opioid response suggesting a graded physiological system. Reversal of the isolation-induced reactions was also time- and stimulus-dependent. The most salient and immediate reversing stimulus was an anesthetized female rat, a finding suggesting "comfort contact" as a calming agent. Moreover, nest odors were sufficient to change the isolates' behavioral profile, although in a delayed fashion. Similarly, Alberts (1981) found a preference to huddle with objects bearing the dam's odors.

One important factor becomes apparent in the demonstration of stress reversal with these biological stimuli; isolation stress reduction does not seem to be mediated by the opioid system. Pain sensitivity returns to control levels, and although crying is eliminated or relatively low, opioid antagonism does not induce or elevate the levels. Whether endogenous opioid relese simply ceases with calming stimuli or another system counteracts it remains to be studied. The dorsomedial thalamus and periventricular gray are central areas in which to seek these interactions (Herman and Panksepp, 1981). Certainly, the serotonergic system (Spear *et al.,* 1985) and the catacholaminergic system (Panksepp *et al.,* 1980) are implicated in neonatal affective behaviors and must be considered.

One of the most interesting implications of these developmental studies is the interaction of the positive and negative systems. Under natural circumstances, biological stimuli are presented to the isolated pups while they are still experiencing an elevated endogenous opioid level. Is the opioid state that is brought about by the isolation positively reinforcing to the neonate, as that promoted by morphine has proved to be (Kehoe and Blass, 1986a)? It seems possible that a dose–response relationship may exist, in that high levels of opioids for particular periods of time may produce a positive state, whereas lower levels attenuate a negative state. The coincidence of the events that produce such a biochemical, physiological, and psychological state and then its reversal should prove to be a fertile area for the further study of associative affective learning.

REFERENCES

Akil, H., and Watson, S. J. Beta-endorphin and biosynthetically related peptides in the central nervous system. In L. Iverson, S. D. Iverson, and S. Snyder (Eds.), *Handbood of psychopharmacology,* Vol. 16. New York: Plenum Press, 1983.

Akil, H., Madden, J., Patrick, R. L., and Barchas, J. D. Stress-induced increase in endogenous opiate peptides: Concurrent analgesia and its partial reversal by naloxone. In H. W. Kosterlitz (Ed)., *Opiates and endogenous opioid peptides.* Amsterdam: Elsevier, 1976a.

Akil, H., Mayer, D. J., and Liebeskind, J. C. Antagonism of stimulation-produced analgesia by naloxone, a narcotic antagonist. *Science* 1976b, *191,* 961–962.

Akil, H. Watson, S. J., Young, E., Liewis, M. E., Khachaturian, H., and Walker, J. M. Endogenous opioids: Biology and function. *Annual Review of Neuroscience,* 1984, *7,* 223–255.

Alberts, J. R. Ontogeny of olfaction: Reciprocal roles of senation and behavior in the development of perception. In R. N. Aslin, J. R. Alberts, and M. R. Petersen (Eds.), *The development of perception: Psychobiological perspectives.* New York: Academic Press, 1981.

Allin, J. T., and Banks, E. M. Functional aspects of ultrasound production by infant albino rats (Rattus norvegicus). *Animal Behavior,* 1972, *20,* 175–185.

Amir, S., and Amit, Z. Endogenous opioid ligands may mediate stress-induced changes in the affective properties of pain related behavior in rats. *Life Science,* 1975, *23,* 1143–1152.

Amir, S., and Bernstein, M. Endogenous opioids interact in stress-induced hyperglycemia in mice. *Physiology and Behavior,* 1982, *28,* 575–577.

Amir, S., Brown, Z. W., and Amit, Z. The role of endorphins in stress: Evidence and speculations. *Neuroscience Biobehavioral Reviews,* 1980 *4,* 77–80.

Arbilla, S., and Langer, S. Z. Morphine and beta-endorphin inhibit release of noradrenaline from cerebral cortex but not of dopamine from rat striatum. *Nature,* 1978, *271,* 559–560.

Auguy-Valette, A., Cros, J., Gouarderes, C., Gout, R., and Pontonnier, G. Morphine analgesia and cerebral opiate receptors: A developmental study. *British Journal of Pharmacology,* 1978 *63,* 303–308.

Bardo, M. T., and Hughes, R. A. Exposure to a nonfunctional hot plate as a factor in the assessment of morphine-induced analgesia and analgesic tolerance in rats. *Pharmacology Biochemistry Behavior,* 1979, *10,* 481–485.

Bardo, M. T., Bhatnagar, R. K., and Gebhart, G. F. Differential effects of chronic morphine and naloxone on opiate receptors, monoanimes, and morphine-induced behaviors in preweanling rats. *Developmental Brain Research,* 1982, *4,* 139–147.

Barr, G. A. Paredes, S. W., Erickson, K. L., and Zukin, R. S. Evidence for K-receptor mediated analgesia in the developing rat. *Society for Neuroscience Abstracts,* 1983, *9,* 328.

Basbaum, A. I., and Fields, H. L. Endogenous pain control systems: Brainstem spinal pathways and endorphin circuitry. *Annual Review of Neuroscience,* 1984, *7,* 309–338.

Bayon, A., Shoemaker, W. J., Bloom F. E., Mauss, A., and Guillemin, R. Perinatal development of the endorphin- and enkephalin-containing systems in the rat brain. *Brain Research*, 1979, *179*, 93–101.

Belenky, G. L., and Holaday, J. W. Repeated electroconvulsive shock (ECS) and morphine tolerance: Demonstration of cross-sensitivity in the rat. *Life Sciences*, 1981, *19*, 553–563.

Belluzzi, J. D., and Stein, L. Enkephalin may mediate euphoria and drive reduction reward. *Nature*, 1977, *266*, 556–558.

Blasig, J., Holit, V., Bauerle, U., and Herz, A. Involvement of endorphins in emotional hyperthermia of rats. *Life Sciences*, 1978, *23*, 2525–2532.

Blass, E. M., Fitzgerald, E., Synder E., and Kehoe, P. Sucrose or milk inhibit distress vocalizations in 10-day-old rats. *Society of Neuroscience Abstracts*, *11*, 1985, 912.

Bloom, F., Battenberg, E., Rossier, J., Ling, N., and Guillemin, R. Neurons containing B-endorphin in rat brain exist separately from those containing enkephalin. Immunocytochemical studies. *Proceedings of the National Academy of Sciences*, 1978, *75*, 1591–1595.

Bodnar, R. J. *Neuropharmacological and neuroendocrine substrates of stress-induced analgesia*. Presentation at the New York Academy of Sciences Conference on Stress-Induced Analgesia, New York, 1985.

Bolles, R. C., and Fanselow, M. S. A perceptual defensive-recuperative model of fear and pain. *Behavioral and Brain Science*, 1980, *3*, 291–323.

Brake, S. C. Suckling infant rats learn a preference for a novel olfactory stimulus paired with milk delivery. *Science*, 1981, *211*, 506–508.

Brown, D. R., and Holtzman, S. G. Suppression of deprivation-induced food and water intake in rats and mice by naloxone. *Pharmacology Biochemistry and Behavior*, 1979, *11*, 567–573.

Bugnon, C. *Étude des neurones immunoreactifs à un immunserum anti-b-endorphine chez le foetus humain et l'homme adult*. Colloque de Neuroendocrinologie Expt., Geneve, 1978.

Cannon, W. B. Organization for physiological homeostasis. *Physiological Reviews*, 1929, *9*, 399–431.

Carr, K. D., and Simon E. J. The role of opioids in feeding and reward elicited by lateral hypothalmic electrical stimulation. *Life Sciences*, 1983, *33*, 563–566.

Caza, P. A., and Spear, L. P. Ontogenesis of morphine-induced behavior in the rat. *Pharmacology Biochemistry Behavior*, 1980, *13*, 45–50.

Chance, W. T. Autoanalgesia: Opiate and non-opiate mechanisms. *Neuroscience Biobehavioral Reviews*, 1980, *4*, 55–67.

Chance, W. T., White, A. C., Krynock, G. M., and Rosecrans, J. A. Autoanalgesia: Behaviorally activated antinociception. *European Journal of Pharmacology*, 1977, *44*, 283–284.

Chang, K. J., and Cuatrecasas, P. Multiple opiate receptors: Enkephalins and morphine bind to receptors of different specificity. *Journal of Biological Chemistry*, 1979, *254*, 2610–2618.

Chang, K. J., and Cuatrecasas, P. Heterogeneity and properties of opiate receptors. *Federation Proceedings*, 1981, *40*, 2730–2734.

Chavkin, C., and Goldstein, A. Specific receptor for the opioid peptide dynorphin: Structure-activity relationships. *Proceedings of the National Academy of Science USA*, 1981, *78*, 6543–6547.

Chavkin, C., Bakhit, C., and Bloom F. E. Evidence for dynorphin-A as a neurotransmitter in rat hippocampus. *Life Sciences*, 1983, *33*, 13–16.

Chesher, G. B. and Chan, B. Footshock induced analgesia in mice: Its reversal by naloxone and cross tolerance with morphine. *Life Sciences*, 1977, *21*, 1569–1574.

Clark, W. G. Influence of opiods on central thermoregulatory mechanisms. *Pharmacology Biochemistry Behavior*, 1979, *10*, 609–613.

Clendeninn, N. J., Petraitis, M., and Simon, E. J. Ontological development of opiate receptors in rodent brain. *Brain Research*, 1976, *118*, 157–160.

Cohen, M. S., Rudolph, A. M., and Melmon, K. L. Responses to morphine in the pregnant ewe. *Pediatric Research*, 1978, *12*, 403.

Cohen, M. S., Rudolph, A. M., and Melmon, K. L. Antagonism of morphine by naloxone in pregnant ewes and fetal lambs. *Developmental Pharmacological Therapy*, 1980, *1*, 58–60.

Cooper, S. Naloxone: Effects on food and water consumption in the non-deprived and deprived rat. *Psychopharmacology*, 1980, *71*, 1–6.

Coyle, J. T., and Compochaiaro, P. Ontogenesis of dopaminergic cholinergic interactions in the rat striatum: A neurochemical study. *Journal of Neurochemistry*, 1976, *27*, 673–678.

Coyle, J. T., and Pert, C. B. Ontogenetic development of 3H-naloxone binding in rat brain. *Neuropharmacology*, 1976, *15*, 555–560.

D'Amour, F. E., and Smith, D. L. A method for determining loss of pain sensation. *Journal of Pharmacology and Experimental Therapeutics*, 1941, *72*, 74–79.

Davis, W. M., and Lin, C. H. Prenatal morphine effects on survival and behavior of rat offspring. *Research Communications on Chemistry Pathology and Pharmacology,* 1972, *3,* 205–214.

Dewey, W. L., and Harris, L. S. The tail-flick test. In S. Ehrenpreis and A. Neidle (Eds.), *Methods in narcotics research.* New York: Marcel Dekker, 1975.

Fanselow, M. S. Shock-induced analgesia on the formalin test: Effects of shock severity, naloxone, hypophysectomy, and associative variables. *Behavioral Neuroscience,* 1984, *98,* 79–95.

Fanselow, M. S. Odors released by stressed rats produce opioid analgesia in unstressed rats. *Behavioral Neuroscience,* 1985, *99,* 589–592.

Fanselow, M. S. and Baackes, M. P. Conditioned fear-induced opiate analgesia on the formalin test: Evidence for two aversive motivational systems. *Learning and Motivation,* 1982, *13,* 200–221.

Fanselow, M. S., and Bolles, R. C. Triggering of the endorphin analgesic reaction by a cue previously associated with shock: Reversal by naloxone. *Bulletin of the Psychonomic Society,* 1979, *14,* 88–90.

File, S. E. Naloxone reduces social and exploratory activity in the rat. *Psychopharmacology,* 1980, *71,* 41–44.

Frederickson, R. C., Burgis, V., and Edwards, J. D. Hyperalgesia induced by naloxone follows diurnal rhythm in resonsivity to painful stimuli. *Science,* 1977, *198,* 756–758.

Friedler, G., and Cochin, J. Growth retardation in offspring of female rats treated with morphine prior to conception. *Science,* 1972, *175,* 654–656.

Goodman, R. R., Synder, S. H., Kuhar, M. J., and Young. W. S. Differentiation of delta and mu receptors localizations by light microscopic autoradiography. *Proceedings of the National Academy of Science USA,* 1980, *77,* 6239–6243.

Grau, J. W., Hyson, R. L., Maier, S. F., Madden, J., IV, and Barchas, J. D. Long-term stress induced analgesia and activation of the opiate system. *Science,* 1981, *213,*1409–1410.

Haber, S. N., and Watson, S. J. The comparison between enkephalin-like and dynorphin-like immunoreactivity in both monkey and human globus pallidus and substantia nigra. *Life Sciences,* 1983, *33,* 33–36.

Handelman, G. E. Neuropeptide administration to neonatal rats regulates sensitivity to peptides in adults. *Neuroendocrinology Letters,* 1983, *5,* 186.

Handelman, G. E., and Quirion, R. Neonatal exposure to morphine increases u opiate binding in the adult forebrain. *European Journal of Pharmacology,* 1983, *94,* 357–358.

Hennessy, M. B., and Kaplan, J. N. Influence of the maternal surrogate on pituitary-adrenal activity and behavior of infant squirrel monkeys. *Developmental Psychobiology,* 1982, *15,* 423–431.

Hennessy, M. B., Kaplan, J. N., Mendoza, S. P., Lowe, E. L., and Levine, S. Separation distress and attachment in surrogate-reared squirrel monkeys. *Physiology and Behavior,* 1979, *23,* 1017–1023.

Herman, B. H., and Panksepp, J. Effects of morphine and naloxone on separation distress and at attachment: Evidence for opiate mediation of social effect. *Pharmacology Biochemistry Behavior,* 1978, *9,* 213–220.

Herman, B. H., and Panksepp, J. Ascending endorphine inhibition of distress vocalization. *Science,* 1981, *211,* 1060–1062.

Hoebel, B. G. The psychopharmacology of feeding. In L. L. Iversen, S. D. Iversen, and S. H. Synder (Eds.), *Handbook of psychopharmacology,* Vol. 8. New York: Plenum Press, 1977.

Holtzman, S. G. Suppression of appetitive behavior in the rat by naloxone: Lack of effect of prior morphine dependence. *Life Sciences,* 1979, *24,* 219–226.

Hunter, G. A., Jr., and Reid, L. D. Assaying addiction liability of opioids. *Life Sciences,* 1983, *33,* 393–396.

Hutchings, D. E. Neurobehavioral effects of prenatal origin: Durgs of use and abuse. In R. H. Schwarz and S. J. Yaffe (Eds.), *Drug and chemical risks to the fetus and newborn, progress in clinical and biological research,* Vol. 36, New York: Alan R. Liss, 1980.

Isom, G. E., and Elshowihy, R. M. Interaction of acute and chronic stress with respiration: Modification by naloxone. *Pharmacology Biochemistry and Behavior,* 1982, *16,* 599–603.

Jacob, J. J., Tremblay, E. D., and Colombel, M. C. Enhancement of nociceptive reactions by naloxone in mice and rats. *Psychopharmacologia,* 1974, *37,* 217–223.

Jaffe, J. H., and Martin, W. R. Narcotic analgesics and antagonists. In L. S. Goodman and A. Gilman (Eds.), *The pharmacological basis of therapeutics,* 5th ed. New York: Macmillan, 1975.

Johannesson, T., and Becker, B. A. The effects of maternally-administered morphine on rat foetal development and resultant tolerance to the analgesic effect of morphine. *Acta Pharmacologica Toxicology,* 1972, *31,* 305–313.

Johannesson, T., and Becker, B. A. Morphine analgesia in rats at various ages. *Acta Pharmacologica Toxicology,* 1973, *31,* 305–313.

Johanson, I. B., and Hall, W. G. Appetitive learning in 1-day-old rat pups. *Science,* 1979, *205,* 419–421.

Katz, R. J. Naltrexone anatagonism of exploration in the rat. *International Journal of Neuroscience,* 1979, *9,* 49–52.

Katz, R. J., and Gormezano, G. A rapid and inexpensive technique for assessing the reinforcing effects of opiate drugs. *Pharmacology Biochemistry Behavior,* 1979, *11,* 231–233.

Katz, R. J., Carroll, B. J., and Baldrighi, G. Behavioral activation by enkephalins in mice. *Pharmacology Biochemistry and Behavior,* 1978, *8,* 493–496.

Kehoe, P. *Behaviorally functional opioid systems in neonatal rats.* Unpublished doctoral dissertation, Johns Hopkins University, Baltimore, 1985.

Kehoe, P., and Blass, E. M. Gustatory determinants of suckling in albino rats 5–20 days of age. *Developmental Psychobiology,* 1985, *18,* 67–82.

Kehoe, P., and Blass, E. M. Behaviorally functional opioid systems in infant rats. I. Evidence for olfactory and gustatory classical conditioning. *Behavioral Neuroscience,* 1986a, *100.* 359–367.

Kehoe, P., and Blass, E. M. Behaviorally functional opioid system in infant rats. II. Evidence for pharmacological, physiological and psychological mediation of pain and stress. *Behavioral Neuroscience,* 1986b, *5,* 624–630.

Kehoe, P., and Blass, E. M., Central nervous system mediation of positive and negative reinforcement in neonatal albino rats. *Developmental Brain Research,* 1986c, *27,* 69–75.

Kehoe, P., and Blass, E. M. Conditioned aversions and their memories in 5-day-old rats during suckling. *Journal of Experimental Psychology: Animal Behavior Processes,* 1986d *12,* 40–47.

Kehoe, P., and Blass, E. M. Opioid-mediation of separation distress in 10-day-old rats: Reversal of stress with maternal stimuli. *Developmental Psychobiology,* 1986e, *19,* 385–398.

Khachaturian, H., Alessi, N. E., Munfakh, N., and Watson, S. J. Ontogeny of opioid and related peptides in the rat CNS and pituitary: An immunocytochemical study. *Life Sciences,* 1983, *33,* 61–64.

Khachaturian, H., Lewis, M. E., Schafer, M. K., and Watson, S. J. Anatomy of the CNS opioid systems. *Trends in Neuroscience,* 1985, *8,* 111–119.

Kirby, M. L. Effects of morphine on spontaneous activity of 18-day rat fetus. *Developmental Neuroscience,* 1979, *2,* 238–244.

Kirby, M. L. Reduction of fetal rat spinal cord volume following maternal morphine injection. *Brain Research,* 1980, *202,* 143–150.

Kirby, M. L. Development of opiate receptor binding in rat spinal cord. *Brain Research,* 1981a, *205,* 400–404.

Kirby, M. L. Effects of morphine and naloxone on spontaneous activity of fetal rats. *Experimental Neurology,* 1981b, *73.* 430–439.

Kirby, M. L. An ultrastructural morphometric study of developing rat substantia gelatinosa. *The Anatomical Record,* 1981c, *200,* 231–237.

Kupferberg, H. J., and Way, E. L. Pharmacologic basis for the increased sensitivity of the newborn rat to morphine. *Journal of Pharmacology adn Experimental Therapy,* 1963, *141,* 105–112.

Lal, H. Miksic, S., adn Smith, N. Naloxone antagonism of conditioned hyperthermia: An evidence for release of endogenous opioid. *Life Science,* 1976, *18,* 971–976.

Lewis, J. W. Cannon, J. T., and Liebeskind, J. C. Opioid nonopioid mechanisms of stress analgesia. *Science,* 1980, *208,* 623–625.

Lewis, J. W., Shavit, Y., Terman, G. W., Nelson, L. R., Gale, R. P., and Liebeskind, J. C. Apparent involvement of opioid peptides in stress-induced enhancement of tumor growth. *Peptides,* 1983, *4,* 635–638.

Lieblich, I., Cohen, E., Ganchrow, J. R., Blass, E. M., and Rergmann, F. Morphine tolerance in genetically selected rats induced by chronically elevated saccharine intake. *Science,* 1983, *221,* 871–873.

Loughlin, S. E., Massamiri, T. R., Kornblum, H. I., and Leslie, F. M. Postnatal development of opioid systems in rat brain. *Neuropeptides,* 1985, *5,* 469–472.

Lubek, M. J., and Wilber, J. F. Regional distribution of leucine enkephalin in hypothalamic and extrahypothalamic loci of the human nervous system. *Neuroscience Letters,* 1980, *18,* 155–161.

Mayer, D. J. *Neural mechanisms of multiple endogenous analgesia systems.* Presentation at the New York Academy of Sciences Conference on Stress-Induced Analagesia, New York, 1985.

Mayer, D. J., Price, D. D., and Rafii, A. Antagonism of acupuncture analgesia in man by the narcotic antagonist naloxone. *Brain Research,* 1977, *121,* 368–372.

McGinty, J. F., and Ford, D. H. The effects of maternal morphine or methadone intake on the growth, reflex development and maze behavior of rat offspring. In D. H. Ford and D. H. Clouet (Eds.), *Tissue responses to addictive drugs.* New York: Spectrum Publications, 1976.

Miller, R. J. The enkephalins. In L. I. Iversen, S. D. Iversen, and S. H. Snyder (Eds.), *Handbook of psychopharmacology,,* Vol. 16. New York: Plenum Press, 1983.

Morley, J. E. The endocrinology of the opiates and the opioid peptides. *Metabolism,* 1981, *30,* 195–209.

Morley, J. E., Levine, A. S., Murray, S. S., and Kneip, J. Peptidergic regulation of norepinephrine-induced feeding. *Pharmacology Biochemistry Behavior,* 1982, *16,* 225–228.

Morley, J. E., Levine, A. S., Yim, G. K., and Lowy, M. T. Opioid modulation of appetite. *Neuroscience and Behavioral Reviews,* 1983, *7,* 281–305.

Mucha, R. F., and Iversen, S. D. Reinforcing properties of morphine and naloxone revealed by conditioned place preferences: A procedural examination. *Psychopharmacology,* 1984, *82,* 241–247.

Mucha, R. F., and van der Kooy, D. Reinforcing effects of intravenous and intracranial opiates revealed by a place preference paradigm. *Neuroscience Abstracts,* 1979, *5,* 657.

Mucha, R. F., van der Kooy, D., O'Shaughnessy, M., and Buceniecks, P. Drug reinforcement studied by the use of place conditioning in rat. *Brain Research,* 1982, *243,* 91–105.

Narayanan, C. H., Fox, M. W., and Hamburger, V. Prenatal development of spontaneous and evoked activity in the rat (*Rattus norwegicus* albinos). *Behavior,* 1971, *40,* 100–134.

Newby-Schmidt, M. B., and Norton, S. Alterations of chick locomotion produced by morphine treatment in ovo. *Neurotoxicology,* 1981, *2,* 743–748.

Ngai, S. H., Berkowitz, B. A., Yang, J. C., Hempstead, J., and Spector, S. Pharmacokinetics of naloxone in rats and in man. *Anestheiology,* 1976, *44,* 398–401.

Noirot, E. Ultrasounds and maternal behavior in small rodents. *Developmental Psychobiology,* 1972, *5,* 371–387.

O'Callaghan, J. P., and Holtzman, S. G. Quantification of the analgesic activity of narcotic antagonists by a modified hot-plate procedure. *Journal of Pharmacology and Experimental Therapeutics,* 1975, *192,* 497–505.

O'Callaghan, J. P., and Holtzman, S. G. Prenatal administration of morphine to the rat: Tolerance to the analgesic effect of morphine in the offspring. *Journal of Pharmacology experimental Toxicology,* 1976, *197,* 533–544.

Panksepp, J. Brain opioids—A neurochemical substrate for narcotic and social dependence. In S. J. Cooper (Ed.), *Theory in psychopharmacology,* London: Academic Press, 1981.

Panksepp, J. and DeEskinazi, F. G. Opiates and homing. *Journal of Comparative and Physiological Psychology,* 1980, *94,* 650–663.

Panksepp, J., Herman, B., Conner, R., Bishop, P., and Scott, J. P. The biology of social attachments: Opiates alleviate separation distress. *Biological Psychiatry,* 1978a, *13,* 607–618.

Panksepp, J., Vilberg, T., Bean, N. J., Coy, D. H., and Kastin, A. J. Reduction of distress vocalization in chicks in opiate-like peptides. *Brain Research Bulletin,* 1978b, *3,* 663–667.

Panksepp, J., Meeker R., and Bean, D. H. The neurochemical control of crying. *Pharmacology Biology and Behavior,* 1980, *12,* 437–443.

Panksepp, J., Siviy, S. M., and Normansell, L. A. Brain opioids and social emotions. In M. Reite and T. Fields (Eds.), *Biology of social attachments.* New York: Academic Press, 1985b.

Panksepp, J., Conner, R., Forster, P., Bishop, P., and Scott, J. P. Opioid effects on social behavior of kennel dogs. *Applied Animal Ethology,* 1983, *10,* 63–74.

Panksepp, J., Jalowiec, J., DeEskinazi, F. G., and Bishop, P. Opiates and play dominance in juvenile rats. *Behavioral Neuroscience,* 1985a, *99,* 441–453.

Panksepp, J., Siviy, S. M., and Normansell, L. A. Brain opioids and social emotions. In M. Reite and T. Fields (Eds.), *Biology of social attachments.* New York: Academic Press, 1985b.

Pasternak, G. W., and Snyder, S. H. Identification of novel high affinity opiate receptor binding in rat brain. *Nature,* 1975, *253,* 563–564.

Pasternak, G. W., Zhang, A., and Tecott, L. Developmental differences between high and low affinity opiate binding sites: Their relationship to analgesia and respiratory depression. *Life Sciences,* 1980, *27,* 1185–1190.

Patey, G., de la Baume, S., Gros, C., and Schwartz, J. C. Ontogenesis of enkephalinergic systems in rat brain: post-natal changes in enkephalin levels, receptors and degrading enzyme activities. *Life Sciences,* 1980, *27,* 245–252.

Pedersen, P. E., Williams, C. L., and Blass, E. M. Activation and odor conditioning of suckling behavior in 3-day-old albino rats. *Journal of Experimental Psychology Animal Behavior Processes*, 1982, *8*, 329–342.

Pert, A., and Yaksh, T. L. Sites of morphine-induced analgesia in the primate brain: Relation to pain pathways. *Brain Research*, 1974, *80*, 135–150.

Quirion, R., Weiss, A. S., and Pert, C. B. Comparative pharmacological properties and autoradiographic distribution of (3H) ethylketocyclazocine binding sites in rat and guinea pig brain. *Life Sciences*, 1983, *33*, 183–186.

Rossi, N. A., and Reid, L. D. Affective states associated with morphine injections. *Physiological Psychology*, 1976, *4*, 269–274.

Roth, K. A., and Katz, R. J. Stress, behavioral arousal and activity—A reexamination of emotionality in the rat. *Neuroscience and Biobehavioral Reviews*, 1979, *3*, 247–263.

Rudy, J. W., and Cheatle, M. D. Ontogeny of association learning: Acquisition of odor aversions by neonatal rats. In N. E. Spear and B. A. Campbell (Eds.), *Ontogeny of learning and memory*, Hillsdale, NJ: Erlbaum, 1979.

Sadee, W., Richards, M. L., Grevel, J., and Rosenbaum, J. S. "In vivo" characterization of four types of opioid binding sites in rat brain. *Life Sciences*, 1983, *33*, 187–189.

Satoh, M., Kawajiri, S., Yamamoto, M., Makino, H., and Tagaki, H. Reversal by naloxone of adaptation of rats to noxious stimuli, *Life Sciences*, 1979, *25*, 685–690.

Selye, H. *Stress in health and disease.* Woburn, MA: Butterworths, 1976.

Sherman, J. E., and Liebeskind, J. C. An endorphinergic, centrifugal, substrate of pain modulation: Recent findings, current concepts, and complexities. In J. J. Bonica (Ed.), *Pain.* New York: Raven Press, 1980.

Sherman, J. E., Proctor, C., and Strub, H. Prior hot plate exposure enhances morphine analgesia in tolerant and drug-naive rats. *Pharmacology Biochemistry Behavior*, 1982, *17*, 229–232.

Sherman, E. J., Strub, H., and Lewis, J. W. Morphine—Analgesia: Enhancement by shock-associated cues. *Behavioral Neuroscience*, 1984, *98*. 293–309.

Simon, E. J., and Hiller, J. M. Multiple opioid receptors. In J. Hughes, H. O. J. Collier, M. J. Rance, and M. B. Tyers (Eds.), *Opioids past present and future.* Philadelphia, PA: Taylor & Francis, 1984.

Sircar, R., and Zukin, S. R. Ontogeny of sigma opiate/phencyclidine binding sites in the brain. *Life Sciences*, 1983, *33*, 255–258.

Slotkin, T. A., Seidler, F. J., and Whitmore, W. L. Precocious development of sympatho-adrenal function in rats whose mothers received methadone. *Life Sciences*, 1980, *26*, 1657–1663.

Smith, G. J., and Spear, N. E. Effects of the home environment on withholding behaviors and conditioning in infant and neonatal rats. *Science*, 1978, *202*, 327–329.

Smotherman, W. P., and Robinson, S. R. The uterus as environment: The ecology of fetal experiences. In E. M. Blass (Eds.), *Developmental psychobiology and behavioral ecology.* New York: Plenum Press, 1987.

Smotherman. W. P., Hunt, L. E., McGinnis, L. M., and Levine, S. Mother-infant separation in group-living rhesus macaques: A hormonal analysis. *Developmental Psychobiology*, 1979, *12*, 211–217.

Snyder, S. H. Drug and neurotransmitter receptors in the brain. *Science*, 1984, *224*, 22–31.

Sobrian, S. K. Prenatal morphine administration alters behavioral development in the rat. *Pharmacology Biochemistry Behavior*, 1977, *7*, 285–288.

Spain, J. W., Bennett, D. B., Roth, B. L., and Coscia, C. J. Ontogeny of benzomorphan-selective (K) sites: A computerized analysis. *Life Sciences*, 1983, *33*, 235–238.

Spain, J. W., Roth, B. L., and Coscia, C. J. Differential ontogeny of multiple opioid receptors (mu, delta, and kappa), *Journal of Neuroscience*, 1985; *5*, 584–588.

Spear, L. P., Enters, E. K., Aswad, M. A., and Louzan, M. Drug and environmentally-induced manipulations of the opiate and serotonergic systems alter nociception in neonatal rat pups. *Behavioral and Neural Biology*, 1985, *44*, 1–20.

Steele, W. J., and Johannesson, T. Effects of morphine infusion in maternal rats at near-term on ribosome size distribution in foetal and maternal rat brain. *Acta Pharmacologica Toxicologica*, 1975, *36*, 236–242.

Stickrod, G., Kimbel, D. P., and Smotherman, W. P. Methionine-enkephalin effects on associations formed in utero. *Peptides*, 1982, *3*, 881–884.

Stoloff, M. L., Kenny, J. T., Blass, E. M., and Hall, W. G. The role of experience in suckling maintenance in albino rats. *Journal of Comparative and Physiological Psychology*, 1980, *94*, 847–856.

Ternes, J. W., Ehrman, R. N., and O'Brien, C. P. Nondependent monkeys self-administer hydromorphone. *Behavioral Neuroscience,* 1985, *99,* 583–588.

Tsang, D., and Ng, S. C. Effect of antenatal exposure to opiates on the development of opiate receptors in rat brain. *Brain Research,* 1980, *188,* 199–206.

Tsang, D., Ng, S. C., Ho, K. P., and Ho, W. K. K. Ontogenesis of opiate binding sites and radioimmunoassayable b-endorphin and enkephalin in regions of rat brain. *Developmental Brain Research,* 1982, *5,* 257–261.

VanRee, J. M., and Niesink, R. S. M. Low doses of beta-endorphin increase social contacts of rats tested in dyadic encounters. *Life Sciences,* 1983, *33,* 611–614.

Vertes, Z., Melegh, G., Vertes, M., and Kovacs, S. Effect of naloxone and D-met2- pro5-enkephalinamide treatment on the DNA synthesis in the developing rat brain. *Life Sciences,* 1982, *31,* 119–126.

Watson, S. J., and Barchas, J. D. Anatomy of the endogenous opioid peptides and related substance: The enkephalins, beta-endorphin, beta-lipotropin and ACTH. In R. F. Beers and E. G. Bassett (Eds.), *Mechanism of pain and analgesic compounds,* New York: Raven Press, 1979.

Watson, S. J., Akil, H., Khachaturian, H., Young, E., and Lewis, M. E. Opioid systems: Anatomical, physiological and clinical perspectives. In J. Hughes, H. O. J. Collier, M. J. Rance, and M. B. Tyers (Eds.), *Opioids past, present and future.* Philadelphia, PA: Taylor and Francis, 1984.

Whiteside, D. A., and Devenport, L. D. Naloxone, preshock, and defensive burying. *Behavioral Neuroscience,* 1985, *99,* 436–440.

Yaksh, T. L., and Rudy, T. A. Analgesia mediated by direct spinal action of narcotics. *Science,* 1978, *192,* 1357–1358.

Zagon, I., and McLaughlin, P. Morphine and brain growth retardation in the rat. *Pharmacology,* 1977, *15,* 276–282.

Zagon, I., and McLaughlin, P. Increased brain size and cellular content in infant rats treated with an opiate antagonist. *Science,* 1983, *221,* 1179–1180.

Zamir, N., Simantov, R., and Segal, M. Pain sensitivity and opioid activity in genetically and experimentally hypertensive rats. *Brain Research,* 1980, *184,* 229–310.

Zhang, A. Z., and Pasternak, G. W. Opiates and enkephalins: A common binding site mediates their analgesic actions in rats. *Life Sciences,* 1981, *29,* 843–851.

Zimmerberg, B., Charap, A. D., and Glick, S. D. Behavioral effects of in utero administration of morphine. *Nature,* 1974, *247,* 376–377.

10

Exploiting the Nursing Niche

The Infant's Sucking and Feeding in the Context of the Mother–Infant Interaction

STEPHEN C. BRAKE, HARRY SHAIR, AND MYRON A. HOFER

INTRODUCTION

Altricial mammals are born into an extremely supportive and nurturing environment. For days, or even weeks, this environment consists primarily of the mother. Her role is usually cast as provider and protector of the relatively helpless young. Although this is undeniably true, mother–infant interactions are much more complex, much more subtle and elegant, than often portrayed. The behavior of the mother serves not only to nurture the young, but to provide them with cues that guide their behavior. The responses of the young, in turn, elicit contingent responses from the mother, so that even the highly dependent offspring manipulate aspects of the mother's behavior and physiology to contribute substantially to their own growth and development.

Over the past few years, considerable time and effort have been devoted to studying the rat as a model for these interactions. Few infants appear to be as dependent on the mother as the newborn rat, and yet the results of recent studies suggest that the young of this species play a large role in shaping the mother–infant interactions of which they are a part. For example, when a pup is isolated and cold, it can summon the dam with ultrasonic vocalizations (Allin and Banks, 1971, 1972; Hofer and Shair, 1978, 1980; Okon, 1972), or it can find its own way back to the

STEPHEN C. BRAKE, HARRY SHAIR, AND MYRON A. HOFER   Department of Developmental Psychobiology, New York State Psychiatric Institute, College of Physicians and Surgeons, Columbia University, New York, New York 10032.

nest (Fleischer and Turkewitz, 1979). It can even learn to approach cues that, once unfamiliar, now signal the presence of the mother and the nest (Brake, 1981; Pedersen, Williams, and Blass, 1982; Sullivan, Brake, Hofer, and Williams, 1986).

A number of interlocking control systems involving the active participation of both mother and offspring have been described since the early 1970s. These systems are designed to regulate cardiovascular function (Hofer, 1983); thermoregulation (Alberts, 1976; Leon, Adels, and Coopersmith, 1985); fluid balance (Alberts and Gubernick, 1983); olfactory behavior (Leon, 1974; Rosenblatt, 1983; Singh and Hofer, 1978; Teicher and Blass, 1976); isolation-induced activity (Hofer, 1983); and distress vocalization (Hofer and Shair, 1980; Oswalt and Meier, 1975). In each system, the infant plays a major role in initiating and maintaining the interactions that ultimatley affect its survival and well-being.

Perhaps the most important of the infant's independently initiated behavioral sequences involves locating a nipple, attaching to it, and withdrawing milk. Collectively known as *suckling*, these actions are among the infant's first fully developed and coordinated responses. They constitute the only means by which essential nutrient is transferred from mother to infant. And yet, despite the importance of these behaviors, our understanding of neonatal feeding has lagged far behind our understanding of the regulation of feeding in adults. Studies that focus on how the infant rat attaches to the nipple (Blass, Hall, and Teicher, 1979b; Hall and Williams, 1983) and how the dam releases milk (Drewett, 1983; Henning, 1980; Lincoln, 1983) have shed some light on the development of neonatal feeding processes, but many questions have remained unanswered and many new ones have been raised. Chief among these are questions that focus on the extent to which the infant can control the amount of milk it consumes and the extent to which it can contribute to its own subsequent growth and development. These issues have been a source of some disagreement over the years.

In this chapter, we focus on an aspect of neonatal feeding that we have studied since the mid-1970s and that is reviewed for the first time here. This work has centered on the structure and function of the rat pup's sucking responses. We believe these investigations have the potential to bring together several lines of work into an integrated picture of how suckling works, and of why suckling is a prime example of how the infant has been equipped by evolution to contribute to its own development.

Selective Review of Recent Research Developments and Controversy

Studies of milk intake by infant rats were frustrated for many years by the baffling unwillingness of the young of this species to suckle artificial nipples. A clue to this mystery was provided in the late 1960s by the work of Ethel Tobach and colleagues, who first demonstrated that infant rats require functional olfactory systems to nurse and, indeed, die if made anosmic soon after birth (Tobach, Rouger, and Schneirla, 1967). This discovery led to a series of studies (Singh and Hofer, 1978; Singh, Tucker, and Hofer, 1976; Teicher and Blass, 1976, 1977) that demonstrated that the presence of an odor near the dam's teats attracts the pups to the teats and elicits the sequence of paw, head, and mouth movements that signal the beginning of the pup's attempts to attach to the nipple. Later studies (Hofer, Fisher, and Shair, 1981) demonstrated that sensory information conveyed by nerve endings in the pup's snout are necessary in pinpointing the nipple's precise location and actually grasping it in the mouth. These surprising special sensory requirements of the infant rat made the study of milk intake from artificial sources very difficult and shifted attention away from how the infant obtains milk to the parameters that affect the infant's avid attraction to the nipple.

And so, by the mid-1970s, it was widely assumed that the only way the infant could regulate its intake was by varying the latency to attach to a nipple or the length of time it remained attached. Even this degree of control seemed to be beyond the capabilities of younger pups. Hall, Cramer, and Blass (1977) showed that pups separated from the dam for several hours attach much more quickly to the teats of an anesthetized dam than nondeprived pups, but only if they are 10 days old or older. Although this was one of the first demonstrations that suckling-deprived pups might be more motivated to approach the dam than their sated litter-mates, attention remained focused on the invariant behavior of the younger pups.

It was generally thought that there was little else the hungry pup could do to maximize intake in any case, as the mother limited the amount of milk the pup might consume. For example, Friedman (1975) showed that the dam's finite supply of milk restricted the amount of nutrient that hungry pups could consume during a bout. And in 1978, Leon, Croskerry, and Smith (1978) found that the dam tends to end a bout and leave the nest whenever the heat generated by the pups at her ventrum increases beyond a certain point. (Later, they found that rate of rise of maternal hypothalamic brain temperatures is most closely linked to bout termination; Leon *et al.,* 1985). Given these limitations, the pup's regulation of its intake by sucking was thought to be minimal. Sucking and swallowing were regarded as simple reflexes elicited by the presence of milk.

This notion was further reinforced when Lincoln and Drewett and their coworkers in England began publishing studies on the neurohormonal basis of milk letdown in the mother rat (see Drewett, 1983; Lincoln, 1983, for reviews). A primary message of their work was that the episodic pattern of milk ejection, mediated by the pulsatile release of oxytocin from the pituitary, seemed to be set in motion by the continuous stimulation provided by suckling pups, though it was not influenced by acute changes in their behavior. In fact, milk ejections seemed to occur most often when pups were quietly attached to the teat. The ejections were immediately followed by what appeared to be a reflex response sequence. The pups arched their backs, opened their mouths, and, presumably, swallowed. (Some of Lincoln's findings actually support the idea that infants may be able to influence the pattern of milk ejections, as will be described below, but this possibility was not then apparent to many of us working in the area.) On the whole, these findings furthered the idea that the pup's sucking was invariant and that all or most regulation of intake came from the dam.

This comfortable view was upset by two striking findings. The first of these was contained in a report by Houpt and Epstein (1973), which actually predated much of the work cited above. This report, which many of us had lost sight of, demonstrated that even the youngest of pups, when deprived of the dam for a few hours, would respond by actively withdrawing more milk from the dam during their next nursing opportunity. Houpt and Epstein (1973), and later Houpt and Houpt (1975), showed not only that deprived pups consumed more than nondeprived littermates, but that pups given various gastrointestinal preloads, regulated their intake according to the volume and content of the loads. Subsequently, similar studies were reported by Friedman (1975) and Drewett (1978). More recently, Lorenz, Ellis, and Epstein (1982) and Lorenz (1983) went on to show that this regulation of intake by gastric fill is mediated by afferents in the vagus and splanchnic nerves.

Lorenz and Epstein also reported that intake is adjusted independent of the pup's latency to attach to the nipple or the duration of time the pup remains attached. In a way, this finding had been anticipated years before when Hall and colleagues (Hall *et al.*, 1977) showed that pups younger than 10 days of age rarely left the nipple. Cramer, Blass, and Hall (1980) showed that these younger pups would remain attached to the teat for hours even if they received no milk.

All of this might have initiated a search to discover how pups manage to adjust intake while attached to the teat. Instead, attention became focused on a relatively short but startling description contained in the Hall and Rosenblatt (1977) report. It related that pups younger than 10 days of age that were repeatedly provided with milk from a cannula placed at the back of the tongue (where the tip of the teat normally rests) continued to consume the milk until they were unable to breath because of severe distention of the gut. This demonstration of life-threatening stomach engorgement seemed to reinforce the idea that pups could not control intake once attached to the nipple, even though these results appeared to directly contradict the earlier findings gathered under more natural conditions. It soon became clear (as we discuss below) that, if milk is delivered forcibly or very rapidly (as when injected through a tongue cannula), the adjustments of intake that the pup is capable of displaying may be bypassed. For example, Cramer and Blass (1983) demonstrated that 5- and 10-day-olds will seriously overdistend their stomachs even when milk is derived from the mother's own mammary ducts, but only if prolonged and repeated milk ejections are elicited by frequent injections of oxytocin, and only if pups are provided with a second and third milk-laden dam in nursing bouts lasting 2–3 h. As the authors reported in the same paper, more normal bout durations and numbers of milk ejections allow pups to adjust their milk intake according to their level of deprivation.

Thus, what was known about neonatal feeding when we began our work suggested that pups may be able to adjust their intake in response to privation (as Hall's later work on independent feeding also suggested; Hall, 1979b; Hall and

Bryan, 1980). However, three crucial questions remained to be answered. First,

351

EXPLOITING THE
NURSING NICHE

how do individual pups do this, given the constraints imposed by the mother (e.g., limited suckling opportunities and milk supply) and the pups' own reluctance to leave the nipple? Second, can entire litters of pups alter the constraints imposed by the dam to change the amount of milk she makes available? And third, what other environmental contingencies may affect the pup's feeding behaviors? We believed an answer to each of these questions could be found in an analysis of the pups' sucking behavior. And it is to a description of this behavior, the processes controlling its patterned expression, and its contribution to the pup's growth and well-being that this chapter is addressed.

How Feeding Is Embedded within the Mother–Infant Interaction

The Discovery of Different Sucking Patterns

When we began our work in the late 1970s, quite a bit was known about the structure of sucking in human newborns and how it was influenced by hunger, taste, and other motivational factors (Crook, 1979; Lipsitt, 1977). However, the difficulty encountered in isolating and manipulating these factors had led some to study animal models of sucking. In the mid 1970s, Drewett, Wakerley, and their colleagues published a series of studies that described sucking in rat pups (e.g. Drewett, Statham, and Wakerley, 1974; Wakerley and Drewett, 1975). Using an ingenious procedure for inserting a recording cannula into the rat dam's teat, they reported that pups did not seem to display the prolonged, deep, and repetitive sucking that occurs during feeding in human infants (so-called nutritive sucking). Instead, they appeared to suck in brief and erratic spurts both during and between milk ejections. Further, these spurts seemed to occur only when the pups readjusted their posture or moved their limbs (also see Drewett, 1978). These findings appeared to be compatible with those of Wolff, who in 1968 had described the sucking responses of several mammalian infants that he fed from bottles using artificial nipples (the rat was not among them). Wolff concluded that only human infants suck in two distinct patterns: the "nutritive" pattern, consisting of the deep and regularly spaced sucks observed during feeding, and a "nonnutritive" pattern, consisting of the brief and shallow sucks seen when a pacifier (or thumb) is placed in the baby's mouth (Wolff, 1968). All of these findings seem to suggest that non-human mammals display only one pattern of sucking, even while feeding, and that this pattern resembles "nonnutritive" sucking.

We found it surprising that hungry pups would engage only in such short-lived and irregular bursts of sucking, and only in conjunction with gross body movements, as if sucking were a by-product of this behavior. Our first step in attempting to investigate these phenomena further was to use the procedure that Drewett and colleagues had pioneered for recording negative pressure from a cannulated nipple. The procedure provided useful information but, in our hands, proved cumbersome as well. It often altered the shape and firmness of the teat, with the result that many pups would not attach to it or would not remain attached for very long. As a solution to this problem, we developed a procedure that allowed the identification of different facets of sucking by recording the electromyographic (EMG) activity of the pup's digastric muscle, a jaw muscle that opens the mouth and supports the tongue (Brake, Wolfson, and Hofer, 1979). Thin silver electrodes were inserted into the muscle tissue during brief surgery, and shortly thereafter, pups (3–13 days of age in these first studies) were allowed to suck on the teats of an anesthetized dam while EMG activity was recorded on a polygraph.

The EMG patterns observed were reliably associated with changes in intraoral negative pressure (sucking) as recorded from the dam's cannulated teats but were much easier to obtain (also see Brake, Tavana, and Myers, 1986). Soon, we abandoned the cannulated-teat procedure and for 5 years used the EMG as our only measure of sucking. We continued to use an anesthetized dam preparation because anesthesia blocks the naturally occurring milk-ejection cycle, allowing us to control milk delivery either by administering intravenous oxytocin to the dam, or by delivering milk directly via a cannula seated in the posterior portion of the pup's mouth, near the intermolar eminence where the tip of the nipple usually rests during suckling (Hall and Rosenblatt, 1977; Martin and Alberts, 1979).

Two major and unexpected findings emerged from our first studies (Brake *et al.,* 1979; Brake and Hofer, 1980). Both demonstrated that sucking does not consist merely of a single, rigidly fixed response pattern. First, we found that pups did, after all, engage in "nutritive" sucking (long episodes of deep and regularly spaced sucks) similar to that of human infants. Surprisingly, however, "nutritive" sucking often appeared in the complete absence of milk delivery. To avoid confusion, we decided to call this pattern *rhythmic sucking* (RS) and defined it as several sucks (at least three, but usually many more) of similar magnitude (or EMG intensity) and duration, with each individual series of sucks lasting 5 sec or more (we later discovered that RS actually consists of at least two different subtypes, as discussed below).

We also found that pups engaged in the brief, erratic type of sucking that others had called *nonnutritive sucking,* and that this form of sucking seemed to occur only in the absence of milk. Nevertheless, to avoid confusion, we relabeled this type of sucking *arrhythmic sucking* (AS) and defined it as bursts of sucks that vary in duration and magnitude and that last for 2–10 s. Examples of RS and AS are provided in Figure 1 and a description of sucking types is provided in Table 1.

Contrary to the suggestions of others, we found that body movements and the occurrence of sucking were not always correlated. In fact, RS usually occurred while the pups were extremely quiescent (only a slow opening and closing of the mouth could sometimes be seen). Almost half of all AS occurred in the absence of body movement as well. We called these episodes of AS *bursts,* and we called the AS that was accompanied by forelimb movement *treadles* (because the limb movement looked like a swimming or water-treading motion; see Table 1). It was true, however, that either treadles or RS occurred every time the pup moved.

The second finding was that sucking, particularly RS, was extremely labile.

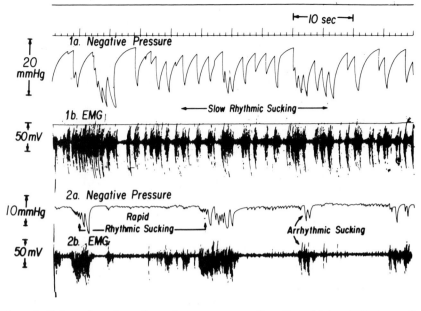

Figure 1. Polygraph tracings of negative pressure recordings (1a and 2a) and EMG recordings (1b and 2b) illustrating rhythmic and arrhythmic sucking.

This was evidenced in several different ways. For example, pups that had been made hungry by being separated from the dam for several hours displayed much more RS when later allowed to attach to the teats of an anesthetized dam than did pups deprived for shorter periods. This was true of pups as young as 3 days of age (and later, we found, as old as 18 days of age), even though they received no milk

TABLE 1. DESCRIPTIONS OF SUCKING

	EMG characteristics		Negative pressure characteristics
Rhythmic sucking, (RS)	Regularly alternating increases and decreases in signal; peak-to-peak interval: 0.5–2 s; duration of episodes: 5 s–5 min	Rapid rhythmic sucking, (RRS)	Frequency: > 1 Hz; Amplitude: 5–50 mmHg Burst duration: 5–10 s
		Slow rhythmic sucking (SRS)	Frequency: < 1 Hz; Amplitude: 5–20 mmHg Burst duration: 5 s–5 min
Arrhythmic sucking, (AS)			
Bursts	Discrete signal bursts lasting 2–5 s		Frequency: 0.5–2 Hz Amplitude: 5–15 mmHg Burst Duration: 3–5 s
Treadles	Movement artifact signal lasting 2–5 s		Frequency: 0.5–2 Hz Amplitude: 5–15 mmHg Burst duration: 3–60 s

from the anesthetized dam (Figure 2). In fact, pups deprived for 20–24 h spent as much as 85% of their time engaged in RS (some episodes lasting as long as 5 min without interruption), whereas pups which had been deprived for 2–6 h engaged in very little RS (all pups displayed occasional bursts of AS).

We also found that RS decreased dramatically as deprived pups continued to suckle in the absence of milk delivery. This, also, was true in pups as young as 3 days of age and as old as 18 days of age. Within an hour of being allowed to attach to a nipple, deprived pups were spending less than 50% of their time sucking, and very little of it was RS (Figure 2). It appeared that these pups feverishly attempted to withdraw milk from the teat when first reunited with the dam but then gave up after failing to get milk. If, however, the pups were provided with just a few brief pulses of milk (commercially available half-and-half, delivered through a posterior tongue cannula) during this period, the incidence of RS quickly returned to a high level and remained elevated for up to half an hour. This energizing effect of milk delivery has been observed in other circumstances. Hall (1979a) noted that pulses of milk delivered to pups through a tongue cannula while they are away from the teat elicit exaggerated body movements. That effect dissipates rather quickly, however, whereas the enhanced sucking that we observed persisted for several minutes.

These data provided the first real evidence that sucking is not a fixed response pattern; instead it is quite malleable. At this point, the temptation was almost irresistible to attribute the surprising responsiveness in sucking to the pup's motivation to feed (or its frustration at being prevented from feeding). This temptation was strengthened by our knowledge that deprived rat pups as young as 10 days old would expend a great deal of energy running in alleyways and mazes in order to suckle (Amsel, Letz, and Burdette, 1977; Brake, 1978; Kenny and Blass, 1977; later, in 1979, Johanson and Hall would show that 1-day-old pups would manipu-

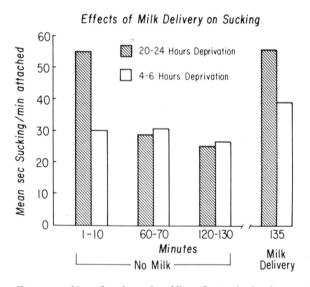

Figure 2. The effects on sucking of prolonged suckling of a teat in the absence of milk delivery in 11–13-day-old pups deprived for 20–24 h and 4–6 h.

late a lever to obtain milk). But we also knew that suckling-age pups would run alleys in order to suckle a dry nipple, and that, in fact, they didn't seem to prefer milk-laden teats to dry ones until sometime between 10 and 17 days of age (Kenny, Stoloff, Bruno, and Blass, 1979; Letz, Burdette, Gregg, Kittrell, and Amsel, 1978). So, although it was clear that deprived pups sucked differently than sated ones, it wasn't clear whether such behavior was due to an increased incentive to feed or simply to an increased incentive to attach to and suck on a teat.

Two Motivational Systems

The finding that sucking is enhanced by deprivation when pups are reunited with a dam, but that it diminishes in the absence of milk delivery, may reflect the increased hunger resulting from the absence of nutrient and the frustration incurred when feeding is blocked. Alternatively, enhanced sucking may reflect changes in the pup's motivation to seek oral contact with the teat in and of itself, and the decline in sucking over time may indicate that the pup gradually habituates to the presence of the nipple in its mouth.

In order to determine whether sucking is under nutritive control, nonnutritive control, or both, 11-to-13-day-old pups were allowed to suckle an anesthetized dam after being maternally deprived for 20–24 h (Brake, Sager, Sullivan, and Hofer, 1982a). Pups were treated in one of three different ways before the assessment of nipple attachment and sucking. For a third of the pups, a 5% body-weight preload of nutrient was delivered to the gut by gavage over a 1–2 min period 30 min before the suckling test ("gastrointestinal satiation"). As in other experiments, the nutrient we used was half-and-half milk creamer, which is similar to rat's milk in the percentage of fat and water it contains. The purpose of this manipulation was to provide a source of satiety cues, including those due to a distension of the gut and postabsorptive effects (Houpt and Epstein, 1973; Lorenz et al., 1982). Another third were allowed to suckle a dam that provided no milk during the 20-to-24-h deprivation period ("oral satiation"). The purpose of this manipulation was to provide pups with oropharyngeal stimulation during maternal separation. The final third received a 5% preload of milk (half-and-half) delivered through a posterior tongue cannula over a 2½ h period, ending 30 min before the test ("gustatory stimulation"). This procedure was intended to provide a prolonged period of gustatory stimulation (but little gastric distension; much of the preload would have emptied from the gut by the time testing began).

We also believed that these manipulations might differentially affect sucking, depending on whether the pups received milk while attached to the dam's teats during the suckling test. So, for half of the pups, milk was made continuously available during the test by connecting the free end of a posterior tongue cannula to a reservoir of milk. Under these conditions, a small amount of milk (about 0.01 ml/min) siphoned to the pup's mouth if it engaged in little or no sucking, but the amount could be increased (up to 0.03 ml/min) by vigorous sucking. The remaining half of the pups received no milk.

As can be seen in Figure 3, the three treatments exerted very different influences on sucking and the amount of time that the pups spent attached to the teat. Further, these effects were quite different when milk was available during the test compared to when it was not.

Gastrointestinal preloads had absolutely no effect on sucking if the pup did not receive milk during the test, but they decreased sucking noticeably if the pup had access to milk (compare the "24-None" and "24-GI" groups in both conditions). That is, the preloads seemed to eliminate the marked increase in sucking that usually occurs when a suckling-deprived pup encounters milk. Thus, gastric preloads seemed to inhibit feeding, probably because of gastric distention (e.g., Drewett and Cordall, 1976), but did not affect nonnutritive sucking. GI fill also had no apparent affect on nipple attachment behaviors. It induced no changes in the pup's latency to attach to a nipple or in the amount of time pups spent attached to a teat.

The effects of oral satiation were also quite different depending on whether pups received milk during the test or not. Oral satiation decreased sucking in the absence of milk but had no affect on sucking if milk was available (compare the "24-None" and "24-Oral" groups in both conditions). In addition, oral satiation decreased the amount of time pups spent attached to the dry teat but had no affect on nipple attachment time if milk was available during the test. Thus, oral satiation seemed to inhibit nonnutritive sucking and nipple attachment but did not affect sucking responses associated with feeding.

The effects of gustatory stimulation were perhaps the most interesting because they revealed the complex interplay of nutritive and nonnutritive factors in the control of feeding. Milk delivered via the pup's tongue cannula before the test

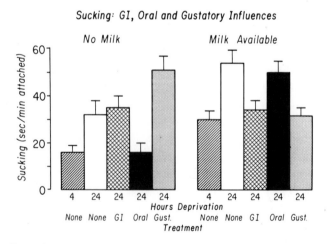

Figure 3. The effects of various pretreatments on sucking when milk was available and when it was not. "GI" indicates stomach preload; "Oral" indicates extended suckling of a dry teat, and "Gust" indicates infusions of milk to the mouth.

dramatically increased sucking if the pup had no access to milk during the test. If the pup had access to milk during the test, however, then sucking was decreased substantially (compare the "24-None" and "24-Gust" conditions). Thus, gustatory stimulation seemed to energize nonnutritive sucking, but it inhibited feeding, as if postabsorptive satiety factors had begun to affect intake. These differences in sucking were observed without any corresponding change in nipple attachment time.

Taken together with other work (Cramer and Blass, 1983; Gisel and Henning, 1979; Houpt and Epstein, 1973; Lorenz *et al.*, 1982), these findings illustrate two important points. First, suckling appears to be mediated by two different motivational systems. One may be called the *feeding system*. It seems to be influenced by nutritive factors such as GI fill and gustatory stimulation. The other may be called the *suckling system*. It seems to be influenced by nonnutritive factors such as perioral sensation. The second point is that, although sucking and nipple attachment behaviors come under the control of both systems, sucking is more influenced by the feeding system, and nipple attachment is more influenced by the suckling system.

Most of our own data supporting these conclusions were derived from studies of pups 11–13 days of age. However, other data suggest that the same holds true for pups as young as 3 days of age (Houpt and Epstein, 1973; Lorenz *et al.*, 1982). Although it is true that pups younger than 10 days of age will sometimes hold the teat in their mouths even after they have received unusually large volumes of milk (Cramer and Blass, 1983; Hall and Rosenblatt, 1977), the findings of Epstein, Lorenz, and others (see Epstein, 1986, for a review) suggest that, under more normal conditions, even newborns can control the rate at which they withdraw milk, depending on their level of privation. Thus, the feeding system is active, even though pups of this age may not exhibit control over the amount of time they remain attached to the teat, and therefore, under certain conditions, they will ultimately over-consume (see Cramer and Blass, 1983).

Remaining attached to the teat at the risk of being flooded with milk is probably adaptive. First, it is quite unlikely that pups will receive too much milk from the dam. Second, as milk delivery is intermittent and unpredictable, it would seem advantageous for the younger pup to remain attached and attempt to withdraw the maximum amount of milk that the mother makes available, rather than to detach quickly following milk delivery and run the risk of being away from the nipple at the time of the next milk ejection. Older pups, on the other hand, are more mobile and so can leave the nipple more readily. They can shift from nipple to nipple, searching for new milk stores, and still reattach before the next milk ejection.

In summary, the two separate but interlocking systems interact in an elegant way to control ingestion. Each contributes to the ultimate goal of removing milk from the teats. As the satiation of suckling does not necessarily result in the satiation of feeding, the pup's willingness to attach to the teat does not always reflect its willingness to suck. Ordinarily, however, the two systems function in harmony and allow the pup a surprising degree of control over its intake, as we discuss in more detail below.

The two interacting motivational systems controlling intake can be studied individually. Feeding may be studied in the absence of nipple attachment (e.g., Hall, 1979b; Hall and Bryan, 1980), and nipple attachment may be studied in the absence of milk delivery. But these behaviors ordinarily occur simultaneously, and so, when the pup is deprived of the opportunity to attach to the teat, it is also deprived of food. Similarly, when it has been nursed by the dam for a long period of time, it is likely to be sated nutritionally as well as for suckling. Under natural circumstances, then, the control of intake depends on an intricate intertwining of these behavioral systems. In other ways, however, the control of ingestion seems to be simpler in infants than in adults. For example, although pups reduce intake as a function of gastrointestinal fill, the nutritive value of the fill seems to be largely irrelevant to the decrement in feeding (e.g., Drewett and Cordall, 1976; Houpt and Houpt, 1975). Further, cholecystokinin (CCK) does not seem to inhibit the withdrawal of milk by young pups in a way analogous to the way it inhibits adult feeding (Blass, Beardsley, and Hall, 1979a), nor does 2-deoxyglucose (2DG) stimulate the withdrawal of milk as 2DG stimulates adult feeding (Houpt and Epstein, 1973).

This is not to say that these or similar neurochemical systems are altogether absent in pups. Epstein and his colleagues (see Epstein, 1986) have elegantly demonstrated that feeding away from the teat is regulated by neurochemical mechanisms similar to those found in the adult, in contrast to the withdrawal of milk from the teat, which apparently has a different neurochemical basis. Norepinepherine, for example, increases independent feeding (consumption of milk delivered through a tongue cannula, away from the teat) in pups younger than 10 days old but does not stimulate withdrawal of milk from the dam. Similarly, Raskin and Campbell (1981) found that amphetamine decreased feeding in 5-day-old pups away from the teat but did not affect intake while suckling. Data such as these lead Epstein (1986) to suggest, as we do, that ingestion is the result of competing motivational systems. Others question whether ingestion during suckling is analogous to adult ingestion or homologous with it (e.g., Blass and Cramer, 1982; Hall and Williams, 1983).

Still, as we have seen, pups of all ages manage to adjust their intake of milk from the dam as a function of privation. How do they do this? As mentioned above, one way is to vary the amount of time they remain attached to the teat, or by shifting from teat to teat, searching for one that has not yet been drained. The notion that nipple shifting serves this purpose is supported by the finding that the continued availability of appreciable amounts of milk at each teat decreases shifting (Brake *et al.*, 1982a; Cramer *et al.*, 1980). It is also true that the incidence of nipple shifting increases as pups grow older and approach the age of weaning. This activity presumably reflects the emergence of adultlike feeding and the attenuation of the pup's motivation to suckle. But as already discussed, nipple shifting alone cannot explain increased ingestion following deprivation (e.g., Lorenz *et al.,* 1982). Several investigators have shown that deprived pups consume more milk from a dam than do nondeprived pups or pups given gastrointestinal preloads, even if all pups are suckling from the same dam and do not vary the amount of time they spend attached to the teat (Drewett and Trew, 1978; Gisel and Henning, 1979; Houpt and Epstein, 1973; Houpt and Houpt, 1975). These pups must vary the parameters of their sucking to adjust their intake.

There are two ways in which pups may adjust intake by sucking: (a) individual pups may adjust intake directly by varying the frequency, the amplitude, or the rate of sucking during and shortly after milk ejection, and (b) entire litters of pups may adjust intake indirectly by varying the vigor of sucking between milk ejections, thus communicating a message to the dam that results in changes in the volume or frequency of subsequent milk ejections. Both of these possibilities were thought unlikely only a few years ago; now, evidence suggests both may occur.

In order to demonstrate how individual pups may adjust intake, Brake, Shindledecker, and Hofer (in preparation) examined sucking during a series of milk deliveries in 10-to-12-day-old pups. In the first experiment of the series, the EMG technique was used to examine RS before and after three milk pulses delivered via a posterior tongue cannula. Each pulse was of fixed volume (0.10 ml), so that the total volume of milk delivered was roughly equivalent to that delivered by the dam during natural milk delivery over a comparable period of time. Two groups of pups were studied. Pups in both groups were separated from the dam 24 h before testing, but one group received a 5% preload of milk (half-and-half) 30 min before the suckling test, and one did not.

The goal of this experiment was to determine how the pups' responses to a given volume of milk varied with satiation as produced by gastrointestinal preload. We believed it was necessary to study sucking in response to milk delivered through a cannula before studying sucking during normal milk ejection because the volume of milk released by the dam during any given milk ejection is difficult to determine. Thus, any differences in the pup's responding following naturally occurring milk ejections could be due to a variation in the volume of milk made available at each teat, and not to a variation in the pup's privational status. As the volume of milk delivered to the two groups of pups in this experiment was identical, any differences in responding between pups given preloads and those given none must be due to privation.

The results clearly indicated that pups that had received a preload engaged in less RS following milk delivery than pups given no preload (Figure 4). During the 5 min following each pulse, pups that had received preloads continued to suck at the rate they had displayed before milk delivery, but pups that had not received preloads increased their sucking substantially. These pups spent 45 s of each minute sucking, an increase of about 50%, due mostly to an increase in RS. This finding suggests that pups may be able to adjust intake according to privation by varying the amount of sucking they display in the minutes after milk ejection. Pups that engage in more sucking during this time could stand a better chance of withdrawing all of the milk that was released into the mammary ducts during the preceding milk ejection. They may also withdraw more milk from an unsuckled teat, should they encounter one after leaving the teat they have just been attached to.

A more likely possibility is that hungry pups consume more milk because they suck with more force during the milk ejection itself. As the EMG measure was not sensitive to changes in the amplitude of intraoral negative pressure, we needed a new measure in order to determine the extent to which this possibility could be true. This new measure was obtained by directly recording changes in intraoral negative pressure with a cannula inserted in the posterior portion of the pup's mouth (at the level of the intermolar eminence). Connecting the free end of the cannula to a pressure transducer and a polygraph allowed recordings of the waves of negative pressure created by the pup as it sucked (see Brake *et al.*, 1986; Pelchat and Brake, 1987). This new device provided an accurate measure of the force of sucking and proved to be a better measure of the duration of sucking as well.

This advance in the sensitivity of our measure led to an important new discovery about RS. We found that RS actually occurs in two different modes. We called one *slow rhythmic sucking* (SRS) and the other *rapid rhythmic sucking* (RRS). SRS can be characterized as a series of relatively long-duration (1 suck every 1–2 s), forceful (5–20 mm Hg) sucks. It constitutes about 75% of RS and tends to occur in the intervals between milk deliveries (particularly in deprived pups). RRS, on the other hand, can be characterized as shorter periods of much more rapid sucking (2–3 sucks every second). The range in amplitude within a period of RRS can vary from 5 mm Hg to 50 mm Hg. RRS occurs most often during milk delivery and while the pup first attaches to the nipple. Examples are presented in Figure 5 (also see Table 1).

Using the negative pressure technique, we examined SRS and RRS during and immediately after three milk ejections elicited in anesthetized dams by the intravenous administration of oxytocin (Brake, Shindledecker, and Hofer, in preparation). As in the first study, all pups were deprived, but only half received preloads before the sucking test. Three important findings emerged from this study. First, hungry pups (those not receiving preloads) engaged in significantly longer episodes of SRS following the second and third milk deliveries of the sequence than sated pups (those receiving preloads). Thus, even when the volume of milk delivered to the pups is variable, hungry pups engage in more sucking (SRS) following milk

PERCENT TIME SUCKING AFTER MILK-EJECTION

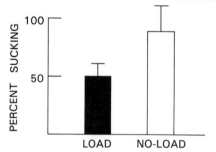

Figure 4. The percentage of time pups spent sucking following milk ejections. "Load" indicates pups received a stomach preload; "No-Load" indicates that they didn't.

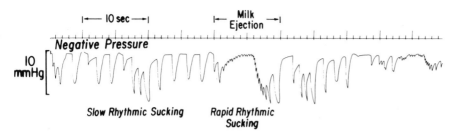

Figure 5. Polygraph tracing of a negative pressure recording illustrating slow and rapid rhythmic sucking before, during, and after a milk ejection.

delivery than sated pups. Second, the force of sucking during the second and third milk deliveries was, on the average, greater in hungry pups than in sated pups (Figure 6).

These two findings clearly indicate that pups may adjust intake by varying the force of sucking during the milk ejection as well as the amount of sucking following it. Interestingly, it appears that differences due to privation are more likely to emerge later in the feeding sequence rather than earlier. Pups did not differ in the force of their sucking during the first milk ejection, but they did differ significantly during the second and third, as if sated pups respond eagerly to the first pulse of a feeding bout but then lose interest.

The third finding of the study, however, cautions against drawing conclusions too quickly about how privation may affect sucking and ingestion. Although the average differences between the rate and the amplitude of sucking between hungry and sated pups were substantial, they were only marginally significant because of the enormous between-subject variability displayed by the hungry pups. In fact, the variance in the amplitude and the rate of sucking in hungry pups was three times that of sated pups, a highly significant difference. In other words, when pups are subjected to a serious environmental challenge (lengthy maternal separation), some are able to compensate quite well by sucking vigorously, whereas others compensate less well (or not at all) and suck weakly.

A final experiment in this series underscored these findings. The sucking responses of three groups of 10-day-old pups were recorded with the intraoral can-

SUCKING PRESSURE DURING MILK-EJECTION

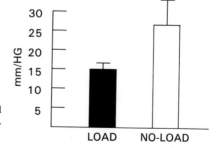

Figure 6. Amplitude of sucking that occurred during milk ejection in pups that were given preloads and pups that weren't.

nula during a single milk ejection that was elicited from an anesthetized dam by iv administration of oxytocin. One of these groups of pups was deprived for 20–24 h before the test, one was deprived for the same length of time but was given a 5% GI preload before the test, and one was deprived for a shorter length of time (4–6 h) and was given no preload. All pups were removed from the teat immediately following the milk ejection and were weighed in order to assess the volume of milk they had consumed. The amount of milk consumed by the pups in all three conditions during the 10- to 20-s milk ejection was extremely variable, ranging from none to 0.62 ml, even though the pups from all three groups were suckling the same dam at the same time. Indeed, the variance was so large that no reliable differences in intake were observed among the groups, in contrast to what others have reported concerning the greater intake of hungry pups during a 2- to 4-h suckling bout. (Group differences in our study were probably less likely to be detected because we allowed the pups to consume for only a few seconds; remember that, in the previous study, no differences in intake were observed between hungry and sated pups during the first milk ejection). The force of the pups' sucking during the milk ejection was also quite variable, ranging from 10 to 70 mm Hg, and again no reliable group differences were detected.

The results of the study clearly illustrate that at least three sources of variance contribute to the amount of milk consumed by suckling pups. First, there are individual differences among pups in the force and rate of their sucking, independent of privation. Second, sucking among pups varies as a function of privation, and it varies in some pups more than in others. Third, the amount of milk released by the dam is variable from one milk ejection to another, and it may even vary from one teat to another during the same milk ejection.

Despite these different sources of variation, however, we found that the force of a pup's sucking during any given milk ejection contributes substantially to the amount of milk it consumes. Strong and reliable correlations were obtained between the amplitude ($r(71) = .40$, $p < .007$) and duration ($r(71) = .57$, $p < .001$) of the sucking episodes displayed during the milk ejection and the amount of milk the pup consumed during that milk ejection.

In summary, the volume of nutrient consumed while suckling depends on several factors, including (a) the amount of time pups remain attached to the teat; (b) the frequency with which pups shift from depleted teats to teats replete with milk; (c) the force of the pups' sucking during milk ejection; (d) the amount of milk released during milk ejection; and, possibly, (e) the rate of the pups' sucking following milk ejection. Perhaps the most variable of all of these factors is the pups' ability to generate negative pressure during milk ejection. Some pups suck harder than others and thus consume more milk. Further, extended deprivation accentuates these individual differences. This finding suggests that some pups may be more competent feeders and may grow more rapidly than their less competent littermates, a possibility explored below.

One of the possible sources of the individual variability in sucking lies in the cycles of sleep–wake states experienced during suckling, particularly around the time of milk ejection. The next section describes these sleep–wake states and some of the surprising results we obtained when we studied sucking patterns in relation to sleep states.

The Relationship of Sleep to Feeding

We have known for some time that sleep–wake states and feeding behavior are related in an intricate way (Kleitman, 1963; Mouret and Bobillier, 1971; Siegel, 1975). In adults, it seems that food deprivation increases wakefulness, and that stomach fill leads to periods of sleep (Danguir and Nicolaïdis, 1979; Jacobs and McGinty, 1971; Rubenstein and Sonnenshein, 1971), and some evidence suggests the same may be true of infants (Gaensbauer and Emde, 1973; Wolff, 1972; Yogman and Zeisel, 1983). This descent into sleep following a meal is generally regarded as part of a postprandial satiety sequence (Antin, Gibbs, Holt, Young, and Smith, 1975; Mansbach and Lorenz, 1983). However, our own series of studies (Shair, Brake, and Hofer, 1984; in preparation) has revealed the existence of unexpected relationships between sucking and sleep that may shed further light on how sated and deprived rat pups differ in their style of feeding.

We first recorded sleep–wake states (by EEG, neck muscle EMG, and respiration) and simultaneous sucking behavior (by digastric EMG) from nondeprived rat pups, each in its home cage with littermates and dam. In these experiments, the dam was not anesthetized, nor were her movements restricted. Each dam nursed its litter for the duration of at least one bout (about 15–20 min) during a 2-h test, and most nursed for several bouts.

Contrary to our expectations, the pups fell asleep very quickly after attaching to a teat and were asleep for about 70% of each nursing bout (a typical example is shown in Figure 7). In fact, the idea that infants sleep primarily following feeding

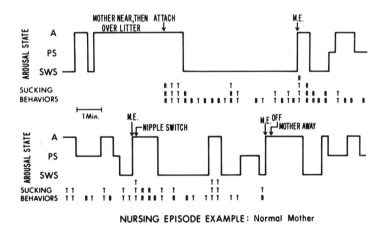

Figure 7. An example of sleep–wake states and sucking during a typical nursing bout. "A" indicates awake, "PS" indicates paradoxical sleep, "SWS" indicates slow-wave sleep, "R" indicates rhythmic sucking, "B" indicates bursts, "T" indicates treadles, and "ME" indicates milk-ejection. The height of the column containing R, B, and T indicates the relative amount of each type of sucking that was occurring at that time.

bouts, when the dam leaves the litter, was not supported by our data. Pups spent about the same amount of time sleeping during the feeding bout, while attached to the teat, as they did following it (Figure 8). The amount of time pups spent asleep did not even change from the first to the second half of the nursing bout, as the pups consumed more and more milk.

We also found that the pups sucked in all three sleep–wake states (slow-wave sleep, or SWS; paradoxical sleep, or PS; awake, or A; Figure 7). In addition, the occurrence of sucking was not limited to the few seconds during which the pup was awake following milk delivery. Considerable amounts of sucking also occurred between milk ejections when the pup was usually asleep. Of all sucking, 14% occurred while the pups were in PS, 33% while they were in SWS, and the remaining 53% when the pups were awake. However, one sucking type (bursts) actually occurred more frequently in SWS than at any other time.

The patterning of sleep and sucking that occurred around the times of milk ejection was distinctive. In all 33 cases observed, the pups were asleep before milk ejection, were awakened by the ejection, and remained awake for a variable (but usually short) amount of time thereafter (Figure 9). Milk ejection also stimulated corresponding increases in RS and treadling (the type of AS that occurs with forelimb movement and that appears to be the pup's attempts to "knead" the nipple). In short, release of milk from the dam awoke the pup and stimulated sucking and milk withdrawal. As the pup fell asleep, within seconds of the termination of milk delivery, rhythmic sucking and treadling returned to baseline levels.

These results suggest that sleep–wake states and feeding behavior are closely linked. However, the relationships are not as straightforward as was once thought. Sleep is not a simple indicator of postprandial satiety. Instead, except for the period immediately following milk ejection, sleep seems to be evenly distributed throughout long nursing bouts. In addition, the pup is just as likely to sleep when attached to the teat as when it is away from the dam.

To obtain a better understanding of these relationships, we examined several 22-h-deprived 2-week-old pups after being reunited with their dam. They fell

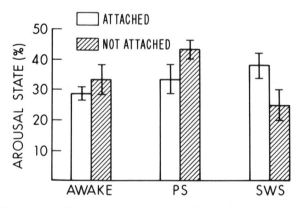

Figure 8. Percentage of time spent in each sleep–wake state when attached to the teat and when not attached.

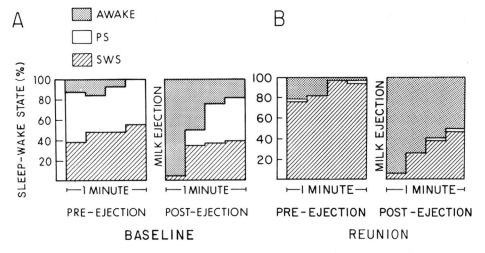

Figure 9. Percentage of time spent in each sleep–wake state in the minutes immediately before and after milk ejection on (A) baseline and (B) reunion days.

quickly asleep after attaching to a teat, just as they had before deprivation, and they slept during most of each nursing bout. However, they were awake a greater percentage of the time and were in PS a smaller percentage of time than they had been before deprivation. This was true even though they were not stimulated to be awake more often by receiving a greater number of milk deliveries than they had before deprivation. In fact, similar changes in sleep–wake percentages have been found following deprivation in pups tested away from the dam (Hofer and Shair, 1982).

We also observed an increase in the time spent in RS and treadles. However, these increases in sucking were not due to increased rates of sucking within each sleep–wake state. Rather, they were due to increased time spent awake and decreased time spent in PS. The rate of sucking within each state remained the same. In other words, sucking increased because the pups spent more time in the states associated with the highest levels of sucking (awake) and less time in the state associated with the lowest level of sucking (PS). A similar phenomenon was seen in the minutes immediately following milk delivery. Deprived pups remained awake longer following milk ejections than sated pups (see Figure 9) and also engaged in more sucking at this time. Thus, the effects of privation on intake may be mediated through changes in sleep–wake behavior. Changes in sucking may also influence milk release in the dam, as will be discussed shortly.

We also found, however, that sleep–wake-state distribution was extremely variable following deprivation, and that some pups remained awake much longer than others. This finding means that individual differences in sucking and intake following deprivation may be linked to individual differences in sleep–wake cycling. Are the pups that are awake the most also the ones that suck the most?

The answer appears to be yes. We found a significant correlation ($r = .41$) between the amount of sucking displayed by deprived pups and the amount of time these pups stayed awake following milk ejection. And again, surprisingly, the incidence of sucking did not increase (or decrease) during a given amount of time in a sleep state. Instead, increases (or decreases) of sucking were accomplished by lengthening (or shortening) the amount of time spent in a given state. Thus, it appears that individual differences in feeding competence may be due to the amount of time the pup remains awake following milk delivery.

Sucking may also serve functions other than the immediate withdrawal of milk, particularly during the intervals between milk ejections when the pup is sleeping. A clue to these other functions of sucking is provided by the fact that pups that have been deprived for long periods of time remain awake longer during these intervals and engage in significantly more slow rhythmic sucking than sated pups (see also Figure 4). It may be that pups continue to suck on the chance that they may be able to withdraw residual amounts of milk from the ducts of the teat. In other work, we have shown that pups attached to the teats of an anesthetized dam can withdraw small amounts of milk from a reservoir connected to their cannulas if they suck hard enough (Brake, et al., 1982a). Pups can even ingest small amounts (< 0.01 ml) of milk in this way while they are asleep (Shair, Gottschalk, Brake, and Hofer, 1983). Continued sucking, whether during sleep or while awake, may also be the pups' way of maintaining a secure grip on the teat. This could be highly advantageous because the occurrence of milk ejections is unpredictable. A pup that continued to suck with some force throughout the interval between milk ejections might be in a better position to withdraw milk when it is secreted into the mammary ducts. Sucking may also help stimulate digestion and absorbtion. Finally, continued sucking may also serve a purpose that is of an entirely different nature: it may be the litter's way of communicating with the dam.

SUCKING AND ADJUSTMENT OF INTAKE: INDIRECT CONTROL BY THE LITTER

Milk ejection in the dam is a response initiated by the pups. Their presence on the teats provides a constant source of stimulation that seems to act on the supraoptic and paraventricular areas of the dam's hypothalamus (Lincoln and Wakerley, 1974; Wakerley and Drewett, 1975). After some length of time (5–20 min), a bolus of oxytocin is released from the pituitary that acts on contractile tissue about the mammary cisterns to release milk into the mammary ducts. Thus, milk ejections occur intermittently.

It isn't entirely clear what determines the length of the interval between milk ejections. It would seem to depend, at least in part, on the nature of the stimulation provided by the pups. Perhaps the only signal that is required is the tactile sensation provided by the contact of the pup's mouth with the epitheal tissue near the teat. After some minimum (though variable) amount of time, a threshold for stimulation may be reached, and oxytocin may be released. However, constant contact with the teat is a form of stimulation to which the dam may easily habituate. It may be that a more discrete and recurring signal is required. And yet, we know that the dam must be asleep in order for milk ejection to occur (Voloschin and Tramezzani, 1979), so although this stimulus must register in the central nervous system, it must not awaken her. If the dam wakes from sleep, the next milk ejection would be canceled. A stimulus that seems to meet all of these requirements is the intermittent sucking that occurs between milk ejections, when the pups are quietly asleep and are not disturbing the dam.

Perhaps, too, the rate and amplitude of the pups' sucking provides additional information. As mentioned above, deprived pups engage in more vigorous sucking between milk ejections than nondeprived pups, possibly because of changes in their sleep–wake states. This increased sucking may convey to the dam the privational status of the litter. This, in turn, could result in a longer or more voluminous release of oxytocin. This notion is supported by evidence suggesting that the sensory tissue surrounding the nipple is extraordinarily sensitive. Although no correlation between an individual pup's sucking and milk release has been demonstrated, the magnitude of the neural response that mediates oxytocin release has been shown to vary as a function of the number of pups suckling the dam (Lincoln, 1983; Lincoln and Wakerley, 1974). Further, milk ejections are less likely to occur during the initial portions of a nursing bout (Shair *et al.*, 1984), as if a requisite amount of stimulation must be received by the dam before the process can begin. Thus, variations in the frequency and the duration of sucking may also exert some influence on milk release.

In general, then, suckling-deprived rat pups may have two methods of maximizing intake. First, as individuals, they may ingest more of the milk that is made available by the dam. They can do this by remaining attached to a teat for longer periods of time, or by shifting more often from dry teats to teats with residual amounts of milk, or by increasing the vigor of their sucking during and immediately following milk ejection. Second, as a litter, deprived pups may induce more frequent or more voluminous milk ejections by increasing the amount of sucking they display between the ejections. All of these behaviors are intricately bound by the sleep–wake cycling of both mother and offspring. In fact, both pups and dam are asleep throughout much of the nursing bout. How might such interactions have evolved?

Norway rats cache their young in burrows. The mother cannot depend solely on fat stores to supply the nutrient that she must make available to her young. Instead, she must forage for food and water. This activity can involve large amounts of time. This time, combined with the time required for nursing, leaves little time for sleep. As a result, evolutionary pressure may have arisen to combine the activities of nursing and sleeping. A dam that manages to do both simultaneously may be better rested and more capable of foraging successfully. And so, those dams whose milk ejections were elicited during slow-wave sleep by the suckling of the pups may have benefited. At the same time, pups that were able to signal changes in privational status to the dam by increased sucking in the intervals between milk letdowns may also have benefited because they may have received more milk. This embedding of feeding within sleep is just one example of how behaviors eventually become tied to sleep–wake states. Variations in heart rate, thermoregulation, and hormone release (see Borbely and Valatx, 1984, for review) have all been linked to the cycling of arousal states. Feeding interactions are particularly interesting because the behavior of both the dam and her litter are symbiotically woven around sleep-state cycling.

ADJUSTMENT OF SUCKING AND INTAKE IN RESPONSE TO ENVIRONMENTAL AND DEVELOPMENTAL VARIATION

We have seen how periods of maternal separation can lead to changes in the behavior of both the dam and the pups. Lengthy separation causes pups to respond to the dam's next visit to the nest with enhanced activity. They attach to the teats more rapidly, suck more vigorously, and remain awake for longer periods of time. These behaviors maximize the pups' chances of withdrawing the milk the dam has to offer. At the same time, the dam is more likely to release milk following long periods of separation from her litter. The increased sucking of the pups and the weight of accumulated milk in the cisterns causes the dam to release more milk during milk ejections. This rids her of the excess of milk she has stored and allows the pups the opportunity to compensate for their inability to ingest in the dam's absence. This release of extra milk, in turn, stimulates even more vigorous sucking, and so on, until the pups become sated, their sucking diminishes, and the milk release is attenuated.

Of course, variations on this theme are abundant. We have found that environmental factors can influence sucking and nipple attachment in highly specific ways. For example, specific differences in the frequency with which the dam releases milk to the pup can have very different effects on the vigor of the pup's sucking, as can variations in the taste of her milk. The pup's patterns of sucking and nipple attachment behaviors also change with age. And as we have already noted, some pups are simply more competent feeders than others. Such pups are more likely to compensate for periods of separation from the dam by maximizing intake, and therefore, they may grow at a faster rate than their littermates. In this section, we explore these issues, concluding with a discussion of how certain environmental contingencies may result in the acquisition of conditioned feeding behaviors.

LONG-LASTING EFFECTS OF DIFFERENT MILK-DELIVERY SCHEDULES

The frequency of the dam's visits to the nest and the frequency and duration of her milk deliveries during a feeding bout are parameters that can vary a great deal during the 3–4 weeks in which she nurses pups. Feeding bouts can last as long as 3 h or may end after only 10 min. Milk ejections may occur within 2 min of each other or may be separated by as much as 30 min. The volume of milk delivered during each ejection can vary from 0.1 to 0.4 ml. There is even the possibility that dams separated from the litter for relatively long periods of time are so milk-laden on their return to the nest that small amounts of milk seep into the terminal galactaphores of the teat, so that the pups have access to milk in the absence of a milk ejection. Finally, these parameters change during development; feeding bouts become more shorter and more infrequent, and the volume of milk supplied by the mother lessens (e.g., Lau and Henning, 1984).

Some of these changes in milk availability probably mirror changes in the pup's needs for milk. For example, as pups grow older and more reliant on solid food, they also seek to suckle less frequently. In any case, pups must respond to both long-term and transient changes in milk availability in order to maintain an optimum consumption of nutrient. We've already seen that pups of all ages do, indeed, compensate in their sucking for variations in the length of the dam's absence from the nest. Perhaps pups also compensate for variations in the quantity or spacing of milk ejections. In order to begin to address this issue, we exposed suckling pups to extreme variations in the frequency and duration of milk delivery (Brake, Sullivan, Sager, and Hofer, 1982b). During the suckling tests, dams were anesthetized to prevent natural milk letdown, and milk was delivered to the suckling pups via a posterior tongue cannula. We asked whether experience with a particular milk delivery schedule on one day can affect the way pups suck on the following day.

In the first experiment, 11 to 13-day-old pups were exposed to different schedules for 2 h. One group received a 10-s pulse of milk every 15–20 min, a periodic schedule resembling that associated with freely moving lactating dams. Another group received no milk during the 2 h, an extremely long interval for pups to be suckling in the absence of milk. Still another group received a slow, continuous infusion of milk during the 2 h. This last procedure meant that the amount of milk these pups received was contingent on the vigor of their sucking (this may be an important point in interpreting the data, as will be discussed shortly). The total volume of milk received by the pups in the periodic-delivery group was yoked to the volume received by this last group of pups. Other pups received a continuous infusion of water, and others received a 2-h infusion of milk while they were away from the teat. Following these treatments, the pups were isolated (but kept warm) for an additional 24 h, and then they were returned to an anesthetized dam and allowed to suckle for 1 h. On this second day, none of the pups received milk.

The results revealed that these very different schedules of milk delivery had dramatic effects on sucking on both the first and second days of the experiment. On the first day, the pups that received milk continuously also sucked continuously (Figure 10; almost all of this sucking was RS). This extremely high rate of sucking was greater than that seen in the pups receiving milk on a more normal intermittent schedule and was clearly due to the activating or incentive value of constant gustatory stimulation (and not simply to the need to clear milk from the mouth; the volume received was determined by the vigor of sucking). The pups that received no milk, on the other hand, began the session by sucking vigorously but soon displayed significantly less RS than any of the other pups.

Interestingly, continuously available water seemed to depress RS rather than to enhance it. These pups engaged in as little RS as the pups that received no fluid. Water, it seems, is not an excitatory stimulus to 2-week-old pups (e.g., Kehoe and Blass, 1984; Kenny and Brake, in preparation; Pelchat and Brake, 1987; see below).

Continuous delivery of both milk and water also affected the pup's tendency

STEPHEN C. BRAKE
ET AL.

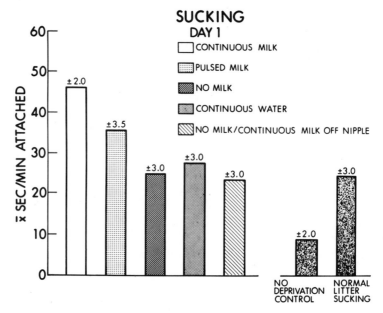

Figure 10. Amount of sucking displayed by different groups of pups receiving milk on different schedules.

to remain attached to a teat, though in opposite ways. Pups receiving milk continuously never left the nipple, whereas pups that received water continuously were away from the teat almost 45% of the time. Clearly, there is something extremely salient or rewarding about continuously available milk to 2-week-old pups, and something equally aversive about continuously available water.

These results reveal the pup's remarkable ability to alter RS, as well as the amount of time it spends attached to the teat, according to what and how it is being fed. But it was the pups' behavior 24 h later that was truly surprising (Figure 11). Pups that had received milk continuously on the first day again engaged in significantly more RS than pups in any of the other groups, even though they were not receiving milk on this second day. Similarly, pups that had received no milk on the first day of the experiment again engaged in significantly less RS 24 h later than pups in any of the other groups.

Even though the schedules used in this experiment were extreme and are not likely to occur under normal circumstances, the results were exciting because they demonstrated, for the first time, that the way milk is delivered to pups during a single feeding bout can have effects on sucking behavior that last for a full day.

It is tempting to speculate that the pups that received milk continuously on the nipple might have learned to suck more vigorously than usual because they were rewarded for doing so. Similarly, the pups that didn't receive milk may have extinguished their responding because they had learned that they would not be rewarded. Such speculation is strengthened by our knowledge that pups can learn new associations while receiving milk at the teat (Brake, 1981; Pelchat and Brake,

1982; see below). In this case, the presence of an anesthetized dam may have served as a contextual conditioned stimulus for such learning. However, some of the data cannot easily be explained in this way. Pups that had received water continuously on the first day did not continue to display the extremely low rates of sucking they had displayed then; instead, they sucked at a rate comparable to that shown by pups that had received milk intermittently on the first day. What was even more perplexing, pups that had received continuous oral infusions while away from the dam on the first day engaged in more sucking on the second day than did untreated control pups; yet these pups could not have associated milk delivery with sucking. These results remain to be explained and indicate how much we have still to learn about the adaptation of sucking patterns to previous experience.

In an effort to see if repeated exposures to the two extreme conditions (no milk and continuous milk) would produce even more pronounced effects over longer periods of time, the study was repeated, this time beginning at 14 days of age and continuing until the pups were 18 days old. Once each day, the pups were allowed to suckle an anesthetized dam for 2 h while receiving milk continuously or while receiving no milk at all. These 2 h were the only suckling experiences the pups received on that day. During the intervening hours, they were fed a wet mash, which most of them readily consumed. Other groups of pups received only a single 2-h experience with continuous milk, or no milk, on Day 18. All pups were then tested at 19 days of age, 24 h after their last suckling experience. Normally reared 19-day-old pups (nondeprived) were also tested at this time.

Some of the results are shown in Figure 12, along with data obtained from the

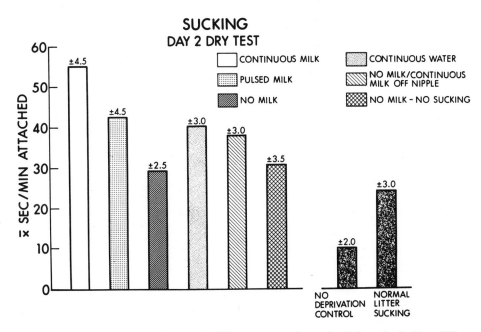

Figure 11. Amount of sucking displayed by different groups of pups that had received milk on different schedules the day before (none of the pups were receiving milk on this day).

younger pups of the previous experiment. First, notice that the normally reared 19-day-old pups (the controls) spent less time attached to a teat and engaged in less sucking than their 12-day-old counterparts. This finding suggests that, as weaning age approaches and the dam's accessibility and supply of milk wane, pups do not attempt to suckle as vigorously. However, as in the previous experiment, pups that received milk continuously during the 2-h suckling sessions, as well as pups that received no milk at all, displayed very different sucking profiles. In this experiment, they also displayed very different tendencies to attach to the teat. The 19-day-old pups that had received milk continuously during a 2-h period for 4 days, or even on just 1 day, engaged in significantly more sucking than did the other 19-day-old pups. On the other hand, 19-day-olds that had received no milk during the treatment periods spent considerably more time away from the nipple than did other 19-day-olds.

The data suggest that the onset of weaning can be delayed by a pup's recent feeding experience. The aspect of this experiment that may be the most important is the consistency with which the pups receive milk. It appears that experience with continuous milk delivery "protected" pups from the early weaning that results from restricted access to the dam. These pups continued to show interest in the teat and to suck vigorously. These findings are supported by recent work of Cramer, Pfister, and Blass (1986) that showed that pups 40 days of age and older continued to suckle avidly if they had been raised by younger, milk-laden dams whose

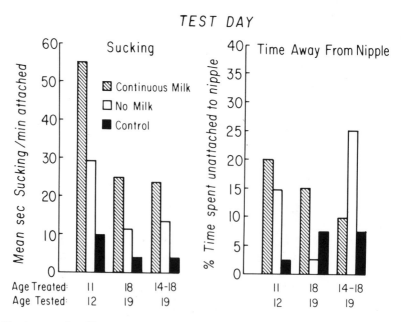

Figure 12. Amount of sucking and time spent away from the teat at 12 or 19 days of age ("Test Day"). Test followed 24 h after treatment. Treatment consisted of a 2-h exposure to either continuous milk or no milk, for 1 day or for 5 days. "Control" indicates behavior of nondeprived, nontreated pups on the test day.

own litters were 15–21 days of age. (This effect was achieved by rotation among litters.)

373

EXPLOITING THE
NURSING NICHE

The findings suggest that pups compensate for strikingly aberrant changes in feeding schedule by altering their sucking and, in some cases, the time they spend attached to the teat. Whether they do so in response to more moderate variations is unknown. However, it should be mentioned that, because pups are capable of learning new associations in the suckling context (Amsel, 1979; Brake, 1978, 1981; Kehoe and Blass, 1986; Kenny and Blass, 1977; Smith and Spear, 1978), it is possible that some part of the changes in sucking and nipple attachment that occur in response to variations in feeding schedule may also be learned.

The Importance of Taste

The results of the studies described above also provide a clue about the importance of taste in the control of feeding. Pups that were presented with milk while attached to the teats of an anesthetized dam engaged in more sucking and remained attached to the nipple longer than pups presented with water. Understanding how pups respond to the taste of the dam's milk is important because pups may experience a variety of tastes in the wild. Rat dams may sample and subsist on a variety of different foodstuffs (Calhoun, 1962). The taste of these foods is passed along to the suckling young in her milk (Galef, 1982; Galef and Henderson, 1972). This means that variations in her diet could result in rather sudden changes in the taste of the milk she feeds to the litter. In addition, the constitution of her milk changes during development (Chalk and Bailey, 1979), and this change, too, may cause the taste of the milk to change.

In 1969, Jacobs and Sharma demonstrated that, beginning around 10 days of age, pups responded to bitter-tasting quinine solutions presented to the front of their mouths by vigorously attempting to turn away from the tube that was used to deliver these solutions. In contrast, pups attempted to lick and consume sweet-tasting solutions (sucrose, lactose, or saccharin). Later, Hall and Bryan (1980) extended these findings by showing that pups older than 5 days of age will consume sucrose-adulterated water presented to the fronts of their mouths through a tongue cannula but will reject quinine-adulterated water. In 1984, Kehoe and Blass examined how pups respond to different tastes when they are attached to the teats of an anesthetized dam. These authors found that pups older than 5 days of age will leave the nipple when presented with quinine-adulterated water and ammonium chloride. They also found that pups' responses to taste depend on where on the tongue the fluids are delivered, and that taste sensitivity increases with age.

In an attempt to determine how bitter-tasting fluids may affect sucking as well as nipple attachment behaviors, Pelchat and Brake (1987) presented 2-week-old pups with milk (half-and-half) or water adulterated with varying concentrations of quinine. Pulses of the fluids (0.1 ml) were delivered through one posterior tongue cannula while sucking was recorded through a second. These authors found that pups that received either a moderate (6×10^{-4} M) or strong (3×10^{-3} M) concentration of quinine in milk decreased the amount of RS they displayed by about

25%. Those receiving the stronger concentration reduced the amplitude of their sucking by almost 50% during the first pulse (Figure 13) and then spent most of the remainder of the test session away from the teat (Figure 14).

These findings indicate that suckling pups possess a full range of responses that can be used to reject unpalatable substances. They can refuse to remain attached to the teat, can decrease the frequency of their sucking, or can decrease the force of their sucking. In short, the 2-week-old pup is not obligated to consume the fluid it is offered. Although it is unlikely that a 2-week-old pup could be discouraged from suckling altogether, decreased intake may be advantageous should an unpleasant taste signal a toxic substance in the milk. Within a day or 2, these pups would be old enough to consume significant amounts of solid food to make up for nutrient lost by avoiding the dam and could even survive without suckling (e.g., Ackerman and Shindledecker, 1978). But what of younger pups that cannot consume solid foods? Do they also have the capacity to avoid unpleasant tastes?

Several investigators have reported that taste bud papilla continue to mature and grow in number until about 5 days after the rat pup's birth (Farbman, 1965; Henderson and Smith, 1977). These reports suggest that taste sensitivity is not fully developed until that time. Further, it seems that the maturation of the taste buds on the posterior portion of the tongue, which are sensitive to bitter tastes, occurs earlier than the maturation of the taste buds sensitive to sweet tastes on the anterior portion of the tongue (Jacobs and Sharma, 1977; Mistretta, 1972). These findings are consistent with the behavioral data as we know them. At about 5 days of age, pups begin to reject bitter-tasting solutions, and at about 10 days of age, they begin to prefer sweet-tasting solutions (Hall and Bryan, 1980; Jacobs and Sharma 1977; Kehoe and Blass, 1984).

Data collected recently by Kenney and Brake (in preparation) have extended

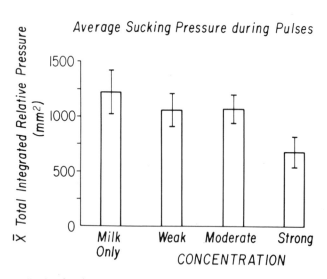

Figure 13. Amplitude of sucking during presentation of milk varying in the degree of quinine concentration (weak = 1.6×10^{-4} M; moderate = 6×10^{-4} M; strong = 3×10^{-3} M).

these findings by providing information about the ontogeny of the pup's sucking in response to bitter and sweet tastes. These authors examined the sucking and nipple attachment responses to pulses of milk adulterated with either quinine or sucrose (presented through a posterior tongue cannula) in pups ranging in age from 3 to 18 days. They discovered that neonates (3- to 5-day-old pups) maintain high levels of sucking when delivered pulses of milk adulterated with either taste. In fact, compared to the amount of sucking displayed by neonates presented with unadulterated milk, it appears that they had a tendency to increase their sucking slightly when presented with either the bitter or the sweet taste. Older pups, on the other hand, made more appropriate discriminations. By 10 days of age, pups decreased the amount of their sucking and left the nipple when presented with bitter tastes (replicating earlier findings), but they increased their sucking and the amount of time they spent on the nipple when presented with sweet tastes.

By the time weaning begins (around 18 days of age), deprived pups will not suck for more than a few seconds when presented quinine-adulterated milk and will not return to the nipple after tasting it, even if allowed an hour to do so. On the other hand, presentations of sucrose-adulterated milk elicit significantly more sucking and longer nipple attachment times than do presentations of unadulterated milk. Further, in a striking reversal of the behavior typical of pups just a few days younger, 18-day-old pups seem to prefer water to milk. This preference may reflect an increasing need for older pups to consume additional amounts of water in order to maintain hydrational balance. (These pups consume large amounts of solid food and so need more water.)

Taken together, the results indicate that 3- to 5-day-old pups, unlike older ones, make little effort to avoid aversive tastes, tastes that may signal the presence of toxic substances in the milk. Nor do these pups seem to increase responding

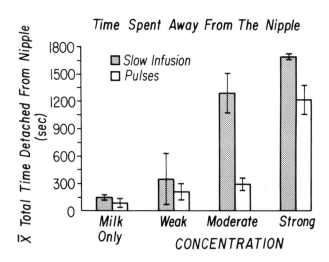

Figure 14. Amount of time spent detached from the nipple in pups receiving weak, moderate, or strong concentrations of quinine.

when presented with flavored milk that older pups find preferable to plain milk. Thus, although young pups can adjust intake on the basis of privational status, they do not seem to do so in response to taste. Thus, interactions between mother and infant during the first days of life seem to be designed to maintain the infant's proximity to the dam.

How Sucking and Feeding Strategies Change during Development

We are now able to piece together a picture of how feeding strategies change during the course of development. In general, the incidence of sucking decreases with age. The 18-day-old pups, whether sated or hungry, engage in less than half as much sucking as younger pups, although 12-day-old pups seem to engage in as much sucking as 3-day-old pups (Brake and Hofer, 1980; Brake *et al.,* 1982b). Older pups, however, suck with more force than younger ones. The sucking of both 12-day-old pups and 18-day-old pups is of greater amplitude than that of 3-day-olds, both during and between milk deliveries (Kenny and Brake, in preparation).

Only one aspect of sucking does not seem to change as the pup grows from neonate to weanling, and that is its susceptibility to deprivation. Maternal deprivation elicits increased sucking regardless of whether pups are 2 days old or 20 days old. This finding, as mentioned previously, stands in contrast to what we know about the effects of privation on nipple attachment behaviors. That is, prior deprivation has little effect on the rapidity with which a pup younger than 10 days old will grasp the nipple, nor on the amount of time it will remain attached. Pups of this age, even when quite sated, quickly attach to the teat and remain there. In general, this stragegy seems to serve the newborn pup very well. It ensures that the pup will always be in proximity to the dam, and it also allows the pup a way of maximizing intake by sucking vigorously.

The amount of control that neonates can exert at the teat is somewhat limited. Pups less than 10 days of age tend to overconsume when large quantities of milk are made available to them at frequent intervals (Cramer and Blass, 1983; Hall and Rosenblatt, 1977). But young pups' control over ingestion is also limited by their inability to detect or reluctance to respond to changes in the taste of the dam's milk. It seems as if the potential benefit of restricting the intake of milk containing a potentially toxic substance is outweighed by the fact that reduced intake could lead to growth retardation or death. In older pups, the risks incurred by decreasing intake or leaving the nipple are less severe, and beginning around 10 days of age, the pup will use both strategies and avoid unpleasant tastes.

The younger pup's tendency not to avoid bad-tasting solutions may also be reflected in what may be a failure to express conditioned taste aversions while suckling, at least under certain conditions. Alberts and colleagues (Gubernick and Alberts, 1984; Martin and Alberts, 1979; Melcer, Alberts, and Gubernick, 1985) have shown that pups younger than 19 days of age disregard the information that the conditioning has provided them and continue to suckle in the presence of a taste associated with subsequent poisoning. This finding is remarkable when one considers that the findings of Kenny and Brake (in preparation), and those of Kehoe and Blass (1984), suggest that pups 5 days of age and older are capable of avoiding unpleasant tastes. Further, Kehoe and Blass (1986) reported that pups as young as 5 days of age are capable of displaying conditioned taste aversions that were acquired while suckling. These authors suggested that the findings of Alberts and colleagues, which seem to indicate that learning was blocked in suckling pups, may be due to the fact that the distinctively flavored milk that the pups received during the conditioning trials may have been delivered too far back in the young pups' mouths to be detected as the taste that was to serve as a conditioned stimulus. Gubernick and Alberts (1984), however, believe that the delay in expressing a conditioned avoidance of taste is somehow determined by the pup's experience with solid food. If access to solid food is delayed for a few days beyond when it would ordinarily occur, the pup's tendency to display conditioned taste aversions while suckling is also delayed.

Experience with solid food also seems to contribute to the attenuation of suckling in the absence of aversive postingestive consequences. Williams, Hall, and Rosenblatt (1980) reported that 25-day-old pups that were denied access to solid food were much more likely to attach to a dam's teats and suckle than pups that had access to solid food. As discussed above, our own data (Brake *et al.*, 1982b), and those of Cramer *et al.* (1986) provide evidence that the reverse is also true. That is, by providing weanling-age pups with more readily available milk than they would ordinarily receive from their own dams, the onset and termination of weaning seem to be delayed. Taken together, these findings suggest that the pup's environment plays a large role in determining how rapidly it will forsake suckling. In general, it seems that pups make the most of their situation; if solid food is to be found in abundance, they begin to feed, but if the dam is likely to continue providing adequate milk, they will, in addition, continue to obtain nutrient from suckling.

FEEDING COMPETENCE AND LONG-TERM GROWTH

We have seen that individual pups can maximize their intake in three ways; they may: (a) increase the force of their sucking during milk ejection; (b) increase the rate of their sucking immediately following milk-ejection; and (c) remain attached to a nipple for longer periods of time. It stands to reason that pups that are able to do all of these things better than their littermates may grow more rapidly. This may be particularly true if they evidence superior feeding competence during the first days of life, as this period is an especially important one in the normal growth and development of mammalian infants (Dobbing, 1976). Periods of milk restriction during this time can lead to permanently stunted growth (Knittle and Hirsch, 1968; Levine and Otis, 1958; McCance, 1960; Winick, 1969). Even when the milk supply is abundant, however, some pups fall off the growth curve or die within the first days of life, though they do not appear to be smaller or less viable than their littermates at birth. Are these pups incompetent feeders?

In our own studies, we have found that the number of naturally occurring fatalities in apparently healthy pups after 5 days is about 1%–2%, and that another 1%–2% have fallen significantly behind in their rate of growth by then. We have also found that the incidence of stunted growth increases significantly in litters in which one-half of the pups are separated from the dam (but are kept warm) at 2 days of age for just 4–6 h (Brake and Kenny, in preparation). Interestingly, this interruption of normal mother-infant interactions seems to affect as many of the pups left with the dam as pups removed from the dam. That is, approximately 15% to 20% of pups left with the dam and 15% to 20% of pups removed from the dam subsequently show signs of retarded growth. These findings are striking because they suggest that some neonates may be particularly susceptible to growth-retardation if conditions in the litter are altered for only a few hours.

It isn't clear which factors are most responsible for growth retardation. Delays of growth may be due to some alteration of the dam's behavior toward her litter, or to some physiological disturbance, such as disruption in the release of growth hormone (e.g. Schanberg, Evonuik, and Kuhn, 1984). It may also be true that the brief interruption of mother–pup interactions disrupts the feeding behavior of some of the pups. These pups may be less able than others to gain weight because they suck or compete for nipples less effectively.

In the first of a series of studies planned to evaluate these possibilities, Brake and Kenny (in preparation) began to examine how sucking is altered by deprivation and how this alteration may contribute to growth. They correlated the vigor of sucking displayed by 2-day-old pups with their rate of growth over the subsequent 14 days (when they began to consume solid food). Each pup was deprived for 6 h before the sucking test and three infusions of equal volume were delivered via a tongue cannula. Preliminary analyses suggested that the amplitude of sucking during these infusions on Day 2 predicted how fast the pups would grow over the next 10 days ($r = .62$). Pups that engaged in vigorous sucking during the three infusions gained more weight during this time than their littermates. This was true even of pups from the same litter with access to the same amount of milk. Thus, these differences in weight could not be due to differences in the amount of milk made available to the pups. Nor were the differences due to differences in weight at the time the sucking recording was made.

It is possible, of course, that pups that are poor feeders also absorb nutrient inefficiently. Still, to our knowledge, this is the first demonstration that the pup's feeding behavior at very young ages may be a valid predictor of its subsequent growth and development. It seems possible, then, that factors that influence RS, such as variations in the dam's milk delivery schedule and in the taste of her milk, may also affect the pup's rate of growth.

THE ROLE OF CONDITIONING

Many of the data reviewed in this chapter suggest that feeding competence may be determined, in part, by the pup's feeding history. For example, we have shown that specific milk delivery schedules can have long-lasting effects on sucking and nipple attachment and can even affect the onset of the behavioral signs of weaning (Brake *et al.,* 1982b). Similarly, Cramer *et al.* (1986) showed that suckling may be prolonged for weeks by providing pups with dams that are replete with milk and continue to nurse. In concluding our review, we discuss the roles that learned associations may play in mother–infant interactions as a way of illustrating that we have only begun to understand the flexibility inherent in the pup's responses to its environment.

Rat pups are capable of a remarkable degree of associative and instrumental learning. Within the first few days of life, they can learn to press a lever in order to receive a pulse of milk (Johanson and Hall, 1979) or a period of intracranial stimulation of the brain (Lithgow and Barr, 1984; Moran, Lew, and Blass, 1981). They can also acquire preferences or aversions for odors and tastes in one situation and display them in another (Brake, 1981; Galef, 1982; Gemberling, Domjan, and Amsel, 1980; Johanson and Teicher, 1980; Pedersen *et al.,* 1982; Rudy and Cheatle, 1979; Sullivan, Hofer, and Brake, 1986; Sullivan, Brake, Hofer and Williams, 1986; Johanson and Tomy, Chapter 7). They even seem capable of acquiring aversions for certain odors *in utero* (Stickrod, Kimbel, and Smotherman, 1982; Smotherman and Robinson, Chapter 5). By the time pups are a week or 10 days of age, they can be taught to negotiate mazes and alleyways for the opportunity to suckle (Amsel *et al.,* 1977; Brake, 1978; Kenny and Blass, 1977), and they will display conditioned consummatory (mouthing) responses to odors paired with milk infusions (Johanson, Hall, and Polefrone, 1984). So, even though certain learning mechanisms or systems seem to mature earlier in development than others (Amsel and Stanton, 1980; Campbell and Ampuero, 1985; Hyson and Rudy, 1984; Vogt and Rudy, 1984a,b), it is clear that many of the components involved in approaching the teat and consuming milk can be conditioned within the first week of life (Pederson *et al.,* 1983). Whether such learning occurs as a natural consequence of suckling, however, is largely unknown.

Brake (1981) and Pelchat and Brake (1982) have suggested that pups may acquire positive associations while suckling. These authors showed that preferences for previously aversive odors were acquired by pups that were exposed to those odors for only a few minutes while attached to the teat of an anesthetized dam. This finding suggests that suckling alone is a reinforcing event, and that pups assign positive value to an odor associated with suckling. However, these authors also showed that pups that withdrew milk from a reservoir while attached to the teat, by sucking vigorously (a tongue cannula was connected to the reservoir), acquired an even greater preference for the odor (Brake, 1981; Pelchat and Brake, 1982; Figure 15). Control procedures in which the CS (odor) and the US (milk) were presented in a backward fashion, and in which the value of the US was devalued following conditioning by toxicosis, demonstrated that the preferences depended on the simultaneous presentation of the CS and the US and were not due to differential attention or habituation.

These studies were among the first to show that pups could learn new associations based on milk reward received while suckling and that the learned associations could influence behavior hours or even days later in a completely different situation. More recently, Kehoe and Blass (1986) demonstrated that taste aversions can also be acquired by suckling pups, if the fluid serving as the CS is delivered to the middle or anterior portion of the pup's tongue (Kehoe, Chapter 9). All of these results are quite compatible with those of Galef and his colleagues (Galef and Clark, 1972; Galef and Sherry, 1973), who demonstrated that pups display preferences for the taste of their own dam's (palatable) diet, possibly as a result, of being repeatedly exposed to it in the dam's milk. Thus, the pup's earliest preferences (or aversions) for food tastes or odors may be acquired while suckling.

These findings also suggest that some sucking or suckling responses themselves could be elicited through acquired associations. For example, Papousek (1967) and Blass, Ganchrow, and Steiner (1984) found that human newborns will turn their heads toward a stimulus that signals the availability of milk or a sweet taste and will also display anticipatory sucking responses to such stimuli. Though we have not yet investigated this possibility in animals, it seems within reason that the pup could learn to suck more vigorously in the presence of a particular cue or could learn to suck as a function of being differentially reinforced for doing so. This notion is supported by our finding that making the delivery of milk contingent on RS results in vigorous and robust levels of sucking, even 24 h later (Brake *et al.*, 1982b). It is also supported by findings of Johanson and colleagues (Johanson *et al.*, 1984) that show that pups display anticipatory mouthing responses to stimuli that were previously paired with infusions of milk delivered away from the teat.

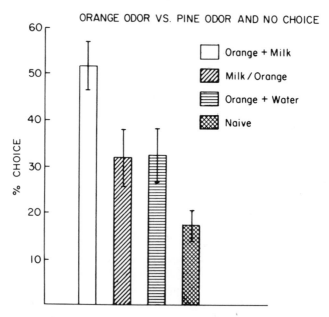

Figure 15. Percentage of time 11–14-day-pups spent over orange odor in a two-odor choice test following experience with various contingencies while suckling. "Orange + Milk" indicates simultaneous pairing of orange odor with milk delivery while suckling, "Milk/Orange" indicates presentation of milk delivery followed by presentation of orange odor, "Orange + Water" indicates simultaneous pairing of orange odor with delivery of water, and "Naive" indicates that pups recieved no experimental treatments before the test.

It is likely that neonatal feeding, like adult feeding, is a behavior subject not only to primary motivation, but also to incentive or acquired motivation. That is, a certain degree of the infant's competence as a feeder may be learned. Contingencies may be embedded within the natural suckling context that could influence a pup's disposition to feed from the teat. For example, imagine that pups are awakened immediately before milk ejection (e.g., Shair *et al.*, 1984) by the engorgement of the teat in their mouths. Repeated occurrences of this sequence may lead to an association between the swelling of the teat and the delivery of milk, so that waking and vigorous sucking precede the delivery of milk by a second or 2, thus maximizing the pup's chances of withdrawing all that is made available. Changes in the tactile properties of the teat may occur at other times, as well, such as when the dam shifts position without delivering milk. This less-than-perfect correlation between changes in the tactile properties of the teat and delivery of milk define a partial reinforcement condition, vis-à-vis milk. Thus, one might expect pups to be extremely persistent in displaying preparatory sucking responses, just as adult animals persist in instrumental and operant tasks following partial reinforcement.

These are only speculations, but it should be noted that pups as young as 11 days of age display response persistence following partial reinforcement in other contexts (Letz *et al.*, 1978). Further, Brake (1978) found that response persistence learned as a consequence of approaching the dam to suckle is retained for at least 10 days and can influence the animal's performance when it is being taught to run in the alley for food reward. Thus, it is conceivable that behavior patterns learned as a consequence of suckling even affect the tenacity with which the animal forages after weaning.

Environmental contributions to acquired behaviors in pups may not be limited to feeding. In fact, feeding may be only one of several mother–infant interactions that have the potential to impart to the pups important information through learning processes. The intriguing suggestion has also been made that neonatal pups are even more likely to learn certain contingencies than are older ones (Pedersen *et al.*, 1982; Sullivan, Hofer, and Brake, 1986). This idea, reminiscent of the concept of *imprinting*, is based on the finding that newborns seem to regard many more stimuli as rewarding than do older pups. For example, Pedersen *et al.* (1982) reported that the tactile sensation of being stroked along the flank seems to be regarded as a reinforcing stimulus by newborns. Novel odors paired with such stimulation come to be preferred odors and will even elicit nipple attachment.

According to Sullivan, Hofer, and Brake (1986) and Sullivan, Brake, Hofer, and Williams (1986), previously novel odors can elicit a wide range of behaviors in 3- to 5-day-old pups simply by having been paired with vigorous stroking, or with being pinched on the tail, or with being exposed to the odor of maternal saliva. For example, pups that had been stroked in the presence of a novel cedar odor and were later exposed to that odor in the presence of milk on the floor of the test container consumed significantly more milk than pups that did not receive the earlier pairings (Figure 16).

The findings suggest that stroking, tail-pinching, and exposure to maternal saliva serve as reinforcers for young rat pups. The one characteristic that all of these forms of stimulation have in common is their ability to elicit robust behavioral activation in newborns. Like pulses of milk, these stimuli initiate a series of gross motor behaviors indicative of intense arousal, such as rolling, stretching, reaching, paw treading, head waving, and mouthing (Hall, 1979a), a pattern of responding that is not seen in older pups. Thus, a form of conditioned arousal, or positive affect, may be associated with a novel cue (odor) paired with these events. That cue may then elicit conditioned arousal, which may enhance the performance of many of the pups' other behaviors (such as feeding). As a result, the infant rat may learn a great number of such associations as a natural consequence of being moved about in the nest or preparing to suckle. Saliva, for example, is encountered whenever the pup attempts to attach to the teat, and tactile stimulation similar to stroking is continuously provided by the dam as she licks and positions the pups. Thus, the pup's affinity for the teat and other characteristics of the dam and the nest (particularly their odor; e.g., Rosenblatt, 1983) may reflect acquired associations.

Finally, much of what we are discovering about how the first behaviors of rat pups may be learned as a natural consequence of suckling may be applicable to human infants as well. Their capacity for learning about contingencies that attend their interactions with the mother is great. A good deal of evidence suggests that human infants can learn to alter their sucking according to reinforcement schedules (Brown, 1972; Crook, 1979; Kaye, 1967; Kobre and Lipsitt, 1972; Kron, 1968; Lipsitt and Kaye, 1964). Sucking is also affected by taste (Desor, Maller, and Turner, 1973), and the performance of instrumental (Crook and Lipsitt, 1976; Lipsitt, 1977) or anticipatory (Blass *et al.,* 1984) sucking responses can be made contingent on the presentation of sweet taste. Further, human newborns learn to perform head-turning responses in order to feed (Papousek, 1967). Human newborns also seem to acquire preferences for odors that they associate with the mother (Cernoch and Porter, 1985; MacFarlane, 1975) and for the sound of their own mother's voice (DeCaspar and Fifer, 1980). In brief, it seems that the learning processes we have begun to identify in lower newborn animals may also be at work in human newborns. A thorough understanding of how such learning is embedded within the context of mother–infant interactions may lead to important discoveries about how the infant's first behaviors are shaped, and about how these early behaviors are modified in later life.

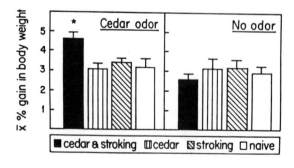

Figure 16. Amount of body weight gained during independent feeding tests in the presence of cedar odor or no odor following different treatment contingencies. "Cedar & Stroking" indicates the simultaneous presentation of cedar odor and stroking, "Cedar" indicates a presentation of odor alone, "Stroking" indicates stroking alone, and "Naive" indicates no treatment.

Six themes have emerged from the work reviewed in this chapter. Each emphasizes that suckling interactions play a significant role in the way the pup interacts with its environment. First, pups can exert a certain degree of control over their intake, individually and perhaps in litters, by adjusting specific sucking patterns. Second, adjustments of sucking and intake are linked to the occurrence of sleep–wake states. Third, pups that suck vigorously following privational challenges also tend to grow more rapidly than those that do not. Fourth, changes in the occurrence and force of sucking—and therefore, intake and growth—are influenced by a number of factors that the pups are likely to experience naturally, such as changes in privation, the taste of the dam's milk, and the timing of milk release. Fifth, pups' sucking patterns change during ontogeny, partly in response to the dam's changing physiology and behavior, partly in response to the pups' changing needs. And sixth, many of the changes in the pup's early suckling and feeding behaviors may be due to associations learned as a natural consequence of mother–infant interactions.

These findings dispel the notion, widely held up to the mid-1970s, that sucking in the infant rat is a simple relfex or a fixed action pattern largely unaffected by motivational states, sensory feedback, or previous experience, or that it is a behavior that takes place in the awake state and subsides as the infant falls asleep. Instead, the infant's sucking appears to have several different output patterns, each adapted to respond sensitively to environmental change, to be integrated with basic sleep–wake rhythms, and to participate in associative and instrumental learning contingencies, much as is the case with other behaviors. The mother, previously cast as the chief actor in the mammalian nursing interaction, must now share the spotlight with her offspring.

REFERENCES

Ackerman, S. A. and Shindledecker, R. A method for artificial feeding of motherless 2-week-old rat pups. *Developmental Psychobiology*, 1978, *11*, 385–391.

Alberts, J. R. Olfactory contributions to behavioral development in rodents. In R. L. Doty (Ed.), *Mammalian olfaction, reproductive processes and behavior*. New York: Academic Press, 1976.

Alberts, J. R., and Gubernick, D. J. Reciprocity and resource exchange: A symbiotic model of parent-offspring relations. In H. Moltz and L. A. Rosenblum (Eds.), *Symbiosis in parent-offspring interactions*. New York: Plenum Press, 1983.

Allin, J. T., and Banks, E. M. Effects of temperature on ultrasound production by infant albino rats. *Developmental Psychobiology*, 1971, *4*, 149–156.

Allin, J. T., and Banks, E. M. Functional aspects of ultrasound production by infant albino rats. *Animal Behaviour*, 1972, *20*, 175–185.

Amsel, A. The ontogeny of appetitive learning and persistence in the rat. In N. E. Spear and B. A. Campbell (Eds.), *Ontogeny of learning and memory*. Hillsdale: Erlbaum, 1979.

Amsel, A., and Stanton, M. Ontogeny and phylogeny of paradoxical reward effects. In J. S. Rosenblatt, R. A. Hinde, C. Beer, and M. Busnel (Eds.), *Advances in the study of behavior*. New York: Academic Press, 1980.

Amsel, A., Letz, R., and Burdette, D. R. Appetitive learning and extinction in 11-day-old rat pups: Effects of various reinforcement conditions. *Journal of Comparative and Physiological Psychology*, 1977, *91*, 1156–1167.

Antin, J., Gibbs, J., Holt, J., Young, R. C., and Smith, G. P. Cholecystokinin elicits the complete behavioral sequence of satiety in rats. *Journal of Comparative and Physiological Psychology*, 1975, *89*, 783–790.

Blass, E. M., and Cramer, C. P. Analogy and homology in the development of ingestive behavior. In A. R. Morrison and P. L. Strick (Eds.), *Changing concepts of the nervous system*. New York: Academic Press, 1982.

Blass, E. M., Beardsley, W., and Hall, W. G. Age-dependent inhibition of suckling by cholecystokinin. *American Journal of Physiology*, 1979a, *236*, E567–E570.

Blass, E. M., Hall, W. G., and Teicher, M. H. The ontogeny of suckling and ingestive behaviors. *Progress in Psychobiology and Physiological Psychology*, 1979b, *8*, 243–299.

Blass, E. M., Ganchrow, J. R., and Steiner, J. E. Classical conditioning in human newborns 2–48 hours of age. *Infant Behavior and Development*, 1984, *2*, 223–236.

Borbely, A., and J. Valatx (Eds.). *Sleep mechanisms: Experimental brain research*. New York: Springer-Verlag, 1984.

Brake, S. C. Discrimination training in infant, preweanling and weanling rats: Effects of prior learning experiences with the discriminanda. *Animal Learning and Behavior*, 1978, *6*, 435–443.

Brake, S. C. Suckling infant rats learn a preference for a novel olfactory stimulus paired with milk delivery. *Science*, 1981, *211*, 506–508.

Brake, S. C., and Hofer, M. A. Maternal deprivation and prolonged suckling in the absence of milk alter the frequency and intensity of sucking responses in neonatal rat pups. *Physiology and Behavior*, 1980, *24*, 185–189.

Brake, S. C., and Kenny, P. Predicting the incidence of growth deficits in infant rats following brief maternal separations. In preparation.

Brake, S. C., Wolfson, V., and Hofer, M. A. Electromyographic patterns associated with non-nutritive sucking in 11–13-day-old rat pups. *Journal of Comparative and Physiological Psychology*, 1979, *93*, 760–770.

Brake, S. C., Sager, D. J., Sullivan, R.,. and Hofer, M. A. The role of intra-oral and gastrointestinal cues in the control of sucking and milk consumption in rat pups. *Developmental Psychobiology*, 1982a, *15*, 529–541.

Brake, S. C., Sullivan, R., Sager, D. J., and Hofer, M. A. Short- and long-term effects of various milk-delivery contingencies on sucking and nipple attachment in rat pups. *Developmental Psychobiology*, 1982b, *15*, 543–556.

Brake, S. C., Tavana, S., and Myers, M. M. A method for recording and analyzing intra-oral negative pressure in suckling rat pups. *Physiology and Behavior*, 1986, *36*, 575–578.

Brake, S. C., Shindledecker, R., and Hofer, M. A. Feeding competence in rat pups: Effects of deprivation on sucking and consumption of milk. In preparation.

Brown, J. Instrumental control of the sucking response in human newborns. *Journal of Experimental Child Psychology*, 1972, *14*, 66–80.

Calhoun, J. B. *The ecology and sociology of the Norway rat*. Monograph 1008, U.S. Department of Health, Education and Welfare. Washington: U.S. Government Printing Office, 1962.

Campbell, B. A., and Ampuero, M. X. Dissociation of autonomic and behavioral components of conditioned fear during development in the rat. *Behavioral Neuroscience*, 1985, *99*, 1089–1102.

Cernoch, J. M., and Porter, R. H. Recognition of maternal axillary odors by infants. *Child Development*, 1985, *56*, 1593–1598.

Chalk, P. A., and Bailey, E. Changes in the yield and carbohydrate, lipid and protein content of milk during lactation in the rat. *Journal of Developmental Physiology*, 1979, *1*, 61–79.

Cramer, C. P., and Blass, E. M. Mechanisms of control of milk intake in suckling rats. *American Journal of Physiology*, 1983, *245*, 154–159.

Cramer, C. P., Blass, E. M., and Hall, W. G. The ontogeny of nipple-shifting behavior in albino rats: Mechanisms of control and possible significance. *Developmental Psychobiology*, 1980, *13*, 165–180.

Cramer, C. P., Pfister, J. F., and Blass, E. M. Suckling in rats extended by continuous living with dams and their preweanling litters. *Animal Behaviour*, 1986, *34*, 415–420.

Crook, C. K. The organization and control of infant sucking. *Advances in Child Development*, 1979, *14*, 209–252.

Crook, C. K., and Lipsitt, L. P. Neonatal nutritive sucking: Effects of taste stimulation upon sucking rhythm and heart rate. *Child Development*, 1976, *47*, 518–522.

Danguir, J., and Nicolaidis, S. Dependence of sleep on nutrient's availability. *Physiology and Behavior*, 1979, *22*, 735–740.

DeCaspar, A. J., and Fifer, W. P. Of human bonding: Newborns prefer their mother's voices. *Science,* 1980, *208,* 1174–1176.

Desor, J. A., Maller, O., and Turner, R. Taste in acceptance of sugars by human infants. *Journal of Comparative and Physiological Psychology,* 1973, *84,* 496–501.

Dobbing, J. Vulnerable periods in somatic growth. In D. F. Roberts and A. M. Thomson (Eds.), *The biology of human fetal growth.* London: Taylor & Sons, 1976.

Drewett, R. F. Gastric and plasma volume in the control of milk intake in suckling rat pups. *Quarterly Journal of Experimental Psychology,* 1978, *30,* 755–764.

Drewett, R. F. Sucking, milk synthesis, and milk ejection in the Norway rat. In R. W. Elwood (Ed.), *Parental behavior in rodents.* New York: Wiley, 1983.

Drewett, R. F., and Cordall, K. M. Control of feeding in suckling rats: Effects of glucose and of osmotic stimuli. *Physiology and Behavior,* 1976, *16,* 711–717.

Drewett, R. F., and Trew, A. M. The milk ejection of the rat, as a stimulus and a response to the litter. *Animal Behaviour,* 1978, *26,* 982–987.

Drewett, R. F., Statham, C., and Wakerley, J. B. A quantitative analysis of the feeding behavior of suckling rats. *Animal Behaviour,* 1974, *22,* 907–913.

Epstein, A. N. The ontogeny of ingestive behaviors: Control of milk intake by suckling rats and the emergence of feeding and drinking at weaning. In R. Ritter, S. Ritter, and C. D. Barnes (Eds.), *Neural and humoral controls of food intake.* New York: Academic Press, 1986.

Farbman, A. I. Electron microscope study of the developing taste bud in rat fungiform papilla. *Developmental Biology,* 1965, *11,* 110–135.

Fleischer, S. F., and Turkewitz, G. Effect of neonatal stunting on development of rats: Large litter rearing. *Developmental Psychobiology,* 1979, *12,* 137–149.

Friedman, M. I. Some determinants of milk ingestion in suckling rat pups. *Journal of Comparative and Physiological Psychology,* 1975, *89,* 636–647.

Gaensbauer, T., and Emde, R. Wakefulness and feeding in human newborns. *Archives of General Psychiatry,* 1973, *28,* 894–897.

Galef, B. G. Studies of social learning in Norway rats: A brief review. *Developmental Psychobiology,* 1982, *15,* 279–296.

Galef, B. G., and Clark, M. M. Mother's milk and adult presence: Two factors determining initial dietary selection by weaning rats. *Journal of Comparative and Physiological Psychology,* 1972, *28,* 213–219.

Galef, B. G. and Henderson, P. W. Mother's milk: A determinant of the feeding preferences of weanling rat pups. *Journal of Comparative and Physiological Psychology,* 1972, *78,* 213–219.

Galef, B. G., and Sherry, D. F. Mother's milk: A medium for the transmission of cues reflecting the flavor of mother's diet. *Journal of Comparative and Physiological Psychology,* 1973, *93,* 374–378.

Gemberling, G. A., Domjan, M.,. and Amsel, A. Aversion learning in 5-day-old rats: Taste-toxiosis and texture-shock aversion learning. *Journal of Comparative and Physiological Psychology,* 1980, *94,* 734–745.

Gisel, E. G., and Henning, S. J. Demonstration of a quiescent period for feeding controls in the developing rat. *Journal of Developmental Physiology,* 1979, *1,* 437, 452.

Gubernick, D. J., and Alberts, J. R. A specialization of taste aversion learning during suckling and its weaning-associated transformation. *Developmental Psychobiology,* 1984, *17,* 613–628.

Hall, W. G. Feeding and behavioral activation in infant rats. *Science,* 1979a, *205,* 206–209.

Hall, W. G. The ontogeny of feeding in rats. I. Ingestive and behavioral responses to oral infusions. *Journal of Comparative and Physiological Psychology,* 1979b, *93,* 977–1000.

Hall, W. G. and Bryan, T. E. The ontogeny of feeding in rats. IV. Taste development as measured by intake and behavioral responses to oral infusions of sucrose and quinine. *Journal of Comparative and Physiological Psychology,* 1980, *95,* 240–251.

Hall, W. G., Cramer, C. P., and Blass, E. M. Ontogeny of suckling in rats: Transitions toward adult ingestion. *Journal of Comparative and Physiological Psychology,* 1977, *91,* 1141–1155.

Hall, W. G., and Rosenblatt, J. S. Suckling behavior and intake control in the developing rat. *Journal of Comparative and Physiological Psychology,* 1977, *91,* 1232–1247.

Hall, W. G., and Williams, C. L. Suckling isn't feeding, or is it? A search for developmental continuities. *Advances in the Study of Behavior,* 1983, *13,* 219–253.

Henderson, P. W., and Smith, G. K. Developmental changes in rat fungiform papilla populations. In J. M. Weiffenbach (Ed.), *Taste and development: The genesis of sweet preference.* Bethesda, MD: U.S. Department of Health, Education and Welfare, 1977.

Henning, S. J. Maternal factors as determinants of food intake during the suckling period. *International Journal of Obesity,* 1980, *4,* 329–332.

Hofer, M. A. The mother-infant interaction as a regulator of infant physiology and behavior. In L. A. Rosenblum and H. Moltz (Eds.), *Symbiosis in parent/offspring interactions.* New York: Plenum Press, 1983.

Hofer, M. A., and Shair, H. Ultrasonic vocalization during social interaction and isolation in 2-week-old rats. *Developmental Psychobiology,* 1978, *11,* 495–504.

Hofer, M. A., and Shair, H. Sensory processes in the control of isolation-induced ultrasonic vocalization by 2-week-old rats. *Journal of Comparative and Physiological Psychology,* 1980, *94,* 271–279.

Hofer, M. A., and Shair, H. Control of sleep-wake states in the infant rat by features of the mother-infant relationship. *Developmental Psychobiology,* 1982, *15,* 229–243.

Hofer, M. A., Fisher, A., and Shair, H. Effects of infraorbital nerve section on survival, growth, and suckling behaviors of developing rats. *Journal of Comparative and Physiological Psychology,* 1981, *95,* 123–133.

Houpt, K. A., and Epstein, A. N. Ontogeny of controls of food intake in the rat: GI fill and glucoprivation. *American Journal of Physiology,* 1973, *225,* 58–66.

Houpt, K. A., and Houpt, T. R. Effects of gastric loads and food deprivation on subsequent food intake in suckling rats. *Journal of Comparative and Physiological Psychology,* 1975, *88,* 764–772.

Hyson, R. L., and Rudy, J. W. Ontogenesis of learning. II. Variation in the rat's reflexive and learned responses to acoustic stimulation. *Developmental Psychobiology,* 1984, *17,* 263–283.

Jacobs, B., and McGinty, D. Effects of food deprivation on sleep and wakefulness in the rat. *Experimental Neurology,* 1971, *30,* 212–222.

Jacobs, H. L. and Sharma, K. N. Taste vs. calories: Sensory and metabolic signals in the control of food intake. In J. P. Morgane (Ed.), *Neural Regulation of food and water intake. Annals of the New York Academy of Science,* 1969, *157,* 1084–1125.

Johanson, I. B., and Hall, W. G. Appetitive learning in 1-day-old rat pups. *Science,* 1979, *205,* 419–421.

Johanson, I. B., and Teicher, M. H. Classical conditioning of an odor preference in 3-day-old rats. *Behavioral and Neural Biology,* 1980, *29,* 132–136.

Johanson, I. B., Hall, W. G., and Polefrone, J. M. Appetitive conditioning in neonatal rats: Conditioned ingestive responding to stimuli paired with oral infusions of milk. *Developmental Psychobiology,* 1984, *17,* 357–382.

Kaye, H. Infant sucking behavior and its modification. *Advances in Child Development and Behavior,* 1967, *3,* 1–52.

Kehoe, P., and Blass, E. M. Gustatory determinants of suckling in albino rats 5–20 days of age. *Developmental Psychobiology,* 1984, *18,* 67–82.

Kehoe, P., and Blass, E. M. Conditioned aversions and their memories in 5-day-old rats during suckling. *Journal of Experimental Psychology: Animal Behavior Processes,* 1986, *12,* 40–47.

Kenny, J. T., and Blass, E. M. Suckling as an incentive to instrumental learning in preweanling rats. *Science,* 1977, *196,* 898–899.

Kenny, P. and Brake, S. C. Ontogeny of sucking in response to taste in rats. In preparation.

Kenny, J. T., Stoloff, M. L., Bruno, J. P., and Blass, E. M. Ontogeny of preference for nutritive over nonnutritive suckling in albino rats. *Journal of Comparative and Physiological Psychology,* 1979, *93,* 752–759.

Kleitman, N. *Sleep and wakefulness.* Chicago: University of Chicago Press, 1963.

Knittle, J. L., and Hirsch, J. Effect of early nutrition on the development of rat epididymal fat pads: Cellularity and metabolism. *Journal of Clinical Investigation,* 1968, *47,* 2091–2098.

Kobre, K. R., and Lipsitt, L. P. A negative contrast effect in newborns. *Journal of Experimental Child*

Kron, R. E. The effect of arousal and of learning upon sucking behavior in the newborn. *Recent Advances in Biological Psychiatry,* 1968, *10,* 302–313.

Lav, C., and Henning, S. J. Regulation of milk ingestion in the infant rat. *Physiology and Behavior,* 1984, *33,* 809–815.

Leon, M. Maternal pheromone. *Physiology and Behavior,* 1974, *13,* 441–453.

Leon, M., Croskerry, P. G., and Smith, G. K. Thermal control of mother-infant contact in rats. *Physiology and Behavior,* 1978, *21,* 793–811.

Leon, M., Adels, L., and Coopersmith, R. Thermal limitation of mother-young contact in Norway rats. *Developmental Psychobiology,* 1985, *18,* 85–105.

Letz, R., Burdette, D. R., Gregg, B., Kittrell, M. E., and Amsel, A. Evidence for a transitional period for the development of persistence in infant rats. *Journal of Comparative and Physiological Psychology,* 1978, *92,* 856–866.

Levine, S., and Otis, L. The effects of handling before and after weaning on the resistance of albino rats to later deprivation. *Canadian Journal of Psychology,* 1958, *12,* 103–108.

Lincoln, D. W. Physiological mechanisms governing the transfer of milk from mother to young. In L. A. Rosenblum and H. Moltz (Eds.), *Symbiosis in parent-offspring interactions.* New York: Plenum Press, 1983.

Lincoln, D. W., and Wakerley, J. B. Electrophysiological evidence for the activation of supraoptic neurosecretory cells during the release of oxytocin. *Journal of Physiology,* 1974, *242,* 533–554.

Lipsitt, L. P. Taste in human neonates: Its effect on sucking and heartrate. In J. M. Weiffenbach (Ed.), *Taste and development: The gensis of sweet preference.* Bethesda, MD: U.S. Department of Health, Education and Welfare, 1977.

Lipsitt, L. P., and Kaye, H. Conditioned sucking in the human newborn. *Psychonomic Science,* 1964, *1,* 29–30.

Lithgow, T., and Barr, G. A. Electrical self-stimulation in 7- and 10-day-old rats. *Behavioral Neuroscience,* 1984, *98,* 479–486.

Lorenz, D. N. Effects of gastric filling and vagotomy on ingestion, nipple attachment, and weight gain by suckling rats. *Developmental Psychobiology,* 1983, *16,* 483–496.

Lorenz, D. N., Ellis, S., and Epstein, A. N. Differential effects of upper gastrointestinal fill on milk ingestion and nipple attachment in the suckling rat. *Developmental Psychobiology,* 1982, *15,* 309–330.

MacFarlane, A. Olfaction in the development of social preferences in the human neonate. In *Parent-infant interaction.* Amsterdam: Ciba Foundation Symposium, *33,* 1975.

Mansbach, R., and Lorenz, D. Cholecystokinin (CCK-8) elicits prandial sleep in rats. *Physiology and Behavior,* 1983, *30,* 179–183.

Martin, L. T., and Alberts, J. R. Taste aversions to mother's milk: The age-related role of nursing in acquisition and expression of a learned association. *Journal of Comparative and Physiological Psychology,* 1979, *93,* 430–445.

McCance, R. A. Severe undernutrition in growing and adult animals. I. Production and general effects. *British Journal of Nutrition,* 1960, *14,* 59–73.

Melcer, T., Alberts, J. R., and Gubernick, D. J. Early weaning does not accelerate the expression of nursing-related taste aversions. *Developmental Psychobiology,* 1985, *18,* 375–382.

Mistretta, C. M. Topographical and histological study of the developing rat tongue, palate, and taste buds. In J. F. Bosma (Ed.), *Third symposium on oral sensation and perception.* Springfield, IL: Charles C Thomas, 1972.

Moran, T. H., Lew, M. F., and Blass, E. M. Intracranial self-stimulation in 3-day-old rat pups. *Science,* 1981, *214,* 1366–1368.

Mouret, J. and Bobillier, P. Diurnal rhythms of sleep in the rat: Augmentation of paradoxical sleep following alterations of the feeding schedule. *International Journal of Neuroscience,* 1971, *2,* 265–270.

Okon, E. E. The temperature relations of vocalization in infant Golden hamsters and Wistar rats. *Journal of Zoology,* 1972, *164,* 227–237.

Oswalt, G. L., and Meier, G. W. Olfactory, thermal, and tactual influences on infantile ultrasonic vocalization in rats. *Developmental Psychobiology,* 1975, *8,* 129–135.

Papousek, H. Experimental studies of appetitional behavior in human newborns and infants. In H. W. Stevenson, E. H. Hess, and H. L. Rheingold (Eds.), *Early behavior: Comparative and developmental approaches.* New York: Wiley, 1967.

Pedersen, P., Williams, C. L., and Blass, E. M. Activation and odor conditioning of suckling behavior in 3-day-old albino rats. *Journal of Experimental Psychology: Animal Behavior Processes,* 1982, *8,* 329–341.

Pelchat, M. L., and Brake, S. C. *Aromatic associations: Studies of olfactory conditioning in suckling rat pups.* Presented at the Annual Meeting, International Society for Developmental Psychobiology, Minneapolis, 1982.

Pelchat, M. L., and Brake, S. C. Sapid savvy in sucklings: The effect of quinine hydrochloride on intraoral negative pressure and intake by 11- to 13-day-old rat pups. *Developmental Psychobiology,* 1987, *20,* 261–275.

Raskin, L. A., and Campbell, B. A. The ontogeny of amphetamine anorexia: A behavioral analysis. *Journal of Comparative and Physiological Psychology*, 1981, *95*, 425–435.

Rosenblatt, J. S. Olfaction mediates developmental transition in the altricial newborn of selected species of mammals. *Developmental Psychobiology*, 1983, *16*, 347–376.

Rubenstein, E., and Sonnenschein, R. Sleep cycles and feeding behavior in the cat: Role of gastrointestinal hormones. *Acta Cientifica Venezolana (Suppl.)*, 1971, *22*, 125–128.

Rudy, J. W., and Cheatle, M. D. Ontogeny of association learning: Acquisition of odor aversions by neonatal rats. In N. E. Spear and B. A. Campbell (Eds.), *Ontogeny of learning and memory*. Hillsdale, NJ: Erlbaum, 1979.

Schanberg, S. M., Evonuik, G., and Kuhn, C. M. Tactile and nutritional aspects of maternal care: Specific regulators of neuroendocrine function and cellular development. *Proceedings of the Society of Experimental and Biology and Medicine*, 1984, *175*, 135–146.

Shair, H., Brake, S. C., and Hofer, M. A. Suckling in the rat: Evidence for patterned behavior during sleep. *Behavioral Neuroscience*, 1984, *96*, 366–370.

Shair, H., Brake, S. C., and Hofer, M. A. The effects of maternal separation on sleep and sucking in the rat pup. In preparation.

Shair, H., Gottschalk, S., Brake, S. C., and Hofer, M. A. *Two-week-old rat pups can ingest small quantities of milk while asleep*. Paper presented at the Annual Meeting of the International Society for Developmental Psychobiology, Hyannis, MA, 1983.

Siegel, J. REM sleep predicts subsequent food intake. *Physiology and Behavior*, 1975, *15*, 399–403.

Singh, P., and Hofer, M. A. Oxytocin reinstates maternal olfactory cues for nipple orientation and attachment in rat pups. *Physiology and Behavior*, 1978, *20*, 385–389.

Singh, P., Tucker, A. M., and Hofer, M. A. Effects of nasal $ZnSO_4$ irrigation and olfactory bulbectomy on rat pups. *Physiology and Behavior*, 1976, *17*, 373–382.

Smith, G. J., and Spear, N. E. Effects of the home environment on withholding behaviors and conditioning in infant and neonatal rats. *Science*, 1978, *202*, 327–329.

Stickrod, G., Kimbel, D. P., and Smotherman, W. P. In utero taste/odor aversion conditioning in the rat. *Physiology and Behavior*, 1982, *28*, 5–7.

Sullivan, R. M., Brake, S. C., Hofer, M. A., and Williams, C. L. Huddling and independent feeding of neonatal rats can be facilitated by a conditioned change in behavioral state. *Developmental Psychobiology*, 1986, *19*, 625–635.

Sullivan, R. M., Hofer, M. A., and Brake, S. C. Olfactory-guided orientation in neonatal rats is enhanced by a conditioned change in behavioral state. *Developmental Psychobiology*, 1986, *19*, 615–623.

Teicher, M. H., and Blass, E. M. Suckling in newborn rats: Eliminated by nipple lavage, reinstated by pup saliva. *Science*, 1976, *193*, 422–425.

Teicher, M. H., and Blass, E. M. First suckling response of the newborn albino rat: The roles of olfaction and amniotic fluid. *Science*, 1977, *198*, 635–636.

Tobach, E., Rouger, Y., and Schneirla, T. C. Development of olfactory function in the rat pup. *American Zoologist*, 1967, *7*, 792–793.

Vogt, M. B., and Rudy, J. W. Ontogenesis of learning. I. Variation in the rat's reflexive and learned responses to gustatory stimulation. *Developmental Psychobiology*, 1984a, *17*, 11–33.

Vogt, M. B., and Rudy, J. W. Ontogenesis of learning. IV. Dissocation of memory and perceptual-alerting processes mediating taste neophobia in the rat. *Developmental Psychobiology*, 1984b, *17*, 601–611.

Voloschin, L. M., and Tramezzani, J. H. Milk ejection reflex linked to slow wave sleep in nursing rats. *Endocrinology*, 1979, *105*, 1202–1207.

Wakerley, J. B., and Drewett, R. F. Pattern of sucking in the infant rat during spontaneous milk ejection. *Physiology and Behavior*, 1975, *15*, 277–281.

Williams, C. L., Hall, W. G., and Rosenblatt, J. S. Changing oral cues in suckling of weaning-age rats: Possible contributions to weaning. *Journal of Comparative and Physiological Psychology*, 1980, *94*, 472–483.

Winick, M. Malnutrition and brain development. *The Journal of Pediatrics*, 1969, *74*, 667–679.

Wolff, P. H. Sucking patterns of infant mammals. *Brain, Behavior and Evolution*, 1968, *1*, 354–367.

Wolff, P. H. The interaction of state and nonnutritive sucking. In J. F. Bosma, (Ed.), *Third annual symposium on oral sensation and perception: The mouth of the infant*. Springfield, IL: Charles C Thomas, 1972.

Yogman, M., and Zeisel, S. Diet and sleep patterns in newborn infants. *New England Journal of Medicine*, 1983, *309*, 1147–1149.

11

Kinship and the Development of Social Preferences

WARREN G. HOLMES

INTRODUCTION

In behavioral interactions between conspecifics, the identities of the individuals are rarely random because some social partners are sought out whereas others are ignored or avoided. Thus, social preferences are exhibited when unequal amounts of time, energy, or other resources are allocated to some individuals (or classes of them) rather than others. Examples include parental care given to related rather than unrelated young (Holmes, 1984a), long-term social bonds and alliances maintained only with certain group members (Hinde, 1983), and mate selection by individuals of one sex based on traits that differ among individuals of the opposite sex (examples in Bateson, 1983). Social preferences are critical to many topics studied by psychobiologists and behavioral ecologists, including the development of individual differences, social relations and mating patterns in groups, and the direction and rate of behavioral evolution. Thus, it is worthwhile to examine the determinants of social preferences and to explain their ontogeny.

Tinbergen (1963) emphasized the distinction between two kinds of explanations for behavior. First, proximate explanations stress the immediate causes (e.g., the physiological basis and the role of experience) or the development of behavior. Second, ultimate explanations stress the survival value and the reproductive consequences of behavior or its evolution across generations. The distinction between proximate and ultimate levels of analysis is relevant to social preferences because

WARREN G. HOLMES   Department of Psychology, University of Michigan, Ann Arbor, Michigan 48109.

of the ease with which the two can be confused when trying to explain such preferences, as exemplified by the following cases.

Genetically related individuals are more likely to assist each other or to avoid competing with each other than are unrelated individuals in several species. In over 300 bird species, for instance, adults provide care to young that they did not produce, and in the vast majority of cases, these "helpers" are grown offspring that assist their parent(s) to rear full or half siblings (review in Emlen, 1984). Preferences for grooming partners in several Old World primate species vary as a function of kinship, among other factors (Seyfarth, 1980, 1983). Finally, female paper wasps (genus *Polisites*) frequently usurp nests built by other females (Gamboa, 1978), and females *(P. fuscatus)* are more likely to destroy the broods in nests of unrelated females than in nests of related females (Klahn and Gamboa, 1983). In each of these examples, one could ask whether the special treatment of kin is due to prior association with relatives *or* whether it is due to the reproductive advantages that may be gained by assisting relatives. However, such a question is inappropriate and misguided because it pits one level of explanation (proximate) against another (ultimate) rather than viewing them as parallel and complementary.

My purpose here is to examine from both proximate and ultimate perspectives the role of genetic relatedness in the development and expression of social preferences. The existence of a preference implies that stimuli can be discriminated on the basis of cues that differ between them (although the absence of a preference in one situation does not mean that discrimination is impossible under other circumstances). Accordingly, I will stress the discrimination or recognition component that frequently underlies the preferential treatment of genetic relatives. I will focus on discriminations that seem to have biological validity in that they have been observed in species-typical circumstances and presumably contribute to the reproductive survival of the individuals that exhibit them. Since the early 1970s, research on many free-living species has revealed the pivotal role of kinship in social relations, and various evolutionary explanations for favoring kin have been proposed. More recently, experimental studies, frequently conducted in the laboratory, have begun to unravel the proximate basis for the preferential treatment of kin. By considering some of these field and laboratory studies, I hope to demonstrate how they complement each other and how the richest explanations of behavior incorporate both proximate and ultimate factors in their development (Tinbergen, 1963).

THE ULTIMATE BASIS OF SOCIAL PREFERENCES

INCLUSIVE FITNESS AND KIN SELECTION

Social preferences presumably evolved because they enhanced the reproductive success of the individuals that exhibited them. Two general evolutionary explanations have been proposed to explain why genetic relatedness and social preferences are associated. The first was developed in a landmark series of papers by William D. Hamilton (1964, 1972, 1975), who introduced the concept of *inclusive fitness.* Hamilton argued that an individual could channel its reproductive efforts in two directions: toward descendant kin (e.g., offspring and grandoffspring) or toward nondescendant or collateral kin (e.g., siblings, nieces, and nephews). Because relatives are individuals that share genes that are identical by immediate descent, reproductive investment in descendant *and* in nondescendant kin can affect an individual's genetic representation in subsequent generations. Thus, inclusive fitness is calculated as the total number of descendant offspring produced by an individual during its lifetime *plus* the individual's effects on offspring production by its relatives, each offspring being weighted by the appropriate coefficient of relatedness. The coefficient of relatedness, r, measures the probability that two individuals share a copy of the same allele at a particular locus, which they inherited from a recent shared ancestor (i.e., alleles that are identical by immediate descent). Closely related individuals (e.g., parent–offspring $r = \frac{1}{2}$; siblings $r = \frac{1}{2}$) are more likely to share an allele than are more distantly related kin (e.g., aunt–niece $r = \frac{1}{4}$; cousin $r = \frac{1}{8}$), so that cooperative or aid-giving behavior directed preferentially to close relatives rather than to distantly related or unrelated conspecifics will have the greatest impact on a donor's inclusive fitness, all other things being equal (see below). From an evolutionary perspective, then, one very general answer to the question of why genetic relatedness or kinship affects social preferences is that individuals have evolved to maximize their inclusive fitness, which is often manifested in favoritism shown to relatives (i.e., nepotism).

Because the inclusive fitness theory is central to the evolution of social preferences, it is useful to examine some misconceptions about the theory and its implications (see extensive discussions in Dawkins, 1979, and Grafen, 1984). First, although two individuals may share more than 90% of their genes because they are members of the same species, genetic similarity in this "uncorrelated" portion of the genome does not bear on the coefficient of relatedness between the individuals. This is true because r refers only to the "correlated" portion of the genome (i.e., genes inherited from a *recent common ancestor*). Differential treatment of individuals will not affect relative gene frequencies in the uncorrelated portion of the genome because all members of a population are almost genetically alike. However, individuals do differ genetically in the correlated portion of the genome, so that differential treatment affecting these genes can produce changes in relative gene frequencies as a function of r.

Second, inclusive fitness theory does not require that animals possess a mental concept of kinship or that they be able to calculate coefficients of relatedness; the theory requires only that they *behave as if* they have such a concept and can make such calculations. Considerable empirical evidence, reviewed throughout this chapter, verifies that, indeed, many organisms do behave as if they can calculate genetic relatedness, and these behaviors are based on several kin recognition mechanisms, which are discussed below.

Finally, the theory does not predict that kin should be favored in all circumstances or that close kin should always be favored over distant kin. In addition to r, the evolution of a behavior depends on the costs and benefits it imposes on a donor and a recipient, respectively, with cost and benefit measured ultimately by offspring production. Because the costs and benefits of an act vary, depending on the identity of the interactants (e.g., their sexes, ages, and physical conditions), one cannot rely on genetic relatedness alone to predict behaviors that will augment inclusive fitness (Altmann, 1979; Schulman and Rubenstein, 1983; West Eberhard, 1975). Indeed, preferential treatment and cooperation do not always vary directly with r (Hoogland, 1986; Sherman, 1981), and in some instances, close kin may be an individual's most severe competitors (Hoogland, 1985).

OPTIMAL MATE CHOICE

The second evolutionary explanation that connects relatedness and preference is genetic compatibility between mates. Regardless of the nature or extent of the parental investment (Trivers, 1972) made by the sexes, females and males should choose as mates individuals whose genes will enhance the survival and reproductive ability of their own offspring. A primary factor affecting genetic compatibility is the degree of consanguinity between prospective mates, because breeding between close relatives depresses many components of fitness (e.g., reduced fecundity and reduced viability of young; Ralls, Brugger, and Ballou, 1979; Shields, 1982, Ch. 4), so that one expects the evolution of proximate mechanisms that will reduce the likelihood of inbreeding (e.g., Hoogland, 1982). Similarly, extreme outbreeding may reduce fitness (although, compared with inbreeding, the empirical support for this claim is weak), a notion that leads to the hypothesis that there exists some optimal balance between inbreeding and outbreeding (Bateson, 1983; Shields, 1982).

Another factor affecting genetic compatibility is the presence of particular alleles in the genomes of prospective mates that may influence offspring survival. For instance, during mate preference tests, both male and female house mice *(Mus musculus)* avoided individuals that carried various *t* alleles at the *T* locus, because in the homozygous condition, these alleles are generally lethal, and in the heterozygous condition, they often cause sterility (Lenington, 1983). Alleles at another locus, the major histocompatibility complex, which control the body's immune system in mammals, can also play a role in mate choice. Both male and female laboratory mice generally prefer mates whose genetic makeup at the major histocompatibility complex differs from their own (review in Boyse, Beauchamp, and Yamazaki, 1983). These preferences result in greater heterozygosity in the major histocompatibility complex of offspring, which may enhance their survival and reproduction through greater resistance to disease.

Although I have linked genetic relatedness to social preferences on the basis of two evolutionary functions, nepotism and mate choice, relatedness is not always the primary evolutionary factor that accounts for preferences (Axelrod and Hamilton, 1981; Wasser, 1982; Wrangham, 1982). For example, in some polygynous mating systems, female preference for mates is based almost exclusively on environmental resources controlled by males (review in Partridge and Halliday, 1984). Similarly, social alliances in which partners provide aid to each other may not involve relatives (Packer, 1977; Smuts, 1985). On the other hand, kinship is a factor that influences many social relationships, whether kin are likely recipients of social assistance or whether they are avoided as potential mates, and it is important to understand the ontogeny of this favoritism, as well as its evolutionary basis.

ASSESSING SOCIAL PREFERENCES

THE MEANING OF SOCIAL PREFERENCE

For my purposes, a *social preference* is a construct inferred when individuals exhibit nonrandom and reliable responses to one social stimulus rather than another. Social stimuli include individual conspecifics or heterospecifics (or groups of either) or their phenotypic attributes, such as odors or auditory signals. Social preferences are manifested when individuals respond differentially to two or more social stimuli that are simultaneously or sequentially available. (The importance of the simultaneous versus the sequential presentation of stimuli is apparent in Evan's work, 1970, on the ring-billed gull, *Larus delawarensis*. Chicks 3–5 days old do not respond selectively to calls of their parents and other adults presented sequentially, but when the two kinds of calls are presented almost simultaneously, the chicks orient to their parents' calls.) Because preferences are inferred from behavioral responses, it is not possible to explain their sensory or neural basis simply by observing their existence. Whether preferences are mediated by perceptual filtering at the receptor level, a more central coding–decoding process, or some other mechanism, can be ascertained only by further experimentation. In addition, preferences can reflect an attraction to one stimulus, avoidance of another, or both.

LABORATORY STUDIES

In laboratory tests, various criteria and methods have been used to search for social preferences. Typically, subjects are presented two or more individuals (or their phenotypic attributes), and the behavior elicited by the stimuli is recorded. For example, infant squirrel monkeys *(Saimiri sciureus)* spend more time near and in contact with their own anesthetized mother than with an age-mate's anesthetized mother (Kaplan, Cubicciotti, and Redican, 1977); juvenile coho salmon *(Oncorhynchus kisutch)* are more likely to swim toward a water source in which their siblings were housed than toward water conditioned by nonsiblings (Quinn and Busack, 1985); and female cowbirds *(Molothrus ater)* exhibit greater copulatory responsiveness to males of their own subspecies than to males of other subspecies (King, West, and Eastzer, 1980).

FIELD STUDIES

Nonrandom associations between individuals occur regularly in nature and imply that social preferences exist. For instance, adult male olive baboons *(Papio anubis)* have preferred partners with whom they form temporary coalitions during aggressive encounters with other males in their troop (Packer, 1977; Smuts, 1985). Female Belding's ground squirrels *(Spermophilus beldingi)* behave less aggressively toward their sisters than toward unrelated females, even when the sisters and the unrelated females have lived as neighbors of the target females for up to 4 years (Sherman, 1981). Paper wasp queens *(P. fuscatus)* destroy the broods of unrelated females and leave untouched those of their sisters (Klahn and Gamboa, 1983). However, in these and other examples of free-living animals, it may be necessary to observe the development of associations if one wishes to understand their relationship to social preferences. This is true because one must know which potential partners were available when the associations were formed. For example, the opportunity to associate with opposite-sexed siblings in adulthood is often precluded in mammals and birds as a result of philopatry by one sex and dispersal from the natal area by the other so that brothers and sisters live apart (reviews in Moore and Ali, 1984; Waser and Jones, 1983).

Even if attractive partners are available temporally and spatially, they may not be accessible because social choices are constrained by competition among individuals seeking access to the same partner. For instance, female vervet monkeys *(Cercopithecus aethiops)* prefer to groom females positioned high in the dominance hierarchy, which may increase the likelihood that high-ranking females will support them during aggressive interactions with other troop members. However, Seyfarth (1980) hypothesized that, because females may face the most competition when they try to groom high-ranking females, they groom females of similar rank. These examples emphasize the point that, in nature, one individual's preferences are often affected by another's, so that investigators must interpret with caution those nonrandom social associations whose development has not been observed.

THE PROXIMATE BASIS OF SOCIAL PREFERENCES

REARING ASSOCIATION AND FAMILIARITY

The link between relatedness and preference is often clarified by examining the social environment in which individuals are reared. In many taxa, preferences are affected by the interactions that individuals have in rearing environments (nests, burrows, or other places in which early development occurs), so that, when they are adults, former rearing associates are treated differently from nonrearing associates. Rearing associates are individuals that encounter each other regularly in species-normal rearing environments, and they may be the same age (e.g., siblings born together) or different ages (e.g., parents and their offspring). In various species of rodents, for example, individuals avoid as mates those conspecifics with which they were reared (Boyd and Blaustein, 1985; Dewsbury, 1982). Adult female paper wasps *(P. metricus)* associate preferentially with former nestmates rather than with nonnestmates when constructing new nests (Ross and Gamboa, 1981). And in many species of mammals (Holmes, 1984a) and birds (Falls, 1982), adults behave amicably toward young they have reared and aggressively toward young they did not rear.

Why has natural selection produced organisms that respond differently to rearing associates? In an evolutionary context, the answer is that, in many situations, rearing associates are relatives that can influence each other's inclusive fitness (e.g., Davis, 1984; Gamboa, 1978; Sherman, 1977), thus making it reproductively advantageous to treat them uniquely. In a proximate sense, individuals become familiar with their rearing associates through repeated exposure to them (e.g., Beer, 1970; Bekoff, 1981). If rearing environments are structured so that only relatives share them, then discrimination between familiar conspecifics (rearing associates) and unfamiliar conspecifics (nonrearing associates) will result in the discrimination of kin. Stated differently:

> When relatives predictably interact in unambiguous social contexts where kinship is not likely to be confounded by the mixing of unequally related individuals, recognition [of kin] may be based on the timing, rate, frequency, or duration of such interactions. . . . Rearing environments . . . provide ideal settings for a mechanism of this kind. (Holmes and Sherman, 1983, p. 47)

Thus, by learning to identify rearing associates as "familiar" and treating them preferentially, individuals come to treat their relatives favorably, which may enhance their inclusive fitness. (Those instances in which kin are not reared together or in which rearing associates are not kin or are unequally related kin are discussed in the next section.)

This view of the relation between rearing association and kinship differs sharply from that presented by some other authors. For example, in a discussion of whether kin selection is a useful explanatory principle, Snowdon (1983) wrote, "Thus, many of the activities that appear to be kin selected, may in fact be due to mere exposure or familiarity" (p. 69). This argument fails to distinguish between proximate and ultimate explanations for kin preferences, and it fails to explain why exposure or familiarity should affect preferences in the first place.

Three predictions can be made based on the hypothesized relationship between exposure to associates in rearing environments and subsequent social preferences:

1. *In those species whose rearing environments regularly separate unequally related individuals, kin and nonkin will be treated similarly if they are reared together.* By manipulating the composition of a brood or a litter that shares a rearing environment, various investigators have examined this prediction. For example, Holmes (1984b) cross-fostered newborn thirteen-lined ground squirrels *(Spermophilus tridecemlineatus)* so that the rearing environments (nest boxes) included related and unrelated young. Later, in dyadic-encounter tests, juveniles reared together engaged in fewer exploratory interactions than juveniles reared apart, whether pairs were composed of kin or nonkin (Figure 1.) Similarly, Porter and his colleagues report that cross-fostered spiny mice *(Acomys cahirinus)* prefer to huddle with rearing associates independently of relatedness (Porter, Wyrick, and Pankey, 1978; Porter, Tepper, and White, 1981). Finally, Boyd and Blaustein (1985) found that gray-tailed voles *(Microtus canicaudus)* reared together, whether related or unrelated, produced fewer litters than individuals reared apart.

A corollary to the rearing-association prediction is that, when individuals do not share a common rearing environment, they will not distinguish each other

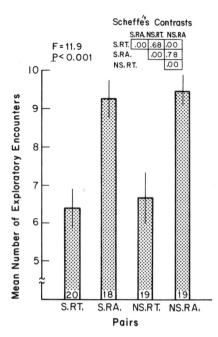

Figure 1. Evidence for sibling recognition in captive thirteen-lined ground squirrels. The frequency (mean $\pm SE$) of exploratory interactions between juvenile *S. tridecemlineatus* during 5-min paired-encounter tests. When pups were cross-fostered shortly after birth, four kinds of pairs could later be tested: siblings reared together (S.RT.); siblings reared apart (S.RA.), nonsiblings reared together (NS.RT.), and nonsiblings reared apart (NS.RA.). The *F* value is based on a one-way ANOVA, and *p* values for comparisons between particular groups are based on Scheffé's test. For example, there was no significant difference ($p < .68$) in the frequency of exploratory interactions for S.RT. compared with NS.RT. The number of pairs tested is shown inside bars. Sibling recognition in *S. tridecemlineatus* seems to be based on familiarity established by direct association during rearing because young reared together, whether related or not, treat each other differently from young reared apart. (From W. G. Holmes, "Sibling Recognition in Thirteen-Lined Ground Squirrels: Effects of Genetic Relatedness, Rearing Association, and Olfaction," *Behavioral Ecology and Sociobiology*, 1984, *14*, 225–233. Copyright (1984) by Springer-Verlag. Reprinted by permission of the publisher and the author.)

based on kinship. Thus, in both thirteen-lined ground squirrels (Figure 1), spiny mice (Porter *et al.,* 1978), and gray-tailed voles (Boyd and Blaustein, 1985), when siblings were separated at birth their interactions during later tests were like those of unrelated young reared apart.

It is important to note that Prediction 1 applies only to those species in which unequally related individuals are kept separate in their *species-normal rearing environments.* Thus, it excludes cases in which members of one species rear the young of another species, like avian brood parasites (Rothstein, 1982), cases in which multiple insemination of a female results in broods or litters of mixed paternity (Cole, 1983; Hanken and Sherman, 1981), cases in which young are reared cooperatively (review in Emlen, 1984), and cases in which young produced by several females share a common rearing environment (Blaustein and O'Hara, 1982; O'Hara and Blaustein, 1982; Waldman, 1982, 1984). Under these circumstances, relatives may or may not be favored, but if they are, favoritism is not likely to be based on simple rearing association.

2. *Preferences for rearing associates will first appear coincident with or just before the time in development when nonrearing associates are initially encountered.* In other words, the initial expression of preferences will coincide temporally with the need to distinguish rearing associates from other individuals. For instance, female feral goats *(Capra hircus)* separate from the herd shortly before parturition and give birth to a kid that remains hidden from the herd for 2–3 days, during which time the mother returns periodically to nurse her kid (Rudge, 1970). The mother can distinguish between her own and another female's young (Klopfer, Adams, and Klopfer, 1964), and this discrimination seems to be based on an olfactory "label"

that is transferred by a combination of licking the kid and the kid's ingesting milk (Gubernick, 1981). In his review, Gubernick (1981) pointed out that, because the kid is hidden for 2–3 days, the mother–kid attachment is solidified (although interactions during the first few hours postpartum are particularly important), so that "by the time feral goat kids join and follow their mother in the herd they already recognize each other" (p. 286).

The co-occurrence of the ability to discriminate kin with the need to discriminate them is also evident in avian research (review in Falls, 1982). In crested terns (*Sterna bergii;* Davies and Carrick, 1962), ring-billed gulls (Miller and Emlen, 1975), bank swallows (*Riparia riparia;* Beecher, Beecher, and Nichols, 1981), and pinon jays (*Gymnorhinus cyanocephalus;* McArthur, 1982), parents first discriminate between their own and alien young near the time when the young become mobile and mixing between broods becomes likely, although empirical support for this timing effect has been questioned in some cases due to methodological problems (Shugart, 1977).

A similar timing effect was revealed by parallel field (Holmes and Sherman, 1982) and laboratory studies (Holmes, 1984a) on the ontogeny of dam–young discrimination in Belding's ground squirrels. *S. beldingi* females rear their litters alone in underground burrows for about 25 days after birth and defend their natal burrow against intrusions by conspecifics (Sherman, 1981). In the field, Sherman found that a dam would retrieve unrelated young placed near her burrow and rear them, but only if the aliens were less than 25 days old and the dam's own litter had not come aboveground (Figure 2). In the laboratory, Holmes discovered that the

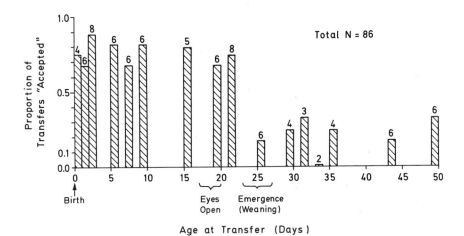

Figure 2. Evidence for the timing of the development of dam–offspring discrimination in free-living Belding's ground squirrels. The proportion of young *S. beldingi* that were "accepted" into foster burrows (that were retrieved into a natal burrow by the resident dam and remained with the resident litter for at least 1 week after they first came aboveground). Age at transfer is the age of young when they were cross-fostered, which matched the age of the target dam's own litter. The numbers above the bars indicate the number of young in which cross-fostering was attempted. (From W. G. Holmes and P. W. Sherman, "The Ontogeny of Kin Recognition in Two Species of Ground Squirrels," *American Zoologist*, 1982, *22*, 491–517. Copyright (1982) by the American Society of Zoologists. Reprinted by permission of the publisher and the authors.)

times taken by a dam to retrieve young she had reared (familiar young) and those she had not (unfamiliar young) were similar until the young reached 22 days of age, when familiar young were retrieved faster than unfamiliar young (Figure 3). Although the difference between mean retrieval times for familiar and unfamiliar 22-day-old young was small, the existence of the difference indicates that dam–young discrimination occurred. Morever, in another type of discrimination test (paired encounters in an arena) when young reached 29 days of age, agonistic interactions in unfamiliar pairs were five times as common as they were in familiar pairs (Holmes, 1984a, Fig. 3). Thus, in both the field and the laboratory, dams first responded preferentially to young they had been rearing when the young reached the age at which they would mix with offspring belonging to other females in their natural environment.

It is important to recall that preferential treatment of kin and the ability to

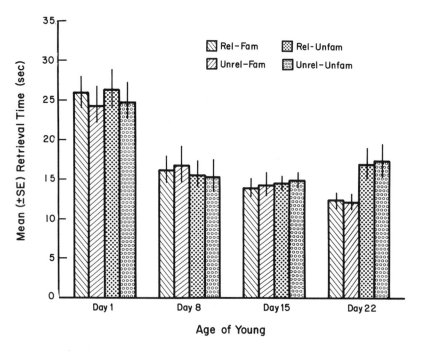

Figure 3. Evidence for the timing of dam–offspring discrimination in captive Belding's ground squirrels. The time (mean $\pm SE$) taken by dams ($n = 8$) to retrieve young back into nestboxes at four times (age in days) during the development of young. Pups were cross-fostered at birth (Day 1), so that during subsequent retrieval tests, dams could be presented four kinds of young simultaneously: related familiar (Rel-Fam), unrelated familiar (Unrel-Fam), related unfamiliar (Rel-Unfam), and unrelated unfamiliar (Unrel-Unfam). *Related* indicates whether the dam was the pup's biological mother, and *familiar* indicates whether the dam reared the pup (after cross-fostering). Retrieval times for the four kinds of young were similar until Day 22, when the dams retrieved familiar young significantly faster ($p < .001$) than unfamiliar young, independently of true relatedness. Both the field (Figure 2) and the laboratory (Figure 3) data indicate that dam–offspring discrimination is first observed at 22–25 days of age, which coincides with the age when free-living young first come aboveground to mingle with other litters. (From W. G. Holmes, "Ontogeny of Dam-Young Recognition in Captive Belding's Ground Squirrels *(Spermophilus beldingi)*," 1984, *98*, 246–256. Copyright (1984) by the American Psychological Association. Reprinted by permission of the publisher and the author.)

recognize kin are not synonymous (cf. Hoogland, 1986). In addition, the first man-ifestation of a kin preference cannot be used to infer when kin are first recogniz-able. For example, retrieval tests revealed that *S. beldingi* dams did not distinguish between familiar and unfamiliar young until young were 22 days old (Figure 3), yet, when 15-day-old young were placed in dams' home cages, dams spent more time sniffing and contacting unfamiliar young than familiar young (Holmes, unpublished data). Preferential treatment of rearing associates may initially appear about the time in development when nonrearing associates are likely to be encoun-tered for the first time, especially in species-typical environments; but rearing asso-ciates may actually be discriminable at an earlier time (Shugart, 1977).

3. *When preferences for kin are mediated by exposure to them in rearing environments, the maintenance of these preferences may or may not depend on repeated exposure to kin outside the rearing environments.* For example, if preferences develop because of uninterrupted association and frequent encounters in a rearing environment, then as adults individuals may have to interact repeatedly or their special treatment of each other may disappear. Thus, in young spiny mice, siblings that preferred to huddle with each other after having been reared together no longer exhibit this preference after they have been separated 8 days (Porter and Wyrick, 1979). Stud-ies of inbreeding avoidance in various species of rodents also report that the inhi-bition from mating with rearing associates disappears if associates are separated for some period of time (Dewsbury, 1982).

On the other hand, if preferences are based on experiences during a brief sensitive period, then the maintenance of these preferences may not depend on frequent and repeated interactions. For instance, paper wasp gynes (potential queens) of *Polistes fuscatus* and *P. metricus* that have been isolated from other wasps for up to 46 days and 99 days, respectively, retain their preference to associate with former nestmates over nonnestmates when tested following isolation (review in Gamboa, Reeve, and Pfennig, 1986).

As shown by the examples above, kin preferences based on prior association are widespread taxonomically, and these preferences, based proximately on learned familiarity, may be among the most common in nature. However, estab-lishing a causal link between prior association and preference is only the first step in elucidating the proximate basis of social preferences. The three hypotheses offered above represent an effort to clarify at the behavioral level the meaning of the term *familiarity*. To suggest that familiarity "explains" social preferences and to stop there is to reify familiarity and to gloss over such important issues as species differences in the effects of prior association.

PHENOTYPE MATCHING

To this point, I have considered how direct interactions with rearing associates (or their phenotypic traits) result in a learned familiarity that mediates later social favoritism. By extension, exposure to certain individuals early in development may influence social preferences for other individuals encountered later by a process called *phenotype matching*. If Individual A encounters an unknown (with respect to relatedness) conspecific, B, then A might treat B favorably if B's phenotype were similar to that of one of A's former rearing associates or even to A's own phenotype. Thus, in the process of phenotype matching, "an individual learns and recalls its relatives' phenotypes or its own phenotype, and compares phenotypes of unfamiliar conspecifics to this learned 'template'" (Holmes and Sherman, 1982, p. 509; see "Comparing Phenotypes" in Alexander, 1979).

Before examining the empirical evidence for phenotype matching, four issues concerning the kin template are considered. Each assumes that rearing associates are models for template formation. First, if the template is to reflect kinship accurately, then rearing associates must share a phenotypic trait or combination of traits that distinguishes them from nonrearing associates. More generally, phenotypic and genotypic similarity must correlate to a greater degree for rearing associates than for nonrearing associates, at least for those traits that influence the template. It is immaterial whether variation in these traits is primarily of genetic origin, environmental origin, or both (Gamboa *et al.*, 1986), as long as rearing associates are more phenotypically similar than other individuals (e.g., Bateson, Lotwick, and Scott, 1980; Carter-Saltzman and Scarr-Salapatek, 1975; Scarr and Grajeck, 1982).

Second, the kin template should be acquired in a context (social and locational) and at a time when the phenotypes of nonkin or unequally related kin would not compromise it. This argument suggests that a sensitive period may exist for template formation (e.g., before leaving the nest in some bird species) and that the template should be resistant to modification once it develops.

Third, under some circumstances, the template itself may limit the degree to which phenotype matching can be used reliably to assess relatedness. Genetic and environmental constraints on development may hold down phenotypic variation in a population so that kin templates do not always differ sharply among different kin groups. These constraints suggest that templates based on several traits rather than just one may evolve, and that templates should be based on traits that show high variation and high heritability in the population relative to other traits that do not influence the template (Beecher, 1982; Gamboa *et al.*, 1986; Lacy and Sherman, 1983).

Finally, there may be specificity in template formation. That is, the acquisition of a template may be selectively constrained as regards the phenotypes that can influence it. If several models were available to influence template formation, and if these models varied in the degree to which they accurately reflected kinship, then selective responsivity to some models rather than others might be adaptive. For example, all phenotypes might not be equally potent models if template formation were mediated by a selective filtering device. Marler (1976) made this point for song acquisition in birds:

> While the auditory template for song of an untrained male white-crowned sparrow is thought of as only an elementary specification of species-specific song, . . . it may nevertheless be sufficient to serve as a kind of filter for external auditory stimuli. (p. 325)

There is, of course, no *a priori* reason to think that sensory templates for bird song and kin templates for phenotype matching share similar ontogenies or proximate controls. However, it is important to recall that some models may more likely influence template formation in phenotype matching than others, and that the malleability of a template during its development may vary from one species to the next.

One way to investigate phenotype matching is to expose individuals to various rearing associates whose phenotypes differ and later, in a test situation, to present to subjects unfamiliar conspecifics whose phenotypes do or do not match those of the subjects' former rearing associates. According to the matching hypothesis, unfamiliar conspecifics that share traits (quantitatively or qualitatively) with the subjects' previous rearing associates should be treated more favorably than unfamiliar individuals whose phenotypes differ from those of rearing associates. For instance, Buckle and Greenberg (1981) created laboratory nests of sweat bees *(Lasioglossum zephyrum)* and later presented different categories of unfamiliar bees (bees with whom guards were not reared) at nest entrances to determine whether the guards would allow the intruders to enter the nest. (In nature, guards allow only their nestmates to enter.) The guards were reared under one of three conditions before the tests: with only their sisters, with equal numbers of their sisters and of unrelated nestmates, or with only nestmates related to each other but unrelated to the guard. When tested, the guards admitted only those intruders whose phenotypic traits (probably odors) matched those of their former nestmates: the guards reared with their sisters admitted only their unfamiliar sisters; the guards reared with both their sisters and unrelated nestmates admitted their unfamiliar sisters *and* their unrelated nestmates' unfamiliar sisters; finally, the guards reared only among unrelated nestmates rejected their own sisters but allowed entry to sisters of their unrelated nestmates.

Phenotype matching can also occur in spiny mice. *A. cahirinus* littermates reared together to weaning and then individually isolated did not manifest a preference to huddle with each other as they had before being isolated (Porter and Wyrick, 1979). However, if two littermates that had been separated from each other were each housed with another of their littermates, then the two huddled with each other preferentially when reunited: "The phenotype of familiar littermates appears to be a significant factor in the development of social preferences" (Porter, Matochik, and Makin, 1983, p. 978), and "familiar social odours can influence interactions among *A. cahirinus* weanlings by serving as a learned standard against which odours of conspecifics are compared" (p. 982).

Phenotype matching seems to underlie the ability of female Belding's ground squirrels to identify their unfamiliar sisters (Holmes, 1986a). Shortly after birth in captivity, pups were cross-fostered so that, as yearlings, they could be observed in paired-encounter tests. All test partners (two females tested together) were unfamiliar (reared apart) and were either sisters or unrelated females. Additionally, test partners either were reared with one another's siblings (i.e., indirectly exposed to each other's phenotype) or were not reared with each other's siblings. (Male–male and male–female pairs were not tested because only sisters manifest the ability to identify each other when reared apart; Holmes and Sherman, 1982.)

In the arena, test partners indirectly exposed to each other were less agonistic (with each other) than those not indirectly exposed to each other, regardless of whether the females were related (Figure 4). That unrelated test partners reared with each other's siblings were less agonistic than unrelated test partners not so reared indicates that agonism between unfamiliar females was not based on pre-natal learning, early postnatal learning before cross-fostering, or some kind of genetically mediated mechanism that was independent of learning. This inference about agonism is suggested because unrelated females did not share a pre- or post-natal environment, nor did they share genes identical by descent. However, unre-lated females in the "indirectly exposed" group were reared with their test part-ner's siblings and may have learned something from their nestmates' phenotypes that influenced their discrimination ability in the arena. On the other hand, expo-sure to nestmates' phenotypes cannot explain all aspects of the differential treat-ment during the tests because unfamiliar *sisters* reared with each other's siblings were even less aggressive than unfamiliar *nonsisters* reared with each other's siblings (Figure 4). Something in addition to cues from nestmates' phenotypes seems to influence the identification of kin by females.

One likely source of additional cues is a female's own phenotype, and it appears that *S. beldingi* females can rely on their own phenotype as a template in the matching process. This inference is based on how litter composition during rearing seemed to affect discrimination: some females in the "sisters indirectly

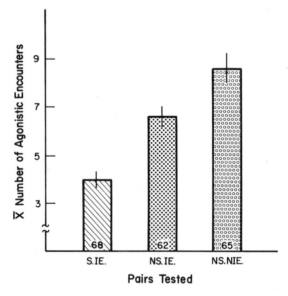

Figure 4. Evidence for discrimination between unfamiliar (reared-apart) female Belding's ground squir-rels by the process of phenotype matching. The frequency (mean $\pm SE$) of agonistic interactions during paired-encounter tests in captivity involved sisters indirectly exposed to each other (S.IE.), nonsisters indirectly exposed to each other (NS.IE.), and nonsisters not indirectly exposed to each other (NS.NIE.). *Indirectly exposed* means that two females tested together were each reared with their test partner's siblings. The number of pairs tested is shown inside the bars. (From W. G. Holmes, "Kin Recognition by Phenotype Matching in Female Belding's Ground Squirrels," *Animal Behaviour*, 1986b, *34*, 38–47. Copyright (1986) by Baillière Tindall. Reprinted by permission of the publisher and the author.)

exposed" group were reared only with unrelated nestmates, whereas others were reared with both their sisters and unrelated nestmates. Unfamiliar sisters were equally nonaggressive whether they had been reared with both related and unrelated nestmates or only with unrelated nestmates (Figure 5). For instance, females reared only with three nonkin were no more aggressive with their unfamiliar sisters than were females reared with three nonkin *and* two siblings. It may be that, when confronted by unfamiliar sisters, females relied primarily on their own phenotypes as models to identify their unfamiliar kin.

When traits used in phenotype matching are genetically specified, an advantage of using a self template is that one's own phenotype would usually provide an accurate kin referent, whereas a template based on the phenotypes of rearing associates might not if the associates were not all equally related. For instance, *S. beldingi* litters routinely contain full siblings and maternal half siblings because females mate with two or more males during their single annual estrus (Hanken and Sherman, 1981). Because female littermates seem able to distinguish full sisters and their maternal half sisters as yearlings in nature, Holmes and Sherman (1982) hypothesized that, if phenotype matching mediated this discrimination, a self template would have to be involved because a template based on the phenotypes of nestmates would be compromised by the presence of two categories of kin. That cross-fostered females reared only with nonkin are able to distinguish their unfamiliar sisters supports the hypothesis that females can use their own phenotype as a standard for comparisons (Holmes, 1986a).

Earlier in my discussion of phenotype matching, I suggested that one method of studying the phenomenon involves exposing individuals to various rearing asso-

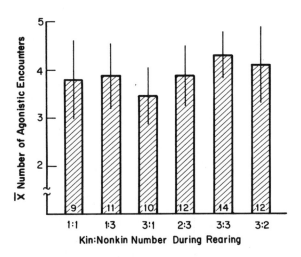

Figure 5. Evidence that female Belding's ground squirrels can use their own phenotype as a kin template in phenotype matching: The frequency (mean $\pm SE$) of agonistic interactions during paired-encounter tests between sisters reared apart from each other. The "Kin:Nonkin Number" is the number of related phenotypes, including her own, and nonrelated phenotypes, respectively, that a female was exposed to throughout rearing. (The rearing dam's phenotype is not included in the number.) For instance, 1:3 indicates that a female was exposed to one related phenotype (her own) and three unrelated phenotypes (three nestmates unrelated to her). The number of pairs tested is shown inside bars.

ciates whose phenotypes differ and later determining whether such exposure affected the subjects' preferences. This method was the basis for the studies on sweat bees, spiny mice, and Belding's ground squirrels described above. Two limitations of this method are that (a) the trait(s) used in the matching is unknown, and (b) the investigator must *assume* that whatever trait(s) is involved, it is more similar among relatives than among nonrelatives. Both of these limitations can be overcome with another method, although it, too, is not without shortcomings.

In the second method of studying phenotype matching, the investigator labels animals artificially with some phenotypic marker and later determines whether the marker influenced preferences for unfamiliar but similarly marked animals (Salzen and Cornell, 1968). For example, besides the experiment on spiny mice reported above, Porter *et al.* (1983) applied artificial odorants (musk oil, oil of clove, lemon-lime, or cherry) to spiny mice weanlings and later presented unfamiliar age-mates (never encountered before testing) whose odorant did or did not match the subject's. Weanlings preferred to huddle with unfamiliar age-mates whose artificial ordorant matched their own and that of their littermates. Porter and his colleagues cautioned, however, that the odorants they used could have been more intense or distinctive than the odors produced by the spiny mice themselves. In other words, investigators can manipulate phenotypes to search for the *possibility* of matching and thus control the trait that may be involved in the matching process, but this technique reveals only what is possible within the context of the manipulation. It cannot reveal whether phenotype matching mediates preferences in species-normal environments, nor can it reveal the sensory modalities or phenotypic traits normally involved in matching, if it occurs.

Paternal half siblings provide a useful opportunity to study the proximate basis of social preferences, in general, and phenotype matching, in particular (Holmes, 1986b). This is true because a shared prenatal environment, which can influence several kinds of preferences, cannot influence the preferences of paternal half siblings for each other because these half siblings develop in separate uteri. (Smotherman and Robinson present in Chapter 5 several examples of how prenatal experience can affect postnatal preferences.) Wu and her colleagues were the first to report a preference for unfamiliar paternal half siblings in a vertebrate, the pig-tailed macaque *(Macaca nemestrina),* and the investigators noted that phenotype matching (against a monkey's own phenotype) may explain the preference (Wu, Holmes, Medina, and Sackett, 1980). More recently, however, Fredrickson and Sackett (1984) claimed to have replicated the original study and suggested that their results contradict the original findings. Interestingly, results from the two investigations are similar *if* one compares the appropriate experimental groups, that is, those in which relatedness and familiarity were matched properly.

Monkeys in Wu *et al.*'s Experiment I and Fredrickson's and Sackett's Group 7 were presented two social stimuli simultaneously, during 600-s preference tests in the laboratory: their unfamiliar paternal half sibling (never encountered before testing) and an unfamiliar and unrelated conspecific matched with the half sibling for age, sex, and body weight. In both studies, the monkeys spent considerably more time near their half sibling than near the unrelated conspecific, although the difference in the Fredrickson and Sackett study was not statistically significant (Figure 6). Comparisons between the two must be made cautiously because (a) Wu *et al.* tested an equal number of males and females ($N = 16$ animals total), whereas Fredrickson and Sackett tested only females ($N = 13$), and (b) the monkeys used in the initial study averaged 5.8 months of age, whereas those in the later study averaged 22.8 months. Social preferences vary with both sex and age in *Macaca* (Suomi, Sackett, and Harlow, 1970).

These differences notwithstanding, at issue is whether choice times (Figure 6) represent "biologically significant" preferences that reflect the ability of monkeys reared apart from their kin to distinguish related from unrelated animals. Contrary to what Fredrickson and Sackett suggested, whether familiarity (rearing association) can influence preferences independently of relatedness does not bear directly on the issue of preferences in the *absence* of familiarity or whether preferences for unfamiliar kin may be based on phenotype matching. Indeed, phenotype matching was proposed (Holmes and Sherman, 1982, 1983) to account for kin recognition when cues based on rearing association were unavailable (e.g., paternal half siblings reared apart) or when rearing-association cues did not correlate accurately with relatedness (e.g., multiple insemination producing full and maternal half siblings that are reared together).

Gouzoules (1984) reviewed the degree to which nonhuman primate social behavior is kin-correlated, and she cited numerous cases in which the "patterns of cooperative behavior in many primate species can be accounted for largely by kinship" (p. 126). Behaviors that vary with kinship include "rates of agonism, coalitions and alliances, and alarm calling, as well as . . . grooming, traveling and feeding together, and alloparenting and infant defense" (p. 112). Busse (1985) discussed father–offspring discrimination in primates and emphasized that, in contrast to earlier views, intimate male–infant affiliations occur in several species that have a multimale social organization, especially the savanna-dwelling baboons (*Papio*

Figure 6. Preferences (mean time in proximity) for unfamiliar paternal half siblings exhibited during 10-min tests of captive pigtail macaques that were reported by (A) Wu *et al.* (1980) or (B) Fredrickson and Sackett (1984). Unfamiliar half siblings elicited more "choice time" than unfamiliar nonkin in both studies. Choice times were statistically different ($p = 0.05$) only in the Wu *et al.* study. (From (A) H. M. H. Wu, W. G. Holmes, S. R. Medina, and G. P. Sackett, "Kin Preference in Infant *Macaca nemestrina*," *Nature*, 1980, *285*, 225–227. Copyright (1980) by Macmillan Journals Ltd. Reprinted by permission of the publisher and the authors. (B) W. T. Fredrickson, and G. P. Sackett, "Kin Preferences in Primates *(Macaca nemestrina):* Relatedness or familiarity?" *Journal of Comparative Psychology*, 1984, *98*, 29–34. Copyright (1984) by the American Psychological Association. Adapted by permission of the publisher and the authors.)

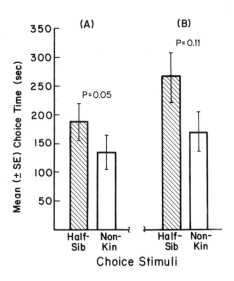

spp.). If males are caring preferentially for their own offspring in these cases, at least two mechanisms may come into play. First, males may recall past social and sexual relations with an infant's mother and may affiliate with infants produced by these females (referred to as *mediated recognition*—Holmes and Sherman, 1982, 1983—and one componenet of Alexander's "social learning model," 1979; for a possible example, see Berenstain, Rodman, and Smith, 1981). Second, phenotype matching could underlie the special male–infant affiliations. Unfortunately, as Gouzoules (1984) wrote, "studies which have actually examined the abilities of primates to discriminate kin have lagged far behind those on other taxa" (p. 99). Thus, research on primate kin recognition is badly needed, especially on those categories of relatives that cannot typically rely on familiarity to identify each other, such as paternal half siblings and father–offspring dyads.

Besides providing an avenue for nepotism, phenotype matching may affect mate preferences. Female laboratory mice reared with their father preferred males (actually their odors) of another strain as opposed to their own strain, but when the fathers were absent during rearing, the females exhibited no male preference (Mainardi, 1964). Gilder and Slater (1978) suggested that female mice prefer as mates males that differ slightly from those with which the females are either very familiar or very unfamiliar, and that familiarity is established by social experience with rearing associates early in development. In various domesticated bird species, individuals of one color morph that are exchanged and reared by parents of another color pair with mates whose color matches that of their rearing parents rather than their own (see Immelmann, 1975, on sexual imprinting). Cooke, Finney, and Rockwell (1976) also reported that mate choice by adult lesser snow geese (*Anser caerulescens*) depends on the color of the parents and silbings with which they were reared.

Although the studies just outlined suggest that the phenotypes of rearing associates can affect mating preferences at a general level (e.g., one color morph or strain over another), none demonstrates that animals use phenotype matching to make fine-grained discriminations among individuals that share several but not all phenotypic traits. A more direct link between matching and mate choice may involve an inbreeding avoidance study in which litters were divided so that brothers and sisters were reared with some of their siblings, but not others. Unfamiliar siblings would be avoided as mates in adulthood if exposure to other siblings during rearing produced a kin template that influenced mate preference.

CONCLUDING REMARKS

INCLUSIVE FITNESS THEORY AND WORKING HYPOTHESES

Laboratory studies of social recognition in spiny mice (Porter *et al.*, 1978), sweat bees (Greenberg, 1979), toad tadpoles (Waldman and Adler, 1979), and pigtail macaques (Wu *et al.*, 1980) were among the first to approach kin recognition explicitly in the context of Hamilton's theory of inclusive fitness (1964). These studies and others considered above have produced several important findings regarding the relationship between kinship and social preferences, as I have outlined here. First, the research has shown that the kinship preference relationship is widespread taxonomically and independent of neural complexity or cognitive ability, as indicated by work on an array of species discussed in recent reviews of kin recognition (Fletcher and Michener, 1987; Gamboa *et al.*, 1986; Sherman and Holmes, 1985). Second, no single proximate mechanism or ontogenetic pathway can account for all cases in which preferred social partners are kin. For instance, rearing association and phenotype matching both mediate learned preferences for kin, but what is learned under the two mechanisms usually differs and the circumstances in which they would be used also differ, as presented in the preceding section. Finally, evolutionary theories (inclusive fitness theory and mate choice theory) that account for the preferential treatment of kin at one level of analysis are now being joined with proximate explanations for kin preferences, and the combination provides the most complete analysis of behavior (Tinbergen, 1963).

Despite recent successes in understanding the kinship-preference relationship, I want to raise two cautionary notes in closing. First, if the primary goal of a research program is to describe and explain social preferences in an adaptive or evolutionary context, then knowledge of the behavior and ecology of individuals living in their natural evironment is essential to both designing experiments and interpreting their results. Recent papers on sibling recognition by laboratory rats discuss discrimination abilities in the context of inclusive fitness theory (Hepper, 1983; Hopp, Owren, and Marion, 1985; Wills, Wesley, Sisemore, Anderson, and Banks, 1983). Although good descriptive studies of free-living rats *(Rattus norvegicus)* are available (Calhoun, 1962; Telle, 1966), little is known about the frequency, context, or manner in which various classes of kin interact in free-living populations. A similar difficulty arises when one tries to examine evolutionarily the kin recognition abilities of strains of laboratory mice (Kareem, 1983; Kareem and Barnard, 1982). Inclusive fitness theory may be used to formulate testable "working hypotheses" about kinship and social preferences in domesticated species maintained in the laboratory, and the behavior of these species may accord well with predictions from the theory. However, a concordance between predicted and observed behavior does not mean that the theory used to generate the prediction can be offered as an explanation for the behavior. Galef (1984) made this point in a discussion of taste aversion learning in rats: "In the absence of information as to the problems posed by environments with which rats have evolved to interact, explanations of behaviors in terms of their adaptive functions are working hypotheses and not explanations" (p. 485). Thus, the goal of one's research program constrains, to some degree, the species that one can study most profitably.

THE MEANING OF GENETIC RECOGNITION

My second point concerns the term *genetic recognition* (or *innate recognition*) and its use in the literature on kinship and social favoritism. To clarify the meaning, it is useful to recall that the discrimination process depends on two components:

(a) the production of phenotypes that make individuals or classes of them unique and (b) the discrimination of those phenotypes by individuals attempting to identify conspecifics (Beecher, 1982). The term *genetic* (or *innate*) can be applied to either component, although investigators have used the term most often to refer to the production component rather than the discrimination component. For instance, Getz and Smith (1983) published an article entitled, "Genetic Kin Recognition: Honey Bees Discriminate Full and Half Sisters," in which they described differential treatment of full and maternal half sisters by female honeybees *(Apis mellifera)*, despite both categories of kin having been raised in neighboring cells of the same hive. The meaning of *genetic kin recognition* is clarified as follows:

> Thus workers are using genetically based labels . . . to discriminate between their full and half-sisters, but it is not clear whether this ability is based on habituation to the labels of their co-group or whether they use their own set of labels as a cue. (Getz and Smith, 1983, p. 148)

The first half of this quotation indicates that the production of phenotypes is genetically specified, whereas the second half suggests that the discrimination of phenotypes is based on some kind of learning process. The title of Greenberg's paper, "Genetic Component of Bee Odor in Kin Recognition" (1979), also refers to the production component rather than to the discrimination component.

Regarding the discrimination component of the recognition process, Hamilton (1964) posited four proximate mechanisms that may allow for the special treatment of kin. One of these is based on a "supergene" that affects (a) some unique phenotypic trait; (b) the perception of the trait in others; and (c) the behavioral responses to individuals that possess the trait (p. 25). Discussions of Hamilton's "genetic recognition mechanism" or "recognition alleles," in which preferential treatment of kin occurs by a process that is independent of learning, have been largely theoretical (Alexander and Borgia, 1978; Blaustein, 1983; Dawkins, 1982; Ridley and Grafen, 1981; Rothstein and Barash, 1983). Sherman and Holmes (1985) proposed that an empirical search for a "genetic recognition" mechanism would be problematic because of the need to control all environmental and experiential cues that could facilitate an acquired ability to distinguish kin, including experiences with an individual's own phenotype. Alexander (1979) even suggested:

> I would regard the onus of proof to be on the investigator who argues that among birds or mammals no social learning opportunities have been involved in nepotistic or reciprocal interactions in which individuals are treated differently. (p. 119)

A major hinderance to empirical research on "recognition alleles" is that, other than Hamilton's general statements (1964), there is no formal model that can be used to generate testable predictions.

SUMMARY

In summary, social preferences for genetically related conspecifics are widespread in nature. From a proximate perspective, these preferences often reflect a familiarity with rearing associates based on direct interactions with them in a rearing environment (e.g., a burrow or a nest) that excludes unrelated conspecifics. Individuals that share phenotypic traits or individuals that have traits like those of former rearing associates may also receive special treatment, based on a process of phenotype matching. From an evolutionary perspective, the preferential treatment of relatives may have evolved in the context of kin favoritism or nepotism or in the context of optimal mate choice. By combining laboratory and field research and by thinking in both a proximate and an ultimate framework, psychobiologists and behavioral ecologists have started to understand why kinship and social preferences are often linked.

Acknowledgments

For editorial help and comments on this chapter, I thank E. Blass, R. Porter, and B. Smuts. My thinking about kin recognition profited from numerous conversations with P. Sherman during our collaborative research on Belding's ground squirrel kin-recognition. For assistance in acquiring, maintaining, and testing ground squirrels, I thank D. Bushberg, R. Caldwell, D. DiMario, D. Gelfand, S. Glickman, B. Grimm, M. Redfearn, C. Rowley, L. Shellberg, and I. Zucker. My research on grounds quirrel kin-recognition was supported with funds from the Office of the Dean of the College of Literature, Science, and the Arts, the Office of the Vice President for Research, a Rackham Faculty Research Grant, and the Department of Psychology, all at the University of Michigan.

REFERENCES

Alexander, R. D. *Darwinism and human affairs.* Seattle: University of Washington Press, 1979.

Alexander, R. D., and Borgia, G. Group selection, altruism, and the levels of organization of life. *Annual Review of Ecology and Systematics,* 1978, *9,* 449–474.

Altmann, S. A. Altruistic behaviour: the fallacy of kin deployment. *Animal Behaviour,* 1979, *27,* 958–959.

Axelrod, R., and Hamilton, W. D. The evolution of cooperation. *Science,* 1981, *211,* 1390–1396.

Bateson, P. Optimal outbreeding. In P. Bateson (Ed.), *Mate choice.* Cambridge: Cambridge University Press, 1983.

Bateson, P., Lotwick, W., and Scott, D. K. Similarities between the faces of parents and offspring in Bewick's swan and the differences between mates. *Journal of Zoology, London,* 1980, *191,* 61–74.

Beecher, M. D. Signature systems and kin recognition. *American Zoologist,* 1982, *22,* 477–490.

Beecher, M. D., Beecher, I. M., and Hahn, S. H. Parent-offspring recognition in bank swallows *(Riparia riparia).* II. Development and acoustic basis. *Animal Behaviour,* 1981, *29,* 95–101.

Beer, C. G. Individual recognition of voice in the social behavior of birds. In J. S. Rosenblatt, C. Beer, and R. Hinde (Eds.), *Advances in the study of behavior,* Vol. 3. New York: Academic Press, 1970.

Bekoff, M. Mammalian sibling interactions: Genes, facilitative environments, and the coefficient of familiarity. In D. J. Gubernick and P. H. Klopfer (Eds.), *Parental care in mammals.* New York: Plenum Publishing Corporation, 1981.

Berenstain, L, Rodman, P. S., and Smith, D. G. Social relations between fathers and offspring in a captive group of rhesus monkeys *(Macaca mulatta). Animal Behaviour,* 1981, *29,* 1057–1063.

Blaustein, A. R. Kin recognition mechanisms: Phenotypic matching or recognition alleles? *American Naturalist,* 1983, *121,* 749–754.

Blaustein, A. R., and O'Hara, R. K. Kin recognition in *Rana cascadae* tadpoles: Maternal and paternal effects. *Animal Behaviour,* 1982, *30,* 1151–1157.

Boyd, S. K., and Blaustein, A. R. Familiarity and inbreeding avoidance in the gray-tailed vole *(Microtus canicaudus)*. *Journal of Mammalogy*, 1985, *66*, 348–352.

Boyse, E. A., Beauchamp, G. K., and Yamazaki, K. The sensory perception of genotypic polymorphism of the major histocompatability complex and other genes: Some physiological and phylogenetic implications. *Human Immunology*, 1983, *6*, 177–183.

Buckle, G. R., and Greenberg, L. Nestmate recognition in sweat bees *(Lasioglossum zephyrum)*: Does an individual recognize its own odour or only odours of its nestmates? *Animal Behaviour*, 1981, *29*, 802–809.

Busse, C. D. Paternity recognition in multi-male primate groups. *American Zoologist*, 1985, *25*, 873–881.

Calhoun, J. B. *The ecology and sociology of the Norway rat*. United States Department of Health, Education, and Welfare, 1962, Bethesda, MD.

Carter-Saltzman, L., and Scarr-Salapatek, S. Blood group, behavioral, and morphological differences among dizygotic twins. *Social Biology*, 1975, *22*, 372–374.

Cole, B. J. Multiple mating and the evolution of social behavior in the Hymenoptera. *Behavioral Ecology and Sociobiology*, 1983, *12*, 191–201.

Cooke, F. Finney, G. H., and Rockwell, R. F. Assortative mating in lesser snow geese *(Anser caerulescens)*. *Behavior Genetics*, 1976, *6*, 127–140.

Davies, S. J. J. F., and Carrick, R. On the ability of crested terns, *Sterna bergii*, to recognize their own chicks. *Australian Journal of Zoology*, 1962, *10*, 171–177.

Davis, L. S. Kin selection and adult female Richardson's ground squirrels: A test. *Canadian Journal of Zoology*, 1984, *62*, 2344–2348.

Dawkins, R. Twelve misunderstandings of kin selection. *Zeitschrift für Tierpsychologie* 1979, *51*, 184–200.

Dawkins, R. *The extended phenotype*. Oxford: W. H. Freeman, 1982.

Dewsbury, D. A. Avoidance of incestuous breeding between siblings in two species of *Peromyscus* mice. *Biology of Behavior*, 1982, *7*, 157–169.

Emlen, S. T. Cooperative breeding in birds and mammals. In J. R. Krebs and N. B. Davies (Eds.), *Behavioural ecology an evolutionary approach*, Sunderland, MA: Sinauer, 1984.

Evans, R. M. Imprinting and the control of mobility in young ring-billed gulls *(Larus delawarensis)*. *Animal Behaviour Monograph*, 1970, *3*, 193–248.

Falls, B. Individual recognition by sounds in birds. In D. H. Kroodsma and E. H. Miller (Eds.), *Acoustic communication in birds*, Vol. 2. New York: Academic Press, 1982.

Fletcher, D. J. C., and Michener, C. D. (Eds.). *Kin recognition in animals*. London: Wiley, 1987.

Fredrickson, W. T., and Sackett, G. P. Kin preferences in primates *(Macaca nemestrina)*: Relatedness or familiarity. *Journal of Comparative Psychology*, 1984, *98*, 29–34.

Galef, B. G., Jr. Reciprocal heuristics: a discussion of the relationship of the study of learned behavior in laboratory and field. *Learning and Motivation*, 1984, *15*, 479–493.

Gamboa, G. J. Intraspecific defense: Advantage of social cooperation among paper wasps foundresses. *Science*, 1978, *199*, 1463–1465.

Gamboa, G. J., Reeve, H. K., and Pfennig, D. W. The evolution and ontogeny of nestmate recognition in social wasps. *Annual Review of Entomology*, 1986, *31*, 431–454.

Getz, W. M., and Smith, K. B. Genetic kin recognition: Honey bees discriminate between full and half sisters. *Nature*, 1983, *302*, 147–148.

Gilder, P. M., and Slater, P. J. B. Interest of mice in conspecific male odours is influenced by degree of kinship. *Nature*, 1978, *274*, 364–365.

Gouzoules, S. Primate mating systems, kin associations, and cooperative behavior: Evidence for kin recognition? *Yearbook of Physical Anthropology*, 1984, *27*, 99–134.

Grafen, A. Natural selection, kin selection and group selection. In J. R. Krebs and N. B. Davies (Eds.), *Behavioural ecology an evolutionary approach*. Sunderland, MA: Sinauer, 1984.

Greenberg, L. Genetic component of bee odor in kin recognition. *Science*, 1979, *206*, 1095–1097.

Gubernick, D. J. Parent and infant attachment in mammals. In D. J. Gubernick and P. H. Klopfer (Eds.), *Parental care in mammals*. New York: Plenum Press, 1981.

Hamilton, W. D. The genetical evolution of social behaviour, I, II. *Journal of Theoretical Biology*, 1964, *7*, 1–52.

Hamilton, W. D. Altruism and related phenomena, mainly in social insects. *Annual Review of Ecology and Systematics*, 1972, *3*, 193–232.

Hamilton, W. D. Innate social aptitudes of man: An approach from evolutionary genetics. In R. Fox (Ed.), *Biosocial anthropology*. New York: Wiley, 1975.

Hanken, J., and Sherman, P. W. Multiple paternity in Belding's ground squirrel litters. *Science*, 1981, *212*, 351–353.

Hepper, P. G. Sibling recognition in the rat. *Animal Behaviour,* 1983, *31,* 1177–1191.

Hinde, R. A. (Ed.). *Primate social relationships.* London: Blackwell Scientific Publications, 1983.

Holmes, W. G. Ontogeny of dam-young recognition in captive Belding's ground squirrels. *Journal of Comparative Psychology,* 1984a, *98,* 246–256.

Holmes, W. G. Sibling recognition in thirteen-lined ground squirrels: Effects of genetic relatedness, rearing association, and olfaction. *Behavioral Ecology and Sociobiology,* 1984b, *14,* 225–233.

Holmes, W. G. Kin recognition by phenotype matching in female Belding's ground squirrels. *Animal Behaviour,* 1986a, *34,* 38–47.

Holmes, W. G. Identification of paternal half-siblings by captive Belding's ground squirrels. *Animal Behaviour,* 1986b, *34,* 321–327.

Holmes, W. G., and Sherman, P. W. The ontogeny of kin recognition in two species of ground squirrels. *American Zoologist,* 1982, *22,* 491–517.

Holmes, W. G., and Sherman, P. W. Kin recognition in animals. *American Scientist,* 1983, *71,* 46–55.

Hoogland, J. L. Prairie dogs avoid extreme inbreeding. *Science,* 1982, *215,* 1639–1641.

Hoogland, J. L. Infanticide in prairie dogs: Lactating females kill offspring of close kin. *Science,* 1985, *230,* 1037–1040.

Hoogland, J. L. Nepotism in prairie dogs *(Cynomys ludovicianus)* varies with competition but not with kinship. *Animal Behaviour,* 1986, *34,* 263–270.

Hopp, S. L., Owren, M. J., and Marion, J. R. Olfactory discrimination of individual littermates in rats *Rattus norvegicus. Journal of Comparative Psychology,* 1985, *99,* 248–251.

Immelmann, K. Sexual and other long-term aspects of imprinting in birds and other species. In D. S. Lehrman, R. A. Hinde, and E. Shaw (Eds.), *Advances in the study of behavior,* Vol. 4. New York: Academic Press, 1975.

Kaplan, J. N., Cubicciotti, D., III, and Redican, W. K. Olfactory discrimination of squirrel monkey mothers by their infants. *Developmental Psychobiology,* 1977, *10,* 447–453.

Kareem, A. M. Effect of increasing periods of familiarity on social interactions between male sibling mice. *Animal Behaviour,* 1983, *31,* 919–926.

Kareem, A. M., and Barnard, C. J. The importance of kinship and familiarity in social interactions between mice. *Animal Behaviour,* 1982, *30,* 594–601.

King, A. P., West, M. J., and Eastzer, D. H. Song structure and song development as potential contributors to reproductive isolation in cowbirds *(Molothrus ater). Journal of Comparative and Physiological Psychology,* 1980, *94,* 1028–1039.

Klahn, J. E., and Gamboa, G. J. Social wasps: Discrimination between kin and nonkin brood. *Science,* 1983, *221,* 482–484.

Klopfer, P. H., Adams, D. K., and Klopfer, M. S. Maternal imprinting in goats. *Proceedings of the National Academy of Science, USA,* 1964, *52,* 911–914.

Lacy, R. C., and Sherman, P. W. Kin recognition by phenotype matching. *American Naturalist,* 1983, *121,* 489–512.

Lenington, S. Social preferences for partners carrying "good genes" in wild house mice. *Animal Behaviour,* 1983, *31,* 325–333.

Mainardi, D. Relations between early experience and sexual preferences in female mice (a progress report). *Atti Associazione Genetica Italiana,* 1964, *9,* 141–145.

Marler, P. Sensory templates in species-specific behavior. In J. C. Fentress (Ed.), *Simpler networks and behavior.* Sunderland, MA: Sinauer, 1976.

McArthur, P. D. Mechanisms and development of parent-young vocal recognition in the piñon jay *(Gymnorhinus cyanocephalus). Animal Behaviour,* 1982, *30,* 62–74.

Miller, D. E., and Emlen, J. T., Jr. Individual chick recognition and family integrity in the ringbilled gull. *Behaviour,* 1975, *52,* 124–144.

Moore, J., and Ali, R. Are dispersal and inbreeding avoidance related? *Animal Behaviour,* 1984, *32,* 94–112.

O'Hara, R. K., and Blaustein, A. R. Kin preference behavior in *Bufo boreas* tadpoles. *Behavioral Ecology and Sociobiology,* 1982, *11,* 43–49.

Packer, C. Reciprocal altruism in *Papio anubis. Nature,* 1977, *265,* 441–443.

Partridge, L., and Halliday, T. R. Mating patterns and mate choice. In J. R. Krebs and N. B. Davies (Eds.), *Behavioural ecology an evolutionary approach.* Sunderland, MA: Sinauer, 1984.

Porter, R. H., and Wyrick, M. Sibling recognition in spiny mice *(Acomys cahirinus):* Influence of age and isolation. *Animal Behaviour,* 1979, *27,* 761–766.

Porter, R. H., Wyrick, M., and Pankey, J. Sibling recognition in spiny mice *(Acomys cahirinus). Behavioral Ecology and Sociobiology,* 1978, *3,* 61–68.

Porter, R. H., Tepper, V. J., and White, D. M. Experiential influences on the development of huddling preferences and "sibling" recognition in spiny mice. *Developmental Psychobiology*, 1981, *14*, 375–382.

Porter, R. H., Matochik, J. A., and Makin, J. W. Evidence for phenotype matching in spiny mice *(Acomys cahirinus)*. *Animal Behaviour*, 1983, *31*, 978–984.

Quinn, T. P., and Busack, C. A. Chemosensory recognition of siblings in juvenile coho salmon *(Oncorhynchus kisutch)*. *Animal Behaviour*, 1985, *33*, 51–56.

Ralls, K., Brugger, K., and Ballou, J. Inbreeding and juvenile mortality in small populations of ungulates. *Science*, 1979, *206*, 1101–1103.

Ridley, M., and Grafen, A. Are green beard genes outlaws? *Animal Behaviour*, 1981, *29*, 954–955.

Ross, N. M., and Gamboa, G. J. Nestmate discrimination in social wasps *(Polistes metricus*, Hymenoptera: Vespidae). *Behavioral Ecology and Sociobiology*, 1981, *9*, 163–165.

Rothstein, S. I. Successes and failures in avian egg and nestling recognition with comments on the utility of optimality reasoning. *American Zoologist*, 1982, *22*, 547–560.

Rothstein, S. I., and Barash, D. P. Gene conflicts and the concepts of outlaw and sheriff alleles. *Journal of Social and Biological Structure*, 1983, *6*, 367–380.

Rudge, M. R. Mother and kid behaviour in feral goats *(Capra hircus* L.). *Zeitschrift für Tierpsychologie*, 1970, *27*, 687–692.

Salzen, E. A., and Cornell, J. M. Self-perception and species recognition in birds. *Behaviour*, 1968, *30*, 44–65.

Scarr, S., and Grajeck, S. Similarities and differences among siblings. In M. E. Lamb and B. Sutton-Smith (Eds.), *Sibling relationships*. Hillsdale, NJ: Erlbaum, 1982.

Schulman, S. R., and Rubenstein, D. I. Kinship, need, and the distribution of altruism. *American Naturalist*, 1983, *121*, 776–788.

Seyfarth, R. M. The distribution of grooming and related behaviours among adult female vervet monkeys. *Animal Behaviour*, 1980, *28*, 798–813.

Seyfarth, R. M. Grooming and social competition in primates. In R. Hinde (Ed.), *Primate social relationships*. Oxford: Blackwell Scientific, 1983.

Sherman, P. W. Nepotism and the evolution of alarm calls. *Science*, 1977, *197*, 1246–1253.

Sherman, P. W. Kinship, demography, and Belding's ground squirrel nepotism. *Behavioral Ecology and Sociobiology*, 1981, *8*, 251–259.

Sherman, P. W., and Holmes, W. G. Kin recognition: Issues and evidence. In B. Hölldobler and M. Lindauer (Eds.), *Experimental behavioral ecology and sociobiology*. Stuggart: G. Fischer Verlag, 1985.

Shields, W. M. *Philopatry, inbreeding, and the evolution of sex*. Albany: State University of New York Press, 1982.

Shugart, G. The development of chick recognition by adult caspian terns. *Proceedings of the Colonial Waterbird Group*, 1977, *1*, 110–117.

Smotherman, W. P., and Robinson, S. R. The uterus as environment: The ecology of fetal experience. In E. Blass (Ed.), *Developmental psychobiology and behavioral ecology, Vol. 9: Handbook of behavioral neurobiology*. New York: Plenum Press, 1987.

Smuts, B. B. *Sex and friendship in baboons*. Hawthorne, NY: Aldine, 1985.

Snowdon, C. T. Ethology, comparative psychology, and animal behavior. *Annual Review of Psychology*, 1983, *34*, 63–94.

Suomi, S. J., Sackett, G. P., and Harlow, H. F. Development of sex preference in rhesus monkeys. *Developmental Psychology*, 1970, *3*, 326–336.

Telle, H. J. Bietrag zur Kenntnis der Verhaltensweise von Ratten, vergleichend dargestellt bei, *Rattus norvegicus* und *Rattus rattus. Zeitschrift für Angewandte Zoologie*, 1966, *53*, 126–196. (Available in English as Technical Translation 1608, Translation Section, National Science Library, National Research Council of Canada, Ottawa, Ontario, Canada.)

Tinbergen, N. On aims and methods of ethology. *Zeitschrift für Tierpsychologie*, 1963, *20*, 410–433.

Trivers, R. L. Parental investment and sexual selection. In B. Campbell (Ed.), *Sexual selection and the descent of man 1871–1971*. Chicago: Aldine, 1972.

Waldman, B. Sibling association among schooling toad tadpoles: Field evidence and implications. *Animal Behaviour*, 1982, *30*, 700–713.

Waldman, B. Kin recognition and sibling association among wood frog *(Rana sylvatica)* tadpoles. *Behavioral Ecology and Sociobiology*, 1984, *14*, 171–180.

Waldman, B., and Adler, K. Toad tadpoles associate preferentially with siblings. *Nature*, 1979, *282*, 611–613.

Waser, P. M., and Jones, W. T. Natal philopatry among solitary mammals. *Quarterly Review of Biology,* 1983, *58,* 355–390.

Wasser, S. K. Reciprocity and the trade-off between associate quality and relatedness. *American Naturalist,* 1982, *119,* 720–731.

West Eberhard, M. J. The evolution of social behavior by kin selection. *Quarterly Review of Biology* 1975, *50,* 1–33.

Wills, G. D., Wesley, A. L., Sisemore, D. A., Anderson, H. N., and Banks, L. M. Discrimination by olfactory cues in albino rats reflecting familiarity and relatedness among conspecifics. *Behavioral and Neural Biology,* 1983, *38,* 139–143.

Wrangham, R. W. Mutualism, kinship and social evolution. In King's College Sociobiology Group (Eds.), *Current problems in sociobiology.* Cambridge, England: Cambridge University Press, 1982.

Wu, H. M. H., Holmes, W. G., Medina, S. R., and Sackett, G. P. Kin preference in infant *Macaca nemestrina. Nature,* 1980, *285,* 225–227.

12

DEVELOPMENT OF INSTINCTIVE BEHAVIOR

AN EPIGENETIC AND ECOLOGICAL APPROACH

DAVID B. MILLER

INTRODUCTION

In 1966, the comparative psychologist T. C. Schneirla wrote that "behavioral onto-genesis is the backbone of comparative psychology" (p. 284). An accurate compre-hension of other aspects of behavior (e.g., behavioral evolution, behavioral genet-ics, and social psychology) depends on understanding how behavior develops within the individual organism. According to Schneirla, shortcomings in the study of behavioral development will inevitably handicap other lines of investigation. Thus, if Schneirla was correct (and I shall adopt the position that he was), we must appreciate how behavior develops and must also be able to assess the soundness of the developmental data base, both conceptually and methodologically.

The Nobel Prize–winning ethologist Nikolaas Tinbergen (1963) advocated that ontogeny be considered one of four major aims in the study of animal behav-ior, along with immediate causation, survival value (i.e., function), and evolution. In a later statement, Tinbergen (1968) argued that the proper study of behavioral development (including the prenatal period) renders the distinction between innate and acquired behavior patterns considerably less sharp than had been believed by classical ethologists (i.e., advocates of innateness), on the one hand, and experimental psychologists (i.e., advocates of modifiability), on the other.

Tinbergen's and Schneirla's views represent a radical departure from classical

DAVID B. MILLER   Department of Psychology, University of Connecticut, Storrs, Connecticut 06268.

ethological thinking (cf. Lorenz, 1965) because they emphasize the importance of incorporating behavioral embryology into the study of behavioral development.[1]

My aim in this chapter is to argue for a developmental approach to the study of instinctive behavior—behavior that is species-typical and that has some adaptive function; behavior that classical ethologists (not to mention some contemporary scientists spanning several disciplines) would be apt to label *genetically determined.* My approach here is epigenetic and ecological, as it has been in my own research on early parent–offspring vocal-auditory interactions in ducks. I describe this research and compare it to other areas of inquiry (i.e., imprinting and critical periods) that, although developmental, are largely nonepigenetic[2] and nonecological. Finally, I discuss the implications of epigenetic and ecological thinking for understanding certain key relationships between development and evolution.

WHAT IS EPIGENESIS?

Historically, the concept of *epigenesis* has been the subject of considerable confusion (e.g., Kitchener, 1978; Lerner, 1980). This concept has been discussed extensively in scholarly reviews by Needham (1959), Gottlieb (1970, 1983), and Oppenheim (1982), so I shall not enter into that discussion here.

Basically, epigenesis is a point of view of development that emerged in opposition to preformationism. Preformationists believed that a fully formed adult exists *in utero,* and that all that takes place in the course of development is a growth or an expansion of preexisting structures. Proponents of epigenesis, on the other hand, maintain that the essence of development is differentiation and change over time rather than mere growth or maturation. Different contemporary schools of epigenesis reflect the relative importance of genetic and experiential factors. As described by Gottlieb (1970, 1983), predetermined epigenetic theories assume that experience (i.e., sensory and/or motor function) does not play a constructive role in the course of development. Rather, genes are "deterministic," and the nervous system matures in a predetermined fashion, giving rise to "innate" behavior. Probabilistic epigenetic theories, on the other hand, maintain that experience plays a crucial role in inducing, guiding, altering, and sustaining the developmental trajectory of the organism. An essential difference between the predetermined and probabilistic epigenetic views is that, in the former, genes control or guide devel-

---

[1]Tinbergen and Schneirla, of course, were by no means the first to advocate the study of prenatal behavior. Wilhelm Preyer (1885) is considered the father of behavioral embryology. In this century, such people as Carmichael (1926), Kuo (1932), Hooker (1952), Hamburger (1963), and Gottlieb (1976) and their students and colleagues empirically demonstrated the importance of beginning the study of behavioral development in the prenatal period.

[2]My use of the term *nonepigenetic* here and throughout this chapter does not imply preformationism. All modern-day developmental theories are epigenetic (along the predetermined-probabilistic continuum; Gottlieb, 1970). My use of *nonepigenetic* means that the criteria for the epigenetic approach set forth by Kuo (1967) and endorsed in this chapter have, in some way, been violated.

opment, whereas in the later, they are influential, along with other controlling factors.

Zing-Yang Kuo (1967) advocated a probabilistic epigenetic approach to the study of behavioral development. It is specifically to Kuo's epigenetic view that I refer throughout this chapter. Kuo emphasized the continuous interaction between a developing organism and its internal and external environments. He believed that, at every point throughout development, this continuous interaction (or what Sameroff, 1975a,b, called a "transaction") establishes a new relationship between the organism and its environment, so that the organism is no longer the same organism and the environment is not the same environment as in the previous moment. Both the organism and the environment are in a continuous state of flux because of this transaction. In other words, changes in the environment produce changes in behavior, which, in turn, modify the environment. This transaction *is* development.

Kuo's epigenetic view dictates further that any behavioral act is the "functional product" of the combined effects of five kinds of determining factors: morphology, biophysical and biochemical factors, stimulating objects in the immediate environment, the developmental history of the organism, and the environmental context in which the behavior is taking place.

Unfortunately, some of these determining factors, especially the environmental context and the ecological validity of the stimulating objects, are often neglected or taken for granted and are regarded as unimportant in many developmental studies. The importance of the environmental context in species-typical behavior has been demonstrated repeatedly (e.g., Brookhart and Hock, 1976; Lombardi and Curio, 1985; McClintock, 1981; Miller, 1977b; Vestal and Schnell, 1986; Wallen, 1982; Whitney, 1986); yet, premature conclusions are often drawn without an adequate consideration of the impact of the immediate setting (e.g., Lorenz, 1940, as compared to Miller, 1977b; Zuckerman, 1932, as compared to Kummer, 1968; Hrdy, 1977, as compared to Curtin and Dolhinow, 1978). The importance of the nature of stimulating objects in species-typical behavior has also been documented (e.g., Gray and Jahrsdoerfer, 1986; Horn and McCabe, 1984; Johnston and Gottlieb, 1981). Yet, again, it is not uncommon to find investigators using unusual (i.e., species-atypical) stimuli—perhaps for mere convenience— when attempting to study species-typical behavior, such as the use of colored leg bands in assessing conspecific mating preferences in zebra finches (Burley, Krantzberg, and Radman, 1982; cf. Immelmann, Hailman, and Baylis, 1982); the use of pure tones when assessing the development of reflexive versus learned responses to auditory stimuli in rats (Hyson and Rudy, 1984; Rudy and Hyson, 1984); dangling a female deer mouse by forceps over the cage of a juvenile male to assess male reproductive development as a function of exposure to the aggressive behavior of the dangling female (Whitsett and Miller, 1985); and countless studies of imprinting in which organisms are exposed to all sorts of unusual objects in an effort to assess their subsequent preferences for these objects (reviewed by Hess, 1973).

DAVID B. MILLER

Like *epigenesis,* the term *ecological* has been applied in a variety of contexts. Of course, ecology is a branch of biology in its own right. The term has often been used as a descriptor in psychology, although in a wide variety of specific applications (e.g., developmental psychology—Bronfenbrenner, 1977; Valsiner and Benigni, 1986; social psychology—Barker and Wright, 1955; environmental psychology—Altman, 1975; sensation and perception—Brunswik, 1955; Gibson, 1966, 1979; Shaw, Turvey, and Mace, 1982; learning—Johnston, 1981; Johnston and Pietrewicz, 1985; Johnston and Turvey, 1980). What is common among the ecological approaches within each of these areas of psychology is the assumption that an animal must be studied in relation to the environment(s) that it inhabits. When we combine this approach with the *ethological* tradition, the environment cannot be an artificial one (such as a laboratory cage); rather, it must be a naturalistic one—an environment in which the species has evolved and continues to evolve, insofar as we are interested in natural rather than artificial selection. I do not claim that evolution has ceased in artificially selected domestic strains of rats and mice. Indeed, it proceeds, and sometimes at an unusually rapid rate (Fitch and Atchley, 1985). However, the evolution of such strains or breeds becomes interesting only when considered comparatively or in relation to that of the wild progenitor, which has *not* evolved in captivity (e.g., Boice, 1977, 1981; Güttinger, 1985; Miller, 1977b; Miller and Gottlieb, 1981; Price, 1984).

The ecological approach that I am advocating has three necessary steps (Miller, 1985): first, naturalistic observation across contexts; second, what Johnston (1981) called "task description"; and, third, experimental manipulation. Studies that are nonecological either ignore or minimize the importance of the first two steps. For example, most studies of animal learning involve only the experimental manipulation of variables that bear little or no resemblance to the organism's natural environment; nor do such studies tap into the kinds of problems that animals face in the real world. (Arguments that criticize, as well as defend, this approach appear in Johnston and Pietrewicz, 1985.) Although animal learning represents a large body of literature, it is not the only area in which nonecological studies can be found. For example, studies that fail to address ecological factors include those on audiogenic seizures in mice (e.g., Fuller, 1985; Henry, 1985); the alternation of distress calls in ducklings (e.g., Gaioni, 1982; Gaioni, Applebaum, and Goldsmith, 1983), and most of the imprinting literature (see the discussion below), to name just a few.

NATURALISTIC OBSERVATION ACROSS CONTEXTS

An important link between the ecological approach and Kuo's conception of behavioral epigenesis (1967) is the significance of the impact of environmental context on behavior. The ecological approach dictates that the proper starting point for behavioral investigation is in the species-typical environment. Unfortunately, this approach is no easy task, as some species inhabit a range of habitats so diverse as to defy their being characterized as "species-typical." Pigeons are equally at home in lofts, on ledges of buildings, and in trees. Rhesus monkeys occupy jungles as well as cities in India. Rats live in alleys, junk yards, barns, and burrows. These diverse environments all qualify as being "natural" for the respective species, if we denote a natural environment as "a habitat in which the species is usually found, one that is self-selected by the species and therefore relatively unrestrained and conducive for reproduction and rearing young" (Miller, 1981, p. 60). Thus, it is important to observe animals across environmental contexts, for failure to do so can lead to artifactual or, at least, incomplete information.

The importance of environmental contexts has been documented in several studies on primate behavior. Urban rhesus monkeys, for example, differ from their jungle counterparts in feeding and sleeping habits, level of aggressiveness, and other social behaviors (Singh, 1969). Langur monkeys exhibit different levels of infanticide in disturbed versus undisturbed jungle settings. Hrdy (1977) wrote that infanticide in male gray langurs is a species-typical strategy or an adaptation in competition for females. Curtin and Dolhinow (1978), on the other hand, argued that the langurs observed by Hrdy were overcrowded and greatly disturbed by agriculture and urbanization, and that infanticide occurs rarely in habitats undisturbed by humans. The pendulum, however, continues to swing on this issue, as Newton (1986) found infanticide by langurs to be associated with a predominantly one-male troop structure, and not with high population density. This observation, however, remains only a partial test of the criticisms raised by Curtin and Dolhinow (1978), who hypothesized that the actual physical structure of the environment induces abnormal behavior (i.e., in habitats that have been altered by humans, such as by deforestation). Newton's observations were made in an undisturbed forest.

TASK DESCRIPTION

Task description (Johnston, 1981) entails extensive observational and quantitative analyses of animals in their species-typical habitats. Task description identifies and describes the kinds of behaviors used in adjusting to particular environments. These "tasks" form the basis for further study.

One way of conceptualizing the process of task description is to consider the distinction between two types of questions that reflect different conceptual strategies in behavioral study: "can" questions and "does" questions (McCall, 1977; Miller, 1981, 1985). "Can" questions address the animal's capabilities, whereas "does" questions directly involve task description by asking how animals normally go about adapting to species-typical environmental situations.

Animals are equipped with a high degree of plasticity, exhibiting capabilities that far outreach the limits of the species-typical behavioral repertoire. I have previously referred to this kind of plasticity as "inductive malleability" (Miller, 1981, 1985). "Can" questions tap into this realm of behavioral potentials. Thus, "can" questions are not at all useless. However, one must be careful in understanding that answers to "can" questions may have no relationship to answers to "does questions across environmental contexts. I shall return to this point in my discussion of imprinting.

EXPERIMENTAL MANIPULATION

In order to understand what actually *causes* development to occur in the way that it does, one must do experiments. Experimental manipulation, whether it takes place in the lab or in the field, involves imposing on animals varying degrees of species-atypical conditions in an attempt to identify the causative factors underlying species-typical behavioral development. Studying "normal" behavioral development by creating "abnormal" conditions is not necessarily antithetical to an ecological approach, *as long as the manipulation has some demonstrable relationship to the natural behavior patterns of the species* as revealed by the task description phase of the investigation (Lehrman, 1970).

Our ultimate task, then, is to discover the particular factors that affect the development of species-typical behavior and how these factors exert their influence. Developmental trajectories are plastic; that is, the course of normal development varies as the organism is affected by and adapts to a constantly fluctuating environment. But there is a limit to this plasticity beyond which the trajectory swerves from a normal to an abnormal course. (This limit can be ascertained only by naturalistic observations across contexts.) Sometimes, the limits that maintain a normal trajectory are amazingly narrow. Experimenting outside the limits can greatly alter the course of normal development and can thereby render a distorted picture of the species-typical developmental process. One phenomenon in which this seems to have been the case is imprinting.

IMPRINTING: A NONEPIGENETIC, NONECOLOGICAL APPROACH TO DEVELOPMENT

Imprinting studies often use stimulus objects that bear little or no resemblance to the kinds of stimuli that the animal is likely to encounter in nature. The arbitrary selection of stimulus objects in imprinting experiments has been assumed to be of no importance because the processes and mechanisms underlying the formation of attachment to such artificial objects must be the same as those underlying the attachment formation to conspecifics. There are, however, data that argue against this sort of generality, thereby pointing to the importance of adopting an ecological approach to the study of such developmental processes.

The data come from two studies, each of which shows important differences in the imprinting process when natural, rather than artificial, stimuli are used. First, Johnston and Gottlieb (1981) were able to successfully imprint young mallard ducklings to a familiar object when the preference test for imprinting involved either one or two *artificial* objects. However, when the preference test involved two *natural* stimuli, the ducklings showed no preference for the familiar object (with the exception of one group in which a reliable preference was found). These data provide grounds for questioning the assumption that visual species identification is accomplished by the imprinting process. As the authors stated:

> It is important to keep the problem of species identification, which young birds encounter and typically solve in the course of their normal ontogeny, conceptually separate from the process of imprinting, which is a laboratory paradigm hypothesized to be part of the solution to the species-identification problem. If, as seems reasonable, we define the problem of species identification to include making discriminations between waterfowl of different species, then our results provide grounds to question the hypothesis that imprinting, as conventionally formulated, is the means by which this problem is solved. (p. 1097)

The second line of evidence that questions the ecological significance of imprinting comes from a neuroanatomical study by Horn and McCabe (1984). They found that lesions to a specific region of the domestic chick brain (the intermediate and medial part of the hyperstriatum ventrale, or IMHV) significantly impaired imprinting to artificial stimuli but had no effect when natural stimuli were used. Among the possible explanations for this result is that different neural mechanisms mediate the development of preferences for artificial versus natural stimuli. The behavioral data of Johnston and Gottlieb (1981; see also Johnson, Bolhuis, and Horn, 1985) and the neuroanatomical data of Horn and McCabe (1984) raise further concern about the generality-of-mechanism assumption.

The study of imprinting can be criticized for its lack of concern about the environmental context. This has been a problem especially in studies of sexual imprinting, which usually use simple two-stimulus choice tests. Using such an experimental situation, Walter (1973) was unable to demonstrate imprinting in female zebra finches and therefore concluded that females identify male conspecifics on an innate basis. However, by altering the environmental context of the testing situation, Sonnemann and Sjölander (1977) found that female zebra finches do imprint. Specifically, instead of offering females a two-stimulus choice task within a 30-min test session, these authors devised a multiple-choice situation involving eight stimulus males in a 72-h test session. Under these conditions, female zebra finches clearly exhibited behavioral preferences that indicated that imprinting had taken place.

The imprinting concept has been extended rather successfully to other forms of early learning. Immelmann (1975), for example, noted that imprintinglike processes seem to be involved in the development of food preferences, the selection of a home area, habitat preferences, and host selection in some parasitic animals. He classified these kinds of effects of early experience as "ecological imprinting," and there are excellent examples of each of these phenomena that demonstrate an ecological, epigenetic approach. Like filial and sexual imprinting, these forms of ecological imprinting entail a very early and rapid form of learning involving nonsocial aspects of the animal's ecology. For example, Pacific salmon recognize the water from the stream in which they were hatched by "olfactory imprinting." Chemical cues in the water allow the salmon to return successfully to their home stream (i.e., the stream in which they were hatched) to spawn (Hasler and Scholz, 1983).

Some investigators have attempted to explain how imprinting may be involved in the recognition of individuals rather than of species (e.g., Bateson, 1966, 1978; Miller, 1979, 1980a). Lorenz (1937) explicitly stated that not individual features, but supraindividual characteristics, are learned in the imprinting process. Yet, several investigations have demonstrated how imprinting may operate in the context of *individual* recognition, as, for example, in the recognition of kin as a possible incest avoidance mechanism (e.g., Bateson, 1978, 1980, 1983; Pusey, 1980).[3] Thus, rather than providing a means by which an organism learns the characteristics of the particular species with which to mate, sexual imprinting may, in fact, provide a mechanism for enabling an animal to recognize the characteristics of particular individuals of its own species with which to *avoid* mating, such as close relatives.

CRITICAL PERIODS: DO THEY EXIST?

According to Lorenz (1937), imprinting is a rapid form of learning that must occur within a critical period of an organism's life. Taken literally, this means that if a stimulus object is encountered outside of this critical period, the animal will not develop a preference for that object. Studies on the reversibility of imprinting (e.g., Mason and Kenney, 1974; Salzen and Meyer, 1967; Suomi, Harlow, and Novak, 1974) and on the extension of such a period of maximal sensitivity into later life (e.g., Brown, 1974) have demonstrated rather convincingly that so-called critical periods for the development of attachments or preferences for imprinting objects are not so critical after all. Moreover, the delineation of critical periods can be affected greatly by procedural factors attendant on experimental conditions, for example, the use of conceptional, or developmental age rather than posthatching age (Gottlieb, 1961); the amount and quality of stimulation, the particular behaviors being measured, and the animal's experience between the initial stimulation and the time of testing (Denenberg, 1964, 1968); the developmental status of the animal at the time of isolation, the duration of the isolation, and the developmental status of the stimulus animal at the time of testing (Cairns, Hood, and Midlam, 1985); and, the environmental context (Kroodsma and Pickert, 1984).

Yet another issue concerning the concept of imprinting and critical periods pertains to a confound that often arises between the experimental effects of early

---

[3]I presented my reformulation of Lorenz's original imprinting question at the Seventeenth International Ornithological Congress in Berlin, West Germany, in 1978 (see Miller, 1980a, for the published version of this presentation). As stated, the reformulation was that "one can further refine the initial question posited by Lorenz by asking how organisms that instinctively prefer to mate with conspecifics come to prefer certain individuals over others. . . . If, in the next 40 years, we hope to come closer to elucidating the original concept of imprinting as posited by Lorenz than we have in the past 40 years, we must extend our experimental paradigms beyond sexual imprinting as it has been studied interspecifically and attempt to identify the intraspecific parameters underlying the development of sexual preferences" (p. 846). Lorenz attended this presentation, and in the discussion period, he stated that he was "absolutely enthusiastic" about the reformulation (much, I should add, to my surprise, yet, nonetheless, to my delight).

experience and the time interval between the experience and the time of testing (or, in other words, the age of the animals when tested; Cairns *et al.,* 1985). When attempting to delineate critical periods, investigators stimulate animals in different groups at different times and then test them at the *same* age to assess the effectiveness of the stimulation. For example, one group of chicks may be exposed to an imprinting stimulus from 0 to 24 h after hatching, and another group between 24 and 48 h after hatching. Then, the usual practice would be to test chicks from both groups at, for example, 72 h of age. The problem with this methodology is that the stimulation-to-testing interval for one group is 48 h, and for the other group it is 24 h. This is no easy matter to resolve, for if the test time were to be advanced to 96 h for the chicks that were stimulated from 24 to 48 h, testing would now occur at different ages, even though the stimulation-to-testing intervals would now be equal (i.e., 48-h intervals).

This methodological issue, which has been largely ignored, was found to be important in a study by Gottlieb (1981) on the effects of prenatal versus postnatal experience on the development of species identification in ducklings. Gottlieb stimulated devocalized (i.e., muted) birds with a recording of a species-typical duckling call either during the late embryonic period or during the early postnatal period. Then, he tested all ducklings at 48 h to assess their preferences for the species-typical maternal assembly call with notes pulsed either at the normal rate of 3.7 notes/s or at a slowed rate of 2.3 notes/s. (Normal, vocal ducklings prefer the 3.7-notes/s call, and unstimulated devocal ducklings prefer either call; the purpose of this study was to see whether and when normally occurring auditory stimulation could reinstate a species-typical preference for the normal, 3.7-notes/s call.) Only the group of ducklings stimulated prenatally showed a preference for the 3.7-notes/s call, a finding suggesting the existence of a prenatal, but not a postnatal, critical period. However, Gottlieb proceeded to test another group of postnatally stimulated ducklings at 65 h (rather than 48 h). Surprisingly, these ducklings showed a preference for the normal, 3.7-notes/s call. Gottlieb interpreted his data as showing that there is a "consolidation period" (or latency) of about 48 h between the termination of exposure to stimulation and the behavioral effect of the stimulation. It is methodologically important to realize that, had he not tested the postnatally stimulated birds at a later age, the seemingly erroneous conclusion would have been reached that prenatal stimulation is important and postnatal stimulation is not, at least within the limits of this experiment.

A further twist was added to this story in two subsequent studies by Gottlieb (1982, 1985a). In the study described above on the existence of a consolidation effect, the stimulation had an unnatural aspect; namely, the notes of the duckling call were pulsed at a constant rate of 4.0 notes/s. Although this is the modal rate of these embryonic contact–contentment notes, it does not encompass the normally occurring range of variability in repetition rates. Although psychologists normally attempt to reduce or eliminate variability from experimental designs, Gottlieb (1982, 1985a) actually incorporated species-typical variability in his design. The range of variability of repetition rates is greater during the embryonic period (2.0–6.0 notes/s) than it is after hatching (2.0–4.0 notes/s).

Gottlieb (1982) found that a 48-h consolidation period is *not* necessary if embryos are stimulated with the normally occurring range of variation in repetition rates. That is, prenatally stimulated ducklings now showed a preference for the 3.7-notes/s assembly call at 24 h rather than at 48 h. Moreover, Gottlieb (1985a) found that *hatchlings* stimulated postnatally with a range of repetition rates extending from 2.0 to 4.0 notes/s (typical of the postnatal period) or from 2.0 to 6.0 notes/s (typical of the prenatal period) failed to show a preference for the 3.7-notes/s maternal call at either 24 or 48 h, a finding suggesting once again the existence of a prenatal critical period for stimulation with the range of repetition rates. But what about the possibility of a postnatal 48 h consolidation period similar to that reported in the earlier study (Gottlieb, 1981) for ducklings stimulated with a range of repetition rates? Gottlieb (personal communication, August 8, 1985) did, in fact, retest at 65 h 61 ducklings that had been stimulated postnatally (Day 26–27 for 7 min/h) with a range of repetition rates consisting of 2, 4, and 6 notes/s, and that had been tested previously at 48 h. Of the 35 ducklings that responded, 14 preferred the normal 3.7-notes/s call, and 21 preferred the 2.3-notes/s call. In other words, even at 65 h, there was no group preference for the normal call. Thus, the 48-h consolidation effect for prenatally or postnatally stimulated birds seems to be an artifact of stimulation at an invariant repetition rate. When incorporating species-typical variability into the nature of the stimulation process (which is rare in experimentation), an embryonic critical period emerges for the effect of normally occurring experience on the development of species-typical behavior, independent of a period of consolidation.

As Gottlieb's experiments increased in their degree of naturalness (i. e., from stimulation with a modal repetition rate to stimulation with the normally occurring range of repetition rates, along with the modal rate), the clearer was the demonstration of a critical period, independent of a consolidation effect. Given the experimentally compelling demonstration, it does appear that normally occurring embryonic stimulation is necessary for the development of the response that Gottlieb was measuring. The validity of the prenatal critical period demonstrated by Gottlieb hinges on the fact that his methodology, which epitomizes the epigenetic, ecological approach advocated in this chapter, was based on events that were anchored in the natural history of the species.

DEVELOPMENT OF ALARM CALL RESPONSIVITY IN MALLARD DUCKLINGS

One line of research that my colleagues and I have pursued has as its main objective explaining how instinctive behavior develops. Our concern is primarily with how subtle, or nonobvious, forms of experience affect the developmental trajectory, rather than theorizing on "ultimate" adaptive functions of presumed behavioral "end points." The first step toward this goal (following naturalistic observation and task description) was to assess the physical structure of the stimulus (the alarm call) and to identify the particular structural properties (the acoustic features) to which ducklings are particularly sensitive.

To augment his research program on the development of species identification in ducklings, Gottlieb and I observed parent–young interactions of several bird species on nests in the field (e.g., Miller, 1977a, 1980b; Miller and Gottlieb, 1976, 1978, 1981). For now, I shall restrict the discussion to our observations of nesting mallard ducks *(Anas platyrhynchos).*

Mallards, like most waterfowl, are ground nesters. They usually lay their 8- to 12-egg clutch in a shallow crevice that they line with vegetation and down feathers. At our field station (located near Raleigh, North Carolina), they also used ground-nest boxes. After the last egg is laid, the hen begins incubation, which lasts for about 25 days. Two to three days before hatching, the embryo moves its head into the air space of the egg and begins vocalizing. About 24 h later, the embryo pips the outer shell and takes about another 24 h to cut its way around the shell and to hatch. The young hatch somewhat synchronously, usually within several hours of one another (Bjärvall, 1967; Hess and Petrovich, 1973; Miller and Gottlieb, 1978). The hen continues to brood the ducklings on the nest for about 12–24 h and then calls them off the nest—an event we refer to as the *nest exodus.*

During the late incubation period and while brooding her young on the nest, the hen utters several types of vocalizations, two of which have the highest frequency of occurrence. The vocalization uttered most often is the assembly call (Figure 1). This is the same call that the hen uses during the nest exodus to lead her young away from the nest. The assembly call has an excitatory effect on the ducklings' behavior; that is, they typically approach the source of the call (be it either a real hen or a loudspeaker, as shown in Figure 4), and they vocalize in return.

The other main type of call that the hen utters is the reconnaissance, or alarm,

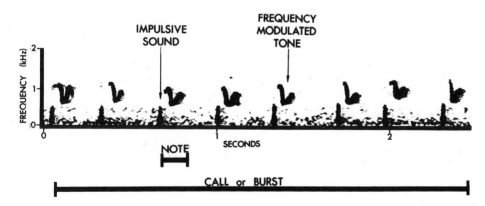

Figure 1. A narrow-band sound spectrogram of a mallard maternal assembly call. The call is composed of a burst of notes, and each note is composed of a low-frequency impulsive sound followed by a frequency-modulated tone. (From "Maternal Vocal Control of Behavioral Inhibition in Mallard Ducklings *(Anas platyrhynchos),*" by D. B. Miller, *Journal of Comparative and Physiological Psychology,* 1980, *94,* 612. Copyright 1980 by the American Psychological Association, Inc. Reprinted by permission.)

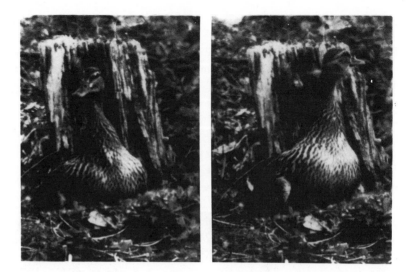

Figure 2. The reconnaissance posture of a mallard hen on sighting a potential predator near the nest. While in this posture, the hen utters the maternal alarm call. (From "Maternal vocalizations of mallard ducks *(Anas platyrhynchos),*" by D. B. Miller and G. Gottlieb, *Animal Behaviour,* 1978, *26,* 1180. Copyright 1978 by Bailliére Tindall. Reprinted by permission.)

call. When potential predators come within the vicinity of the nest, the hen adopts a seemingly wary or alert posture (Figure 2). The low-amplitude alarm call (Figure 3) that the hen utters while in this posture inhibits duckling behavior. Specifically, the ducklings stop vocalizing immediately and crouch down (Figure 4). This is typical of the "freezing" response that occurs in many species. (This behavior can be traced at least to the writings of Douglas Spalding, 1873.)

As is the case with the assembly call, the ducklings' responsiveness to the alarm call is highly robust. Depending on the nature of the test and the age of the ducklings, between 80% and 95% of the thousands of ducklings that we have tested over the past eight years exhibited instantaneous and prolonged freezing when the call was broadcast. The "task description" of our research, therefore, is freezing by ducklings on hearing the maternal alarm call, which typically occurs on *initial* exposure to the alarm call.

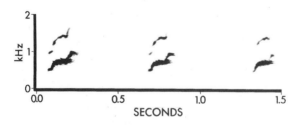

Figure 3. A narrow-band sound spectrogram of a mallard maternal alarm (or reconnaissance) call. (From "Alarm Call Responsivity of Mallard Ducklings. I. The Acoustical Boundary Between Behavioral Inhibition and Excitation," by D. B. Miller, *Developmental Psychobiology,* 1983, *16,* 188. Copyright 1983 by John Wiley & Sons, Inc. Reprinted by permission.)

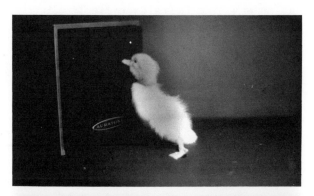

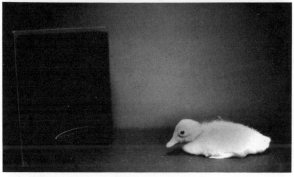

Figure 4. A domestic mallard (Peking) duckling's initial response to the two types of maternal call. *Top:* The duckling approaches the loudspeaker broadcasting the assembly call. *Bottom:* Seconds later, the assembly call is turned off, and the alarm call is broadcast. The duckling instantaneously "freezes" (i.e., crouches down and stops vocalizing). The feathers are sleeked against the body, giving the eyes a bulging appearance, which is typical of the freezing response.

ACOUSTIC FEATURES OF ALARM CALLS

Mallard maternal alarm calls are uttered at very low amplitudes and are undetectable by humans standing farther than about 5–10 feet from the nest; thus, unlike alarm calls of many other species, these are not long-distance signals. During our field observations, we placed a microphone at the nest that enabled us to hear and record these vocalizations.

Alarm calls differ strikingly from assembly calls on all of the acoustic features that we measured (Miller, 1980b; Table 1). The calls are readily distinguished by the manner in which the frequency changes over time (frequency modulation). Alarm notes have ascending frequency modulations (as portrayed in the sound spectrogram in Figure 3), whereas assembly notes are variations of descending frequency modulations (Figure 1). As shown in Figure 1, assembly notes have two parts: a low-frequency impulsive sound and a frequency-modulated tone. Although the anatomical origin (as well as the communicative significance) of the impulsive

TABLE 1. MODAL ACOUSTIC FEATURES OF MALLARD MATERNAL ALARM AND ASSEMBLY CALLS[a]

	Maternal call	
Acoustic feature	Alarm	Assembly
Frequency modulation	Ascending	Descending
Dominant frequency	676 ± 77 Hz	970 ± 337 Hz
Note duration	161 ± 39 ms	112 ± 27 ms
Repetition rate	1.1 ± 0.4 notes/s	3.7 ± 1.1 notes/s
Notes per burst	2.1 ± 1.2	3.5 ± 1.7
Impulsive	9%	85%

[a]The alarm call data are from "Effects of Domestication on Production and Perception of Mallard Maternal Alarm Calls: Developmental Lag in Behavioral Arousal," by D. B. Miller and G. Gottlieb, *Journal of Comparative and Physiological Psychology*, 1981, *95*, 210. Copyright 1981 by the American Psychological Association, Inc. The assembly call data are from "Maternal Vocalizations of Mallard Ducks *(Anas platyrhynchos),*" by D. B. Miller and G. Gottlieb, *Animal Behaviour*, 1978, *26*, 1191. Copyright 1978 by Baillière Tindall. Adapted by permission.

sound is unknown (Miller and Gottlieb, 1978), it was present in 85% of the assembly notes in our sample ($N = 586$). However, only 9% of the alarm notes ($N = 215$) were preceded by this sound.

As shown in Table 1, alarm and assembly notes also differ significantly with regard to dominant frequency, note duration, number of notes per burst, and repetition rate (i.e., the number of notes per second within a given burst). The striking difference in repetition rate (1.1 notes/s for alarm versus 3.7 notes/s for assembly) is particularly important in governing the ducklings' selective responsiveness to the assembly call, both prenatally and postnatally (Gottlieb, 1978, 1979). These factors gave rise to our own experimental analyses of the causal factors underlying alarm call responsivity. We assessed whether variations in repetition rate alone differentially affected behavioral inhibition (i.e., freezing) versus excitation.

EXPERIMENTAL ANALYSIS OF ALARM CALL RESPONSIVITY

GENERAL METHODOLOGY. All of our laboratory experiments involve independent groups, each composed of 30 ducklings. A duckling is never tested twice. The ducklings are domestic mallards (Peking breed). For control of auditory experience, the ducklings are hatched in soundproof incubators in our laboratory under rigorous sound controls. The only sounds, other than incubator fans and doors opening and closing, that the ducklings have heard before testing are their own perinatal vocalizations and those of comparably aged broodmates. On hatching, each duckling is removed from the incubator, is placed in an individual plastic box (for individual identification), and is brooded with other comparably aged, boxed ducklings until the time of testing. Ducklings are tested individually in a circular arena (173 cm in diameter). A loudspeaker is mounted in the side wall of the arena, through which a test call can be broadcast.

maternal calls were used to assess whether variations in repetition rate alone (with

all other acoustic features held constant) differentially affected behavioral inhibition versus excitation. The alarm and assembly calls (Figure 5) were recorded from the same hen on her field nest.

For assessment of the effect of variations in repetition rate, the 1.4-notes/s alarm call was quickened to a rate of 3.7 notes/s by splicing out pieces of tape in between the notes. Likewise, the 3.7-notes/s assembly call was slowed to a rate of 1.4 notes/s by inserting pieces of blank tape in between the notes. Oscillograms of the resulting four test calls (normal, 1.4-notes/s alarm; quickened, 3.7-notes/s alarm; normal, 3.7-notes/s assembly; slowed, 1.4-notes/s assembly) are shown in Figure 6.

Each duckling was given a 6-min test when it reached 24 ± 6 h of age. The test was divided into 2 min of silence (i.e., no broadcast), then 2 min of call broadcast, and, again, 2 min of silence. A control group of 30 ducklings was tested in continuous silence for 6 min. The number of vocalizations (distress calls and contact–contentment calls) uttered by the duckling was counted during each 2-min period. Also, we counted the number of ducklings that exhibited what we call a *full freeze,* which is a total cessation of all vocal and locomotor behavior within 10 s of the broadcast and remaining in the "frozen" state for the duration of the broadcast or (for an even more robust measure of freezing) throughout the 2-min posttest period.

Variations in repetition rate alone can differentially effect behavioral inhibition and excitation. As shown in Figure 7, ducklings exposed to either call pulsed

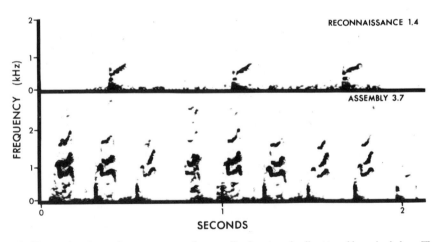

Figure 5. Narrow-band sound spectrograms of two mallard maternal calls uttered by a single hen. These calls (and their altered forms, depicted by oscillograms in Figure 6) were used to assess the effect of variations in repetition rate on behavioral inhibition and excitation. (From "Maternal Vocal Control of Behavioral Inhibition in Mallard Ducklings *(Anas platyrhynchos),*" by D. B. Miller, *Journal of Comparative and Physiological Psychology,* 1980, *94,* 617. Copyright 1980 by the American Psychological Association. Reprinted by permission.)

RECONNAISSANCE   1.4

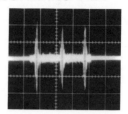

RECONNAISSANCE   3.7

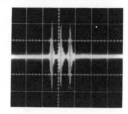

ASSEMBLY   3.7

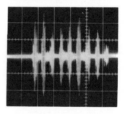

ASSEMBLY   1.4

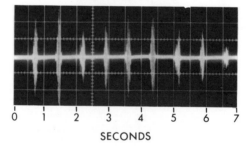

SECONDS

Figure 6. Oscillograms of the two normal (reconnaissance 1.4 and assembly 3.7) calls shown in Figure 5, and the two altered-rate (reconnaissance 3.7 and assembly 1.4) versions of these calls. (From "Maternal Vocal Control of Behavioral Inhibition in Mallard Ducklings *(Anas platyrhynchos),*" by D. B. Miller, *Journal of Comparative and Physiological Psychology,* 1980, *94,* 618. Copyright 1980 by the American Psychological Association, Inc. Reprinted by permission.)

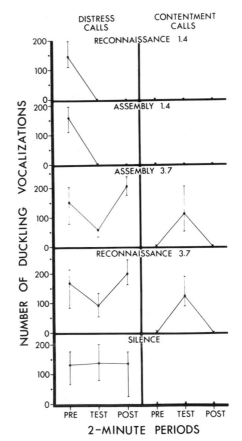

Figure 7. Number of duckling distress and contentment calls uttered in each 2-min period (pretest, test, and posttest) of the 6-min tests designed to assess the effect of repetition rate on inhibiton and excitation. The values plotted are the medians and the first and third quartiles. (From "Maternal Vocal Control of Behavioral Inhibition in Mallard Ducklings *(Anas platyrhynchos),*" by D. B. Miller, *Journal of Comparative and Physiological Psychology,* 1980, *94,* 618. Copyright 1980 by the American Psychological Association, Inc. Reprinted by permission.)

at 1.4 notes/s inhibited their vocal behavior during the broadcast and remained silent throughout the posttest period. However, ducklings tested to either call pulsed at 3.7 notes/s reduced their level of distress calling. Moreover, their level of uttering contentment calls increased dramatically. The ducklings' behavior changed markedly at broadcast termination. They stopped uttering contentment calls and resumed uttering distress calls at a rate exceeding that in the pretest period. Ducklings tested in continuous silence uttered a fairly constant level of distress calls and no contentment calls.

The number of birds exhibiting full freeze was quite high for both slow-rate calls and was virtually absent for both fast-rate calls (Table 2). (Other details of these data are reported in Miller, 1980b).

Repetition rate, therefore, is a critical cue that ducklings extract from the maternal alarm call. Moreover, there is an optimal range of slow repetition rates affecting behavioral inhibition (Miller, 1983a,b). Specifically, the greatest levels of inhibition occur to repetition rates between 0.8 and 1.8 notes/s, with 1.6 notes/s being optimal. Rates that are too slow (0.2 and 0.4 notes/s) are only moderately

TABLE 2. NUMBER OF DUCKLINGS EXHIBITING FULL
FREEZE TO EACH TEST CALL[a]

Call	Frozen throughout broadcast period	Frozen throughout broadcast and posttest periods
Alarm 1.4	25	24
Assembly 1.4	26	21
Assembly 3.7	0	0
Alarm 3.7	0	0

[a]Numbers are based on a total of 30 ducklings tested to each call.

effective. Obviously, fast rates promote behavioral excitation, as discussed above. A relatively sharp "boundary" between behavioral excitation and inhibition exists around 2.6–2.8 notes/s. Rates less than 2.6 notes/s inhibit, and rates above 2.8 notes/s excite (Miller, 1983a). This boundary also reflects call production: assembly calls have rates greater than 2.8 notes/s, and alarm calls have rates less than 2.6 notes/s (Figure 8). The repetition rate of maternal vocal production matches the duckling's auditory perception. Thus, the auditory perceptual specificity necessary for adaptive responsiveness (i.e., freezing) is sharply attuned to normally occurring stimulus features of the natural rearing environment.

THE ROLE OF OTHER ACOUSTIC FEATURES. Although repetition rate is a critical acoustic feature of alarm (and assembly) calls, there are other features that differentiate these call types. Gottlieb (1975a,b,c, 1985b) found that dominant frequency plays a subsidiary role to repetition rate in affecting the preferential responsiveness of ducklings to the assembly call. Frequency modulation appears to play no role (although *some* form of frequency modulation is probably preferable

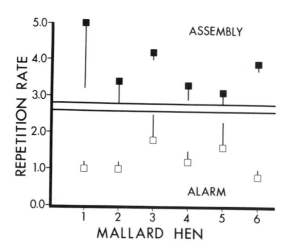

Figure 8. Mean (± *SD*) repetition rates of assembly and alarm calls uttered by six different mallard hens. The horizontal lines demarcate the acoustical "boundary" between behavioral inhibition and excitation (i.e., 2.6–2.8 notes/s). (From "Alarm Call Responsivity of Mallard Ducklings. I. The Acoustical Boundary between Behavioral Inhibition and Excitation," by D. B. Miller, *Developmental Psychobiology*, 1983, *16*, 193. Copyright 1983 by John Wiley & Sons, Inc. Reprinted by permission.

to white noise or a pure tone). The question now is whether any of these other features affect the freezing response.

Charles Blaich and I used variations of natural calls (plus filtered white noise) to assess the effect of note duration, frequency modulation, dominant frequency, and repetition rate on alarm call responsivity (Miller and Blaich, 1986). We found that note duration plays a slight role in affecting alarm call responsiveness; specifically, atypical short notes (i.e., 52 ms) are not quite as effective as the modal 165-ms notes. Frequency modulation, however, does not appear to play any role. Alarm notes played backward (so that the frequency modulation is descending instead of ascending) are just as effective as the normal ascending notes. Filtered white noise is somewhat less effective, bearing out Gottlieb's contention (1985b) that some form (although nonspecific) of frequency modulation bolsters responsiveness. Finally, although the dominant frequency is of some importance (although subsidiary to repetition rate) in the ducklings' responsiveness to the assembly call, we found that this cue plays little or no role in alarm call responsivity.

In summary, it appears that, of all the available acoustical information contained in the alarm call, the repetition rate is of paramount and critical importance. Now that we know the particular feature to which ducklings respond, it is possible to begin a search for the factors that affect the trajectory of this instinctive behavior.

PRENATAL PRECURSORS OF ALARM CALL RESPONSIVITY. Given the robustness of the freezing response at least as early as 12 h after hatching, a developmental analysis must begin prenatally. The auditory system of Peking duck embryos begins to function long before hatching, and the first behavioral response to the maternal assembly call occurs on Day 22, 5 days before hatching (Gottlieb, 1979). This response is a change in the rate of oral activity, or bill clapping. In the normal course of events, the embryo's bill penetrates the inner membrane and moves into the air space of the egg around Day 24.5. At this time, the lungs ventilate as the bird breathes the air in the egg's air space, and the embryo beings to vocalize. It pips the outer shell about 1 day later and takes yet another day to hatch (on Day 27). Thus, the embryo provides itself (and other embryos in the nest) auditory stimulation about 2.5 days before hatching, and it can also hear any vocalizations that the hen may utter (though hens do not usually become very vocal until the eggs are well pipped).

Gottlieb (1979) assessed changes in the rate of bill clapping of embryos at three different ages—Day 22, Day 24, and Day 26—as a function of exposure to four different repetition rates of assembly notes (Table 3.) On Day 22, the only repetition rate that elicited a reliable response was 3.7 notes/s (the modal rate for assembly calls). There was a significant decrease in bill clapping on exposure to this rate. Differential onset of inhibition and excitation to slow and fast repetition rates, respectively, occurs on Day 24. At this age, the 3.7 notes/s call elicits an increase of bill clapping (i.e., excitation), whereas the slower 2.3-notes/s rate causes significant inhibition. By Day 26, the inhibitory and excitatory states are fully differen-

TABLE 3. PRENATAL AGES AT WHICH SIGNIFICANT LEVELS OF
INHIBITION (*I*) AND EXCITATION (*E*) OF BILL-CLAPPING OCCUR AT
DIFFERENT REPETITION RATES OF THE MALLARD ASSEMBLY CALL[a]

Age	Repetition rates (notes/s)			
	1.0	2.3	2.3	3.7
Day 22	—	—	I	—
Day 24	—	I	E	—
Day 26	I	I	E	E

[a]From "Development of Species Identification in Ducklings. V. Perceptual Differentiation in the Embryo," By G. Gottlieb, *Journal of Comparative and Physiological Psychology*, 1979, *93*, 838. Copyright 1979 by the American Psychological Association, Inc. Adapted by Permission.

tiated. Both fast rates (3.7 and 6.0 notes/s) cause excitation, and both slow rates (1.0 and 2.3 notes/s) cause inhibition.

Although bill clapping differs greatly from freezing, Gottlieb's data indicate that differential responsiveness to fast- and slow-rate calls occurs well before hatching. This phenomenon is characteristic of the "anticipatory" nature of development, by which we mean that the capacity to exhibit species-typical behavior develops before the time that an organism actually needs to exhibit such behavior in adapting to its ecological niche (cf. Anokhin, 1964; Carmichael, 1963; Gottlieb, 1983). The particular experiences that contribute to the induction of these phenomena are yet to be explored. We have, however, assessed whether normally occurring auditory experience is necessary to maintain alarm call responsivity.

EFFECT OF EMBRYONIC DEVOCALIZATION. The strategy of this research has been to assess the kinds of normally occurring stimuli that affect the development of alarm call responsiveness. The first obvious stimulus is the hen herself. Must embryos and/or ducklings hear the hen at one point in time in order to respond to her alarm calls at a later time? The answer, based on our past laboratory experiments, is no. As described above in our first series of experiments, ducklings that have been hatched in the laboratory exhibit the freezing response on initial exposure to the alarm call and with no prior contact with a hen.

Perhaps a less obvious form of stimulation is necessary. Perhaps exposure to their own perinatal vocalizations affects the ducklings' response to the hen's alarm call. Gottlieb and Vandenbergh (1968) devised a simple surgical procedure to mute Peking duck embryos. This devocalization operation, when performed on Day 24.5, just before the time that the embryo moves its bill into the air space of the egg and begins to vocalize, successfully eliminates auditory self-stimulation with embryonic and neonatal calls. Following surgery, the embryo is placed in an individual, soundproof incubation compartment, where it is allowed to hatch and is brooded until the time of testing.

In this and all subsequent experiments, the test situation consisted of a 2-min pretest period of silence followed by a 1-min test period during which the modal

1.6-notes/s alarm call was broadcast repeatedly. To score a "full freeze," the duckling had to inhibit all vocal and locomotor activity within 10 s of the broadcast of the call and had to remain in this state for the duration of the test period.

We tested 30 12-h-old vocal communal ducklings (i. e., our usual brooding condition in which birds are placed in plastic boxes and housed together under brooder lamps) and 30 12-h-old devocal isolates. As shown by the first two bars in Figure 9, freezing by devocal ducklings was significantly reduced. Devocal isolates tested at 24 h of age showed an even greater reduction in freezing: 26 of 30 vocal communals froze, whereas only 6 of 30 devocal isolates froze (Miller and Blaich, 1984).

It appears that normally occurring, self- and/or sib-produced auditory stimulation greatly affects the development of alarm call responsivity. Given that inhibition of bill clapping to the slow 2.3-notes/s call is present even before the onset of embryonic vocal activity, it would seem that perinatal auditory experience maintains (rather than induces) this inhibitory behavior. It is conceivable that some ducklings are more susceptible to this experiential influence than are others, which is why freezing is not totally eliminated in devocal isolate birds. Nevertheless, the incidence of freezing is dramatically attenuated.

EFFECT OF REPLACEMENT OF NORMALLY OCCURRING AUDITORY STIMULATION IN DEVOCAL DUCKLINGS. To see whether or not exposure to perinatal duckling calls is the critical experiential factor affecting alarm call responsiveness, we stimulated a group of 30 devocal-isolate ducklings with a recording of an embryonic "long-slow" note (i.e., a two-note call with long note durations and a slow repetition rate of 1.5 notes/s) for 1 min every 2 h from Day 25.5 to testing (12 h posthatch). (We determined this low rate of stimulation by monitoring the vocal activity of ducklings before and after hatching, which revealed a corresponding low incidence of the occurrence of long-slow notes.)

The third column in Figure 9 shows that the high level of freezing typical of vocal-communal ducklings is reinstated in devocal-isolate ducklings that have received normally occurring auditory stimulation. Thus, this form of stimulation is sufficient to maintain the ducklings' freezing response to the maternal alarm call. Given that the devocal ducklings cannot vocalize, it is noteworthy that the impor-

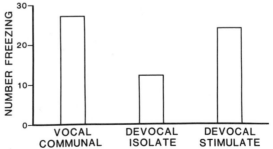

Figure 9. Number of vocal-communal, devocal-isolate, and devocal-stimulate ducklings freezing on exposure to the mallard maternal alarm call ($n = 30$ ducklings per group).

tant aspect of normally occurring auditory stimulation within the limitations of these experiments is of a *social* nature: sib stimulation (provided by a tape recording), as opposed to self-stimulation. This finding has caused us to focus attention on the nature of social rearing with regard to the freezing response.

EFFECT OF SOCIAL REARING ON ALARM CALL RESPONSIVITY. It will be recalled that ducklings in our vocal-communal condition are physically (i.e., visually and tactually) isolated from one another until the time of testing. Nevertheless, they seem to behave normally in that they show a high rate of freezing to the alarm call, as do wild ducklings on natural nests.

In striving to make our rearing conditions as "natural" as possible, we reared a group of ducklings socially in a brood of 12 (i.e., a typical brood size for mallards). Much to our surprise, these ducklings exhibited a significant reduction in alarm call responsivity, as shown in the first two columns of Figure 10 (Blaich and Miller, 1986). Why should making a rearing condition seemingly more natural so greatly attenuate the occurrence of a species-typical behavior?

The answer lies in the amount of vocal stimulation that the ducklings provide one another in the vocal-communal versus the social groups. The incidence of the occurrence of distress calls was significantly greater in the vocal-communal group than in the socially reared birds. To assess the importance of this form of stimulation, Blaich and Miller (1986) stimulated socially reared ducklings in the brooder with a recording of distress calls for 14 min/h from around the time of hatching to an hour or so before testing at 12 h posthatch age. (This rate of stimulation also was determined by monitoring the vocal activity of vocal-communal ducklings.)

As shown by the third column in Figure 10, social-stimulate ducklings exhibited a level of freezing comparable to that of vocal-communal ducklings. Stimulating socially reared ducklings with distress calls provides a form of experience that is necessary for reinstating alarm call responsivity. In fact, we found that stimulating socially reared ducklings with other forms of normally occurring stimuli (i. e., duckling contentment calls and maternal assembly calls) also fosters the reinstatement of freezing (Blaich and Miller, 1986). These forms of stimulation are either attenuated (distress and contentment calls) or eliminated (assembly calls) in laboratory social rearing. Vocal-communal ducklings, however, produce levels of dis-

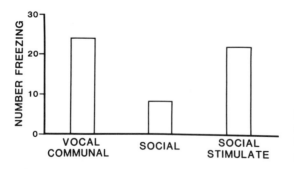

Figure 10. Number of vocal-communal, social, and social-stimulate ducklings freezing on exposure to the alarm call. (n = 30 ducklings per group)

tress and contentment calls that more closely approximate those in a natural nesting situation, thereby promoting normal alarm-call responsiveness. This experiment demonstrates the importance of the epigenetic, ecological approach advocated in this chapter by showing that experiments must be designed with an understanding of all possible sources of stimulation impinging on the organism in its species-typical environment. Such stimuli may, from a human perspective, be subtle or nonobvious, yet crucial for the development of normal instinctive behavior.

Development and Evolution

This chapter has been about behavioral development—how behavior changes (or is maintained) throughout the life span of the individual, and how epigenetic and ecological factors influence ontogenesis. Development is thus concerned with proximal causes. Evolution studies, on the other hand, have focused on ultimate causes that influence the form and function, including the behavior, of transgenerational change. Yet, ontogenesis and phylogenesis cannot be regarded as separate. Each process of change feeds back and affects the other. Selection acts on the animal in its stimulative environment throughout ontogeny. This has to be the case, as our view of development does not accept the existence of developmental end points (except for death; Gottlieb, 1976). Although development and evolution are intertwined, it is usually the case that investigators in either discipline fail to incorporate into their respective areas of inquiry questions associated with the other area. Churchill (1980), for example, stated that "the very success of causally directed embryological research steered embryologists away from a fresh appraisal of the causal connection between phylogeny and ontogeny" (p. 121).

An exception, however, is the idea that developmental differences provide the basis for evolution. Changes in developmental events can affect the subsequent evolutionary trajectory of the species (Cairns, 1976; de Beer, 1958; Goodwin, 1982; Gould, 1977; Ho and Saunders, 1979, 1984; Mivart, 1871).

A few examples will serve to clarify this point. First, the evolution of flightlessness in certain species of birds has been attributed to a slowing down (or even an arrest) of the development of plumage characteristics (de Beer, 1958) and the size and angle of certain bones used in flight (Feduccia, 1980). The adult flightless species have plumage and bone characteristics found in the young of closely related species whose adult forms are capable of flight. (The young cannot fly.) A second example concerns the evolution of species of sand fleas of the genus *Orchestia* (Matsuda, 1982). At one time, sand fleas of this genus were exclusively intertidal. Now, however, some species are freshwater aquatic and even terrestrial. The most evolutionarily recent terrestrial forms have numerous morphological characteristics that suggest early developmental arrest. For instance, terrestrial adults have a reduction in the size of the male gnathopod (used in amplexus), fewer pleopods (appendages), and relatively translucent skin. These are all characteristics of *young stages* of intertidal and/or freshwater aquatic forms, which now are characteristics of the *adult* terrestrial form. A final example, as discussed by de Beer (1958), is the evolution of humans. Many features of adult humans resemble those of embryonic (but not adult) anthropoid apes, a finding suggesting a retardation in the rate of development in the human apelike ancestor. The human big toe, for example, is large and round in both fetus and adult—an apparent adaptation for walking on a flat surface. In apes, however, the large, round big toe in the embryo develops into a narrower structure in the adult, allowing for apposability and, therefore, grasping.

The idea that evolution is subservient to development (rather than vice versa) has had a long "evolutionary" history. In 1866, Ernst Haeckel published his famous "biogenetic law," or "theory of recapitulation," which enjoyed considerable popularity in the decades that followed before it was rejected, at least in its extreme form (Mayr, 1982). According to this principle, which, incidentally, was independently "discovered" by other individuals in the second half of the nineteenth century (Gould, 1977; Mayr, 1982), "ontogeny recapitulates phylogeny." In other words, the evolutionary steps through which an organism has passed are reflected in the developmental stages of individuals of the species. One need only observe the development of descendants to learn the evolutionary origins of the species. According to this view, phylogeny is the cause of ontogeny. Changes in development occur only because evolution has occurred, and these evolutionary changes are added onto the final adult stages of development, thereby "causing" developmental changes to take place in the adult descendants. Although this view fostered some interest in the descriptive or normative study of embryology as investigators tried to reconstruct evolutionary lineages, it clearly placed development secondary to evolution. Taken to its extreme, recapitulationists could well have argued that development is a mere by-product of evolution.

Beginning around the late 1800s, evidence from a number of camps began to accumulate attesting to the untenability of the biogenetic law (see de Beer, 1958, and Gould, 1977, for more elaborate presentations of the rise and fall of recapitulationism). Instead of evolution causing changes in development, the view that began to prevail was that changes in development can lead to evolutionary change. De Beer (1958, previous editions going back to 1930) used the term *heterochrony* to refer to the notion that changes in the timing of developmental events, in either a forward (acceleration) or a backward (neoteny) direction, can cause changes in evolution. It has been only recently, however, that considerable interest in this relationship between ontogeny and phylogeny has been stirred, particularly at the molecular, mechanistic level (e.g., Bonner, 1982; Goodwin, 1982; Raff and Kaufman, 1983).

This recent emergence of interest in ontogeny has important implications for biologists and psychologists alike, working at all levels of organization (e.g., cell biology, neurophysiology, and behavior). One might argue that, in order to understand how evolution proceeds, we must focus our attention on development. The most illuminating studies will be of a comparative nature. How, for example, do the developmental trajectories of two or more closely related species differ? How do different ecological pressures affect these trajectories? What are the actual developmental mechanisms that affect differences in the timing of developmental events among closely related species?

Given the fact that evolutionary change proceeds at a rate that is too slow for us to track, one logical approach to assessing heterochronic effects is to compare the development of domestic breeds with that of their wild progenitors. As noted by Price (1984), although it seems reasonable that domestication has affected the developmental rates of certain biological characteristics, there is a paucity of studies that test this premise, particularly at the behavioral level.

There are two reports of heterochronic effects between lines of domestic animals (rather than between domestic breeds and their progenitors). Fuller and Sjursen (1967) found that certain strains of laboratory mice classified as nonsusceptible to audiogenic seizures when tested at 21 days of age were indeed highly susceptible when tested at 28 days of age. Thus, there is a developmental lag in this form of sensitivity because of artificial selection. In studying the selective breeding of laboratory mice for high and low levels of aggression, Cairns (1976), found significant differences in levels of aggression as early as the first and second generations of selected lines of mice tested at 64 days of age. However, on testing at 180 days of age, the low-aggression line of these mice behaved like the high-aggression line, and the two lines were no longer distinguishable. Thus, rather than selecting for low levels of aggression *per se,* Cairns had selected for a developmental lag in the level of aggressive behavior.

As discussed by Price (1984), a few investigators have suggested that adult domestic dogs often display juvenile behavior patterns, relative to those of the wolf. This, like the above studies on mice, is an example of neoteny—a slowing down of developmental events or, in its extreme form, a retention of juvenile characteristics into adulthood.

Our work on alarm call responsivity in wild and domestic mallard ducklings also provides evidence of a slight deceleration in development consequent on domestication (Miller and Gottlieb, 1981). Although 24-h-old Peking and mallard ducklings exhibited significant levels of inhibition on hearing the alarm call, Pekings had significantly greater levels of inhibition than mallards (Table 4). Mallards also seemed to be more "aroused" (i.e., behaviorally activated) than Pekings, as evidenced by the significantly greater number of distress calls uttered in the pretest period by the wild ducklings (202 ± 72 for mallards; 136 ± 61 for

TABLE 4. NUMBER OF DUCKLINGS FREEZING TO MALLARD
AND PEKING ALARM CALLS[a]

Subject	Age (h)	Alarm call type	
		Mallard	Peking
Mallard	24	16	14
Peking	24	27	27
Peking	72	13	—[b]

[a]Each group was composed of 30 ducklings.
[b]Pekings were not tested to the Peking call at 72 h of age.

Pekings). To assess the possibility of a developmental lag in behavioral arousal due to domestication, we tested a group of Pekings at 72 h of age (Day 3 posthatch) to the maternal alarm call, monitoring their vocal behavior in each 2-min period of the 6-min test and assessing the incidence of freezing. The 3-day-old Pekings uttered significantly more distress calls during the pretest period (231 ± 51) than did the 1-day-old Pekings (136 ± 61), and they were comparable to 1-day-old mallards in this regard. Likewise, Table 4 shows that the incidence of a full freeze in 72-h-old Pekings was comparable to that in 24-h-old mallards, and significantly less than in 24-h-old Pekings. Thus, it appears that domestication had decelerated the development of behavioral arousal and the rate of decline of alarm call responsivity in the ducklings.

Studies such as these on domestic animals illustrate how heterochronic effects can become manifest in a relatively short period of time. Like Darwin, we may be able to use data on artificial selection to better understand the means by which evolution proceeds via natural selection. If this view is correct, we must underscore this chapter's opening quotation by Schneirla (1966) and adopt a developmental perspective.

Acknowledgments

This chapter was prepared in connection with activites supported by Research Grant BNS 83-08459 from the National Science Foundation.

The ontogeny of my own thinking has been affected greatly by two individuals with whom I have had the pleasure to collaborate at different points in time: Gilbert Gottlieb and Charles F. Blaich. Many ideas that I have expressed originated in our interactions, though these views may not always articulate with theirs. I am also grateful to Charles F. Blaich for relieving me of other duties during the preparation of this manuscript and for both his and Gilbert Gottlieb's helpful comments on an earlier draft.

REFERENCES

Altman, I. *The environment and social behavior.* Monterey, CA: Brooks/Cole, 1975.

Anokhin, P. K. Systemogenesis as a general regulator of brain development. In W. A. Himwich and H. E. Himwich (Eds.) *The developing brain.* New York: American Elsevier, 1964.

Barker, R. G., and Wright, H. F. *Midwest and its children: The psychological ecology of an American town.* New York: Harper & Row, 1955.

Bateson, P. Sexual imprinting and optimal outbreeding. *Nature,* 1978, *273,* 659–660.

Bateson, P. Optimal outbreeding and the development of sexual preferences in Japanese quail. *Zeitschrift für Tierpsychologie,* 1980, *53,* 231–244.

Bateson, P. Rules for changing the rules. In D. S. Bendall (Ed.), *Evolution from molecules to men.* Cambridge: Cambridge University Press, 1983.

Bateson, P. P. G. The characteristics and context of imprinting. *Biological Reviews,* 1966 *41,* 177–220

Bjärvall, A. The critical period and the interval between hatching and exodus in mallard ducklings. *Behaviour,* 1967, *28,* 141–148.

Blaich, C. F., and Miller, D. B. Alarm call responsivity of mallard ducklings (*Anas platyrchynchos*): IV. Effects of social experience. *Journal of Comparative Psychology,* 1986, *100,* 401–405.

Boice, R. Burrows of wild and albino rats: Effects of domestication, outdoor raising, age, experience, and maternal state. *Journal of Comparative and Physiological Psychology*, 1977, *91*, 649–661.

Boice, R. Behavioral comparability of wild and domesticated rats. *Behavioral Genetics*, 1981, *11*, 545–553.

Bonner, J. T. (Ed.) *Evolution and development*. Berlin: Springer-Verlag, 1982.

Bronfenbrenner, U. Toward an experimental ecology of human development. *American Psychologist*, 1977, *32*, 513–531.

Brookhart, J., and Hock, E. The effects of experimental context and experiential background on infants' behavior toward their mothers and a stranger. *Child Development*, 1976, *47*, 333–340.

Brown, R. T. Following and visual imprinting across a wide age range. *Developmental Psychobiology*, 1974, *8*, 27–33.

Brunswik, E. Representative design and probabilistic theory in a functional psychology. *Psychological Review*, 1955, *62*, 193–217.

Burley, N., Krantzberg, G., and Radman, P. Influence of colour-banding on the conspecific preferences of zebra finches. *Animal Behaviour*, 1982, *30*, 444–455.

Cairns, R. B. The ontogeny and phylogeny of social interactions. In M. E. Hahn and E. C. Simmel (Eds.), *Communicative behavior and evolution*. New York: Academic Press, 1976.

Cairns, R. B., Hood, K. E., and Midlam, J. On fighting in mice: Is there a sensitive period for isolation effects? *Animal Behaviour*, 1985, *33*, 166–180.

Carmichael, L. The development of behavior in vertebrates experimentally removed from the influence of external stimulation. *Psychological Review*, 1926, *33*, 51–58.

Carmichael, L. The onset and early development of behavior. In L. Carmichael (Ed.), *Manual of child psychology*. New York: Wiley, 1963.

Churchill, F. B. The modern evolutionary synthesis and the biogenetic law. In E. Mayr and W. B. Provine (Eds.), *The evolutionary synthesis*. Cambridge: Harvard University Press, 1980.

Curtin, R., and Dolhinow, P. Primate social behavior in a changing world. *American Scientist*, 1978, *66*, 468–475.

de Beer, G. *Embryos and ancestors* (3rd ed.). London: Oxford University Press, 1958.

Denenberg, V. H. Critical periods, stimulus input, and emotional reactivity: A theory of infantile stimulation. *Psychological Review*, 1964, *71*, 335–351.

Denenberg, V. H. A consideration of the usefulness of the critical period hypothesis as applied to the stimulation of rodents in infancy. In G. Newton and S. Levine (Eds.), *Early experience and behavior: The psychobiology of development*. Springfield, IL: Charles C Thomas, 1968.

Feduccia, A. *The age of birds*. Cambridge: Harvard University Press, 1980.

Fitch, W. M., and Atchley, W. R. Evolution in inbred strains of mice appears rapid. *Science*, 1985, *228*, 1169–1175.

Fuller, J. L. Effects of maturation and priming on audiogenic seizure thresholds in mice. *Developmental Psychobiology*, 1985, *18*, 141–149.

Fuller, J. L., and Sjursen, F. H., Jr. Audiogenic seizures in eleven mouse strains. *Journal of Heredity*, 1967, *58*, 135–140.

Gaioni, S. J. Distress call alternation in Peking ducklings *(Anas platyrhynchos)*. *Animal Behaviour*, 1982, *30*, 774–789.

Gaioni, S. J., Applebaum, S., and Goldsmith, J. The response of young Peking ducklings to sibling distress calls. *Developmental psychobiology*, 1983, *16*, 423–437.

Gibson, J. J. *The senses considered as perceptual systems*. Boston: Houghton-Mifflin, 1966.

Gibson, J. J. *The ecological approach to visual perception*. Boston: Houghton-Mifflin, 1979.

Goodwin, B. C. Development and evolution. *Journal of Theoretical Biology*, 1982, *97*, 43–55.

Gottlieb, G. Developmental age as a baseline for determination of the critical period in imprinting. *Journal of Comparative and Physiological Psychology*, 1961, *54*, 422–427.

Gottlieb, G. Conceptions of prenatal behavior. In L. R. Aronson, E. Tobach, D. S. Lehrman, and J. S. Rosenblatt (Eds.), *Development and evolution of behavior: Essays in memory of T. C. Schneirla*. San Francisco: W. H. Freeman, 1970.

Gottlieb, G. Development of species identification in ducklings: I. Nature of perceptual deficit caused by embryonic auditory deprivation. *Journal of Comparative and Physiological Psychology*, 1975a, *89*, 387–399.

Gottlieb, G. Development of species identification in ducklings: II. Experiential prevention of perceptual deficit caused by embryonic auditory deprivation. *Journal of Comparative and Physiological Psychology*, 1975b, *89*, 675–684.

Gottlieb, G. Development of species identification in ducklings: III. Maturational rectification of perceptual deficit caused by auditory deprivation. *Journal of Comparative and Physiological Psychology,* 1975c, *89,* 899–912.

Gottlieb, G. Conceptions of prenatal development: Behavioral embryology. *Psychological Review,* 1976, *83,* 215–234.

Gottlieb, G. Development of species identification in ducklings: IV. Change in species-specific perception caused by auditory deprivation. *Journal of Comparative and Physiological Psychology,* 1978, *92,* 375–387.

Gottlieb, G. Development of species identification in ducklings: V. Perceptual differentiation in the embryo. *Journal of Comparative and Physiological Psychology,* 1979, *93,* 831–854.

Gottlieb, G. Development of species identification in ducklings: VIII. Embryonic versus postnatal critical period for the maintenance of species-typical perception. *Journal of Comparative and Physiological Psychology,* 1981, *95,* 540–547.

Gottlieb, G. Development of species identification in ducklings: IX. The necessity of experiencing normal variations in embryonic auditory stimulation. *Developmental Psychobiology,* 1982, *15,* 507–517.

Gottlieb, G. The Psychobiological approach to developmental issues. In M. M. Haith and J. J. Campos (Eds,), *Handbood of child psychology:* Vol. 2. *Infancy and developmental psychobiology.* New York: Wiley, 1983.

Gottlieb, G. Development of species identification in ducklings: XI. Embryonic critical period for species-typical perception in the hatchling. *Animal Behaviour,* 1985a, *33,* 225–233.

Gottlieb, G. On discovering significant acoustic dimensions of auditory stimulation for infants. In G. Gottlieb and N. A. Krasnegor (Eds.), *Measurement of audition and vision in the first year of postnatal life: A methodological overview.* Norwood, NJ: Ablex, 1985b.

Gottlieb, G., and Vandenbergh, J. G. Ontogeny of vocalization in duck and chick embryos. *Journal of Experimental Zoology,* 1968, *168,* 307–326.

Gould, S. J. *Ontogeny and phylogeny.* Cambridge, MA: Belknap Press, 1977.

Gray, L., and Jahrsdoerfer, R. Naturalistic psychophysics: Thresholds of ducklings *(Anas platyrynchos)* and chicks *(Gallus gallus)* to tones that resemble mallard calls. *Journal of Comparative Psychology,* 1986, *100,* 91–94.

Güttinger, H. R. Consequences of domestication on the song structures in the canary. *Behaviour,* 1985, *94,* 254–278.

Haeckel, E. *Generelle morphologie der organismen.* Berlin: Georg Reimer, 1866.

Hamburger, V. Some aspects of the embryology of behavior. *Quarterly Review of Biology,* 1963, *38,* 342–365.

Hasler, A. D., and Scholz, A. T. *Olfactory imprinting and homing in salmon.* New York: Springer-Verlag, 1983.

Henry, K. R. Cochlear function and audiogenic seizures: Developmental covariance in the LP/J mouse. *Developmental Psychobiology,* 1985, *18,* 461–466.

Hess, E. H. *Imprinting.* New York: Van Nostrand Reinhold, 1973.

Hess, E. H., and Petrovich, S. B. The early development of parent-young interaction in nature. In J. R. Nesselroade and H. W. Reese (Eds.), *Life-span developmental psychology: Methodological issues.* New York: Academic Press, 1973.

Ho, M. W., and Saunders, P. T. Beyond neo-Darwinism—An epigenetic approach to evolution. *Journal of Theoretical Biology,* 1979, *78,* 573–591.

Ho, M. W. and Saunders, P. T. (Eds.) *Beyond neo-Darwinism.* New York: Acedemic Press, 1984.

Hooker, D. *The prenatal origin of behavior.* Lawrence: University of Kansas Press, 1952.

Horn, G., and McCabe, B. J. Predispositions and preferences. Effects on imprinting of lesions to the chick brain. *Animal Behaviour,* 1984, *32,* 288–292.

Hrdy, S. B. Infanticide as a primate reproductive strategy. *American Scientist,* 1977, *65,* 40–49.

Hyson, R. L., and Rudy, J. W. Ontogenesis of learning. II. Variation in the rat's reflexive and learned responses to acoustic stimulation. *Developmental Psychobiology,* 1984, *17,* 263–283.

Immelmann, K. Ecological significance of imprinting and early experience. *Annual Review of Ecology and Systematics,* 1975, *6,* 15–37.

Immelmann, K., Hailman, J. P., and Baylis, J. R. Reputed band attractiveness and sex manipulation in zebra finches. *Science,* 1982, *215,* 422.

Johnson, M. H., Bolhuis, J. J., and Horn, G. Interaction between acquired preferences and developing predispositions during imprinting. *Animal Behaviour,* 1985, *33,* 1000–1006.

Johnston, T. D. Contrasting approaches to a theory of learning. *Behavioral and Brain Sciences,* 1981, *4,* 125–173.

Johnston, T. D., and Gottlieb, G. Development of visual species identification in ducklings: What is the role of imprinting? *Animal Behaviour*, 1981, *29*, 1082–1099.

Johnston, T. D., and Pietrewicz, A. T. (Eds.) *Issues in the ecological study of learning.* Hillsdale, NJ: Erlbaum, 1985.

Johnston, T. D., and Turvey, M. T. A sketch of an ecological metatheory for theories of learning. In G. H. Bower (Ed.), *The psychology of learning and motivation*, Vol. 14. New York: Academic Press, 1980.

Kitchener, R. F. Epigenesis: The role of biological models in developmental psychology. *Human Development*, 1978, *21*, 141–160.

Kroodsma, D. E., and Pickert, R. Sensitive phases for song learning: Effects of social interaction and individual variation. *Animal Behaviour*, 1984, *32*, 389–394.

Kummer, H. *Social organization of Hamadryas baboons: A field study.* Chicago: University of Chicago Press, 1968.

Kuo, Z.-Y. Ontogeny of embryonic behavior in aves. I. The chronology and general nature of the behavior in the chick embryo. *Journal of Experimental Zoology*, 1932, *61*, 395–430.

Kuo, Z.-Y. *The dynamics of behavior development: An epigenetic view.* New York: Random House, 1967.

Lehrman, D. S. Semantic and conceptual issues in the nature-nurture problem. In L. R. Aronson, E. Tobach, D. S. Lehrman, and J. S. Rosenblatt (Eds.), *Development and evolution of behavior: Essays in memory of T. C. Schneirla.* San Francisco: W. H. Freeman, 1970.

Lerner, R. M. Concepts of epigenesis: Descriptive and explanatory issues. A critique of Kitchener's comments. *Human Development*, 1980, *23*, 63–72.

Lombardi, C. M., and Curio, E. Influence of environment on mobbing by Zebra Finches. *Bird Behaviour*, 1985, *6*, 28–33.

Lorenz, K. The companion in the bird's world. *Auk*, 1937, *54*, 245–273.

Lorenz, K. Durch Domestikation verursachte Störungen arteigenen Verhaltens. *Zeitschrift für angewandte Psychologie und Charakterkunde*, 1940, *59*, 2–82.

Lorenz, K. *Evolution and modification of behavior.* Chicago: University of Chicago Press, 1965.

Mason, W. A., and Kenney, M. D. Redirection of filial attachments in rhesus monkeys: Dogs as mother surrogates. *Science*, 1974, *183*, 1209–1211.

Matsuda, R. The evolutionary process in talitrid amphipods and salamanders in changing environments, with a discussion of "genetic assimilation" and some other evolutionary concerns. *Canadian Journal of Zoology*, 1982, *60*, 733–749.

Mayr, E. *The growth of biological thought: Diversity, evolution, and inheritance.* Cambridge, MA: Belknap Press, 1982.

McCall, R. B. Challenges to a science of developmental psychology. *Child Development*, 1977, *48*, 333–344.

McClintock, M. K. Simplicity from complexity: A naturalistic approach to behavior and neuroendocrine function. In I. Silverman (Ed.), *New directions for methodology of social and behavioral science* (No. 8): *Generalizing from laboratory to life.* San Francisco: Jossey-Bass, 1981.

Miller, D. B. Early parent-young interaction in red junglefowl: Earlobe pecking. *Condor*, 1977a, *79*, 503–504.

Miller, D. B. Social displays of mallard ducks *(Anas platyrhynchos)*: Effects of domestication. *Journal of Comparative and Physiological Psychology*, 1977b, *91*, 221–232.

Miller, D. B. Long-term recognition of father's song by female zebra finches. *Nature*, 1977, *280*, 389–391.

Miller, D. B. Beyond sexual imprinting. In R. Nöhring (Ed.) *Acta XVII congressus internationalis ornithologici*, Vol. 2. Berlin: Verlag der Deutschen Ornithologen-Gesellschaft, 1980a.

Miller, D. B. Maternal vocal control of behavioral inhibition in mallard ducklings *(Anas platyrhynchos)*. *Journal of Comparative and Physiological Psychology*, 1980b, *94*, 606–623.

Miller, D. B. Conceptual strategies in behavioral development: Normal development and plasticity. In K. Immelmann, G. W. Barlow, L. Petrinovich, and M. Main (Eds.) *Behavioral development: The Bielefeld interdisciplinary project.* Cambridge: Cambridge University Press, 1981.

Miller, D. B. Alarm call responsivity of mallard ducklings: I. The acoustical boundary between behavioral inhibition and excitation. *Developmental Psychobiology*, 1983a, *16*, 185–194.

Miller, D. B. Alarm call responsivity of mallard ducklings: II. Perceptual specificity along an acoustical dimension affecting behavioral inhibition. *Developmental Psychobiology*, 1983b, *16*, 195–205.

Miller, D. B. Methodological issues in the ecological study of learning. In T. D. Johnston and A. T. Pietrewicz (Eds.), *Issues in the ecological study of learning.* Hillsdale, NJ: Erlbaum, 1985.

Miller, D. B., and Blaich, C. F. Alarm call responsivity of mallard ducklings: The inadequacy of learning and genetic explanations of instinctive behavior. *Learning and Motivation*, 1984, *15*, 417–427.

Miller, D. B., and Blaich, C. F. Alarm call responsivity of mallard ducklings: III. Acoustic features affecting behavioral inhibition. *Developmental Psychobiology,* 1986, *19,* 291–301.

Miller, D. B., and Gottlieb, G. Acoustic features of wood duck *(Aix sponsa)* maternal calls. *Behaviour,* 1976, *57,* 260–280.

Miller, D. B., and Gottlieb, G. Maternal vocalizations of mallard ducks *(Anas platyrhynchos). Animal Behaviour,* 1978, *26,* 1178–1194.

Miller, D. B., and Gottlieb, G. Effects of domestication on production and perception of mallard maternal alarm calls: Developmental lag in behavioral arousal. *Journal of Comparative and Physiological Psychology,* 1981, *95,* 205–219.

Mivart, G. *On the genesis of species.* London: Macmillan, 1871.

Needham, J. *A history of embryology.* Cambridge: Cambridge University Press, 1959.

Newton, P. N. Infanticide in an undisturbed forest population of hanuman langurs, *Presbytis entellus. Animal Behaviour,* 1986, *34,* 785–789.

Oppenheim, R. W. Preformation and epigenesis in the origins of the nervous system and behavior: Issues, concepts, and their history. In P. P. G. Bateson and P. H. Klopfer (Eds.), *Perspectives in ethology.* Vol. 5. Ontogeny. New York: Plenum Press, 1982.

Preyer, W. *Specielle physiologie des embryo.* Leipzig: Grieben, 1885.

Price, E. O. Behavioral aspects of animal domestication. *Quarterly Review of Biology,* 1984, *59,* 1–32.

Pusey, A. E. Inbreeding avoidance in chimpanzees. *Animal Behaviour,* 1980, *28,* 543–552.

Raff, R. A., and Kaufman, T. C. *Embryos, genes, and evolution: The developmental-genetic basis of evolutionary change.* New York: Macmillan, 1983.

Rudy, J. W., and Hyson, R. L. Ontogenesis of learning. III. Variation in the rat's differential reflexive and learned responses to sound frequencies. *Developmental Psychobiology,* 1984, *17,* 285–300.

Salzen, E. A., and Meyer, C. C. Imprinting: Reversal of a preference established during the critical period. *Nature,* 1967, *215,* 785–786.

Sameroff, A. J. Early influences on development: Fact or fancy? *Merrill-Palmer Quarterly,* 1975a, *21,* 267–294.

Sameroff, A. Transactional models in early social relations. *Human Development,* 1975b. *18,* 65-79

Schneirla, T. C. Behavioral development and comparative psychology. *Quarterly Review of Biology,* 1966, *41,* 283–302.

Shaw, R., Turvey, M. T., and Mace, W. Ecological psychology: The consequence of a committment to realism. In W. Weimer and D. Palermo, (Eds.), *Cognition and the symbolic processes, II.* Hillsdale, NJ: Erlbaum, 1982.

Singh, S. D. Urban monkeys. *Scientific American,* 1969, *221,* 108–115.

Sonnemann, P. and Sjölander, S. Effects of cross-fostering on the sexual imprinting of the female zebra finch *Taeniopygia guttata. Zeitschrift für Tierpsychologie,* 1977, *45,* 337–348.

Spalding, D. A. Instinct, with original observations on young animals. *Macmillan's Magazine,* 1873, *27,* 282–293.

Suomi, S. J., Harlow, H. F., and Novak, M. A. Reversal of social deficits produced by isolation rearing in monkeys. *Journal of Human Evolution,* 1974, *3,* 527–534.

Tinbergen, N. On aims and methods of ethology. *Zeitschrift für Tierpsychologie,* 1963, *20,* 410–429.

Tinbergen N. On war and peace in animals and man. *Science,* 1968, *160,* 1411–1418.

Valsiner, J., and Benigni, L. Naturalistic research and ecological thinking in the study of child development. *Developmental Review,* 1986, *6,* 203–223.

Vestal, B. M., and Schnell, G. D. Influence of environmental complexity and space on social interactions of mice *(Mus musculus* and *Peromyscus leucopus). Journal of Comparative Psychology,* 1986, *100,* 143–154.

Wallen, K. Influence of female hormonal state on rhesus sexual behavior varies with space for social interaction. *Science,* 1982, *217,* 375–377.

Walter, M. J. Effects of parental colouration on the mate preference of offspring in the zebra finch, *Taeniopygia guttata castanotis* Gould. *Behaviour,* 1973, *46,* 154–173.

Whitney, J. F. Effect of medial preoptic lesions on sexual behavior of female rats is determined by test situation. *Behavioral Neuroscience,* 1986, *100,* 230–235.

Whitsett, J. M., and Miller, L. L. Reproductive development in male deer mice exposed to aggressive behavior. *Developmental Psychobiology,* 1985, *18,* 287–290.

Zuckerman, S. *The social life of monkeys and apes.* London: Routledge & Kegan Paul, 1932.

Index